THIRD EDITION

Bennett & Rabbetts' Clinical Visual Optics

This work is dedicated to
Margery Rabbetts
and to the memory of
Winifred Bennett
our respective wives

THIRD EDITION

Bennett & Rabbetts'
Clinical
Visual Optics

RONALD B RABBETTS

MSc, SMSA, FCOptom, DCLP

Practising Ophthalmic Optician, Portsmouth,
Clinical Supervisor, Institute of
Optometry, London

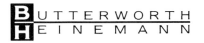

OXFORD   AUCKLAND   BOSTON   JOHANESBURG   MELBOURNE   NEW DELHI

Butterworth-Heinemann
Linacre House, Jordan Hill, Oxford OX2 8DP
225 Wildwood Avenue, Woburn, MA 01801-2041
A division of Reed Educational and Professional Publishing Ltd

 A member of the Reed Elsevier plc group

First published 1984
Reprinted 1987
Second edition 1989
Reprinted 1991, 1992, 1993
Third edition 1998
Reprinted 1999, 2000

British Library Cataloguing in Publication Data

Clinical visual optics – 3rd edn
  1. Man. Eyes, refraction disorders
  I. Title   II. Rabbetts, Ronald B.
  617. 7'55

ISBN 0 7506 1817 5

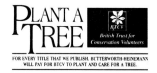

Data manipulation by David Gregson Associates, Beccles, Suffolk
Printed and bound in Great Britain by The Bath Press plc, Bath

Contents

Preface to third edition

The reception accorded to the first two editions of this book has been most gratifying. Although no drastic changes have been needed in this edition, almost all the chapters in the book have been revised to take account of the latest research and instrumentation.

The second edition proposed a replacement for the Gullstrand–Emsley schematic eye and its fellow reduced eye. In this edition, the new schematic and reduced eyes have been adopted throughout, entailing considerable revision, particularly of Chapters 12 and 15. Several of the figures on chromatic aberration are now based on wavenumber rather than wavelength.

The treatment of magnifiers now emphasizes the relationship with the user's eye, while the chapter on objective refraction describes the optical principles of several modern auto-refractors. The chapter on measurement of ocular dimensions has been expanded to include material on videokeratography, while some recent ideas of the development of refractive error are included in the section on the distribution of ametropia.

Sadly, just as we were about to start this revision, my co-author, Arthur Bennett, died (in his early eighties, having retained his remarkable mental abilities right to the end). Since the previous edition, we had kept in constant touch over optical matters; so I hope that he would have been pleased with the revision, including those areas in which he took a special interest.

As the book still, obviously, contains a vast amount of Arthur's original work, and as it has become generally known as 'Bennett and Rabbetts', it continues under the joint authorship.

R.B. Rabbetts

Preface to first edition

This book has been written as a successor to H.H. Emsley's *Visual Optics*. Its aim is to provide an up-to-date text on ocular dioptrics, the various subjective and objective techniques of refraction, and the optical instruments used in the examination of the eye. Other topics include the side-effects of spectacle and contact-lens corrections and the aberrations of the eye. The four chapters on the oculo-motor system and stereopsis are intended to provide a foundation for further study.

As indicated by the title, we have emphasized the clinical relevance of the subject matter. At the same time, we have endeavoured to maintain the high standard set by Emsley in his exposition of underlying principles.

While the majority of readers will be students of optometry, ophthalmology and ophthalmic dispensing, it is hoped that this book will also serve as a reference work for those already in practice, in addition to optical designers, physicists, psychologists and others engaged in visual science.

The great majority of the diagrams have not been drawn to scale so that certain dimensions, particularly small angles, are clear enough to be seen. The arrow heads placed at one end only of dimension lines indicate the direction of measurement according to the sign convention adopted.

To supplement the references at the end of each chapter to authors cited in the text, a bibliography of works suitable for further study has been given at the end of the book. This bibliography is not exhaustive, but includes texts on related subjects such as orthoptics and physiology, which are outside the scope of this work. References to journals are abbreviated to the form adopted by the *World List of Scientific Periodicals.*

A set of exercises can be found at the end of most chapters. These exercises are mainly numerical and answers are given at the end of the book. To economize on space, the exercises include the derivation of some expressions and the extension of certain topics not developed in the text.

Although each of us prepared the initial draft for half the chapters, we both take responsibility for the entire contents, which we have thoroughly discussed.

A.G. Bennett

R.B. Rabbetts

Acknowledgements

The authors gratefully express their thanks to all those who have assisted in various ways in the preparation of this work. In particular, they have greatly profited from helpful discussions with colleagues, especially Mr J.L. Francis, for many years a Senior Lecturer at the Institute of Optometry (London), Dr W.N. Charman of the University of Manchester Institute of Science and Technology, Dr A.R. Hill of the Visual Science Unit, Radcliffe Infirmary, Oxford, Dr C.E. Campbell of Humphrey Instruments, Inc., San Leandro, California and Professor M. Millodot.

Thanks are also due to the authors and publications concerned for permission to reproduce various text figures or photographs. Most of the numerous other figures were first drawn by the authors as a basis for the finished diagrams kindly prepared for reproduction by Mr R. John.

Tables 21.2 to *21.5* were compiled from the data made available to A.G. Bennett by the then Ministry of Health and used in his paper of 1965, cited in the references for Chapter 21.

By kind permission of City University, the exercises include a large number which have been in use for many years in their Department of Optometry and Visual Science.

Information concerning their products was kindly supplied by the following firms:

American Optical Corporation Inc.
Bausch & Lomb
Birmingham Optical Group Ltd
Carl Zeiss Ltd
Clement Clarke International Ltd
Coherent Radiation Inc.
Essilor Ltd
Humphrey Instruments Inc.
IOO Marketing Ltd
Keeler Ltd
Oculus-Optikgeräte GmbH
Rodenstock Instrumente GmbH
Tinsley Instruments Ltd.

The authors are also greatly indebted to Miss J.M. Taylor, Librarian of the British Optical Association Foundation, for her valuable assistance and to those who helped in typing the manuscript, principally Miss Gloria Taylor; also Ronald Rabbetts' wife, Margery, who edited the scanned-in computer file for the third edition.

Finally, the authors are happy to express their sincere gratitude to their respective families for the tolerance shown during the many years of work involved in writing and revising this book.

List of symbols

Geometrical optics

Standard symbols are used, excepting L_s and L'_s (reciprocal of ℓ_s, ℓ'_s respectively) which are used to denote vergences with respect to the spectacle plane.

Static refraction

F_e	Static power of eye in general or power of a given eye
F_o	Reference power of lens or eye (in context)
F_{sp}	Distance spectacle refraction (reciprocal of f'_{sp})
K'	Dioptric length of the eye in general or of a given eye (related to k')
K'_o	Dioptric length of a standard emmetropic eye
K	Distance ocular refraction (reciprocal of k)

Near vision and accommodation

B	Dioptric distance to near point of accommodation, measured from the eye (reciprocal of b)
A	Ocular accommodation in general
A_s	Spectacle accommodation in general
Amp	Maximum amplitude of accommodation
Add	Addition for near vision

Astigmatism

The subscripts α and β denote the two principal meridians of an astigmatic eye or lens.

Ast	Ocular astigmatism, equal to $K_\alpha - K_\beta$
C	Spectacle cylinder in general
C_n	Spectacle cylinder for near vision

Note. We have adopted the rule that α denotes the more powerful *ocular* meridian. On this basis, Ast becomes negative in sign, with the β meridian as the axis of the minus correcting cylinder.

Miscellaneous

d	Vertex distance
g	Pupil diameter
j	Blur-circle diameter
p	Semi intra-ocular distance
PD	Interpupillary distance
SM	Spectacle magnification
RSM	Relative spectacle magnification

Other symbols are defined where they are used and inevitably may carry different meanings in different chapters.

1

General introduction

The visual system

By universal consent, vision is regarded as the most precious of our senses and its loss as catastrophic. It is also the most complex, so that its study involves several different branches of science. The following brief review of related aspects is intended to place the scope of the present work in context.

The eye as a bodily organ

Since the eye is part of the body, it cannot be understood without some knowledge of general anatomy and physiology. It follows, then, that a more detailed study of ocular anatomy and physiology is required. Also, since drugs are often used in eye examination, pharmacology is another related study. Moreover, medically prescribed drugs may have ocular side-effects with which optical practitioners should be familiar.

Since one essential part of a complete eye examination is to detect any condition requiring medical attention, an adequate knowledge of general pathology is a necessary basis for a comprehensive study of abnormal ocular conditions. The presence of various systemic diseases, as well as disorders of the eye itself, may be inferred or suspected from a careful eye examination.

The eye as an optical instrument

Given the integrity of the eye as a bodily organ, we can now consider the main stages in the visual process. First is the normal stimulus to vision, generally known as light. Visible light is radiation within a narrow waveband of the electromagnetic spectrum, from about 380 to 780 nm. Radiations in the neighbouring spectral regions on either side – the ultraviolet and infrared – are also important clinically because of their potentially harmful effects on the eyes.

The eyes of many creatures incorporate an optical system, even if only a pinhole aperture, capable of forming an optical image. In the human eye, the performance of its optical system has almost reached the limit imposed by the nature of light itself. Given good illumination, it should normally be possible to resolve 40 lines per centimetre at a distance of 40 cm.

The eye's optical system, its possible focusing and other defects, and the various means of determining and correcting them form the main subject matter of this book. Other topics include the principles of various optical instruments used in the examination and testing of the eyes.

The eye as a photosensor

The formation of an image of the external scene is only the first step in the visual process. The internal lining, the retina, covers the greater part of the eye and forms a sensitive screen on which the optical image should fall when in sharp focus. No disadvantage arises from the fact that the interior of the eyeball is steeply curved: so is the optical image.

A striking feature of the human eye is that it can operate over an enormous range of brightness levels. This is made possible by the existence of two different sets of retinal receptors, named rods and cones. The rods become fully active at low (scotopic) and the cones at high (photopic) levels of luminance. In a single eye there are an estimated seven million cones and at least ten times that number of rods.

The rod and cone systems can operate simultaneously, but when very low illumination is suddenly encountered, it may take several minutes for the eyes to become 'dark-adapted'.

The next stage in the visual process is a complicated photochemical reaction between the light falling on the retina and chemical light absorbing substances within it. Rod reaction is mediated by the substance known as visual purple. Several different pigments take part in cone reaction, resulting in the radiant energy of the incident light being transformed into electrical impulses which are conveyed to the brain. These impulses are sent either singly or integrated from groups of retinal receptors via the optic nerve. A detailed study of these processes falls within the scope of physiological optics, a subject with ill-defined boundaries.

The quantity of light entering the eye can be regulated by the iris, which controls the pupil diameter. Since this latter also affects the eye's optical performance in various conditions, a balance may need to be struck between conflicting desirabilities.

The eye (and brain) as a data processor

An over-simplified earlier view of the relay from retina to brain suggested a comparison with the arrays of individually connected light bulbs used to display messages. Signals from the retinal receptors of each eye passed to the visual cortex of the brain where a single 'ocular' image was constructed point for point by the 'fusion' of the right and left retinal images. It is now known that the retinal and neural processes are much more complex. Interaction takes place between various groups of retinal receptors and there appear to be specialized neural channels for the detection of horizontal and vertical lines, different spatial frequencies and other important features of the scene viewed. A great deal of current visual research is in this field.

The eyes as a pair

The human frame allows many important organs to occur conveniently in pairs, affording some insurance in the event of injury or disease. A further advantage accrues to the eyes from this arrangement. Thanks to their slightly different viewpoints, additional information can be extracted about the relative positions of objects in space. With one eye closed, judgement of distances becomes unreliable.

Since vision is an integrated sensation, we are seldom conscious of our separate eyes. Various pathological conditions may gradually destroy part of the field of vision of one eye long before the victim notices the loss.

Binocular vision, the simultaneous use of both eyes working in conjunction, occurs in various stages of development in different species, but reaches its highest level of refinement in the primates. One of the factors making it possible is that the retina is not equally sensitive over its entire extent. In a very small central area – the fovea centralis – densely packed with cones only, the visual acuity or sharpness of vision reaches a pronounced peak. Two important advantages result. First, we are enabled to concentrate our visual and mental attention on a small but adequate field. Secondly, the fovea is able to play a key role in monitoring the necessary eye movements, which have to be carried out with great precision. Unless the central object of regard is imaged on the fovea of each eye, diplopia (double vision) results.

A set of six external muscles attached to the eyeball enables it to be moved smoothly in any desired direction. Faults in the system can occur. A squint is an obvious breakdown of co-ordination, but there are other less-pronounced anomalies of binocular vision which may call for relief. The investigation of binocular vision is an important sector of ophthalmic practice.

Visual perception

The manner in which the endless stream of data from our sensory organs becomes transmuted into sensations unique to the individual is largely unknown. A great deal of cerebral editing takes place. In the interests of the whole organism, some information is wholly or partially suppressed, or interpreted so as to conform to previous experience.

There is food for thought in the aphorism of Goethe that the mind seeks harmony and totality. This applies with particular force to vision. We would find it disturbing if the data from two different senses were contradictory. For example, in some contrived experimental situations, the apparent position of a near object varies according to whether or not it is held in the hand. Some people, too, experience disquiet when viewing a drawing of an 'impossible object'. As to totality, a striking feature of visual perception is our constant assumption that every drawing, however crude or simple, is intended to convey a meaning or represent a likeness. Even a very young child, when shown a crudely drawn circle containing two smaller circles above a vertical and a horizontal line, will interpret it as a face.

The familiar 'optical illusions' shed an interesting light on this subject. Many of them could perhaps be described as errors of visual judgement, arising from the data processing of the visual system. Other well-known illusions seem to suggest a visual preference for lines to intersect at right-angles. For example, long straight lines can be made to appear tilted or curved by a succession of short oblique lines drawn through them. The direction in which the line appears to be bent is such as to reduce its obliquity to the intersecting lines.

One of the most important topics of visual perception is colour vision, the mechanism of which figures prominently in physiological optics. The development of colour photography and television has generated considerable research in colour vision, which has an extensive specialized literature of its own.

Although what we finally perceive does not depend on the retinal image alone, this image is still the basis of the visual process. When studying a visual phenomenon or problem, the optics of the situation should always be exhausted before considering other and perhaps more speculative factors.

Visual perception comes under the heading of psychology. Most related research is carried out within this discipline or in collaboration with visual scientists.

Treatment of optics

In this work we have followed the principles, sign convention and symbols adopted jointly in the United Kingdom many years ago by the Applied Optics Department of the former Northampton Polytechnic Institute (now the City University) and the Imperial College. They are also used in Freeman's *Optics*, first published in 1934 as Fincham's *Optics*. The basis of the sign convention is that the direction of the incident light is always positive. Where possible, diagrams are drawn with the incident light coming from the left, so that the Cartesian sign convention for the *x*-axis also applies. When the incident light is from right to left, this becomes the positive direction and the Cartesian convention ceases to apply.

Though this sign convention is in world-wide use, not only in the ophthalmic field but in technical optics generally, other conventions unfortunately persist at a lower level. The great advantage of any convention is that it enables collections of rules for different cases to be replaced by a single algebraic relationship.

Because of its simplicity in optical calculations, extensive use has been made of the 'step-along' method associated with William Swaine and the layout for it devised later by Bennett.

In problems involving an eye looking through a lens or prism, students will find it helpful to follow the two-stage approach. First, the eye is ignored and the position and size of the image formed by the lens or prism are determined by the usual method. Next, this image, wherever it is formed, becomes the object for the eye, real or virtual as the case may be.

The value of diagrams, as distinct from thumbnail sketches, cannot be emphasized too strongly and they seldom need to be drawn to scale. If the diagram is right, the problem is already solved in principle. In making scale drawings, it is often essential to choose a very much larger scale vertically than horizontally. Only the true values of angles are falsified by this procedure.

Relevant standards and organizations

Official standards organizations

In all the countries in which optometry is firmly rooted, there is an official national standards organization. These bodies are mainly concerned with practical standards having industrial and consumer applications. Most of them fall into one of the following categories:

(1) dimension standards,
(2) standards of quality or performance,
(3) standard methods of testing or sampling,
(4) standard nomenclature and symbols,
(5) standard codes of practice.

A great many national standards have been published in the ophthalmic optical field.

International standards are the concern of three bodies working on parallel lines: the International Organization for Standardization (ISO), the International Electrotechnical Commission (IEC) and the Comité Européen de Normalisation (CEN), or European Committee for Standardization. The main object of the ISO is to reach international agreement on industrial standards facilitating commerce. Its membership comprises the official standards bodies of some 60 countries. To further its primary objective, the ISO also promotes the interchange and dissemination of scientific and technical data on standards.

The detailed work of preparing ISO standards is carried out on a voluntary basis by about 160 technical committees, 500 subcommittees and 600 working groups, all composed of nominees of the participating national standards organizations. These organizations can either accept a published ISO ophthalmic standard to which they have assented or incorporate the substance of it in a separate national standard. For Europe, the CEN is generally adopting the relevant ISO ophthalmic standards as official European standards: these automatically must replace any previous national standard.

In 1978, the ISO decided to set up the Technical Committee ISO/TC 172 to be responsible for international standards over a wide range of technical optics as well as ophthalmic optics. Manufacturing standards relating to the broad field of spectacle lenses, spectacle frames and their measurement, contact lenses and materials, and a number of ophthalmic instruments are among those in course of preparation or have been published; for example the two dealing with 'optotypes' (test charts) are briefly summarized in Chapter 3.

In general, even official standards are not mandatory in themselves unless referred to in legal contracts, legislation or statutory regulations. In the European Union, the general requirements for spectacles, contact lenses and ophthalmic instruments are covered by the Medical Devices Directive, published by the European Commission. The simplest way to satisfy this Directive is usually to demonstrate that the product complies with the relevant CEN standard.

Scientific units: the CIPM

Under the terms of the Metre Convention of 1875, to which forty or so countries are now parties, the Comité International des Poids et Mesures (CIPM) is the recognized authority on all scientific matters relating to the metric system, including the fundamental physical units of mass, length and time.

In 1960, the CIPM adopted a rationalized restructuring of the metric system known as SI (Système International d'Unités). The metre (m), kilogram (kg) and second (s) are three of the 'basic units', the remaining four being the ampere (A), the degree Kelvin (K), the candela (cd) and the mole (mol). To these are added the radian (rad) and steradian (sr) as 'supplementary units'. All other units, called 'derived', are defined in terms of the basic units.* Standard symbols are used, and there is a convention governing the choice of subdivisions and multiples of units.

An official translation into English of the Système International d'Unités has been prepared jointly by the National Bureau of Standards (USA) and the National Physical Laboratory (UK). It is published independently by the same body in the USA and by Her Majesty's Stationery Office in the United Kingdom.

Other organizations

There are certain other international bodies concerned with technical or ophthalmic optics.

Commission Internationale de l'Eclairage

The International Commission on Illumination, known in Great Britain by the initials of its French name (CIE) and in the USA as ICI, is the recognized inter-

---

*The unit of focal power, the dioptre, which is defined in the next chapter, has the physical dimensions of, and the official SI abbreviation, m^{-1}. In this text, the symbol D will continue to be employed, partly for historical reasons, partly for brevity, and partly to distinguish power from curvature.

national body concerned with photometry and colorimetry. It has published many standard tables in these fields and was responsible for the CIE chromaticity chart and system of colorimetry. In 1929, the CIPM decided to extend its competence to photometric standards and four years later set up a Consultative Committee on Photometry with which the CIE has fully cooperated. The revised definition of the candela, the unit of luminance adopted by the CIPM in 1967, was put forward by the CIE.

International Commission on Optics (ICO)

This body was set up in 1948 with a number of general aims including that of promoting international agreement on nomenclature, units, symbols, specifications, methods of control and similar subjects. However, since the ISO has entered this field, it is unlikely that the ICO would wish to pursue any separate activities within it.

International Federation of Ophthalmological Societies

At the fourteenth International Ophthalmological Congress, held in 1933, it was decided to set up this Federation to put future activities on a more organized footing. Membership is composed of the national ophthalmological societies of some forty or more countries. Though the Federation had recently shown a renewed interest in formulating an international test chart for visual acuity, it may now be content to pursue this aim through the ISO. Medical bodies are usually well represented on appropriate technical committees of national standards organizations.

Photometric units

Many changes in photometric nomenclature and units were made in the third (1970) edition of the International Electrotechnical Vocabulary, prepared jointly by the IEC and the CIE. In particular, the unit of luminance is now the candela per square metre, replacing the footlambert, millilambert and other former units. For this reason, we have added a scale in cd/m^2 to those diagrams reproduced from earlier writings, in which older units of luminance were employed. The conversion factors to cd/m^2 are 3.426 for footlamberts, 3.183 for millilamberts.

The troland, a special unit of retinal illuminance, is explained on page 24.

Definitions in experimental assessment

In relation to the performance of equipment and the criteria to be adopted for diagnostic purposes, the reader may come across various familiar terms which have acquired a specialized meaning in this context. Although little used in this book, some definitions of them are provided here as they are not otherwise readily available.

Accuracy: a general term describing the ability of an instrument to provide good results. It may be broken down into:

Precision or repeatability: this is the consistency with which repeated measurements are made, and could be related to statistical concepts such as the standard deviation. The official ISO definition is given at the end of this section.

Comparability or validity: this is the ability to measure correctly what is supposed to be measured.

For example, a focimeter (lensometer) would be giving valid results if the mean of several measurements of a +6.00 D lens were +6.00 D, even though the standard deviation was +1.00 D. Conversely, another instrument would be precise if the standard deviation were +0.05 D, even though the mean result of +5.50 D was incorrect (invalid). Neither instrument could be regarded as accurate.

In clinical work, criteria have to be adopted to distinguish or discriminate between normals and abnormals.

Because no instrument or test routine is perfect, some subjects will be incorrectly classified. To take a very simple example, a poor ability to converge the eyes is likely to cause symptoms in near work. If the percentage of the sample population is plotted against the near point of convergence, for both the symptom-free and symptomatic groups, then one might find a result similar to that in *Figure 1.1*. Because of the overlapping of the two curves, any dividing line D is likely to produce four subclassifications, set out in *Table 1.1*.

If the near point of convergence were a reliable and valid predictor of symptoms in near work, there would be no misclassifications of false negative and false positive. In practice, however, these errors in classification are inevitable.

Thus in this example, false negatives are people who should have been identified as having poor convergence. False positives are asymptomatic people that the test has inappropriately identified as abnormal.

Moving the dividing line D towards poorer convergence will reduce the number of false positives, but at the expense of increasing the number of false negatives.

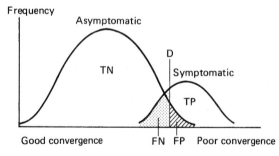

Figure 1.1. Population frequency of a normal (asymptomatic) and an abnormal (symptomatic) population. The dividing line (D) partitions the asymptomatic group into true negatives and false positives (shown hatched), and the symptomatic into false negatives (shown stippled) and true positives. (After Reeves and Hill, 1987, reproduced by kind permission of the editor of *Optician*.)

Table 1.1 Classification of true and false negatives and positives. (The figures in parentheses are used in a numerical example later)

Sample population	Test result	
	Negative (normal convergence)	Positive (poor convergence)
Normal (asymptomatic)	True (1000)	False (15)
Abnormal (symptomatic)	False (10)	True (40)

Two terms used to describe the ability of a test to discriminate between normals and abnormals are sensitivity and specificity.

Sensitivity* is measured by the proportion of abnormals (or true positives) who are identified by the test to the total number of abnormals. Mathematically, it is the ratio:

(true positives)/(true positives + false negatives).

Specificity* relates to the proportion of normals (or true negatives) who pass the test to the total number of normals. Mathematically, it is the ratio:

(true negatives)/(true negatives + false positives).

False positive error rate is the proportion of false positives expressed as a percentage of the total number of positive classifications obtained on the test.

The function (1− specificity) or false alarm rate, indicating the ratio of false positives to all normals, is an alternative concept.

A graph of sensitivity plotted against the false alarm rate is termed an ROC (receiver operating characteristic) curve. An explanation with examples is given by Jenkins *et al.* (1989).

False negative error rate is the proportion of false negative results expressed as a proportion of the total number of negative classifications on the test.

Using the figures in the table, the sensitivity is 40/50, or 80%, while the specificity is 1000/1015, or 98.5%. The false positive error rate is 15/55 or 27.3%, while the false negative error rate is 10/1010 or 1.0%.

An ideal test, whether of an instrument or clinical procedure, will have both high sensitivity and specificity. If an instrument is made too sensitive, it is likely to fail an increased proportion of normals. Conversely, if the specificity is raised, sensitivity usually drops. Hill (1987) demonstrates that two neighbouring dividing lines can be used to give reduced numbers of false positives and false negatives. People whose results lie in the zone of uncertainty between the two cut-off criteria should be further examined by other tests before being classified.

Some official ISO definitions taken from BS ISO 3534-1:1993 *Statistics – Vocabulary and symbols – Part 1: Probability and general statistical terms*, and reproduced with the kind permission of the British Standards Institution† are:

Precision: The closeness of agreement between independent test results obtained under stipulated conditions.
Repeatability: Precision under repeatability conditions.
Repeatability conditions: Conditions where independent test results are obtained with the same method on identical test items in the same laboratory by the same operator using the same equipment within short intervals of time.
Reproducibility: Precision under reproducibility conditions.
Reproducibility conditions: Conditions where test results are obtained with the same method on identical test items in different laboratories with different operators using different equipment.
Reproducibility Standard Deviation, s_R: The standard deviation of test results obtained under reproducibility conditions. (This is a measure of the dispersion of the distribution of test results under repeatability conditions.)
Reproducibility limit, R: The value less than or equal to which the absolute difference between two test results obtained under reproducibility conditions may be expected to lie with a probability of 95%.

Some articles with references to this subject are listed below.

Future developments

Confident predictions are naturally difficult in this era of rapid change. Spectacles have now been in existence for 700 years and seem likely to retain their popularity indefinitely. Although contact lenses have made enormous advances, they are still generally unsuitable for the young and the elderly and there are fears that prolonged or indiscriminate wear may lead to wide-scale damage to the cornea. Various surgical methods of correcting focusing errors by modifying the curvature of the cornea have been devised. Although some successes have been achieved, these methods are at present somewhat inaccurate as well as too drastic for the majority of spectacle wearers, while some techniques are appropriate only for short-sighted people.

As we shall see in Chapters 18 and 19, automation has already established itself in some of the instruments and routines used in eye examination. As a result, certain parts of the examination may become increasingly delegated to assistants without optometric qualifications. Plotting of the visual fields, even by traditional methods, is regarded as one that can be carried out by auxiliary personnel. The scope for automation in the testing of binocular functions is probably limited.

---

* A possible but somewhat clumsy mnemonic for remembering these terms is that seNsitivity is *not* to do with Negatives, while sPecificity is *not* to do with Positives.

† Complete editions of the standards can be obtained by post from BSI Customer Services, 389 Chiswick High Road, London W4 4AL.

It is unlikely to provide information as quickly and conveniently as the simple cover test and fixation disparity test, both described in Chapter 10.

In researches on vision, increasing use is being made of techniques of gaining information from the electrical activity in the visual centres of the brain. Whether these methods will find a use in routine eye examination is open to doubt.

Further reading

ASPINALL, P. and HILL, A.R. (1983) Clinical inferences and decisions – I. Diagnosis and Bayes' theorem. *Ophthal. Physiol. Opt.*, **3**, 295–304

ASPINALL, P. and HILL, A.R. (1984) Clinical inferences and decisions – II. Decision trees, receiver operator curves and subjective probability. *Ophthal. Physiol. Opt.*, **4**, 31–38

ASPINALL, P.A. and HILL, A.R. (1984) Clinical inferences and decisions – III. Utility assessment and the Bayesian decision model. *Ophthal. Physiol. Opt.*, **4**, 251–263

GILCHRIST, J. (1992) QROC curves and kappa functions: new methods for evaluating the quality of clinical decisions. *Ophthal. Physiol. Opt.*, **12**, 350–360

HILL, A.R. (1987) Making decisions in ophthalmology, Ch. 8 in *Progress in Retinal Research*, Vol. 6 (Osborne, N. and Chader, G., eds), Oxford: Pergamon

HOUGH, T., LIVNAT, A., and KEREN, E. (1996) Inter-laboratory reproducibility of toric hydrogel lenses using the focimeter and the moiré deflectometer. *J. Br. Contact Lens Assoc.*, **19**, 117–127

JENKINS, T.C.A., PICKWELL, L.D. and YEKTA, A.A. (1989) Criteria for decompensation in binocular vision. *Ophthal. Physiol. Opt.*, **9**, 121–125

REEVES, B.C. and HILL, A.R. (1987) Practical problems in measuring contrast sensitivity. *Optician*, **193**(5085), 29–34; (5086), 30–34

REEVES, B.C., HILL, A.R. and ROSS, J.E. (1988) Test–retest reliability of the Arden Grating Test: inter-tester variability. *Ophthal. Physiol. Opt.*, **8**, 128–138

2

The eye's optical system

The eye and the camera

Considered as an optical instrument, the eye has certain similarities to a camera, though it would be truer to say that the camera has been copied from the eye. The points of difference are worth noting, the eye being superior on almost every count. It is much more compact, has a wider field of view, operates over a much more extensive range of luminance levels and its resolving power is close to the theoretical limit. Paradoxically – as Helmholtz pointed out – the typical eye nevertheless exhibits aberrations and errors of centration that an optical designer would consider unacceptable in a high-grade man-made system.

The aberrations of the eye are considered in detail in Chapter 15 and so here we shall look at the basic image-forming properties of the eye from the standpoint of simple geometrical optics valid for the paraxial region. Although you are probably familiar with optical principles, an outline of the notation and methods used in this book is given in the following pages. For a more detailed treatment including proofs, the works listed in the bibliography at the end of the book are useful.

Laws of optical image formation

Sign convention

(1) Distances measured in the same direction as that in which the incident light is travelling are regarded as positive in sign; if in the opposite direction, as negative.
(2) Object and image distances, focal lengths and radii of curvature are measured *from* the lens, mirror or surface concerned. The sign follows from (1).
(3) Diagrams are normally drawn so that the incident light travels from left to right.
(4) The vertical distance from the optical axis to a point above it is taken as positive, and to a point below it as negative.
(5) For some purposes, a sign convention for angles is needed. In accordance with accepted mathematical convention, angles measured in an anticlockwise direction are regarded as positive. The angle between a ray and the optical axis is measured from the ray to the axis.

Symbols

Standard symbols for the most important quantities are as follows:

Refractive index	n
Object distance	ℓ
Image distance	ℓ'
First focal length	f
Second focal length	f'
Radius of curvature	r
Object height	h
Image height	h'

The presence of a dash (or 'prime') shows at once that the symbol refers to a quantity after refraction or reflection, the same symbol undashed denoting the corresponding quantity before refraction or reflection.

To denote the reciprocal of a distance, the corresponding capital letter is used. Thus $L = 1/\ell$, $R = 1/r$ and so on.

Letters used as symbols denoting a quantity are normally printed in italic type. On the other hand, letters in Roman capitals denote geometrical points. This helps to distinguish between F (the power of a lens or surface) and F (the first principal focus).

Subscript numerals are helpful in identifying one of a series of successive refractions or reflections. For example h'_2 denotes the image height after the second refraction or reflection.

'Real' and 'virtual'

When refraction or reflection takes place at two or more surfaces in succession, the image formed at the first, whatever its nature, becomes the object for the next. This gives rise to the possibility of 'virtual' objects as well as virtual images. Real and virtual types of object may give rise to either type of image.

Definitions

(1) A real object is one from which incident rays diverge.
(2) A virtual object is one towards which incident rays are converging as the result of a previous refraction or reflection.

(3) A real image is one towards which refracted or reflected rays converge and is therefore capable of being received on a screen.

(4) A virtual image is one from which refracted or reflected rays *appear* to emanate.

Refraction at a spherical surface

Let A be the vertex and C the centre of curvature of a spherical surface, a line through A and C being taken as the 'axis' (*Figure 2.1*).

If the surface is converging (for example, convex, air to glass) the first principal focus F is the real point on the axis giving rise to an image at infinity, the refracted ray being parallel to the axis. The second principal focus F′ is the real image point on the axis corresponding to an object point at infinity, the incident rays being parallel to the axis.

The same definitions apply to a diverging surface, except that in this case F is a virtual object point and F′ a virtual image point (*Figure 2.2*).

In both cases, the distance AF is the first focal length f and AF′ the second focal length $f′$.

Let B be an axial object point giving rise to the image point B′ (*Figure 2.3*). Then, in all possible cases,

$$\ell = AB$$
$$\ell′ = AB′$$
$$r = AC$$
$$n = \text{refractive index of first medium}$$
$$n′ = \text{refractive index of second medium}$$

and

$$\frac{n′}{\ell′} = \frac{n}{\ell} + \frac{n′ - n}{r} \tag{2.1}$$

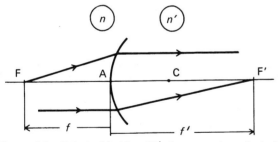

Figure 2.1. Principal foci F and F′ of a converging spherical refracting surface.

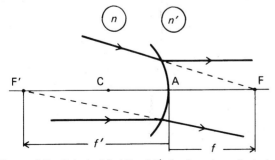

Figure 2.2. Principal foci F and F′ of a diverging spherical refracting surface.

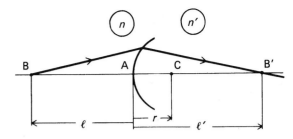

Figure 2.3. Refraction at a converging spherical surface.

For an object at infinity, $n/\ell = 0$ and $\ell′ = f′$. Similarly, for an image at infinity $n′/\ell′ = 0$ and $\ell = f$. Hence

$$\frac{n′}{f′} = \frac{-n}{f} = \frac{n′ - n}{r} \tag{2.2}$$

Power and vergence

For a spherical refracting surface, the power F is given by the relationship

$$F = \frac{n′}{f′} = \frac{-n}{f} = \frac{n′ - n}{r} = (n′ - n)R \tag{2.3}$$

where the curvature R is the reciprocal of the radius of curvature in metres. The unit of curvature is the reciprocal metre (m^{-1}). From equation (2.3) the surface power is seen to be proportional to the *reciprocal* of the focal lengths. The unit of focal power is the dioptre (D), the focal lengths being expressed in metres for this purpose.

The term 'reduced distance' denotes a distance (or thickness of material) traversed by a pencil of rays, divided by the refractive index of the given medium. On this basis, the reciprocal of a reduced object or image distance, such as $n′/\ell′$ in equation (2.1), is traditionally called the 'reduced vergence'. For brevity, however, we shall omit the word 'reduced' from this term. In this work vergence will be used to denote the reciprocal of an object or image distance (in metres) multiplied by the refractive index of the corresponding medium.[*] Like focal power, its unit is the dioptre. Accordingly

Object vergence $L = n/\ell$ (in metres)
Image vergence $L′ = n′/\ell′$ (in metres)

Equation (2.1) can now be rewritten in the more convenient form

$$L′ = L + F \tag{2.4}$$

in which all quantities are in dioptres.

It is a fundamental rule that a positive value of L or $L′$ always denotes convergence, while a negative value always denotes divergence.

Unless otherwise stated, all distances in algebraic formulae throughout this book should be taken to be in metres. If numerical values in millimetres are substi-

---

[*] The term 'vergence' has traditionally been used as a synonym for wavefront curvature, the unit of which is the reciprocal metre, not the dioptre.

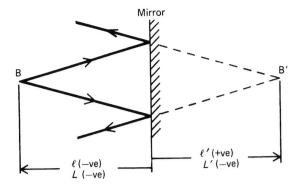

Figure 2.4. Sign convention for reflection.

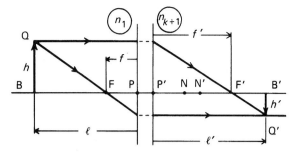

Figure 2.5. The cardinal points and conjugate foci of an unequifocal refracting system.

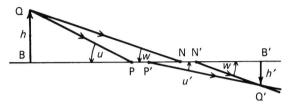

Figure 2.6. Image construction for an optical system using the principal and nodal points.

tuted in such expressions, a compensating factor of 1000 must be introduced.

The thin lens

A thin lens in air has two principal foci F and F′ and two focal lengths f and f', defined exactly as for a spherical refracting surface. In this case, however, the power F of the lens is given by

$$F = 1/f' = -1/f \qquad (2.5)$$

again in dioptres if f' and f are in metres.

The conjugate focus relationship (2.4) applies equally to a thin lens in air.

Reflection

When light is reflected by a mirror (*Figure 2.4*), whether plane or spherical, there is a reversal of direction which upsets the usual correspondence between the signs of ℓ and L'. The same applies to the focal length of a mirror, since the focal length is also an image distance. Consequently, for reflection only we must put (assuming the mirror is in air)

$$L' = -1/\ell'; \qquad \ell = -1/L' \qquad (2.6)$$

and

$$F = -1/f' = \frac{-2}{r}; \quad f' = -1/F \qquad (2.7)$$

There is, however, no change in the relationship $L = 1/\ell$.

The conjugate focus relationship for reflection then assumes the familiar form

$$L' = L + F$$

Theoretically, reflection obeys the same laws as refraction if $-n$ is substituted for n'.

Unequifocal systems

The eye is an example of an unequifocal optical system, one in which the first and last media have different refractive indices. In general, such systems have six cardinal points (*Figure 2.5*) as follows:

(1) F and F′, the first and second principal foci, defined exactly as for a single refracting surface.

(2) P and P′, the first and second principal points.
(3) N and N′, the first and second nodal points.

The cardinal points are always symmetrically positioned such that PP′= NN′ and FP = N′F′.

The system as a whole has an 'equivalent power' F such that

$$F = \frac{n_{k+1}}{f'} = \frac{-n_1}{f} \qquad (2.8)$$

where $f' = $ P′F′, $f = $ PF, $n_1 = $ refractive index of first medium and $n_{k+1} = $ refractive index of last medium, the system having k surfaces.

If the object distance ℓ is measured from P and the image distance ℓ' is measured from P′, the conjugate focus relationship again takes the form

$$L' = L + F$$

where $L = n_1/\ell$ and $L' = n_{k+1}/\ell'$.

Let a ray from an extra-axial object point Q be directed towards P, making an angle u with the optical axis (*Figure 2.6*). The corresponding emergent ray will appear to have passed through P′ making an angle u' with the optical axis such that

$$n_{k+1}u' = n_1 u \qquad (2.9)$$

Let another ray from Q be directed towards the first nodal point N. The corresponding emergent ray will appear to have passed through the second nodal point N′ without undergoing a change of direction. As indicated in *Figure 2.6*, these two pairs of rays can be used to construct the image B′Q′ of an object BQ.

The properties of the two principal foci F and F′ can also be used for this purpose, as shown in *Figure 2.5*.

Transverse magnification

The expression

$$m = h'/h = L/L' \qquad (2.10)$$

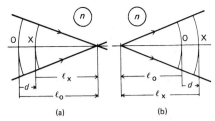

Figure 2.7.   Effectivity: (a) converging bundle, (b) diverging bundle.

in which *m* denotes the transverse magnification, applies equally to refraction and reflection at a single surface, as well as to thin lenses and optical systems. Because this vergence formula for magnification is so general, its use is preferable to the alternative forms, in which vergence is expressed in terms of object and image distances.

Effectivity

Let a pencil of rays (*Figure 2.7*) be travelling in a medium of refractive index *n* and let the distance to the origin (or from the focus) of the pencil be ℓ_o measured at a specific point O. After travelling a distance *d* metres from O to another specified point X, the wavefront is at a distance ℓ_x from its origin or focus. Hence,

$$\ell_x = \ell_o - d$$

and

$$L_x = \frac{n}{\ell_x} = \frac{n}{\ell_o - d} = \frac{n}{(n/L_o) - d}$$

$$= \frac{L_o}{1 - (d/n)L_o} \tag{2.11}$$

This expresses a general effectivity relationship, 'effectivity' denoting a change of vergence as light passes from one surface or reference point to another.

If *d* is relatively small, the above expression can be expanded by the binomial theorem to give the useful approximation

$$L_x \approx L_o \left(1 + \frac{d}{n} L_o + \cdots \right)$$

$$\approx L_o + \frac{d}{n} \cdot L_o^2 + \cdots \tag{2.12}$$

The quantity *d/n* is an example of a reduced distance.

Refractive index

The refractive index of a transparent medium varies with wavelength, and, to a lesser extent, with temperature. Unless the context indicates otherwise, the term should be understood as an abbreviation for 'mean refractive index', namely, the value for a selected wavelength in the brightest part of the spectrum. The d-line of the helium spectrum ($\lambda = 587.6$ nm) is often chosen for this purpose. Measurements are normally made at a temperature in the neighbourhood of 18–20°C.

Angles and prism power

Throughout the text, angles will be expressed in radians, degrees, or prism dioptres (symbol Δ). This last measure, which is of great convenience in ophthalmic optics, was introduced in 1890 by C. F. Prentice (but not given this name by him). If *u* is any angle less than 90°, then

$$u \text{ in } \Delta = 100 \tan u \tag{2.13}$$

Thus, in *Figure 2.6*

$$u = 100(\text{BQ}/\text{BP}) \Delta$$

Thus, in terms of SI units, the prism dioptre is expressed as cm/m.

A disadvantage of this system is that the tangent of an angle does not increase in proportion to the angle itself when other than small values are concerned. For example, 20 Δ is equivalent to $\tan^{-1} 0.20$ or 11.31°, whereas 40 Δ is equivalent to $\tan^{-1} 0.40$ or 21.80°.

For small angles, the formula

$$4° = 7 \Delta \tag{2.14}$$

is an easily remembered and useful approximation.

It also follows from equation (2.13) that for small values the prism dioptre is equivalent to one-hundredth of a radian, since both the sine and the tangent of a small angle are very nearly equal to the angle itself in radian measure.

In the ophthalmic world, the prism dioptre is the accepted unit of prismatic power and deviation. According to the currrent British Standard[*] for ophthalmic trial case lenses, prisms are to be numbered according to the deviation (in Δ) undergone by a ray of wavelength 587.6 nm incident normally at one surface.

The cornea

With this introduction we can now study the various components of the eye's optical system, first in sequence and then the system as a whole.

The cornea (*Figure 2.8*) is a highly transparent structure of meniscus form, approximately 12 mm in diameter and slightly smaller vertically than horizontally.

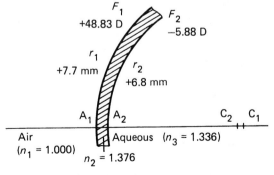

Figure 2.8.   Profile of the human cornea (to scale): average values as adopted in Gullstrand's schematic eye.

---

[*] BS 3162: *Ophthalmic trial case lenses.*

The centre thickness is usually between 0.5 and 0.6 mm.

A thin layer of lacrimal fluid normally covers the anterior surface but it is too thin to affect the power appreciably and may be ignored in this context.

To a first approximation both surfaces may be regarded as spherical, the radii of curvature having values in the neighbourhood of +7.7 mm (anterior) and +6.8 mm (posterior).*

The refractive index of the corneal substance may be taken as 1.376 and that of the aqueous humour, in contact with the back surface of the cornea, as 1.336.* By applying equation (2.3), the two surface powers of the cornea may be found as follows:

(1) *Anterior surface*

$$\text{Power } F_1 = \frac{1000(1.376 - 1)}{+7.7}$$
$$= +48.83 \text{ D}$$

(2) *Posterior surface*

$$\text{Power } F_2 = \frac{1000(1.336 - 1.376)}{+6.8}$$
$$= -5.88 \text{ D}$$

The power of the cornea as a whole is therefore about +43 D, over two-thirds of the total power of the eye.

When the eyes are unprotected under water, the anterior surface of the cornea has its power greatly reduced, the retinal image then becoming inordinately blurred.

The anterior chamber

The anterior chamber is the cavity lying behind the cornea and in front of the iris and crystalline lens. It is filled with a colourless liquid aptly termed the aqueous humour, since its water content is 98%.

The depth of the anterior chamber, measured along the eye's optical axis, is strictly the distance from the posterior vertex of the cornea to the anterior surface of the crystalline, but the term as sometimes used includes the corneal thickness. Excluding this latter, an average value would be about 3.0 mm.

From an optical point of view, the depth of the anterior chamber is important inasmuch as it affects the total power of the eye's optical system. If all other elements remained unchanged, a reduction of 1 mm in the depth of the anterior chamber (through a forward shift of the crystalline) would increase the eye's total power by about 1.4 D. The reverse effect would result from a shift in the opposite direction.

The iris and pupil

The amount of light admitted to the eye is regulated by the pupil, an approximately circular opening in the iris.

In normal conditions the pupils react to:

(1) A change in luminance – the 'direct' reflex
(2) A change in luminance applied to one eye only, also producing a 'consensual' reflex in the fellow eye,
(3) Near fixation, which is accompanied by pupillary contraction.

Failure or anomaly of one or more of these reflexes may be an important pointer to some underlying disorder.

The pupil size decreases with age at an approximately uniform rate which does, however, tend to slow down in later life. Largely because of differences in techniques of measurement, there is only a limited measure of agreement between various published studies. The following diameters can be taken as typical. For the eye in total darkness, 7.6 mm at age 10, 6.2 mm at age 45, and 5.2 mm at age 80. For the light-adapted eye, 4.8 mm at age 10, 4.0 mm at age 45, and 3.4 mm at age 80.

Pupil size can be affected by a number of external or secondary agencies such as drugs, emotions, and sudden changes in the state of mind.

The crystalline lens

The crystalline lens serves the double purpose of supplying the balance of the eye's refractive power and providing a mechanism for focusing at different distances. This latter faculty is called accommodation.

Both anatomically and optically, the lens is a highly complex structure, composed of layers of fibres laid down in an essentially radial pattern that is regular enough to allow a symmetrical diffraction halo to be formed (*see* Chapter 22). The lens continues to grow in bulk throughout life by the formation of fresh layers of fibres on the exterior. As part of the normal process of ageing it is susceptible to various changes impairing its flexibility and transparency. Its centre thickness is thereby increased, while the radii of curvature may become longer.

The lens substance is enclosed in a highly elastic capsule. A structure of suspensory ligaments, called the zonule of Zinn, stretches from the periphery of the capsule to the surrounding ciliary body, holding the lens in position and controlling the curvature of its surfaces through variations in tension produced by the action of the ciliary muscle.

The lens has a diameter of approximately 9 mm and is biconvex in form, the radius of its anterior surface being about 1.7 times that of its posterior surface. When the lens is in its unaccommodated state, the centre thickness has traditionally been taken as 3.6 mm, a figure appropriate to a young adult. As accommodation is brought into play, both surfaces, but especially the anterior, assume a more steeply curved form. The centre thickness thus increases and the vertex of the anterior surface moves forward, reducing the depth of the anterior diameter. The profiles of a typical crystalline in its relaxed and fully accommodated states are shown superimposed in *Figure 2.9* which has

---

* The values assumed by Gullstrand in his schematic eye.

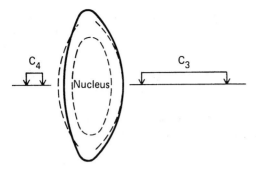

Figure 2.9. Profiles of the human crystalline lens in its relaxed and fully accommodated states.

been drawn to scale. The diagram also indicates the range of positions of the two centres of curvature.

The back surface of the crystalline is in contact with the vitreous humour, a transparent gel which fills the posterior segment of the globe. The vitreous humour has very nearly the same chemical composition as the aqueous and its refractive index may be taken as the same, 1.336.

Because of its onion-like structure and the compression exerted on the innermost layers, the crystalline lens is far from being optically homogeneous. A slit-lamp section reveals several bands of discontinuity. In particular, it is possible to distinguish a central biconvex portion called the nucleus, from the surrounding portion, called the cortex. In the centre of the nucleus, the refractive index reaches its maximum value between 1.40 and 1.41 but diminishes from the centre outwards, being about 1.385 near the poles and about 1.375 near the equator.

It may easily be deduced that a refractive index gradient of this pattern, irrespective of any surface curvatures, must produce a converging effect like a positive lens. Since the velocity of light in a medium is inversely proportional to its refractive index, an incident wavefront would become progressively less retarded from the centre outwards and hence assume a convergent form. By way of confirmation, Ivanoff (1953) crushed a rabbit crystalline between parallel glass plates so that all the surfaces including those of the nucleus were rendered effectively plane. He then found that the element so produced had a power in air of just over $+6$ D.

In his book *Physical Optics*, Wood (1911) described a simple method of making 'pseudo lenses' from discs of gelatine enclosed between glass plates. Immersion in water, which has a lower refractive index, brings about a progressive decline in index towards the periphery, producing positive power up to about $+12$ D. Both Ivanoff (following Bouasse) and Wood have given mathematical analyses, while Fowler and Pateras (1990) give some experimental results.

As a result of this effect, the crystalline lens has a greater power than would be the case if its refractive index were uniform and had the highest value actually found. In fact, it is necessary to assume a fictitious refractive index of about 1.42 to bring the power of a homogeneous crystalline lens up to a typical value in the neighbourhood of $+21$ D.

The assumption that the lens surfaces are spherical is for convenience only. Careful observation reveals a marked degree of peripheral flattening, especially of the anterior surface in its accommodated state. Owing to this, and to the peripheral flattening of the cornea, the eye's spherical aberration is kept within reasonable limits, as we shall see in Chapter 15.

The retina

Anatomically an outgrowth of the brain, the retina is a thin but enormously intricate structure, its functions being much more extensive than was originally supposed. It lines the posterior portion of the globe, extending functionally up to the *ora serrata* close to the ciliary body.

A surprising feature of the retina is that the nerve fibres transmitting impulses from individual or groups of retinal receptors travel across its surface to their exit via the main trunk of the optic nerve. The retina is also supplied with blood vessels which are clearly visible through an ophthalmoscope. Despite these obstructions to the incident light, the efficiency of the system does not appear to suffer. Under certain conditions, however, retinal blood vessels may be seen entoptically by the shadows which they cast (*see* Chapter 22).

As described more fully in Chapter 3, the ability of the retina to distinguish detail is not uniform over its entire extent and reaches a maximum in the macular region. This is an approximately circular area of diameter about 1.5 mm containing a smaller central area, the fovea, populated exclusively by retinal cones. It is at the fovea that the eye attains its maximum resolving power. When an object engages visual attention, the two eyes are instinctively turned so that the image lies on each fovea.

From an optical point of view, the retina could be described as the screen on which the image is formed. It can be regarded as part of a concave spherical surface with a radius of curvature in the neighbourhood of -12 mm.

In cameras and optical instruments generally, it is convenient to have images formed on plane surfaces, but the curvature of the retina has two positive advantages. In the first place, the images formed by optical systems tend to have curved surfaces. The curvature of the retina is of the right order from this point of view (*see* Chapter 15). Secondly, the steeply curved retina is able to cover a much wider field of view than would otherwise be possible.

The schematic eye

General properties

The schematic eye is a theoretical optical specification of an idealized eye, retaining average dimensions but omitting the complications (*see* Chapter 12 for details). The equivalent power of the unaccommodated eye as a whole is $+60$ D and its cardinal points are situated as shown in *Figure 2.10*. The first and second principal

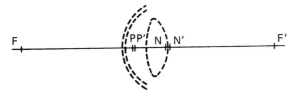

Figure 2.10. The cardinal points of the unaccommodated schematic eye (to scale).

points, P and P′, lie in the anterior chamber at distances of about 1.5 and 1.8 mm respectively from the front surface of the cornea. The nodal points, N and N′, are also separated by 0.3 mm and straddle the back surface of the crystalline lens. The anterior focal length PF is about −16.7 mm and the posterior focal length P′F′ about +22.3 mm.

The general relationships and ray paths indicated in *Figures 2.5* and *2.6* apply in every particular to the schematic eye.

Optical centration

In the schematic eye it is assumed that all the refracting surfaces are coaxial, the cornea and crystalline having a common optical axis. The optical centration of the typical human eye seems to be defective, the crystalline lens being usually decentred and tilted with respect to the cornea. For this reason the eye does not possess a true optical axis. However, as shown in Chapter 12, the principal points of the cornea very nearly coincide as do those of the schematic crystalline lens. Consequently, a line drawn as nearly as possible through these two pairs of points would represent a very close approximation to an optical axis. The use of this term in relation to the eye can be justified on this basis.

Entrance and exit pupils

The real pupil HJ is assumed to lie in the plane of the anterior pole of the crystalline lens (*Figure 2.11*). If its centre at E_o is regarded as an object for the cornea, it will give rise to a slightly magnified image with its

centre at E. This image is called the 'entrance pupil'. Taken as an object for the crystalline lens, the pupil HJ will give rise to another image, the 'exit pupil', with its centre at E′.

It follows from this that an incident pencil of rays directed towards and filling the entrance pupil would pass through the entire area of the real pupil, after refraction by the cornea, and on finally emerging into the vitreous body, would appear to have been limited by the exit pupil.

Further, since a ray directed towards the axial point E appears after refraction to have passed through the axial point E′, these two points must be conjugate with respect to the system as a whole.

On the basis of paraxial theory, it may be shown that the entrance pupil is situated about 3 mm behind the anterior surface of the cornea and is about 13% larger than the real pupil. The exit pupil lies closely behind the real pupil and is only 3% larger.

Because E and E′ are conjugate points, another relationship can be established. If an incident ray directed towards E makes an angle u with the optical axis, the conjugate refracted ray will make an angle u' with the axis such that

$$u'/u = \text{a constant for a given system}$$

For the schematic eye the value of this constant is about 0.82.

The visual axis

It might be reasonable to expect that the fovea would be situated on the retina at its intersection with the optical axis, a point termed the 'posterior pole'. In fact, the fovea is normally displaced temporally and downwards from the expected position. We are therefore led to postulate a 'visual axis' as distinct from the optical axis.

The visual axis has been taken by many writers to be the imaginary line directed towards the first nodal point N such that a parallel line through N′ would pass through the fovea. Apart from a slight displacement due to the separation of the two nodal points, as seen in *Figure 2.6*, an incident ray travelling along this path would be otherwise undeviated. Indeed, it could be assumed without serious error that a mean position of the two nodal points existed and the visual axis could be defined as the line passing through this mean position and the fovea.

However, the present writers share the objection to this concept already voiced by others. The term 'visual axis' ought to mean the axis or chief ray of the actual pencil of rays which enters the pupil and is converged to the fovea. Accordingly, despite the weight of present contrary opinion, the term 'visual axis' will be used here to denote the incident ray path directed towards the centre E of the entrance pupil such that the conjugate refracted ray falls on the fovea, M′ (*Figure 2.12*).

The angle between the optical and visual axis is called the angle alpha, and is considered positive when the visual axis in object space lies on the nasal side of the optical axis. A positive value in the neighbourhood of 5° is commonly found. There seems to be general agree-

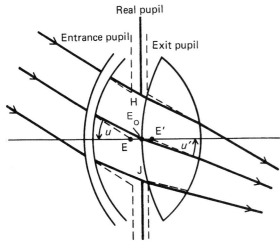

Figure 2.11. The eye's real pupil and its images, the entrance and exit pupils.

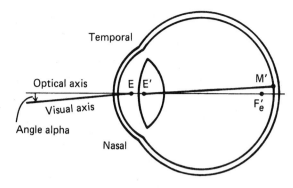

Figure 2.12.   The optical and visual axes of the eye. Its second principal focus F'_e is shown in a position indicating myopia.

ment with Donders' observation that the angle tends to be smaller in myopia and greater in hypermetropia.

As for the vertical plane, the visual axis in object space is generally inclined in an upward direction from the optical axis, the figure commonly quoted being about 2°.

The monocular visual field

The monocular field

On the temporal side, where there are no obstructions, the field of vision extends through more than 90° from the optical axis. The extreme ray entering the eye from this side follows approximately the path indicated in *Figure 2.13*. This diagram also explains why the retina extends so far forwards. It would not need to do so if light could not reach it.

The nose, brow and cheek limit the monocular visual field in other directions, so that its shape is irregular. A more detailed treatment of the visual fields is given in Chapter 8.

One can note here a useful application of the nodal points. If UN and VN in *Figure 2.14* are incident rays enclosing an angle *u*, the conjugate refracted rays will diverge as though from N′, still including the same angle *u*. Suppose these rays meet the retina at U′ and V′. Then, without entering at all into questions of visual

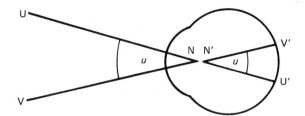

Figure 2.14.   Visual projection through the nodal point.

perception, one may draw the following inference: a linear extent of the retina subtending a known angle at the second nodal point corresponds to an equal angular extent of object space.

The fovea is about 0.3 mm horizontally by 0.2 mm vertically, subtending an angle at the second nodal point of about 0.018 by 0.012 rad. At a typical reading distance of 350 mm, this would cover an area of 6.3×4.2 mm, wide enough for four letters of the size commonly used for newsprint.

The blind spot

At the *papilla*, or optic disc, where the main trunk of the optic nerve leaves the eye, there are no retinal receptors. Consequently there is a corresponding 'blind spot' in the monocular field of vision, first noted by Mariotte in 1668.

The optic disc measures about 2 mm vertically by 1.5 mm horizontally, subtending an angle of some 7° by 5° at the second nodal point. This is also the angular subtense of the blind region in space. It has been pointed out that ten full moons placed side by side could disappear from view within this space.

The centre of the optic disc lies nasalwards from the fovea and slightly upwards from it. The centre of the blind space is accordingly some 15° on the temporal side of the visual axis and 2° below it.

In *Figure 2.15*, the positions on the retina of the macula and optic disc are shown in relation to the posterior pole. Dimensions given in degrees refer to the angular subtense at the second nodal point.

Undoubtedly the most surprising feature of the blind spot is that normally its existence is never noticed. Even if one eye is occluded and the other views a

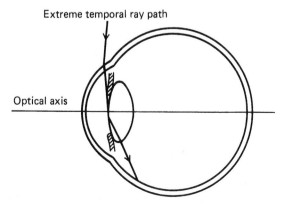

Figure 2.13.   The ray path at the limit of the eye's field of view.

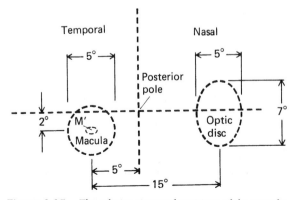

Figure 2.15.   The relative sizes and positions of the macula and optic disc. M′ denotes the fovea.

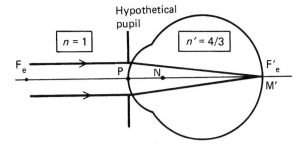

Figure 2.16. The reduced eye and its hypothetical pupil.

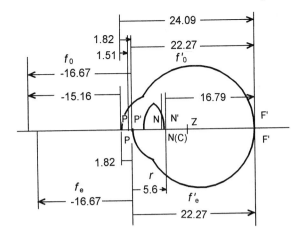

Figure 2.17. Comparison of the Bennett–Rabbetts schematic eye with the simple reduced eye.

strongly patterned or brightly coloured expanse, the observer is still not conscious of any gap. Nevertheless, the blind spot can easily be mapped if suitable fixation and moving test-objects are used.

Although the blind areas of the right and left eyes do not overlap, Bridgman (1964) has pointed out that in certain oblique directions of gaze part of the blind space of one eye is occluded by the nose from the field of vision of the other eye.

The reduced eye

For most purposes, the optical imagery of the eye can be adequately studied on the basis of a simple analogue, called a 'reduced eye'. As shown in *Figure 2.16* it consists of a single convex surface separating air from a medium of refractive index n' similar to that of the vitreous body.

Since convenience and simplicity are basic to the concept of a reduced eye, round figures are entirely appropriate. As in Emsley's (1946) version, we take the power F_e to be exactly $+60\,D$ but the value of n' as 1.336. The two focal lengths, derived from equation (2.3), are

$$f_e = PF_e = -1000/F_e = -1000/+60$$
$$= -16.67\,mm$$

and

$$f'_e = PF'_e = 1000\,n'/F_e = 1336/60$$
$$= +22.27\,mm$$

Equation (2.3) also gives the necessary radius of curvature r of the refracting surface as

$$r = \frac{1000\,(n'-1)}{F_e} = \frac{336}{60} = +5.60\,mm$$

In the case of a single refracting surface, the two principal points coincide with each other and with the vertex of the surface, denoted by P. Similarly, the two nodal points coincide with each other and with the centre of curvature of the surface (now denoted by N). This is logical, since any ray directed toward this point meets the surface normally and is hence undeviated.

The line passing through P and N constitutes the optical axis, and the fovea, denoted by M′, is assumed to be on this line which accordingly becomes the visual axis as well.

If the unaccommodated eye is in focus for distant objects it is said to be 'emmetropic'. In this event its second principal focus F′ coincides with M′.

For convenience, the pupil of the reduced eye is considered to lie at the refracting surface, as shown in *Figure 2.16*. The entrance and exit pupils now coincide with this hypothetical pupil and the principal point P fills the additional role of being the centre of the pupil.

Figure 2.17 sets in juxtaposition the reduced and the Bennett–Rabbetts schematic eye with the second principal focus F′ of each in coincidence.

The principal point of the reduced eye is seen to coincide with the second principal point of the schematic eye. Hence, vergence calculations based on the principal points of the schematic eye and the simple reduced eye will give similar results. If the cornea of the schematic eye is taken as the reference point, then in round figures, the vertex of the reduced eye lies 1.8 mm behind that of the schematic eye. Hence, if a spectacle lens is assumed to be 12 mm from the cornea, its distance from the reduced eye should be reckoned as 13.8 mm. Exercise 2.6 gives a reduced eye due to Davison (pers. comm., 1995), also of power $+60\,D$, but with a similar overall length to that of the Bennett–Rabbetts schematic eye.

The retinal image

Algebraic treatment

The retinal image is inverted – a fact first propounded by Kepler in the early seventeenth century and later demonstrated by Scheiner.

A distinction must be drawn between the retinal image, which may be sharp or blurred according to circumstances, and the optical image. This latter term denotes the sharp image formed by the refracting system of the eye as though the retina were absent. The actual formation of the optical image is, of course, prevented if it lies behind the retina.

Given the necessary data, the position and size of an optical image can be determined from the algebraic formulae already given in this chapter.

Example 1

An object 50 mm high is situated on the optical axis of the standard emmetropic reduced eye at a distance of 250 mm from its principal point. Find the position and size of the optical image.

It is easier to work in terms of vergences. Thus

$$\ell = -250 \text{ mm}$$

$$L = 1000/-250 = -4.00 \text{ D}$$

$$F_e = +60.00 \text{ D}$$

$$L' = L + F_e = +56.00 \text{ D}$$

$$\ell' = \frac{1000n'}{L'} = \frac{1336}{56} = +23.86 \text{ mm}$$

The height h' of the optical image can be found from equation (2.10)

$$h' = hL/L' = \frac{50 \times -4.00}{+56.00} = -3.57 \text{ mm}$$

The minus sign denotes inversion of the image.

Since the image distance in this case (23.86 mm) is greater than the axial length of the eye (22.27 mm), the optical image becomes a theoretical construction only.

Object at infinity

An object at infinity is imaged in the plane of the second principal focus. Its size depends on the angular subtense of the object.

In *Figure 2.18*, rays from the extremity Q of a distant object inclined at the positive angle u to the optical axis are focused at Q' in the plane of F_e. A ray through the nodal point is undeviated. A ray incident at P is deviated towards the axis, the refracted ray making an angle u' with it such that

$$n' \sin u' = n \sin u$$

in accordance with the law of refraction.

In this case $n = 1$ and, if the angle u is small, the last expression can be put in the simpler paraxial form:

$$n'u' = nu = u \tag{2.15}$$

or

$$u' = u/n' \tag{2.16}$$

From the diagram

$$u' = -h'/f_e'$$

and thus

$$h' = -u'f_e' = -uf_e'/n' = -u/F_e \tag{2.17}$$

In this expression, h' is in metres and u in radians.

Example 2

A distant object subtending an angle of 5° is viewed by a reduced eye with a power of +62 D. Find the position and size of the optical image.

$$\ell' = f_e' = n'/F_e = 1336/62 = +21.55 \text{ mm}$$

$$u = 5 \times \pi/180 = 0.0873 \text{ rad}$$

$$h = \frac{-0.0873 \times 1000}{62} = -1.41 \text{ mm}$$

Ray-construction methods

The image formed by a single refracting surface such as the reduced eye can be found by constructing two or more ray paths from the given object point.

Diagrams of this kind are drawn to scale, but different scales may be used for horizontal and vertical dimensions. The refracting surface should be replaced by the tangent to its vertex.

The ray paths commonly used in these constructions are shown in *Figure 2.19*, in which BQ is an object for the eye. The image point Q' is the intersection of any two (or more) of the following refracted rays originating from Q.

Ray 1   Parallel to the optical axis, passing through F_e' after refraction.

Ray 2   Through the first principal focus F_e refracted parallel to the axis.

Ray 3   Through the nodal point, undeviated.

Ray 4   Directed towards the principal point P.

To find the refracted ray path for this last ray, locate the point Y on BQ such that

$$BY = BQ/n' = 0.75 \, BQ$$

(strictly, BY = 0.749 BQ).

The refracted ray path is YP produced. This construction is justified by equation (2.16) which can be written as

$$\tan u' = (\tan u)/n'$$

since it has already been assumed that u is small. It can be most useful to carry out constructions of this kind, verifying the results by calculation. However, it should be borne in mind that they are subject to the same lim-

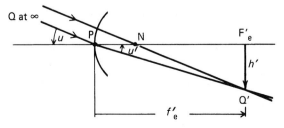

Figure 2.18.   Image construction in the reduced eye: distant object.

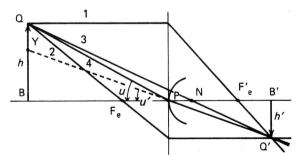

Figure 2.19.   Image construction in the reduced eye: near object.

itations as the approximate expressions on which they are based.

Magnification in visual optics

In optics, transverse magnification is given by the ratio of image to object size, as in equation (2.10). In visual optics, however, magnification is frequently taken as the ratio between any linear dimension of the retinal image when the optical device, e.g. a spectacle lens, magnifier, etc., is in use and the corresponding dimension when the object is viewed without the device.

The object is usually assumed to be in the same position for both conditions, but particularly for magnifying devices, the object is assumed to be positioned initially at the reference seeing distance (formerly termed the 'least distance of distinct vision') of -250 mm from the eye.

Jalie (1995) has pointed out that, in all cases, magnification can be calculated by determining the image size produced by the optical device alone, then calculating its angular subtense at the eye's entrance pupil, and lastly comparing this with the angle the object would subtend without the device.

Nature of mirror imagery

The so-called lateral inversion of the image formed by a plane mirror, notably one's own reflection, still gives rise to perplexity and debate. Arguments from psychological or related grounds tend to be needlessly invoked.

To understand the true nature of mirror imagery demands consideration of an object in three dimensions, not two. For a plane mirror, any object point and its reflected image lie on a common normal to the surface and are equidistant from it. Consequently, the object shown in *Figure 2.20*, representing a central vertical section through the head of an observer, is imaged as depicted. The image is formed as though the object had been pulled through the mirror, and turned inside out in the process. The same would take place in any vertical section parallel to the plane of the diagram. As a result, the left eye of the observer appears as the right eye of the three-dimensional image gazing back at him.

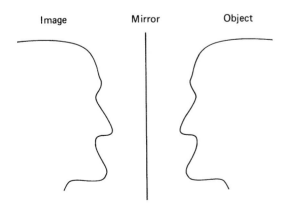

Figure 2.20. Vertical section through the centre of an observer's head and its mirror image. Since imagery of the same type takes place in every plane parallel to that of the diagram, it follows that the left eye of the observer becomes the right eye of the three-dimensional mirror image, and vice versa.

Just as a right-hand glove turned inside out takes the form of a left-hand glove, so the mirror image of one's own right hand appears as a left hand. The same three-dimensional transformation is shown by the virtual images formed by concave and convex mirrors, accompanied by magnification or its opposite.

Clearly, the term 'lateral inversion' does not adequately describe the phenomenon. 'Mirror metamorphosis' is offered as an improvement on the term 'perversion', which has been suggested in the past without gaining effective support.

Exercises

2.1 (a) A pencil of rays emerges from a lens with a vergence of $+6.00$ D. What is its vergence after a travel of 10 mm in air? (b) A pencil of rays emerges from a lens with a vergence of -8.00 D. What is its vergence after a travel of 15 mm in air?

2.2 The macula of an emmetropic reduced eye has a diameter of 1.5 mm. What angle does it subtend at the nodal point and what is the corresponding linear extent of object space at 10 m from the eye?

2.3 A schematic eye has a single-surface cornea of 7.5 mm radius of curvature, an anterior chamber depth of 3 mm and a homogeneous crystalline lens of thickness 3.5 mm, refractive index 1.4 and back surface radius of curvature -6 mm. Both aqueous and vitreous have a refractive index of 1.336. Calculate the position and magnification of the entrance and exit pupils.

2.4 The diagram (not to scale) illustrates the positions P and P$'$ of the principal points of a telephoto lens system formed by two thin lenses of power $+10$ D and -5 D at A$_1$ and A$_2$ respectively. An object point B and its image B$'$ are also shown. From the given measurements, all in mm, determine the following distances, using in each case only distances of stated length and paying strict attention to signs: A$_1$P, A$_2$F$'$, PP$'$, F$'$B$'$ and PB. (Example: FB = FA$_1$ + A$_1$B = $-(-162.5)+(-662.5) = -500$ mm.)

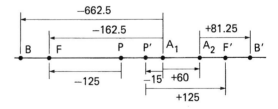

2.5 The diagram illustrates a diverging meniscus lens of thickness t with its first principal point P at a distance e from vertex A$_1$ and its second principal point P$'$ at a distance e' from vertex A$_2$. An object point B is at a distance ℓ from P and its image B$'$ at a distance ℓ' from P$'$. Using only these letter symbols, express the following distances: P$'$A$_1$, A$_2$B$'$, PP$'$, B$'$P and BB$'$. (Example: A$_1$B = A$_1$P + PB = $e + \ell$.)

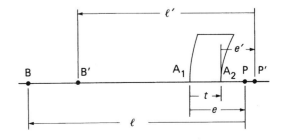

2.6 What are the radii of curvature and refractive index of a simple reduced eye of power +60.00 D and axial length 24.00 mm, which is the overall length of the schematic eye?

References

BRIDGMAN, C.S. (1964) Viewing conditions under which the blind spot is not compensated by vision in the other eye. *Am. J. Optom.*, **41**, 426–428

EMSLEY, H.H. (1946) *Visual Optics*, 4th edn. London: Hatton Press, 34–36

FOWLER, C.W. and PATERAS, E.S. (1990) A gradient-index ophthalmic lens based on Wood's convex pseudo-lens. *Ophthal. Physiol. Opt.*, **10**, 262–270

IVANOFF, A. (1953) *Les Aberrations de l'Oeil*. Paris: Editions de la Revue d'Optique

JALIE, M. (1995) The Arthur Bennett Memorial lecture (unpublished in written form)

PRENTICE, C.F. (1890) A metric system of numbering and measuring prisms. *Arch. Ophthal., N.Y.*, **19**, 64–75, 128–135

WOOD, R.W. (1911) *Physical Optics*, 2nd edn. New York: Macmillan

3

Visual acuity and contrast sensitivity

Introduction

Vision is the process by which an organism sees and includes all the stages from the physical stimulus reaching the eye to the mental perception. The amount of information needed by an organism varies from species to species and the visual system tends to be adapted accordingly. One of the simplest requirements is in the earthworm, *Lumbricus*, where perception of light is all that is needed and thus simple, light-sensitive cells in the epithelium are sufficient. The unicellular aquatic organism, *Euglena gracilis*, has the additional requirement of needing to identify the direction of the incident light. Adjacent to a photosensitive region is a pigment spot which casts a shadow on this region in certain orientations of the cell, enabling it to swim towards the light. The compound eye of insects has a series of minute lenses, each focusing light on to receptor cells. Each individual unit therefore 'sees' only a limited region in space. Although there will be a small amount of overlap between these input regions for neighbouring units, some detail in the outside environment can be obtained. An alternative method of obtaining detailed information about the environment is to form an image of the outside world on an array of receptor elements, using just one lens system or pinhole aperture. The vertebrate eye is of this type, having but a single lens-system.

An order of visual performance

The human eye is capable of many different tasks, involving many different complexities of vision. These tasks may be classified under the following headings:

(1) Light perception, for example, the threshold of vision in the normal eye or the only response of a diseased eye.
(2) Discrimination, or the ability of the visual system to distinguish an object from its background.
(3) Form vision and recognition, such as the ability to identify letters and words.
(4) Resolution or the ability to see detail.
(5) Localization, for example, realizing that an object is situated to one side of another object.
(6) Higher tasks where the visual system stimulates other responses, for example, a motor response in handling something.

The two most important aspects in clinical work are those of form vision and resolution. If the eye views a large letter so that the detail in its retinal image is large with respect to the size of the retinal receptors, it is the general shape of the letter which has to be recognized, no matter whether the retinal image is sharp or blurred. If the size of the letter is progressively decreased with the retinal image remaining in focus, then the eye's ability to resolve detail is used more and more, until the image becomes so small that the visual system can no longer identify the letter. The terms 'vision' and 'visual acuity' in clinical work relate to the detail size of letters that can just be recognized and will be defined on pages 26–27.

Line discrimination

The ability of the eye to perceive that an object is separate from its background depends partly upon the relative luminances of object and ground. If the ground is very dark, the object will be seen, provided that the illumination of its retinal image exceeds the luminance threshold of the eye at that adaptation level. The ability to see a dark object against an illuminated ground is dependent on a different threshold. In these conditions, the contrast in the image of a large object is similar to the contrast in the object (*Figure 3.1*). As the object is reduced in size, so the contrast in the image falls, partly due to imperfections in the eye's optical system.

A dark object will be perceived, provided that the variation in retinal illumination exceeds the luminance difference threshold, $\Delta L/L$. This fraction, known as the Weber–Fechner fraction, varies with the background luminance and reaches a minimum value of about 2% at moderate photopic levels. Thus, provided that the retinal image of a dark object causes an illumination drop on the retina of about 2%, it will probably be seen. Under good conditions, a line subtending as little as 0.5 seconds of arc may be seen, provided that it is sufficiently long (for example, a telephone wire) for its image to cover many receptors. Similarly, a disc of about 30 seconds subtense may be seen.

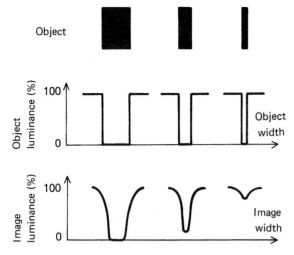

Figure 3.1. Contrast transfer in an optical system. The upper row shows three bar objects of different widths. The middle and lower rows show the luminance across the width of the object and image.

If the object shows a reduced contrast with the background, such as a grey line on a light ground, the variation in retinal illumination must again exceed the luminance difference threshold over a sufficient area for discrimination to result.

Resolution: receptor theory

A brief introduction to the structure of the retina is given here as a background to the discussion on resolution. For a more detailed account, the reader should refer to one of the specialized textbooks on ocular anatomy or physiology.

The retina lies against the pigmented choroid, which provides both a nutrient supply to the outer layers of the retina and a black-out. This absorbs light that may have passed through the sclera and also reduces the amount of light scattered back in a diffuse manner after its initial passage through the retina. The outermost layer of the retina is the pigment epithelium, which also helps to absorb light and contributes greatly to retinal receptor metabolism. Where these layers are deficient in pigment, as in albinos and blonds, the vision may be reduced because the contrast in the optical image is reduced by stray light. Light passing through the sclera and iris and light scattered around inside the eye both contribute to spoiling the quality of the retinal image.

The second layer is the photosensitive or bacillary layer. This consists of the outer and inner segments of two types of cell, the rods and cones, so called because of their shape. The rods provide achromatic vision in the scotopic or low range of luminances. The cones provide colour vision and work in the photopic or high range of luminances. The luminance range in the middle where both types of receptors operate is called the mesopic region. Typical receptors are illustrated in *Figure 3.2*. The population density of the receptors

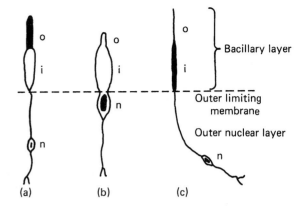

Figure 3.2. Simplified illustration of the retinal receptors, where o represents the outer segment, i the inner segment and n the nucleus: (a) rod, (b) cone, (c) foveal cone.

varies in different areas of the retina. Only near the posterior pole do cones predominate; in the fovea there are only cones. These are, however, much slimmer than the peripheral cones and this enables them to be packed much closer together.

The outer limiting membrane divides the photosensitive areas of the rods and cones from their nuclei in the outer nuclear layer. The endings on these nerve cells synapse with relay cells known as bipolar cells. These in turn synapse with the ganglion cells whose fibres pass across the surface of the retina to the optic nerve head and then via the optic nerve to the lateral geniculate body in the brain. Instead of conducting nerve impulses to the brain, some nerve cells in the relay layers make contact with other cells including rods and cones. Their function may be concerned with processing the neural 'image' and making up for some of the optical defects of the eye. The neural connections in the retina are very complex and in general each ganglion nerve receives impulses from many receptors. Only in the foveal region does the number of cones and ganglion fibres become approximately equal.

With the exception of the pigment epithelium, the retina is transparent and the optical image is formed on the bacillary layer after the light has passed through the nuclear and synaptic layers. Despite the transparency, some degradation of the image occurs, so in the foveal region the majority of the neural elements are tilted away (*Figure 3.2*) so that there is very little tissue in front of the cone layer. Duke-Elder (1958) discusses Wall's suggestion that the deep foveal pit in some birds of prey, taking a cusp-like form, serves the purpose of magnifying the image. The argument is that rays of light incident just off the apex of the cusp are deviated away from it, thus spreading the image over a greater number of retinal cones. Another favourable feature is that there are no blood capillaries in this region to reduce contrast.

In the fovea, the cones have a diameter of about 1.5 μm (microns) and they are separated by an edge to edge space of about 0.5 μm. Thus the effective separation between cone centres is about 2 μm. Suppose the eye were viewing two closely adjacent point sources of light: if their images fell on two neighbouring cones,

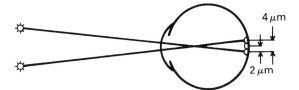

Figure 3.3. Receptor theory of resolution.

they would be perceived as only a single source. If, however, there was one unstimulated cone between those illuminated by the images, then resolution would probably occur. Hence, a separation between the images of 4 μm is required (*Figure 3.3*). Assuming the nodal point to be $16\frac{2}{3}$ mm in front of the retina, this represents a theoretical limit to resolution of about 49 seconds of arc.

This simplified analysis is valid only if each cone can transmit a separate impulse, which means that there is at least one nerve fibre to each foveal cone. In the periphery of the retina, each nerve fibre is stimulated by many receptors and therefore it is the size of the receptor field corresponding to each nerve fibre that is important, rather than the size of the individual receptors. A further complication is that the retina is capable of distinguishing colour, so that some of the nerve fibres must conduct colour information. There is, however, little variation in resolution with wavelength (*see*, for example, Shlaer *et al.*, 1941).

The eye is in constant movement and so any image is passed from cone to cone. This prevents the reduction of contrast by adaptation in the neural 'image' – the Troxler or extinction effect – and also provides for an integration of information received by the various neural components, thus contributing to the eye's good performance. The twinkling of stars, however, is not due to the image falling between receptors or stimulating first one receptor and then its neighbour, but to fluctuations in the light paths through the atmosphere. The eye has appreciable aberrations (*see* Chapter 15) and these spread the optical image of a star so that it falls over several cones. Even if these geometrical aberrations were eliminated, the wave nature of light would still spoil the image.

Resolution: wave theory

The nature of light cannot be explained simply. In terms of stimulating receptors, light appears to act as if it consisted of discrete components or quanta, while image and shadow formation suggests that light has a wave structure.

The wave theory predicts that, even with a perfect optical system, the image of a point object cannot be a point, but must spread to cover a finite area due to diffraction of light at the margins of the optical system. For a circular aperture, this image pattern takes the form of a central bright disc surrounded by much fainter rings, which can be ignored in this context.

The central disc containing about 84% of the light in the entire diffraction pattern is termed the Airy disc. In

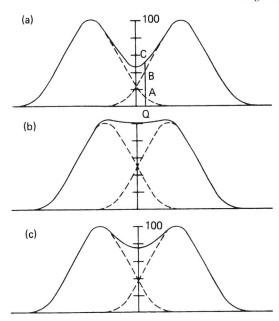

Figure 3.4. Wave theory of resolution: (a) two separated Airy discs, (b) discs too close to be resolved, (c) discs separated by half their width – the Rayleigh criterion.

the eye, its angular subtense ω at the nodal point is given by the expression

$$\omega = \frac{2.44\lambda}{g} \text{ rad} \qquad (3.1)$$

where λ is the wavelength of the light in metres and g the pupil diameter, also in metres.

Thus, for $\lambda = 555$ nm* (555×10^{-9} m) and $g = 3$ mm (3×10^{-3} m),

$$\omega = \frac{2.44 \times 555 \times 10^{-9}}{3 \times 10^{-3}} \text{ rad}$$

$$\approx 93 \text{ seconds of arc}$$

The distribution of light within an Airy disc is strongly peaked at the centre, as shown by the dashed curves in *Figure 3.4*, accurately drawn to scale.

If there are two closely adjacent point sources, there will be two overlapping diffraction patterns, each contributing to the illuminance of the retinal image in the area of overlap. The dashed lines in *Figure 3.4* show the relative illuminance curves for individual Airy discs, while the solid lines show the summation across the area of overlap. For example, at a point Q (*Figure 3.4a*), the illuminance due to the left-hand Airy disc is proportional to QA while that due to the other Airy disc is proportional to QB. The sum of QA and QB is equal to QC, which determines the corresponding point on the summation curve.

If two neighbouring patterns are sufficiently separated, the combined illuminance curve will show two peaks with a dip in between (*Figure 3.4a*). As the point objects approach each other, so will their images and eventually the two peaks will merge together into a

---

* The wavelength corresponding to the brightest (yellow–green) part of the spectrum.

single bright peak. Under these conditions, the eye cannot possibly see the two objects as separate, that is, they are unresolved (*Figure 3.4b*).

Lord Rayleigh suggested that resolution was just obtained if the central peak of the second Airy disc fell on the extreme edge of the first, so that the separation of the geometric images of the point objects was half the diameter of the Airy disc (*Figure 3.4c*). The depression or saddle between the peaks then has a minimum illuminance of about 74% of that of the peaks.

This formulation, known as the Rayleigh criterion, establishes a value for θ_{min}, the minimum angle of resolution of the eye. It is half the angle subtended at the nodal point by a single Airy disc. Hence,

$$\theta_{min} = \frac{1.22\lambda}{g} \text{rad} \tag{3.2}$$

The minimum angle of resolution is often referred to as resolving power, but the authors prefer not to use this term because the smaller value of θ_{min}, the better the eye.

For a 3 mm pupil and $\lambda = 555$ nm, the value of θ_{min} is 47 seconds of arc. The similarity between this theoretical limiting value and the minimum of 49 seconds given by receptor theory is most striking. Other factors influencing resolution are considered on pages 22–26.

Under optimum astronomical conditions, Dawes (1867) found that the minimum angle of resolution could be smaller than Rayleigh's value. The Dawes limit gives θ_{min} the value of

$$\theta_{min} = \frac{1.00\lambda}{g} \text{rad} \tag{3.3}$$

The illuminance in the middle of the trough is then only a few per cent lower than at the peaks of the luminosity curve. For a 3 mm pupil and $\lambda = 555$ nm, the Dawes limit is only 38 seconds of arc. A figure of 1 minute of arc is frequently quoted[*] as the minimum angle of resolution of a good eye. Although this is a lower order of performance than the various theoretical minima, it appears to be unattainable under indoor experimental conditions. The best results obtained by Ogle (1951) were in the neighbourhood of 90 seconds of arc. Much depends on the relative luminance of the point sources and the background.

The cross-section of the diffraction pattern for the image of a single line is very similar to that of a single point but differs slightly in the illuminance of the side stripes. A strip of the retina is stimulated, giving summation effects which possibly make resolution easier if no finer.

This argument is similar to the one involved in line discrimination (page 19), namely, that a dip in retinal illuminance enables a dark object to be perceived, provided that the variation in illuminance exceeds the luminance difference threshold. The same idea can be extended to the receptor theory outlined on pages 20–21. It is not necessary to assume a completely unstimulated central cone. There may be some spread of light over it, but discrimination could still occur, provided that the outer cones were more strongly illuminated. It must be pointed out, however, that the luminance difference threshold for relatively large bipartite fields may not have the same values as for minute areas of the retina.

Grating resolution and acuity

The previous section extended the principle of resolution to the case of two parallel line objects as distinct from two points. In turn, the line objects may be considered as a particular case of the grating which consists of a series of parallel black and white lines (*Figure 3.5a*). Usually, the black lines have the same width as the white lines, and both are of the same width over the whole area of the test pattern. Such a grating is known as a Foucault grating or square-wave grating, since the contrast alters abruptly at the change from black to white and vice versa. Gratings may also be designed where the black line is only half the width, for example, of the white line.

The grating, especially in its sinusoidal form (*see* pages 46–55) is frequently used in psychophysical experiments on vision. In general, it is presented with the stripes vertical or horizontal. Even when the eye's focusing is corrected for irregularities such as astigmatism (*see* Chapter 5), the eye's limit of resolution varies with the angle of presentation of the test grating. The eye performs better with horizontal or vertical gratings than with oblique gratings (*see*, for example, Nachmias, 1960; Campbell *et al.*, 1966; Tootle and Berkley, 1983; Ross, 1992).

The Foucault grating is a simple test to use because the apparent width of the grating element may be varied by rotating the plane of the grating about an axis parallel to the lines (*Figure 3.5b*). The disadvantage of the grating as a test object is that its streaky nature may be appreciated before the actual elements are properly resolved. If the grating is rotated so that its elements become apparently finer, an angle will be reached at which it can no longer be resolved. The rotation being continued a little more, the grating elements may again, under some conditions of observation, become

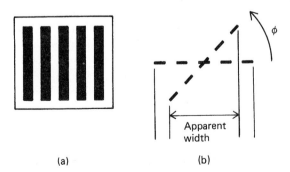

(a)   (b)

Figure 3.5. Foucault grating and the effect of tilt ϕ, on its apparent width, which is reduced by the factor cos ϕ.

apparently visible over a short critical range. This is known as spurious resolution (*see also* pages 50–51).

The limit of resolution for a square-wave grating is traditionally expressed as the angular subtense in seconds of arc of the grating element (one black plus white line). If these are of equal width, the size of the grating element is the same as the centre-to-centre distance of neighbouring black or white lines. A typical value of the limit of resolution of a square-wave grating is 80–90 seconds of arc.

In general, visual acuity is inversely related to the minimum angle of resolution. Hence, if A denotes the angular subtense of the basic detail of the smallest discernible test object – for example, the line width of the test letters or characters on any standard form of test chart – the visual acuity V may be defined as

$$V = k/A \qquad (3.4)$$

where k is an arbitrary constant. This is the basis of the decimal notation for recording visual acuity, in which A is expressed in minutes of arc and the value given to k is unity. A more detailed explanation is given on pages 26–31.

Grating acuity can also be expressed in the form of line-width acuity, the unit being reciprocal minutes. For example, if a subject's limit of resolution for a grating is 90 seconds, the angular subtense A of a single line is 45 seconds or 0.75 minutes of arc. The line-width acuity is therefore $1/0.75$ or 1.33. Expressed in this way, grating acuity can be directly compared with clinical acuity expressed in decimal notation.

Resolution and pupil size

On pages 21–22 we showed that, according to the wave theory of light, diffraction at the pupil margin gives the minimum separable visual angle as an inverse function of pupil diameter (equation 3.2). Thus, at large pupil diameters, the Airy disc is small, and the limit of resolution should also be small. Conversely, small pupil diameters give a larger threshold angle. While the relationship is true for an aberration-free optical system, the eye's aberrations reduce its performance at larger pupil diameters.

Figure 3.6 shows the mean data obtained by Rabbetts from six subjects for grating resolution at constant retinal illumination, the test object luminance being reduced as pupil diameter was increased. The straight line represents the performance predicted by the Rayleigh criterion (equation 3.5). The actual performance of the eye is seen to depart from that of an aberration-free system when the pupil diameter approaches 1.5 mm. The best acuity, equivalent to a limit of resolution of 77 seconds of arc occurred at a pupil diameter of 3 mm, but many authors quote figures of 2.0–2.4 mm. Above the optimum diameter, resolution becomes poorer under photopic conditions, because the effects of aberrations then begin to predominate. Under normal scotopic conditions, an increase in pupil size gives greater retinal illumination, which improves the acuity.

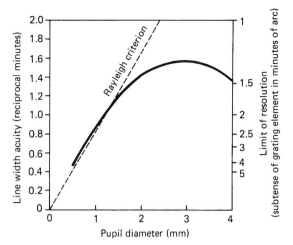

Figure 3.6. Resolution of Foucault grating as a function of pupil size.

Stiles–Crawford and Campbell effects

Named after its discoverers in 1933, the Stiles–Crawford effect relates to the directional sensitivity of the fovea. Rays of light passing through the centre of the pupil are less oblique to the cones after refraction and stimulate them more strongly than rays through peripheral areas of the pupil.

If the Stiles–Crawford effect did not exist, a pupil of smaller size would elicit the same response in terms of apparent brightness than a given actual size in real conditions. Let the respective diameters of the actual and equivalent pupils be denoted by d and d_e and their respective areas by S and S_e. In an extensive treatment of this subject, Le Grand (1948) derived an expression for S_e which is immediately reducible to

$$S_e = (\pi d^2/4)\,[1 - 0.0106\,d^2 + 0.0000417\,d^4]$$

For the actual pupil, $S = \pi d^2/4$. Since the area of a circle is proportional to the square of its diameter, it follows that

$$S_e/S = d_e^2/d^2$$

whence

$$d_e = d\sqrt{\mu} \qquad (3.5)$$

where

$$\mu = 1 - 0.0106\,d^2 + 0.0000417\,d^4 \qquad (3.6)$$

Table 3.1 has been compiled from this basis.

Table 3.1 Stiles–Crawford effect. Relationship between actual and effective pupil diameters

Actual pupil diameter (mm)	Effective pupil diameter (mm)
1	0.99
2	1.96
3	2.86
4	3.67
5	4.36
6	4.92
7	5.33

An associated effect, named after Campbell (1958), refers to the loss in visual acuity when incident rays are restricted to a peripheral area of the pupil. It results not only from the Stiles–Crawford effect, but also from the ocular aberrations attendant on oblique incidence (Green, 1967; Walsh and Charman, 1985).

As reported by Enoch *et al.* (1980), it has been found that the directional sensitivity of the fovea of one eye is significantly reduced if it is occluded by a black patch for several days. The effect takes 3–6 days to reach its maximum, and complete recovery after removal of the patch takes a similar time. Other transient and minor visual effects are described. The bearing of these discoveries on the general question of the alignment of retinal receptors is discussed in some detail.

Resolution and illumination

Fixed pupil size

The retina works more efficiently at higher levels of illumination, making it easier to read in a good light than outside at dusk. However, there are other factors to be considered. The pupil diameter alters with the level of illumination, and so, in scientific measurements, the pupil size is fixed. The eye's own pupil is usually dilated with a drug (mydriatic) and an artificial pupil of a size smaller than the dilated pupil is placed immediately in front of the cornea.

The results found by Shlaer (1937) for a grating and a Landolt ring or C are shown in *Figure 3.7*. The grating acuity results are expressed in terms of line width, as in equation (3.4). The Landolt ring is a circle with a gap (for a full description *see* page 32). The subject has to recognize the orientation of the gap; the reciprocal subtense of the gap width that is just correctly seen is a measure of the acuity.

Retinal illumination is given in trolands. Because the illuminance of the retinal image varies with the square of pupil diameter, it is not sufficient to state the luminance of the test object. Troland suggested a unit based upon an eye with a pupillary area of one square millimetre viewing a surface of luminance one candela per square metre. This unit is now named after him, though it was originally called the photon. The troland is a very convenient measure of retinal illuminance

since five trolands represents five times as much retinal illuminance as one troland, for the same eye, irrespective of whether it is pupil size or object luminance or both that have been altered. It should not be overlooked, however, that the actual retinal illuminance is influenced by the transparency of the eye's media as well as by the Stiles–Crawford effect.

Shlaer's results for the grating show an increase in acuity from 0.8 at 1 troland (log 1 = 0) to 1.3 at 10 trolands.

At higher and lower illumination levels there was a smaller rate of variation. Similar variations plotting as a sigmoid (S-shaped) curve were found with the Landolt ring.

Variable (normal) pupil size

An alternative approach is to allow the pupil to take its natural size as the illumination of the test object is varied. Although this may give less information about the physiology of the retina, it gives a better idea of what happens in normal conditions.

Thus, Foxell and Stevens (1955) measured the ability of the eye to resolve the gap in a Landolt ring as a function of background luminance. The acuity improved steadily with increased luminance up to approximately 3400 cd/m^2, after which resolution became poorer (*Figure 3.8*). They also studied the influence of surround size at various luminance levels. The acuity was found to improve with increased surround size, the improvement being much less marked for surround sizes over 6°.

Foxell and Stevens also investigated the effect of varying the surround illumination over a 120° field with respect to that of a small central field of 0.5° forming the immediate background to the test object. This experiment was repeated for a range of values of the central field luminance from 3.4 to 34 000 cd/m². Their results are shown in *Figure 3.9*. It appears that the best acuity is obtained when the surround luminance is approxi-

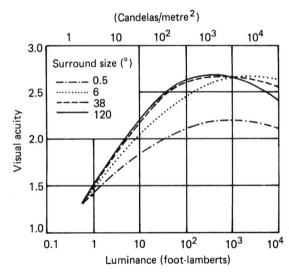

Figure 3.8. Visual acuity as a function of luminance for different diameter surrounds. (Redrawn from Foxell and Stevens, by kind permission of the publishers of *Br. J. Ophthal.*)

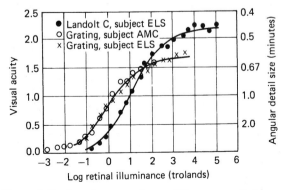

Figure 3.7. Visual acuity and retinal illumination. (Reference from Shlaer, copyright The Rockefeller University Press.)

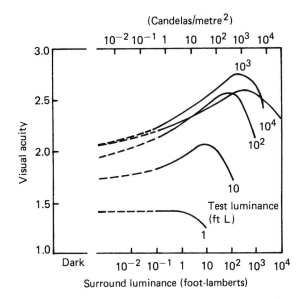

Figure 3.9. Visual acuity as a function of surround luminance for various background luminances. (Redrawn from Foxell and Stevens, by kind permission of the publishers of *Br. J. Ophthal.*)

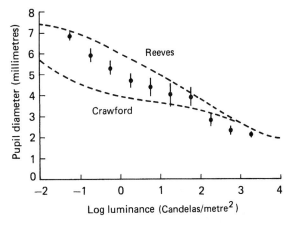

Figure 3.10. Pupil size and illumination. (Campbell and Gregory, 1960. Reproduced by kind permission of the publishers of *Nature.*)

mately equal to that of the central field for values of the latter up to nearly 3400 cd/m^2.

The results of this and similar studies have important clinical implications in the illumination of test charts. For example, if a single letter is shown illuminated on a dark background, as is possible with some test-type projectors, a poorer acuity than with an illuminated surround will be expected for most patients.

Over the range of possible luminances for test charts (40–600 cd/m^2), Sheedy *et al.* (1984) found an almost linear improvement in logMAR acuity (*see* pages 30–31) when plotted against luminance, also on a logarithmic scale. For test letters the logMAR acuity was found to be −0.085 ($V = 1.22$) at 46 cd/m^2, improving to −0.155 ($V = 1.43$) at 563 cd/m^2. The slope of the regression line was approximately −0.06, from which a simple relationship can be derived between a change in test chart luminance and the resulting change in logMAR visual acuity. Sheedy and colleagues deduced that if a variation of ±0.01 of a logMAR unit is permissible, a standard value L for the luminance could be allowed to vary by about 0.17 of a log unit. This would give a tolerance ranging from 0.68 times to 1.47 times the nominal value of L. Landolt ring acuity was found to be less affected by luminance changes than letter acuity.

Pupil size and illumination

The pupil constricts with increasing luminance levels, although most of the adaptation occurs in the retina. An average pupil size as a function of luminance has been determined independently by Reeves (1918) and Crawford (1936), whose results are plotted as the dashed lines in *Figure 3.10*. Similar results from De Groot and Gebhard (1952) and Flamant (1948) are illustrated in Hoover (1987). Campbell and Gregory

(1960) later investigated this relationship in a slightly different manner, by determining for a range of artificial pupil diameters the luminance level most favourable for resolution of a three-bar grating. Their results are plotted as the circles in *Figure 3.10* and are seen to fall within the range between Reeves's and Crawford's results. This suggests that pupil size is adjusted to give optimum visual acuity over a wide range of luminances, a conclusion supported by Laughlin (1992). He also points out that, at any particular illumination level, the optimum diameter is a broad function, so that deviations from the optimum have only a small effect on performance.

Stanley and Davies (1995) demonstrated that the area of the adapting stimulus and its luminance were inversely proportional. Thus pupil contraction would result from increasing either the area of the field of view or its luminance. They suggested that some of the reported differences in pupil size for the same illuminance might therefore be due to differences in the stimulus area. The pupil diameters for all their nine subjects (aged 21–33, mean 27, pers. comm.) could be predicted by a single formula which related diameter g to the product p of the square of the angle subtended by the stimulus diameter and its luminance:

$$g = 7.75 - 5.75 \frac{(p/846)^{0.41}}{(p/846)^{0.41} + 2}$$

The maximum angle they studied was 25°. Since the retina becomes less sensitive towards the periphery, increasing the adapting field size eventually produces a diminishing decrease in pupil size. Thus Stanley and Davies (pers. comm.) found that for a field of 66 cd/m^2, increasing the field size from 25° to 60° decreased the pupil diameter by only 6% as opposed to the 20% predicted by the above formula. Similarly, a 1.6° field at 8000 cd/m^2 presented to the fovea produced a pupil diameter of 4.3 mm, which increased to 5.2 mm when positioned 10° away and 5.55 mm when 20° from the fovea.

Palmer (1966) has found, however, that where the pupil is unable to affect the illumination of the retinal image, it becomes larger than normal. This situation can occur when the eye is used with an instrument, such that all the light passes through an exit pupil smaller than the eye's own pupil.

Pupil diameter and age

The pupil diameter decreases with age. Winn *et al.* (1994) showed that, although there is a large variation between people in any age group, pupils of young subjects dilated much more at low luminances than those of older people. They found average results of 8 mm for 20 year olds viewing a $10°$ diameter adapting field of $9\,cd/m^2$ constricting to $4.5\,mm$ at $1100\,cd/m^2$ compared with 5 mm and 3.5 mm respectively for 80-year-old subjects. The reduction in pupil size with age has the disadvantage of lowering retinal illuminance, hence reducing vision, but, conversely, reducing the deleterious effects of aberrations and light scattered by older lenses (Woodhouse, 1975). Winn and colleagues also found no significant relationship between pupil size and gender, refractive error or iris colour.

Woods (1991) gives an extensive review of ageing and vision, including pupil diameter.

Vernier acuity

An entirely different aspect of vision is involved in vernier acuity, the principle of which is illustrated in *Figure 3.11a*. Two parallel straight lines are displaced fractionally with respect to each other, giving rise to a break in contour. The angular subtense of the least detectable break is a measure of vernier acuity. Where the ends of the lines are close together in the direction of their length, acuity is maximal but discrimination falls as the ends of the lines become separated (French, 1920). For average observers, vernier acuity ranges from 10 seconds of arc upwards, but values as remarkable as 2–5 seconds are not uncommon among skilled observers. Such fine limits are well below the angular subtense of a single foveal cone (about 20 seconds) and much smaller than the limit of resolution for parallel lines.

Because of diffraction and aberrations, the retinal image of a line has somewhat blurred borders. As a result, the transition from a low to a relatively high level of illumination is not abrupt. It takes the form indicated by the two identical curves at (b) in *Figure 3.11*. If the break AB in the line shown at (a) is near the threshold of discrimination, the blurred image of the edge of the line will extend over a relatively longer distance, say from A to A′ above the break and from B to B′ below it. The drop in illumination below the level of the break is represented by the vertical distance between the curves, which is very nearly constant across the whole width of the blurred fringe. In consequence, the retinal cones in the fringe below the break are less strongly stimulated. The effects of summation and inhibition zones within the retina immediately above and below the break are the most probable explanation of the extraordinary level of vernier acuity (*see*, for example, Williams and Essock, 1986; Wilson, 1986). An alternative explanation is that the visual system can determine the 'centre of gravity' of the light distribution in each of the two adjacent sections of the retinal image (Westheimer and McKee, 1977; Watt *et al.*, 1983; Whitaker and Walker, 1988).

In some cases, however, the observer may perceive one line consistently to one side of the other, thus making an alignment error. For a particular observer such errors tend to be similar, but can vary according to whether binocular or right or left monocular viewing is used (Tomlinson, 1969). Emsley (1946) and Carter (1958) found setting errors of up to 0.8–0.9 minutes of arc. At one-third of a metre, this is equivalent to 0.1 mm, a significant error. Even so, the principle of vernier alignment is frequently and successfully used in instruments. It derives its name from Pierre Vernier (1580–1637), the inventor of the scale that bears his name.

A similar type of visual process may be involved in the perception of dot alignment; if three dots are placed in a row, a slight transverse displacement of the centre dot is readily discernible. Vilar *et al.* (1995) suggest this arrangement is preferable to the usual vernier acuity display since it avoids judgement of the vertical. Like others, they found that this test showed no alteration in performance with the observer's age over the range 20 to over 70 years, while there was little difference whether the stimuli were sharp or degraded.

Even if one of the outer dots is removed, the eye is still able to detect a small lateral offset between two vertically separated dots, but the threshold is increased to 20 seconds of arc. The term hyperacuity has been given by Westheimer (1976) to the eyes' ability to perform sensitive tasks of this kind. Hyperacuity tests may also be used to assess retinal function in patients with cataract (*see also* page 45), since they are relatively insensitive to blur. A description of some of these hyperacuities is given in McKee *et al.* (1990) and in the references for the section relating to cataract.

Vision and visual acuity in clinical practice

Introduction

In the previous sections, the resolution of the eye has been considered in relation to a pair of point sources,

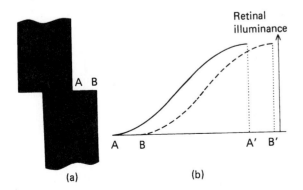

Figure 3.11. (a) Lateral displacement in a line object. (b) Superimposed graphs of retinal illuminance of one side of the retinal image of the two parts of the line.

line gratings and Landolt rings. These make useful test objects for scientific study, but, with the exception of the Landolt rings, are not satisfactory for clinical work. Point sources and gratings do not represent the type of detail that a patient normally views. It is useful to employ, as test objects, characters with which the patient is familiar. If symbols of varying size are used, smaller characters will be seen by people with better vision, while patients with poor sight will need larger characters.

The characters most frequently chosen have been capital letters, but numbers and other symbols have been used. Some of the charts with symbols other than letters will be discussed on page 33.

Letter charts require both recognition of the symbol and resolution of the detail within the letter itself, although studies by Coates (1935) and others show that the overall letter shape is also very important in identification. Thus, instead of the term limit of resolution, clinicians use two other terms as follows:

(1) *Visual acuity*. This is determined from the size of the smallest line of letters or symbols in the test chart that can be read by the patient after any defects of focusing, other than aberrations, have been corrected.
(2) *Unaided vision* (often shortened to *Vision*). This is determined from the size of the smallest line of letters or symbols in the test chart that can be read by the patient with the naked eye.

On pages 19–26, we have assumed that the eye was properly focused, the discussion relating to visual acuity rather than vision. Both vision and visual acuity may be taken for the right and left eyes individually and also binocularly. Except in patients where the co-ordinated use of the two eyes is poor, vision and visual acuity are usually slightly better when determined binocularly.

Distance test charts and acuity

In tests of distance vision, the testing distance should be large enough not to stimulate accommodation. The accepted value in Britain and many other countries is 6 m, but 5 m is commonly used in some European countries. In the USA the standard distance is 20 ft, a little over 6 m. There is, however, a move in that country to institute a reduced testing distance of 4 m, compensating for it by adding -0.25 D to the refractive findings. Other associated proposals are outlined in a later section on the logMAR system (*see* pages 30–31).

If the consulting room is not long enough, the usual solution is to use a 'reverse' or 'indirect' test chart mounted over or to the side of the patient's head, in conjunction with a mirror at 3 m. The mirror must be of good quality and large enough for the patient to see the whole of the chart and some of its surround without moving the head.

Test charts mounted on cards need to be externally illuminated. They have generally been superseded by internally illuminated test cabinets in which the charts are printed on translucent sheet material, or by test

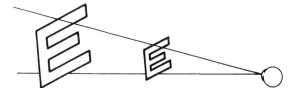

Figure 3.12. Constant angular subtense requires increasing size in proportion to distance.

chart projectors. In this case, a 6 m viewing distance may require a 6 m projection distance, the projector illuminating the screen after reflection in a mirror.

Test charts for literate adults usually present stylized capital letters designed to fit a grid of unit squares. One of the first of such charts was introduced by Snellen in 1862. Although different letter designs and symbols have since been introduced, charts of letters are often called Snellen charts. The term 'letter chart' is also commonly used. Snellen's own term 'optotypes' is now used less frequently, especially in the English-speaking world, but has persisted sufficiently elsewhere to be adopted by the International Organization for Standardization (ISO).

Consider a rectangular letter such as a capital E (*Figure 3.12*). It was assumed by Snellen that this letter could just be seen by the average corrected eye if the thickness of the limbs and of the spaces between them each subtended 1 minute of arc at the eye. The angular subtense of such a letter would therefore be 5 minutes vertically and 4–6 minutes horizontally, depending on the style of type and the particular letter of the alphabet.

As shown in *Figure 3.13*, a conventional test chart contains about 10 lines of letters in a progression of sizes, each designated by the distance at which the overall height of the letter subtends 5 minutes, the detail size or limb width then subtending 1 minute of arc. Thus, the overall height of a 6 m letter subtends 5 minutes at 6 m. Its height should be 8.73 mm, which is the tangent of 5 minutes multiplied by 6000. A 12 m letter subtends 5 minutes at 12 m or 10 minutes at 6 m, so its height is twice that of a 6 m letter and so on.

Visual acuity can be measured in several different ways and various different notations for recording it have been suggested from time to time. The basis of the generally accepted method is shown in *Figure 3.14* in which h is the overall height of the test letter and y the width of a single limb. Let d be the standard testing distance, D the distance at which the limb width subtends an arbitrary angle A_o and A the angular subtense at the standard testing distance of the limb width of the smallest letters that can be read.

The visual acuity V, or 'visus' as Snellen called it, can then be expressed as the ratio A_o/A. That is

$$V = \frac{A_o}{A} = \frac{y/D}{y/d}$$

$$= d/D \tag{3.7}$$

This ratio is known as 'Snellen's fraction' and is the notation most widely used in ophthalmic practice for recording vision and visual acuity. It is written, for example, as 6/18, 20/60.

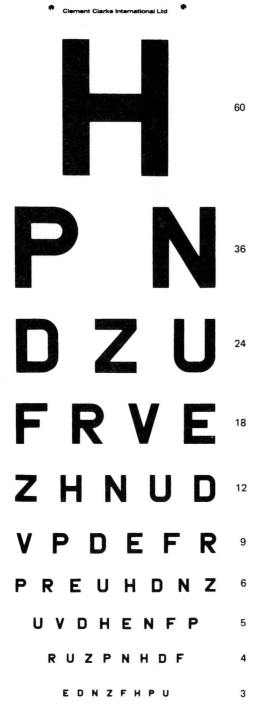

Figure 3.13. A complete Snellen letter chart for use at 6 m, to the full specification of British Standard BS 4274: 1968. Additional figures in larger type have been inserted in the right-hand margin to assist identification of the letter sizes. (Reproduced at about 40% of actual size by courtesy of Clement Clarke International Ltd.)

The relationship $V = A_o/A$ is in line with the general expression $V = k/A$, derived previously in equation (3.4). Following Snellen, the letter sizes on test charts are based on the arbitrary value of 1 minute for the angle A_o. With this substitution, Snellen's fraction in decimal notation becomes equivalent to

$$V = 1/A \text{ (where } A \text{ is in minutes of arc)} \tag{3.8}$$

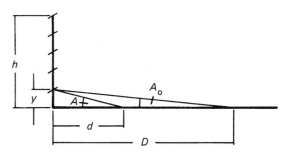

Figure 3.14. Derivation of the Snellen fraction d/D.

Because of the variation in legibility of different letters it is unlikely that most patients will be able to read all the letters on one line and none on the next smaller line. They are more likely to be able to read most of the letters on one line and just one or two on the next. This is recorded as in the example $6/12 + 3$, denoting that the patient could read the whole of the 12 m line and three letters of the next line. Similarly, if all but two letters are read on the 6 m line, the vision is $6/6 - 2$.

If, for some reason, a test chart is not used at the standard distance, the *actual* distance should be given as the numerator of the Snellen fraction.

The Snellen fraction may also be expressed as a decimal: thus, $6/12$ is equivalent to 0.5, $20/80$ to 0.25 and so on. This method of recording acuity, used in a few countries, has been called decimal V notation. For many purposes it is useful to be able to express the acuity in this way, but from the clinical standpoint the disappearance of the testing distance is a disadvantage.

Since a 6 m letter subtends 5 minutes at the standard testing distance of 6 m, the size h' of its retinal image in an eye of power $+60$ D is given by equation (2.17) as

$$h' = -u/F_e = -0.001454/60 \text{ (m)}$$
$$= -0.024 \text{ mm}$$

thus extending over about 12 cones. It is not surprising, therefore, that acuities better than $6/6$ – commonly regarded as a satisfactory standard – are enjoyed by many people, especially in good illumination.

Variation in letter styles and legibility

One of the main distinctions between the different letter styles used in test charts is that between serif and non-serif letters. The term 'serif' denotes an ornamental cross-stroke at the end of a limb (*Figure 3.15*). Although serif letters were employed by Snellen and are still in use, they are giving way to non-serif letters. The latter

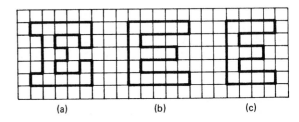

Figure 3.15. Letter styles: (a) 5×5 serif E, (b) 5×5 non-serif E, (c) 5×4 non-serif E.

are more in keeping with bold typefaces of modern design and appear less cluttered as well as being generally easier to read than serif letters.

It can be seen from *Figure 3.15* that non-serif letters appear better proportioned on a 5×4 grid than on a 5×5 grid. On a 5×5 grid, the letter O would have a line width of one unit, the central space being 3 units in diameter. The same letter on a 5×4 grid would have a central space of 2 units, which is still greater than the spaces in a letter E. Because of this variation in the structure of different letters, even if all designed to fit the same grid, their legibility varies. The letters L, T and U, for example, are easier to read than B or G, while letters which are similar in shape tend to be confused, such as C D G O Q and H K M N W.

Many detailed studies of relative legibility have been made. Hartridge and Owen (1922), using letters of 5×4 proportions and probably of non-serif design, ranked them in order of increasing difficulty as follows:

L A J E | N H X P F Z U T D | Y V K C B O R S
          selection
         recommended

A later study by Coates (1935) determined legibility scores for 104 different letters copied from four test charts with letters of different styles or formats. The tests were conducted in sunlight by four young male observers with good acuity, the score being based on the greatest distance at which each letter could be recognized. The figures were then adjusted so as to make the overall mean equal to unity. In the 5×4 non-serif style, the letters E, Z, F, H, P, N, D, V and R (in decreasing order of legibility) had scores within the range 1.1 to 0.9. The easiest letter was L (1.39) and the hardest B (0.67).

The selection of letters for test charts has been the subject of much debate. On one hand it is argued that all the letters used should be of similar legibility, the ideal being that the subject should be able to read all or none of the letters on any line. On the other hand, it has been contended that the test becomes more reliable if every line contains one of the more difficult letters or a pair of letters easily confused such as C G, F P, H N. In fact, the letters F, P, H and N were found in both the investigations just summarized to belong to the group of medium legibility.

Grimm *et al.* (1994), using letters from the Linea-Antiqua typeface which have widths 4.5–5.5 times the limb width, and height 7 times the limb width, selected C, D, E, K, N, P, U and Z because they presented similar difficulty. This typeface was selected for familiarity, being used on road signs in Germany.

The 1968 version of British Standard BS 4274, entitled 'Test charts for clinically determining distance visual acuity', stipulated that letters shall be of 5×4 non-serif construction, the selection being limited to D, E, F, H, N, P, R, U, V and Z, which are all of similar legibility. In general, this 5×4 format is more difficult to read than 5×5, especially in the presence of an uncorrected focusing error or poor vision.

In addition to or instead of letters, numerals can be used in test charts. The last three lines of Snellen's first published test chart each ended with a single numeral.

Later, the numerals 0, 1, 4 and 7 were used in a stylized form for the left-hand half of the 'International Chart' adopted by the Eleventh International Congress of Ophthalmology in 1909. The right-hand half of each row consisted of Landolt rings, but as the selected numerals had been found more legible than Landolt rings of the same size, the dimensions of the numerals were made 20% smaller than Landolt rings for the same acuity grading. Test charts of numerals may be useful in examining illiterates, most of whom can at least read figures.

Progression of sizes

This is another controversial question. Snellen's original test chart was designed for use at 20 Paris feet (approximately 6.5 m), the range of sizes being 20, 30, 40, 50, 70, 100 and 200 ft. The metric equivalent of this progression is 6, 9, 12, 15, 21, 30 and 60 m. This range may have been selected intuitively but it is fairly close to a regular geometrical progression, a mathematical series in which each number bears a constant ratio to the previous one. To start at any number and end with a tenfold increase in 6 steps requires this ratio to be $\sqrt[6]{10}$ or 1.468.

There is a strong consensus of opinion in favour of a geometrical progression of letter sizes, but several different views as to the best ratio to adopt. Two, in particular, have found some distinguished advocates. One is the square root of 2 (1.414) which would result in an exact doubling of the size at every second line. Unfortunately, it would not produce a close approximation to a 200 ft or 60 m line, both enshrined in many legal enactments and regulations. The other is the cube root of 2 (1.260) which would double the size at every third line and produce a size close enough to 200 ft or 60 m. The main objection to this progression is that the intervals are held to be a little too small for normal clinical use.

In the British Standard already mentioned, the range of sizes is 3, 4, 5, 6, 9, 12, 18, 24, 36 and 60 m. The omission of a 7.5 m line, included in some earlier charts, was regretted by some practitioners who felt that the jump from 6/6 to 6/9 was too great for useful clinical distinctions to be made.

Monoyer, who introduced the 5×4 non-serif letter style together with the decimal *V* notation, was also the originator of an entirely different progression of sizes, ranging from $V = 1$ to $V = 0.1$ at intervals of 0.1. This system still has its adherents but it is not a geometrical progression. Starting from the equivalent of a 6 m line, it takes another four lines to arrive at the equivalent of a 10 m line ($V = 0.6$), yet there is nothing to bridge the gap between 6/30 and 6/60.

Test charts for ordinary use are inadequate for assessing the vision of patients with low visual acuity (LVA). To fill this need, Keeler (1956) introduced the A series of 20 types sizes ranging from A1 (equal to 6/6) to A20 (approximately 6/420 or $V = 0.014$). This series forms a strict geometrical progression with a constant ratio of 1.25, very close to $\sqrt[3]{2}$. The Snellen equivalents just quoted are based on the specified viewing distance of 25 cm.

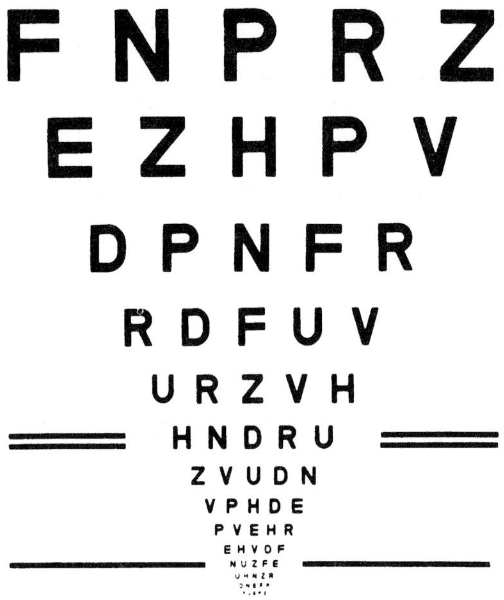

F N P R Z
E Z H P V
D P N F R
R D F U V
U R Z V H
H N D R U
Z V U D N
VPHDE
PVEHR
EHVDF
NUZFE
UHNZR
ZNEF

Figure 3.16. A Bailey–Lovie letter chart for distance vision (about 1/10th actual size). (Reproduced from Edwards and Llewellyn's *Optometry*.)

Table 3.2 The log MAR scale, corresponding minimum angles of resolution, and equivalent decimal *V* and Snellen distance acuities

log MAR steps	Angular size of detail (min of arc)	Corresponding distance acuities		
		Decimal V	at 6 m	at 20 ft
1.3	20.0	0.050	6/120	20/400
1.2	15.8	0.063	6/95	20/320
1.1	12.6	0.079	6/75	20/250
1.0	10.0	0.100	6/60	20/200
0.9	7.9	0.126	6/48	20/160
0.8	6.3	0.158	6/38	20/125
0.7	5.0	0.200	6/30	20/100
0.6	4.0	0.251	6/24	20/80
0.5	3.15	0.316	6/19	20/63
0.4	2.5	0.398	6/15	20/50
0.3	2.0	0.501	6/12	20/40
0.2	1.6	0.631	6/9.5	20/32
0.1	1.25	0.794	6/7.5	20/25
0	1.0	1.000	6/6	20/20
−0.1	0.79	1.259	6/4.75	20/16
−0.2	0.63	1.585	6/3.75	20/12.5
−0.3	0.50	1.995	6/3	20/10

The logMAR scale: Bailey–Lovie and Ferris charts

In his review of the principles and problems of test chart design, Bennett (1965) pointed out that in addition to other suggested geometrical, progressions of letter sizes, a constant ratio of $\sqrt[10]{10}$ or 1.2589 had been advocated by Blaskovics (1923, 1924) and Kettesy (1948). In 1976, this progression was chosen by the Australian optometrists Bailey and Lovie to express visual acuity in terms of the logarithm of the angular limb width (in minutes of arc) of the smallest letters recognized at 6 m. This notation was termed logMAR, 'MAR' standing for minimum angle of resolution. Thus, the 6 m line with its limb subtense of 1 minute of arc is denoted by logMAR 0 and the 60 m line of limb subtense 10 minutes of arc by logMAR 1. The progression of sizes is in 0.1 logMAR intervals. In the Bailey–Lovie test charts (*Figure 3.16*), it extends downwards from logMAR 1 to logMAR 0, continuing with three lines of smaller size having negative logMAR values (−0.1, −0.2, and −0.3) because the angular subtense is less than 1 minute of arc.

The logMAR number, denoted here by L_m can be converted into Snellen acuity by means of equation (3.8). Since $V = 1/A$ in which *A* is the angular limb width in minutes of arc, it follows that

$$\text{decimal } V = 1/\text{antilog } L_m \qquad (3.9)$$

Table 3.2 gives a comprehensive range of logMAR sizes, together with the corresponding angular limb widths, decimal *V* acuity, and the equivalent Snellen acuities for testing distances of 6 m and 20 ft.

It so happens that the logMAR progression is virtually indistinguishable from the $\sqrt[3]{2}$ basis advocated by Green (1868) and others. This gives a constant ratio of 1.2599. A feature of this progression is that the letter size doubles at every third line, from whatever line one

starts. This is seen from *Table 3.2* to apply almost exactly to the logMAR progression.

Certain other features of the Bailey–Lovie chart may be noted. The letters selected, of 5×4 non-serif format, are the 10 specified in the British Standard BS 4724 on the grounds of similar legibility. There are 5 letters on every line, even the biggest. To equalize the possible effects of the crowding phenomenon (*see* page 43), the inter-letter spacing on each line is equal to the letter width, and the inter-row spacing equal to the letter height of the lower row.

For use in the USA, the Bailey–Lovie chart has been modified by Ferris *et al.* (1982) to comply with the stipulations of the Committee on Vision of the National Academy of Sciences – National Research Council. Accordingly, the 10 letters used, C, D, H, K, N, O, R, S, V and Z, are those recommended by Sloan *et al.* (1952). They are of 5×5 non-serif format, of similar legibility, and also comparable in legibility to Landolt rings of the same size. Also, the letter dimensions are scaled down to suit the 4 m testing distance laid down by the Committee.

Used in conjunction with a suitable scoring system, the logMAR charts are demonstrably better suited for research and statistical analysis than the conventional letter charts used in refraction. Their large size – the Bailey–Lovie chart measures approximately 75 cm high by 80 cm wide – would present problems in clinical practice. Suitable methods of illumination have been described by Ferris and Sperduto (1982).

The current draft for revision of BS 4274 Part 1 entitled 'Specification for test charts for clinical determination of distance visual acuity' proposes the Bailey–Lovie layout from the 12 m size downwards, the typical dimensions of consulting room charts necessitating fewer letters for the larger lines. The letter selection suggested is C, D, E, F, H, K, P, R, U, V and Z in a 5×5 format.

As logMAR values decrease with letter size, becoming negative in sign, scoring systems can be complicated, though not unduly so. The first to be published was that of Kitchin and Bailey (1981), but several alternative systems have since been devised. Of these, the simplest is to score 0.02 of a logMAR unit for every letter correctly identified, beginning with the logMAR 1 (6/60 or 20/200) line. Thus, if every letter on each of the fourteen lines of the Bailey–Lovie or Ferris chart were correctly read, the score would be 1.40. The negative values for good acuities can be avoided by subtracting the logMAR acuity from 1. In this case, 6/6 (logMAR 0) becomes 1, 6/60 becomes 0, and 6/3.75 or logMAR −0.2 becomes 1.2.

When the vision is poor, the testing distance can be decreased. By halving it, another three lines of the chart should become legible, and halving it again should make a further three lines legible. In practice, the simplest method would be to choose a reduced distance equal to one-tenth of the denominator *D* of one of the Snellen fractions on the chart, for example, testing at 2.4 m. *Table 3.2* shows the logMAR equivalent of 6/24 to be 0.6. Since this is equivalent to logMAR 1.0 at the reduced distance of 2.4 m, 0.4 should be added to the logMAR size read. For example, if the 15 m line is then read, the apparent score of 0.4 becomes 0.8.

Comparison of acuity notations

Figure 3.17 shows the relationship between the various progressions and notations. A horizontal line placed across the chart gives equivalent values on all the distance acuity scales. Reading test type acuity can be converted into a Snellen distance value only on the basis of the stated viewing distance. For practical purposes, 35 cm and 14 in can be regarded as identical.

Notations for poor vision

If even the largest letter on the test chart cannot be read at the normal distance, a measurement of the vision can possibly be made by walking the patient towards the chart until the largest letter is just recognized. If this occurs at 2 m, for example, the vision is recorded as 2/60. A separate test card can be moved towards the patient if he is not readily mobile. The Bailey–Lovie chart with its five letters on each line, even for the large sizes, lends itself to assessment of poor vision.

Where vision is, say, worse than 0.5/60, an alternative method is to ask the patient to count the number of fingers held up at some specified near distance, say 25 cm. This would be recorded as 'CF at 25 cm'. If the vision merely permits the patient to be aware of a hand moved near the eye, it would be recorded as 'hand

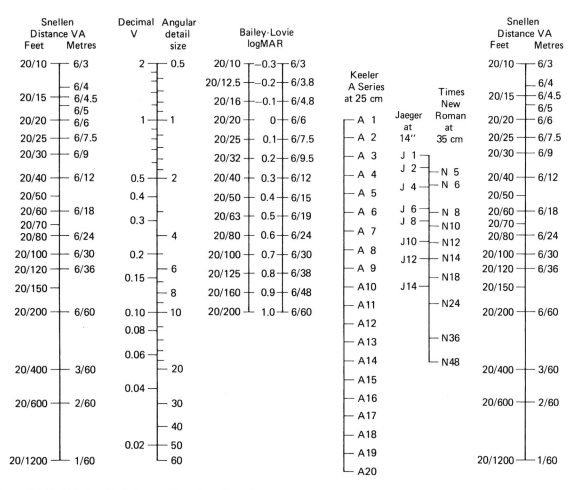

Figure 3.17.   Relationship between different acuity scales.

movements' (HM). An even lower category of vision is the mere perception of light (PL).

Repeatability of measurement

One might expect that the ability to read a few more or fewer letters on the chart would indicate a definite improvement or deterioration in vision. Using Bailey–Lovie charts, both Lovie-Kitchin (1988, 1989) and Reeves *et al.* (1993) found similar mean differences of about 0.03 ± 0.09 logMAR for the test–retest visual acuities. Adopting the criterion of a difference of at least two standard deviations before a change can be assumed to be statistically significant, an acuity of 6/4.8 would have to drop to around 6/7.5 to be meaningful.

Thus the impression of an improvement in visual acuity following an eye examination perhaps should be verified by allowing the patient to compare the original spectacles with the new results.

Brown and Yap (1995), also using Bailey–Lovie charts, compared the visual acuities of the right and left eyes of 72 subjects, finding the standard deviation of the difference to be 0.050 logMAR, or half a line. They concluded that a difference in acuity of more than 5 letters on such a chart indicated that further investigation was needed.

Other clinical tests of visual acuity

Whenever an acuity is measured by means of a chart or method not in normal routine use, or with single letters,* or at a non-standard distance, it is advisable to enter particulars in the patient's records.

The Landolt ring (or C)

The Landolt ring can be described as a letter C on a 5×5 grid, the parallel-sided gap having a width of one grid unit. In clinical practice, this gap is presented in one of four positions: up, down, right, or left. The patient merely has to indicate which one it is. Originally, four oblique presentations were also included, but are not in general use.

Because it does not demand literacy and avoids the difficulties of unsuitable alphabets, the Landolt ring has come into widespread use and is the basis for the internationally standardized test of visual acuity – *see* page 35. Nevertheless, it does have a few minor drawbacks of its own. If uncorrected astigmatism is present, recognition of the gap is easier in some settings than in others. It is less easy to keep in step with the patient's responses, especially if he returns without warning to the beginning of the line to start again. When uncertain of the true position of the gap, some patients have been found to show a guessing bias, often choosing the setting to the right. Any guess has a one in four or eight chance of being correct.

The checkerboard test

A checkerboard pattern of black and white squares makes a convenient test of resolution. It is used in some vision screening instruments, where the test objects take the form of a diamond divided into four smaller diamonds. Three of these are grey or appear grey under the test conditions, while the fourth is a checkerboard. Below resolution, this too appears a neutral grey and is indistinguishable from the rest of the diamond. In a similar test object, the checkerboard is replaced by an array of black circles on a white ground.

Calibration of test objects of this kind in terms of Snellen acuity needs to be determined experimentally.

Children's tests

The illiterate E test

This test, for which we are again indebted to Snellen, uses only the letter E in the normal range of sizes, drawn on a 5×5 grid. The open side, which has to be identified, is presented in the same four settings as the Landolt ring.

The test is particularly useful for children, who can be given a cut-out letter to hold in the same direction as the letter on the chart. If confused by a whole line of letters or symbols, some children respond better if shown only one at a time, especially if it is viewed directly and not in a mirror. From this point of view, a cube with a letter E of a different size on each face is better than a test chart.

Coates found the illiterate E test to have a legibility as high as 1.38 in comparison with the mean figure for test letters. A relative legibility score is not available for the Sjögren hand test which embodies a similar idea.

The Sheridan–Gardiner test

This is also useful for children. The examiner has a book with a conventional range of Snellen letter sizes with one letter on each page. The child is given a reference card showing the selection of letters used and has to match the letter shown with one on the reference card (Sheridan, 1970).

The Cambridge Crowding Cards

These cards, providing a test on similar lines to the Sheridan–Gardiner system, were devised at the Visual Development Unit of Cambridge University. The main difference is that the letter to be identified on each card, at a distance of 3 m, is surrounded by four other letters so that the possible effects of the crowding phenomenon (*see* page 43) can be brought into play.

LogMAR crowded test

These cards,† originally termed the Glasgow Acuity Cards, are bound in a spiral top book for use at 3 m,

---

* Often easier to read than a row of letters (see page 43).

† Obtainable from Keeler Ltd, Clewer Hill Road, Windsor, Berks SL4 4AA.

and present letter sizes in the Bailey–Lovie logMAR progression from the 19 m to the 1.5 m size, i.e. 6/38 to 6/3 equivalent. There are four letters in a line on each card, and to ensure identification of crowding difficulties, the letter spacing is half the letter width, while a border is added at a similar distance above and at the ends of the line. To reduce fatigue or boredom, three screening cards showing four letters each of successively smaller size enable the starting point for measurement to be determined. It is claimed that a maximum of three uniformly sized cards needs to be shown to measure acuity. The reversible letters H, O, U, V, X and Y are used to avoid potential problems with left–right orientation.

The test is described by McGraw and Winn (1993, 1995) in articles providing many useful references.

Stycar tests

Dr Mary Sheridan was also the originator of two tests known as 'Stycar', formed from the initial letters of Sheridan Tests for Young Children and Retardates. One of them, the graded-balls vision test (Sheridan, 1973), is a development of Worth's ivory-ball test introduced in 1903. A set of balls is used, ranging in diameter from 61 to 3 mm. They are rolled across the floor 3 m in front of the infant, whose response is observed. If the ball is seen, the child will follow its movement with his eyes and may even crawl to retrieve it. A 'static' variation of the test is to use a screen so that any ball from the set can be exposed to view and then hidden again. It can be argued that this is a visual field or an awareness test rather than an examination of acuity.

The other Stycar test uses test charts of the conventional type, but no line has more than three letters, selected from A, C, H, L, O, T, U, V and X. These letters were chosen because they can be easily copied by young children (Sheridan, 1963). One chart makes use of only five different letters, another only seven and a third all nine. A three-year-old child can cope with the five-letter chart, and a four-year old with the seven- or even nine-letter chart. As with the Sheridan–Gardiner test, the child is given a key card with the appropriate choice of letter. Whereas the Sheridan–Gardiner test depends on the recognition of isolated letters or symbols, the result obtained with this Stycar test is closer to conventional Snellen acuity.

Ffooks's test

The illiterate E has been criticized as a test for children because recognition of orientation is a visual task presenting difficulties to them. Vertical settings of the E tend to be correctly indicated more often than horizontal.

The test introduced by Ffooks (1965) uses three symbols free from directional bias: a square, a circle and an equilateral triangle. The presentation is by means of a book with two to four symbols on each page or by a cube with a single symbol on each face. Cut-out symbols are given to the child. The similar KOLT test, described in Grimm *et al.* (1994), also includes a + symbol.

Script letters

Young schoolchildren are more familiar with script or lower case letters than with block capitals. Test charts of such letters are available.

Pictorial charts

These show pictures with which the child is familiar, the assumption being that they can be recognized if large enough. These charts are difficult to quantify and confusion may be caused to the child if two objects of greatly different size, for example, a cat and a car, appear on the same line. Tests drawn on Snellen principles are the Allen (1957) and Kay (1983) pictures. Mayer and Gross (1990) added eight crowding bars in an octagonal formation around four of the Allen pictures, and demonstrated about 0.24 logMAR drop in acuity between the simple and crowded picture acuities for amblyopic eyes.

The Sonksen Picture Guide to Visual Function (SPGVF)

A different approach introduced by Sonksen in 1983 is to employ specified pictures from the Ladybird series of children's books. Sonksen and Macrae (1987) calibrated these for difficulty in terms of their recognition distance, as determined by children from a primary school who had been given artificially induced refractive errors. The pictures are generally shown at 3 m, but if a child needs a shorter distance to recognize them, poor vision is indicated. The test is suitable for children from about 21 months. For screening purposes, the six most difficult pictures from their series were recommended.

The Cardiff Acuity Test

The Cardiff Acuity Test,[*] described by Woodhouse *et al.* (1992) and Adoh *et al.* (1992), is a preferential looking test – *see* page 38. While these authors recommend the conventional grating preferential looking test for infants, the Cardiff test has been developed for the toddler age group of about $1-2\frac{1}{2}$ years. Pictures of a fish, car, train, house, boat or duck, selected from Kay's (1983) work, are used to help keep the child's attention.

The picture is positioned at the top or bottom of a grey card. The outline of the figure is drawn with a white line bordered by two black lines of half the width, so that the overall reflectance matches that of the grey card. All the pictures are the same size, so that the acuity test is the perception of the white line; below resolution, the picture merges into the card. The cards are presented at the child's eye level at 1 m, or 50 cm if a better response is obtained or for poorer acuities, while the practitioner observes the child's direction of gaze from the side of the card.

Three cards are available for each acuity level, 6/60 to 6/6 equivalent in 0.1 log steps if employed at 1 m. If the toddler's response is correct for the first two cards

---

[*] Obtainable from Keeler Ltd, Clewer Hill Road, Windsor, Berks SL4 4AA.

of any size, those of the next smaller acuity level are tried. If a wrong estimate of picture position is made, or no definite fixation is observed, then the previous set of cards is again presented using all three cards. The endpoint is where two of the three cards are consistently seen correctly.

Geer and Westall (1996) evaluated these cards, to find that they were not as good at identifying mild amblyopia as a letter chart, presumably because of the lack of crowding. They found them useful for holding the attention of the toddler age group. They also evaluated tests based on the VECR (*see* page 39). Although these performed better and would be suitable for this age group, they are too expensive for routine use.

Computer presentation of subjective charts

Some test chart cabinets and projector charts can provide only a limited range of letter charts, perhaps only one selection of letters of each size. Test charts on visual display units can be provided by the Medmont AT20 and the Mentor B-VAT, while Lenne *et al.* (1995) describe software for measuring visual acuity for research puposes.

The UMIST Eye System* can provide a large range of letter charts, with Bailey–Lovie 5×4 letters, Sloan 5×5 letters, Stycar letters, lower-case letters and symbols. The letters for any line on a particular chart are chosen at random from the selection, so that memorization is not possible. These can all be provided at different contrasts. The software can also provide many other charts for refraction, as well as colour vision and field screening.

In the USA, the TVA system* can provide many similar tests.

Illumination and luminance contrast of test charts

The effects of pupil size and illumination on visual acuity were discussed on pages 24–25. It is essential that test charts should be adequately illuminated at a level where acuity does not alter greatly with change in illumination. The 1968 edition of British Standard BS 4274 specified the following levels:

(1) *Externally illuminated charts*
   Minimum illuminance   480 lux
   For new equipment   600 lux
(2) *Internally illuminated charts*
   Minimum luminance $120 \, \text{cd/m}^2$
   For new equipment $150 \, \text{cd/m}^2$

The current draft British Standard adopts the luminance range of the ISO standard discussed below, namely $80 \, \text{cd/m}^2$ to $320 \, \text{cd/m}^2$.

For internally illuminated charts, Smith (1982b)

showed that the luminance (L) can be estimated with a photographic exposure meter or camera metering system. With the meter set for a given ASA film speed rating, the F/no. and exposure (t in seconds) for correct exposure are noted. The luminance is then found from the formula

$$\text{Luminance} = \frac{13.1 \times (\text{F/no.})^2}{\text{exposure (s)} \times \text{ASA setting}} \, \text{cd/m}^2$$

(3.10)

In this equation, for example, F/4 should be entered as 4. $120 \, \text{cd/m}^2$ is approximately $1/60$ s at F/4 for 100 ASA speed rating. For externally illuminated charts, the luminance is estimated as above after covering the chart with a piece of white blotting paper, which acts as an inexpensive but highly diffusive surface of reflectance ρ about 0.8. The blotting paper must cover the whole field of the exposure meter. If light of illuminance E lux falls on a unit area of reflectance ρ, the flux re-radiated by that area will be ρE lux. Then, if the apparent luminance of the surface is L and it acts as a perfect diffuser, the total flux radiated into a surrounding hemisphere from unit area of the surface is πL lux. Hence,

$$\rho E = \pi L$$

and

$$E = \pi L / \rho \, \text{lux}$$

(3.11)

To avoid glare, the test chart surroundings should be illuminated to a similar level. Also, general room lighting should be left on. The patient's pupil size will then approximate to that in his normal surroundings; few patients need a correction specifically for use in low illumination. Visual acuity is adversely affected by poor contrast as well as by poor illumination. If L_1 denotes the luminance of the white background of a test chart and L_2 the luminance of the black letters, the luminance contrast is defined as $(L_1 - L_2)/L_1$.

This fraction is often expressed as a percentage. The British Standard BS 4274 stipulates a minimum of 0.9 or 90% for all types of test charts. Experience has shown that to attain this figure a really dense black of very low transmittance or reflectance is required. In general, test chart projectors are unable to reach a 90% contrast unless the room is made very dark, which is undesirable for the reason already mentioned. At least one manufacturer, however, has succeeded in meeting the British Standard while ordinary room lighting is in use. The aluminized projection screens required for tests requiring polarized illumination may, however, give reduced contrast with good room lighting. VDU displays, described above, may also have slightly lower luminance than the original BS recommended levels.

The variation in grating acuity with luminance contrast has been studied by (among others) Shlaer (1937) and Arnulf (quoted by Fabry, 1936). In good illumination they found that there was relatively little change in the minimum angle of resolution, and hence in acuity, when the luminance contrast was reduced to 20%. Clinical experience suggests, however, that these findings would not apply to patients with cloudy ocular media or opacities. Poor contrast appears to reduce

---

* Available from Department of Optometry and Vision Sciences, UMIST, PO Box 88, Manchester M60 1QD and Innomed Corporation, Brea, CA 92621, USA respectively.

their acuity much more than in the normal patient with clear media – *see* page 43.

The new ISO standards

Two international standards relating to distance test charts were initially published as ISO standards in 1994, and as British and European standards in 1996:

BS EN ISO 8596: 1996 BS 4274: Part 2: 1996 Visual acuity test types – Specification for Landolt ring optotype for non-clinical purposes

BS EN ISO 8597: 1996 BS 4274: Part 3: 1996 Visual acuity test types – Method for correlating optotypes used for non-clinical purposes.

The purpose of the first of these is to provide a basis for an internationally valid certification of visual acuity to meet official or legal requirements. Understandably, the chosen test characters are Landolt rings, in the logMAR progression to which three sizes larger than 1.0 (6/60) have been added, namely, 1.1, 1.2 and 1.3 logMAR.

As it was not found possible to agree on one standard testing distance, a minimum of 4 m is stipulated, and the actual testing distance is always to be recorded. Also, because of the wide diversity of opinion, the permissible range of test chart luminance is from 80 to 320 cd/m^2. Other lighting requirements are specified in detail.

Because many different alphabets and other test characters are in use throughout the world, ISO 8596 is not intended for use in routine ophthalmic practice. Nevertheless, it may be desirable to correlate national standard test charts to ISO 8596 by experiment. ISO 8597 lays down details of the procedure to be followed when this course is undertaken. Thus Grimm *et al.* (1994) found that their selected letters had to be made 5% smaller than Landolt rings to give similar acuity scores, with individual letters also needing to be made slightly larger or smaller than the average to give equal legibility.

Conversely, Coates (1935) reported the Landolt ring was easier to read than the letter styles he investigated, with the ring having a legibility of 1.13 in relation to the mean legibility of all his test letters.

Near visual acuity: reading-test types

In general, a separate measurement of visual acuity in near vision is seldom required, but scaled-down versions of distance letter charts for use in near vision can be obtained for this purpose. Reading-test types are used mainly to determine the sufficiency of accommodation or the near addition required. They can, nevertheless, be approximately related to Snellen distance acuity, though the reading of words and sentences probably involves slightly different perceptual processes than the recognition of single letters.

In the printing industry, the size of a typeface is currently specified by 'points', e.g. 8 point, one point being 1/72 of an inch. This dimension refers to the 'body' on which the letter is raised or mounted. Since lower case letters vary in height, their actual size is best indicated by the 'x-height', that is to say, the height of letters such as e, m and x which have the same vertical dimension, unlike other letters with ascenders or descenders. Unfortunately, typefaces of the same point size but of different designs may not have the same x-height, which can be found only by measurement.

If the x-height of a particular typeface is known, its angular subtense (in minutes of arc) at a given working distance can easily be determined, from which an approximation to the corresponding Snellen acuity can be made. For example, given an x-height of 1.5 mm (typical for an 8-point type size) and a reading distance of 35 cm, the angular subtense is 14.7 minutes, corresponding to a Snellen acuity of very nearly 6/18. This is the basis on which the scales in *Figure 3.17* representing two different reading-test types in current use were constructed.

The earliest reading types to attain widespread popularity were introduced by Jaeger in 1854 and have still survived. They present short passages of continuous reading matter in a range of available print sizes which are simply numbered for reference with the prefix J, the smallest size being J1. It can be seen from *Figure 3.17* that J1 (at 35 cm) is roughly the equivalent of 6/9 or 20/30. In Britain, the reading types in general current use conform to the recommendations of the Faculty of Ophthalmologists (Law, 1952). The typeface selected, known as Times New Roman, was designed for *The Times* newspaper but subsequently came into more general use. The various sizes are distinguished by a number indicating the point size, prefixed by the letter N. Thus, N6 denotes the 6-point type size. From the scale in *Figure 3.17* it can be seen that the smallest size is N5, the subsequent sizes being 6, 8, 10, 12, 14, 18, 24, 36 and 48 point. Some practitioners deplore the fact that the new series does not include even a near approximation to J1; in fact, J2 is smaller than N5.

The Faculty of Ophthalmologists also recommended that if these test types are used to record a near visual acuity, it should be at a distance of 35 cm.

Sloan and Habel's M notation

A new notation for indicating the x-height of test letters and for recording near visual acuity was described by Sloan and Habel (1956). The x-height is expressed by a number *M* denoting the distance in metres at which it subtends an angle of 5 minutes of arc. The *M* number thus corresponds to the denominator *D* of the Snellen fraction $V = d/D$. Consequently, the height 8.73 mm of the 6 m letters on a standard Snellen chart is 6 M. It follows that size 1.0 M is 8.73/6 or approximately 1.45 mm, which is very close to the x-height of the 8-point type used for the great bulk of newsprint material. The approximate relationship 1.0 M = N8, 2.0 M = N16, and *pro rata*, applies throughout the main range of sizes.

Before the *M* number of a type size can be equated to a visual acuity rating, a specific viewing distance must be assumed, representing *d* in the Snellen fraction. In terms of decimal acuity we can therefore write

decimal $V = d$ (in metres)$/M$ number

For example, if $d = 40$ cm (0.4 m) and the smallest type that can be read at this distance is 0.5 M, then

decimal $V = 0.4/0.5 = 0.8$

equivalent to 6/7.5 or 20/25.

In general, if a reading chart is designed for use at a distance *d* in cm, the *M* size corresponding to 6/6 is $d/100$.

As an aid to prescribing magnification in cases of low visual acuity, a set of test cards was made available with letter sizes of 1 to 10 M. If the ability to read 1.0 M at a given viewing distance is taken as a reasonable standard, but the smallest type which a particular patient can read at this distance is 3 M, a need is clearly indicated for magnification in the neighbourhood of 3×.

A further paper by Sloan and Brown (1963) describes a large chart of test letters for measuring distance visual acuity and a reading chart of Snellen letters designed for use at 40 cm.

The Bailey–Lovie Word Reading Chart

Reading charts using the Times Roman typeface and based on the principles of their logMAR distance chart have been designed by Bailey and Lovie (1980).

Although it was not found practicable to adhere exactly to the strict logarithmic progression, a reasonable approximation to it has been achieved. Those sizes for which no sufficiently close printers' types exist were produced by photographic enlargement or reduction. The 17 sizes in all have x-heights varying from about 14.5 mm (N80) to as little as 0.36 mm (N2). In logMAR units the range is from 1.6 (6/240) to 0.0 (6/6). The Snellen equivalents in parentheses relate to the stipulated reading distance of 25 cm.

For reasons fully detailed, unconnected words have been chosen instead of continuous reading matter. Each line from 1.0 logMAR down to the smallest contains a selection of six words, two each with 4, 7 and 10 letters. As with the distance chart, the inter-word and inter-row spacing have been kept on a uniform basis in relation to the letter size of each row.

Extra-fine reading charts

Jenkins *et al.* (1995) developed the Bradford Near Vision Charts for experiments on the effects of fixation disparity (*see* Chapter 10) on binocular near acuity. These six charts showed five lines of five four- or five-letter words of 3.5 to 1.0 point size to be viewed at 40 cm, giving angular subtenses of 41 to 16 seconds of arc limb width. Their pre-presbyopic subjects managed a mean result of just under 30 seconds of arc. It could be argued that these charts could also be employed for selecting people for very demanding near vision tasks. This was the argument of Vos *et al.* (1994), who investigated the Priegel test, an internally illuminated Landolt ring test with gap sizes from 0.12 to 0.04 mm. The

younger subjects managed the smallest gap, possibly because they could hold the test closer than older subjects.

Visual acuity in the peripheral field

The structure of the retina has been discussed briefly on pages 20–21 in relation to visual acuity. For the reasons explained, the high resolution at the fovea is not maintained in the peripheral parts of the retina. Indeed, it would scarcely be possible or even beneficial to do so. With a mobile eye, the loss of detail in peripheral vision is unimportant. Movements in the peripheral field are readily detected and the eyes or head can quickly be turned to obtain a direct view. In scotopic conditions of illumination, the pre-eminence of the fovea is lost and there is then little difference between central and peripheral acuities.

Many studies of visual acuity in the peripheral field have been made, those of Low (1951) and Millodot (1966) giving reviews. One of the best known and earliest was by Wertheim (1894) who used a grating as test object. The acuity was measured centrally, at 2.5° and 5° from fixation, and at every 5° interval up to 70°. *Figure 3.18* shows the results for the nasal side of the retina, expressed in terms of acuity relative to that at the fovea, the gap in the graph representing the blind spot. Apart from this feature, the corresponding graph for the temporal side of the retina is very similar.

It was pointed out by Low that the shape of this graph with its sharp peak can give a misleading impression. This type of curve is characteristic of a simple reciprocal function and Snellen acuity is the reciprocal of the angular subtense *A* of the smallest detail size recognized. If the curve of *Figure 3.18* is re-plotted in terms of the angle *A* instead of visual acuity, as in *Figure 3.19*, the graph becomes very nearly linear over half its extent.

Studies in the central region up to 85 minutes from fixation were made by Weymouth *et al.* (1928), using a grating of 10 minutes overall width. Over this range the fall in acuity was found to be nearly linear, though slightly greater in the vertical meridian than in the horizontal. In his study, which involved three observers, Millodot (1966) measured the peripheral acuity at 5-

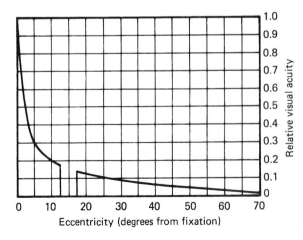

Figure 3.18. Visual acuity as a function of eccentricity in the nasal retina. (Redrawn from Wertheim, 1894.)

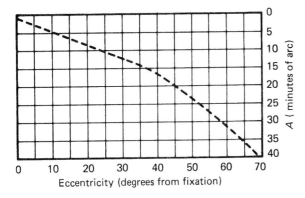

Figure 3.19. Angular detail size *A* in minutes of arc as a function of eccentricity.

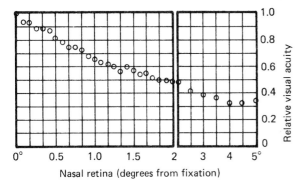

Figure 3.20. Visual acuity as a function of eccentricity in the nasal retina. (Redrawn from Millodot, 1966, by kind permission of the publishers of *Br. J. Physiol. Optics.*)

minute intervals up to 2° and then at 30-minute intervals. A Landolt ring was used as a test object and the results published in the form of the actual acuities, which varied at fixation from 0.85 to 1.25. *Figure 3.20* shows the mean of Millodot's results for the nasal retina, the original data having first been converted into relative acuities for this purpose. Weymouth and colleagues' results up to 85-minute eccentricity are in good agreement, though slightly higher for eccentricities less than 20 minutes.

In round figures, taking the foveal acuity as 6/6 (20/20), the peripheral acuity is 6/9 (20/30) at 1° eccentricity, 6/12 (20/40) from $1\frac{1}{2}$ to 2°, and 6/18 (20/60) from 3° to 5°. These figures have clinical significance when eccentric fixation is in use; for example, in the case of retinal burns, senile macular degeneration and some forms of amblyopia (*see* pages 41–43).

When reading print, the eyes do not fixate each word in turn, certainly not each letter, but make only two or three jumps (saccades) along each line. Cattell, quoted by Low (1951), showed that in the near periphery 'words were three times as recognizable as random series of letters and sentences twice as recognizable as random series of words'.

The factors responsible for the decline in acuity with eccentricity also affect the visibility of an isolated stimulus imaged away from the fovea. In field plotting, for example, it is found that the size of the smallest object visible increases with eccentricity. The locus of all points in the field where a stimulus of a particular size is only just perceived is called an isopter.

Contrast sensitivity (*see* later in this chapter) as a function of eccentricity has been studied by Pointer and Hess (1989, 1990).

Kinetic (or dynamic) visual acuity

The previous sections of this chapter have been concerned with stationary test objects. When visual acuity is measured with moving test stimuli, the result is known as kinetic visual acuity. It is also called 'dynamic visual acuity', but this expression is confusing, since the term 'dynamic' is generally understood by optometrists to refer to the state of the eye when accommodating for a near object.

Kinetic visual acuity or KVA may depend upon several factors:

(1) The static visual acuity or SVA,
(2) The speed of the tracking movements,
(3) The accuracy of the fixation on the moving object.

If the SVA is poor, it is unlikely that the KVA will be good. Long and May (1992) found no correlation between SVA and KVA for their 60 student subjects having binocular SVAs between 6/4 and 6/12.

Westheimer (1954) found that the eyes could maintain fixation up to an angular speed of 30°/s. Brown (1972a), however, found that the eye's pursuit velocity was lower than that of the object. 'Saccades', high-velocity re-fixation movements, were made to regain approximate fixation.

This lag of fixation behind the test object means that the retinal image falls off the fovea and on to a part of the retina possessing intrinsically lower acuity.

KVA was studied first by Ludvigh and Miller (1958) for a test object rotating in a circular path in a plane parallel to that of the face. Their later survey (Miller and Ludvigh, 1962) discusses many of the factors relating to this subject. Brown (1972a) found that the kinetic visual threshold (reciprocal acuity) rose approximately linearly from the static value of 0.75 minute to 3.5 minutes at a velocity of 90°/s. Similar results were also obtained by Miller and Reeder (1965). For a 600 ms exposure time, Long and May (1992) found the KVA to drop from 3 minutes of arc at 60°/s to around 10 minutes at 120°/s. For a 200 ms exposure time, the results increased to around 10 and 25 minutes respectively. They suggest that the following response is saccade dominated for the shorter time interval, saccade and pursuit for the longer exposure. Interestingly, males had slightly better KVA than females.

Measurements of KVA appear to be influenced by learning, practice increasing the acuity. The luminance contrast of the test object is another factor. If it falls below about 23%, Brown (1972b) showed that KVA deteriorates, due to the effect of reduced contrast on static acuity and eye movement control.

Objective determination of vision

While the subjective measurement of vision and visual acuity using letter or similar charts is usually satisfactory, there are cases where an objective determination would be a helpful or even the only method available. Infants, patients who may be unable to co-operate adequately and malingerers are examples.

Because these tests present simpler visual stimuli than the traditional letter chart, and may be monitoring a response from lower in the visual/cerebral system than is required for letter recognition, the acuities recorded may be optimistic in comparison with those which a Snellen chart might give.

Reviews of the objective methods of determining visual acuity have been given by Voipio (1961), Pearson (1966) and Dobson and Teller (1978). Methods (2)–(5) below follow the classification of Voipio.

Methods of determining visual acuity

(1) Forced choice preferential looking (PL) or differential fixation

A young infant in a darkened room is simultaneously shown a plain disc and a patterned disc both of the same size and mean luminance. Provided that the child can see the pattern, it should be more interested to look at the patterned rather than the plain disc. The patterned discs are usually square-wave gratings in a geometrical progression of sizes which can be equated to Snellen acuity on the basis of equation (3.8). A routine system of examination by this technique has been described by Gwiazda *et al.* (1980). When there are no complications, the binocular acuity can be determined in less than five minutes. Monocular acuities also can be measured by this method.

The basis of a simpler method of applying the PL technique, in the form of 'acuity cards', was described by Teller *et al.* (1974). An account of this method in its developed form and of clinical trials with it was given by McDonald *et al.* (1985).

A set of long grey cards has a grating at one end, of the same mean luminance as the card itself. Depending on the version used, the grating frequency increases with each successive card by a factor of $\sqrt{2}$ or 2. The cards are placed behind an aperture in a grey screen. Each has a small central spyhole through which the examiner can note the response of the infant, who is held at a distance of about 36 cm from the card. Successively finer cards are shown until there is no fixation or pointing response from the infant.

A number of additional studies – for example, by Dobson *et al.* (1986) and Thompson and Drasdo (1988) – have found that although this technique is quicker (taking 3–5 min) than the use of twin projectors or visual display units, it is no less accurate.

The technique is reported to work well with infants up to about 18 months, binocular acuities being easier to measure than monocular. Some children dislike having either eye covered. If, however, there is no reluctance to having one particular eye covered, it may be because that eye is amblyopic. Success rates of over 90% are reported. Normative data for the Teller cards have been presented by Salomão *et al.* (1995) and Mayer *et al.* (1995). Both Friendly *et al.* (1990) and Sireteanu *et al.* (1990) caution that the Teller card test appears not to identify the loss in acuity in amblyopes. This may be because the measurement is by a grating rather than letter acuity, since Vernon *et al.* (1990) found that gratings formed by interferometry (*see* page 44) were also poor at identifying amblyopes, because seven of their nine subjects had grating acuities within one octave (i.e. half the frequency) of their better eye, and six showed acuities better than or equal to 6/9 equivalent. More than half their subject's amblyopic eyes with Snellen acuity of 6/18 or worse showed grating acuities indistinguishable from normal. Chandna (1991) suggested that a Teller card acuity difference greater than half an octave between the eyes should be considered abnormal, even though the acuities in any age group varied over ±2 octaves.

The Cardiff Acuity Cards have been described on pages 33–34.

(2) Methods based on evoking an oscillatory motion

If a detailed object is swung back and forth across the field of vision, the eyes will follow it with a pendular motion, provided that the target detail can be resolved.

A checkerboard or vertical grating oscillates horizontally against a background of the same mean luminance so that the edges of the test object cannot be seen as a luminance difference. The subject sits close to the apparatus and the pendular motion of his eyes is monitored through a magnifier or microscope. The observation distance is then increased until this motion ceases. The greatest distance at which response occurs is used to calculate the objective acuity.

If y is the detail size in millimetres and D the greatest observation distance in metres, then the angular subtense A of the detail size becomes

$$A = y/1000D \text{ rad} = 3.444y/D \text{ minutes of arc}$$

Thus from equation (3.6)

$$V = 1/A = D/3.44y \qquad (3.12)$$

Correlation with subjective acuities of up to +0.91 have been reported. Projectors using zoom magnification systems may be used instead of altering the observation distance.

(3) Methods based on evoking an opto-kinetic nystagmus (OKN)

This method is similar to the previous one, except that the test object moves continuously in one direction instead of oscillating. Provided that the detail is resolved, the eyes follow the moving object for a limited rotation and then rapidly swing back. There is thus a slow following phase and a rapid recovery phase and such motion is called nystagmus. Good correlations with subjective acuity have again been recorded. The acuity of neonates can be estimated by this method (Gorman *et al.*, 1957, 1959).

(4) Methods based on arresting opto-kinetic nystagmus

Opto-kinetic nystagmus is produced by a coarse grating. Superimposed on this is a stationary object of fine detail on a background of the same mean luminance. The nystagmus is halted if the patient's fixation is transferred to the test object, which occurs when the detail can be resolved.

Techniques (2)–(4) require careful choice of stimulus and speed of motion.

(5) Methods based on the galvanic skin response

This method was devised by Wagner (1950) and utilizes the galvanic skin response. This is the alteration in resistance of the skin to an electrical voltage when the patient reacts to a conditioned stimulus. In this application, the patient may be shown a series of Snellen letters, of the same size. Following every demonstration of one particular letter of the alphabet, the patient is subjected to a mildly unpleasant stimulus, such as an electric shock or loud noise. In this way, the patient becomes conditioned to react to any viewing of this one particular letter.

After the conditioning process, the patient is shown a series of test letters of decreasing size, including the letter to which he has been conditioned. The skin resistance response is monitored, and when no response is made to the relevant letter, it is assumed that the letter is below threshold. The test can be repeated with increasing letter sizes.

The problems with this technique are the considerable variation from person to person in normal skin resistance and the difficulties in producing a conditioned response. Pearson (1970) repeated this technique using an auditory shock, but without obtaining satisfactory results.

(6) Methods based on the visually evoked cortical response (VECR)

All neural activity is accompanied by electrical effects. Nerve conduction, for example, results from a polarized ionic wave or spike potential passing down the fibre. Stimulation of the retina by light similarly results in potential changes. On animal specimens, electrodes may be placed in the retina or optic nerve, enabling measurements to be taken of the electrical activity in single relay or ganglion cells and their fibres. An averaged response due to a relatively large portion of the retina may be measured at the cornea. A transparent contact lens bearing an electrode is worn on the cornea, while a reference electrode is placed on the cheek. The potential changes, resulting from viewing a flash of light are recorded as an electroretinogram (ERG). It is possible to distinguish between the responses of rod and cone pathways, so that the ERG can be used to determine whether the predominantly cone-populated fovea is functional in patients whose media are too opaque to allow a determination of acuity or ophthalmoscopic examination of the interior of the eye.

The ERG gives an indication of the functioning of the retina, but vision requires satisfactory performance of the whole visual pathways, which end at the occipital cortex. By placing electrodes on the scalp at the appropriate rear part of the head, it is possible to pick up neural activity in the brain. This activity will be related to the visual information, but the electrodes will also pick up stray noise and signals from other parts of the brain. The relevant activity may be extracted by an averaging process. If the eye views a checkerboard pattern which reverses in contrast at regular intervals at about 12 Hz, the cortical response should similarly show cyclic potential changes. The responses to each test object cycle may be added together by electronic recording, while signals due to stray noise and other brain activity should average out to zero. The resultant mean signal is called the visually evoked cortical response or potential (VECR, VECP or just VEP).

Responses were initially determined for stroboscopic flashes of light, but later investigators used patterned stimuli of constant mean luminance, such as the checkerboard pattern, to enhance foveal response.

The VECR may be employed to investigate the performance of the visual pathways in amblyopia (*see* pages 41–43) and retinal or nerve pathway diseases. Thus, a study by Nawratzki *et al.* (1966) with flashes of light showed a difference in latency of the VECR following the stimulus between normal and amblyopic eyes. Fishman and Copenhaver (1967) also used flash illumination and found little difference in latency, but could distinguish an altered response in patients with unilateral macular disease.

Arden *et al.* (1974) used a checkerboard pattern and found a depressed VECR when the eye was amblyopic (less than about 6/18), and also measured a meridional amblyopia in a patient whose eye showed low astigmatism. Ikeda (1976) suggests that the reduced response indicates an organic lesion or functional suppression of the visual pathway.

Although a supra-threshold grating is used, say 5.5 minutes of arc, the amplitude of the VECR is found to correlate well with acuity (Douthwaite and Jenkins, 1987).

The visually evoked response has been used by Millodot and Riggs (1970) to examine the focusing of the eye. The amplitudes of the responses (both VECR and ERG) were shown to produce a marked peak when the image of the checkerboard was in focus on the retina.

Visual efficiency

A normal visual acuity is about 6/6, often slightly better. In terms of the minimum angle of resolution, this is twice as good as 6/12. However, it can also be said that an object only just discernible by a person with 6/12 vision can be seen more easily by someone with better vision. This leads to the concept of visual efficiency, according to which an acuity 6/12 (or 0.5) does not imply that visual capacity in terms of fitness for employment is reduced to one-half.

In 1925 the American Medical Association (AMA) adopted a visual efficiency scale based on the work of Snell and Scott Sterling. A number of identical 'obscurant' glasses were made and the acuity of normal observers measured when looking through first one glass, then two together, three together and so on. Six glasses were found to reduce the vision from 20/20 to 20/400 and each successive glass was considered to reduce the visual efficiency by one-sixth. For example, three glasses, giving an acuity of 20/100 were deemed to represent a visual efficiency of 50%.

The experimental results were found to agree reasonably well with the mathematical relationship whereby visual efficiency E decreases logarithmically as the minimum angular detail size A or the letter size D increases arithmetically. Accordingly, if log E is plotted against A or D, the resulting graph is a straight line. The position of this line can be determined by two points. One has the co-ordinates ($A = 1$, $E = 100\%$), arising from the decision to equate 100% visual efficiency with the 'normal' visual standard of 20/20. The other point, whose co-ordinates are ($A = 10$, $E = 20\%$), is fixed by the decision to equate 20% visual efficiency to exactly 20/200, broadly in line with the experimental results. It then follows that the equation of the line is

$$\log E = -0.0777A + 2.0777 \qquad (3.13)$$

From which

$$A = \frac{2.0777 - \log E}{0.0777} \qquad (3.14)$$

and

$$V = 1/A = \frac{0.0777}{2.0777 - \log E} \qquad (3.15)$$

In 1955, the AMA adopted a report by its Council on Industrial Health, in which modifications to the original

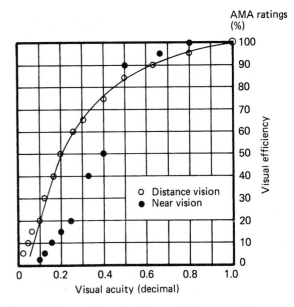

Figure 3.21.   Relationship between AMA visual efficiency and Snellen visual acuity in decimal notation.

visual acuity efficiency scale were proposed. For distance vision, ratings under 20% were related to lower Snellen acuities than before. For example, 10% efficiency was equated to 20/400 instead of 20/280. At the same time, a separate scale of ratings for near vision was introduced. Details of the decimal V equivalents of the 1955 acuity ratings are given in *Table 3.3* and are shown graphically in *Figure 3.21*. The curved line in this diagram represents the original theoretical relationship expressed by equation (3.15), without rounding off.

The big drop in the near vision efficiency ratings between $V = 0.5$ (90%) and $V = 0.4$ (50%) reflects the fact that inability to read J4 or its near equivalent N6 at 14 in would be a considerable handicap in many near visual tasks.

Table 3.3   1955 AMA visual acuity efficiency ratings and their equivalents

AMA efficiency rating (%)	Distance vision				Near vision		
	Snellen VA (feet)	Snellen VA (metres)	Angle A (minutes)		Snellen VA (inches)	Times New Roman* (at 35 cm)	Angle A (minutes)
100	20/20	6/6	1.0		14/18	–	1.3
95	20/25	6/7.5	1.25		14/22	N5	1.6
90	20/32	6/10	1.6		14/28	N6	2.0
85	20/40	6/12	2.0				
75	20/50	6/15	2.5				
65	20/64	6/18	3.2				
60	20/80	6/24	4.0				
50	20/100	6/30	5.0		14/35	N7	2.5
40	20/125	6/36	6.25		14/45	N9	3.2
30	20/160	6/48	8.0				
20	20/200	6/60	10.0		14/56	N12	4.0
15	20/300	6/90	15.0		14/70	N14	5.0
10	20/400	6/120	20.0		14/87	N18	6.2
5	20/800	6/240	40.0		14/112	N24	8.0
2					14/140	–	10.0

* Approximate equivalents

In the 1955 revision, the visual efficiency (VE) of one eye was defined quantitatively as the product of three separate ratings: central visual efficiency (distance and near acuities combined), visual field efficiency and motility efficiency. For example, if the three scores are 70, 30 and 80%, the visual efficiency is $0.7 \times 0.3 \times 0.8$, equal to 0.168 or 16.8%. A score below 10% in any one function is regarded as a total loss of visual efficiency.

Binocular visual efficiency (BVE) is computed from the formula

$$BVE = \frac{3B + P}{4}$$

where B is the visual efficiency of the better (or only) eye and P the visual efficiency of the poorer (or lost) eye. The BVE is thus equal to at least 75% of the better eye's VE.

Detailed procedures are laid down for determining the three components of the VE rating. They are here described only in outline. To assess the central acuity rating, the mean of the distance and near ratings is taken, any necessary refractive correction being supplied by conventional ophthalmic lenses. Special rules apply in aphakia.

The visual field efficiency is assessed on a perimeter with a 3/330 white stimulus (6/330 for uncorrected aphakia). The field of view is measured in degrees in the eight principal directions at $45°$ intervals and the total divided by five. This gives the efficiency rating as a percentage of the total possible score of $500°$, to which the various meridians contribute appropriately.

In assessing motility efficiency, diplopia within $20°$ of the primary position counts as a 100% loss of efficiency. If diplopia occurs within $20°$–$40°$ from fixation, the loss of efficiency is determined by means of a special chart divided into areas with different ratings. Suppression or loss of binocular vision is regarded as a 50% loss of motility efficiency in the eye affected.

The earlier AMA visual acuity ratings have been discussed by Hofstetter (1950) and Sloan (1951), while Luckiesh (1945) has described in detail the test chart based on equation (3.13). Ryan (1962) has provided a comprehensive historical review and a commentary on the 1955 revision and innovations.

The development of visual acuity

In the same way that a baby has to learn to co-ordinate its muscular activity, visual acuity also develops with time. This is partly due to the anatomical development of the fovea itself, which is not completed until a few months after birth.

One of the early estimates of visual acuity in the infant was made by Worth (1903) using a series of five ivory balls (*see* page 33). Another well-known study was made by Chavasse (1939). Curve A in *Figure 3.22* is based on his findings, but is re-plotted here in terms of the useful concept of visual acuity efficiency. An additional scaling gives the acuity in decimal notation.

Several of the more recent techniques described on pages 38–39 have thrown new light on the visual devel-

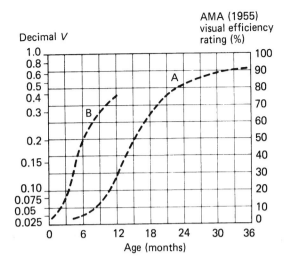

Figure 3.22. Development of visual acuity with age. Curve A: results of Chavasse (1939). Curve B: mean results of recent investigations.

opment of the very young, even the newly born. Without exception, they all indicate a much higher level of acuity than had previously been supposed. A comprehensive review of experimental results for infants up to six months was given by Dobson and Teller (1978). Although the methods of optokinetic nystagmus (OKN) and preferential looking (PL) were shown to produce findings in fair agreement, the results from the method of visually evoked cortical response (VECR) gave appreciably higher acuities.

Curve B in *Figure 3.22* represents the mean results surveyed by Dobson and Teller, together with the later findings of Gwiazda *et al.* (1980) for 30 infants ranging from 2 to 58 weeks of age. At birth, the mean acuity given by the scanty data is about 6/240 (20/800). By one month, it is of the order of 6/120 (20/400), rising to about 6/30 (20/100) at 6 months and about 6/15 (20/50) at 1 year. Chandna (1991), also using Teller Cards over the 6-month to 4-year age span, found results approximately mid-way between curves A and B.

These curves do not include results obtained from the VECR method. Using this technique, Marg *et al.* (1976) found an acuity of about 6/18 (20/60) at 3 months, rising to 6/6 (20/20) by the end of 6 months. Somewhat lower values were found by Sokol and Dobson (1976), but still much higher than those of curve B.

The high acuities revealed in these various studies refer to gratings or checkerboards. They do not imply a parallel development of shape perception and analysis as required for the recognition of test symbols or letters, nor the verbal or motor response.

Amblyopia

Types of amblyopia

Poor unaided vision may be produced solely by a refractive (focusing) error in one or both eyes. In some patients, the *corrected* visual acuity is below normal, for example, 6/9 or less, although there is no pathological cause such as irregularity of the refracting surfaces or media, non-congenital cataract or disorders at the macula or in the optic nerve. Reduced acuity of this type is known as amblyopia.

Amblyopia may be classified under many headings but the most important ones are: congenital, occlusion, refractive and strabismic. The various toxic amblyopias, such as tobacco amblyopia, are not considered here because they are of pathological origin.

Congenital amblyopia

The visual acuity is usually reduced in both eyes by a similar amount and, on examination of the macula with an ophthalmoscope, the fovea may appear to be ill-developed (no foveal reflex). The refractive error is not large. The letters on the test chart do not appear to jumble and fixation is central.

Occlusion amblyopia

If a child is born with cloudy media, as in congenital cataract, the retina is immediately deprived of a clear image and amblyopia results: hence the need for early diagnosis (Jacobson *et al.*, 1981). Prompt surgical intervention and provision of a refractive correction, usually a contact lens, are essential. Occlusion of an eye of a young infant to stimulate development of the fellow eye's vision also entails a rapid loss of acuity. For this reason, the occlusion must be part-time, not constant.

Refractive amblyopia

In general, this arises when there is a large refractive error in one or both eyes, the retina and nervous pathways having been deprived of an adequately detailed stimulus for development.

Discussion of treatment does not fall within the scope of this text, but if the refractive error is corrected before the patient is about 8 years old, there is a good chance that almost normal acuity will be attained. If the error is in one eye only, it is often necessary for the good eye to be covered for a certain length of time in order to stimulate development of the poorer eye's acuity (*see* page 263).

Refractive amblyopia may be divided into three main types: anisometropic, bilateral and meridional.

Anisometropic amblyopia occurs when there is a focusing error of appreciable magnitude in one eye only, in which case vision in the poorer eye is affected. This is less likely to happen if the eye is myopic (short-sighted) only by a moderate amount, enabling it to be used for near vision.

Bilateral refractive amblyopia may arise if both eyes have high myopic errors (rare in the young child), high hypermetropic errors for which the eyes are unable to accommodate or marked astigmatism.*

Meridional amblyopia, a legacy of early uncorrected

astigmatism of relatively marked degree, was first noted in 1890 by Martin (cited in the study by Mitchell *et al.*, 1973). The uncorrected astigmatic eye is able to form sharp images only of lines substantially parallel to its two mutually perpendicular meridians. Moreover, lines in these two orientations cannot be focused on the retina simultaneously. If, in addition, the eye is hypermetropic in both principal meridians, one set of lines will be more out of focus in both distance and near vision. The development of acuity for lines in the favoured meridian will thus be normal, while that for lines in oblique and out-of-focus directions will be hindered. Even when the astigmatism is subsequently corrected, the grating acuity for the out-of-focus meridian, and to a lesser extent oblique meridians, may remain below that of the favoured meridian. The Snellen letter acuity may nevertheless be virtually normal. In myopic astigmatism, it may be possible for one meridian to be in focus (or nearly so) for distance vision, the other for near vision, thus reducing the meridional acuity difference.

Although marked astigmatism seems to be common in young infants, it is usually outgrown by the end of the second year, apparently without lasting effects.

Meridional amblyopia should not be confused with the normal reduction in acuity for gratings in oblique meridians, as mentioned on page 22. This is probably a physiological response to the preponderance of vertical and horizontal lines in our environment, though Charman and Voisin (1993) postulate that this oblique effect may indeed result from meridional out-of-focus effects from the preponderance of even small horizontal and vertical astigmatic errors in the young eye.

Strabismic amblyopia

When the patient has a unilateral squint, the vision in the squinting eye is often poor. Classical ideas suggest that the acuity would have developed normally up to the time of onset of the strabismus, but that the development to be expected in subsequent years would not occur. This was known as amblyopia of arrest. Because the squinting eye does not enter fully into binocular vision, it was thought that following the onset of the squint, the vision might deteriorate: amblyopia of extinction. These two are often grouped together as amblyopia ex anopsia (of disuse).

Although these concepts are useful, current ideas on the functioning of the strabismic eye have led to a revision of the nomenclature. Under earlier and somewhat artificial conditions of examination of the squinting patient's binocular system, the mental image due to the strabismic eye was found to be suppressed. More recent and sophisticated tests, for example Bagolini glasses or the synoptophore with Stanworth's semi-reflecting mirrors, show suppression is often minimal. The strabismic eye may contribute significantly to the binocular percept. The term 'strabismic amblyopia' is preferable to either amblyopia ex anopsia or suppression amblyopia, since it does not imply a specific cause of the poor vision.

As a matter of insurance in case the good eye should be lost or injured, the authors feel that improvement of

---

* These various refractive errors are discussed in Chapters 4 and 5.

the acuity of the patient's amblyopic eye is more important than curing the strabismus. Any significant refractive error in either or both eyes must be corrected and followed by occlusion of the good eye to force the child to use his less efficient eye. The rate at which the acuity improves will depend upon the age of the child both now and at the onset of the strabismus and the amount of amblyopia present before treatment starts. A red filter worn over the poor eye tends to help by stimulating the use of the fovea, especially under relatively low illumination conditions indoors. A suggested explanation is that the red filter absorbs blue and green light to which the rods are more sensitive than the cones under mesopic conditions.

Many readers may find it useful to return to this section after reading Chapter 10 on anomalies of binocular vision.

The crowding phenomenon (separation difficulty)

The crowding phenomenon is a difficulty sometimes shown in separating the letters on a line of type or of a test chart. It particularly affects patients with strabismic amblyopia or macular degeneration .

The end letters of the line may be read but those in the centre are jumbled and the order may be confused. The measured acuity may be higher if the test letters are shown singly. This may be done by screening the remaining letters on the line with white card, by using a Maddox chart which has only one letter on each line, or by using the Sheridan–Gardiner test, a Cube E or Ffooks's symbols (*see* pages 32–33).

The term 'angular acuity' has been used to denote acuity determined by single letters, particularly of the E or Landolt-ring variety, in which only resolution of the critical feature is required. In contrast with this, the term 'morphoscopic', implying recognition of form, has been applied to acuity measured by recognition of letters on a normal chart or rarely, of single unknown letters or symbols.

It is found in practice that when acuity is better for letters or symbols viewed singly, the kind used is immaterial. The authors therefore consider the term 'isolated symbol' or 'monotype' acuity, which also carries its own meaning to be preferable to 'angular acuity'. Indeed, all acuities are based on angular subtenses. The term 'morphoscopic acuity' is better expressed as 'chart acuity' or 'line acuity'.

The crowding phenomenon may arise because the eye is not fixating centrally with the fovea, but is using a region just to one side of it. The reduced acuity is governed by the amount of eccentricity as shown in *Figure 3.18*. The precise position in space corresponding to the true foveal centre may often be determined by utilizing Haidinger's brushes, an entoptic phenomenon described in Chapter 22. Alternatively, the patient may be asked to fixate the centre of the smallest field of the ophthalmoscope. The practitioner can then observe the position of the foveal reflex relative to the illuminated area. More accurate results are obtained if an instrument is used to project a graticule image on to the patient's retina.

Regan *et al.* (1992) have challenged this concept, suggesting that the amblyope's poor chart acuity results from defective control of gaze, or an inability to select the intended direction of gaze. Their evidence came from measuring acuities on a chart where the single test letter was repeated in a regular array in the centre of the chart, the array being surrounded by other letters. In many cases, the amblyopes showed repeat letter acuity similar to or even better than their chart acuity, a result opposite to that predicted by the crowding phenomenon. Subjects with nystagmus, a condition usually giving horizontal oscillations of the direction of gaze, were shown by Simmers *et al.* (1996) to perform better on this test than on Glasgow Acuity Cards logMAR crowded test, confirming Regan's original idea.

Amblyopia is discussed further by Mallett (1969), Schapero (1971), Amos (1977, 1978), Mallett (1988), Nelson (1988), Jennings (1993), Grounds (1996) and in texts on orthoptics.

Poor acuity

Much of the discussion in this chapter on factors affecting visual acuity has assumed a healthy eye. The visual acuity may decline with increased years due to various ageing changes and/or pathological conditions. The causes may lie in the visual pathways or brain; in the retina, especially in the form of macular degeneration; or in cloudy media, most commonly in the crystalline lens. Lens opacities reduce the contrast of the retinal image by increasing the amount of diffusely scattered light within the eye.

A simple test to demonstrate the fall in acuity with scattered light is to introduce a glare source, for example, an Anglepoise light shone into the eye from near the visual axis while the patient is trying to read the test chart. Holladay (1986) introduced a Brightness Acuity Meter for this purpose. It consists of a brightly illuminated hemispherical cup, held over the eye, with a 12 mm aperture through which the patient views the chart. This device not only produces scattered light, but also induces pupil miosis, thus often restricting the light entering the eye to the densest part of a cataract. Although no longer manufactured, the instrument was claimed to demonstrate the handicap suffered out of doors by a patient with cataract. The Tearscope, an instrument intended for viewing the quality of the tear film, may serve the same purpose.

Poor contrast in the object is a hindrance in many such cases. When a low-contrast test chart is used, the authors have found that patients with unclear media show a significant deterioration in acuity. Thus, although the acuity may seem satisfactory when measured with a normal high-contrast test chart, the lower luminance contrast of a newspaper and even poorer contrast of many other objects in daily life may cause much difficulty. Low-contrast charts are described on pages 53–54.

It has been reported by Arden (1978) and others that

in certain pathological conditions the contrast sensitivity of the eye is measurably reduced, even though in some cases the Snellen acuity remains normal. This topic, together with associated clinical tests, is further discussed on pages 51 *et seq.*

Prince (1958, 1959), amongst many other researchers, investigated different styles of print for the patient with poor vision. He recommended a non-serif typeface with slightly increased spacing between the individual letters of each word. In Britain, the first large-scale venture in books designed specially for poor acuity was launched by F. A. Thorpe (Publishing) Ltd of Glenfield, Leicester. Their extensive series of 'Ulverscroft Large Print Books' are printed in 18-point type with specially black ink to ensure good contrast even under magnification. In the USA, a catalogue entitled 'Large Type Books in Print' has been compiled by the R. R. Bowker Company, of 1180 Avenue of the Americas, New York, New York 10036.

Magnification in near vision may be obtained by reading at a closer than normal distance, or by using handheld or stand magnifiers, spectacle magnifiers or telescopic spectacles. The latter may also be designed for distance vision. The optical principles of such devices are discussed in Chapter 13.

For near vision, specially designed lenses with magnifications up to 8× are readily obtainable, as are compound systems magnifying up to 20×. A more sophisticated technique uses close-up photography of the reading material with closed-circuit television. The screen contrast can readily be increased and may even be reversed to give white print on a dark background. This is preferred by a high proportion of patients, especially those with opacities in the media, since there is less light from the screen to be scattered in the eye (Lowe, 1977; Silver and Fass, 1977). Practical aspects of helping the patient with poor visual acuity are discussed on pages 252–254.

Retinal function in cataract

It might seem that a patient with moderate or severe cloudiness of the crystalline lens (cataract) would best be served by an operation to remove the lens, despite the resulting aphakia. The simultaneous presence of degenerative retinal changes would make the operation much less worth while, but the cataract may prevent a satisfactory view of the retina. The electroretinogram discussed previously on page 39 provides a crude measure of the cone and hence the macular response in the eye.

A more recent technique is to produce Young's interference fringes on the retina by imaging two tiny coherent sources within the pupil, the fringe spacing being inversely proportional to the source separation. Provided that the beams can pass through relatively clear areas in the media, high-contrast interference fringes will be formed on the retina. Lotmar (1980) points out that the contrast is not dependent on the intensity of the coherent beams but on their wave amplitude, which is the square root of the intensity. Consequently, a reduction of the intensity of one beam to 1% (0.01) reduces the amplitude to only 10% (0.1), giving a fringe

contrast of 20% of the original. If the patient can distinguish the fringes and their orientation, the retinal resolution can be determined and expressed in terms of an equivalent visual acuity. Should this be good, there is thought to be a favourable prognosis for vision following lens extraction (Rassow and Rätzke, 1978). Halliday and Ross (1983) found, however, that only 45% of their patients saw as predicted after operation. Those with dense cataracts tended to do better, while others with macular changes or possibly with previous amblyopia did worse. The suggestion was made that paramacular acuity falls off with eccentricity more rapidly for Snellen letters than for fine gratings, which thus give a more optimistic prediction.

Most instruments of this type use lasers and some form of beam-splitter, as described, among others, by Rassow and Rätzke (1978) and Smith *et al.* (1979). Lotmar, however, describes an instrument with a tungsten light source and moiré fringes, though he shows that under conditions of Maxwellian view this is equivalent to an interference system. The fringes are achromatic and the double images of the source in the pupil are each 0.2 mm in diameter. Thorn and Schwartz (1990) showed that grating test objects remained much more visible in the presence of blur than letter charts, and explained this by the possibility of spurious resolution (*see* pages 50–51). They consequently questioned whether it was sensible to use gratings for predicting postoperative chart acuity. Thibos *et al.* (1991) point out that the lateral chromatic aberration of the eye will blur white light fringes if they are orientated perpendicular to the displacement of the beam paths in the patient's pupil. They predict a threefold loss in the acuity measurement if the beam is displaced $3\frac{1}{2}$–4 mm from the pupil centre. This may also affect the results from the next two techniques.

An alternative approach, devised by Guyton (Boyd and Guyton, 1983) and termed the Potential Acuity Meter (PAM – no longer manufactured), projects a Snellen chart in Maxwellian view through the pupil. The aerial image of the pinhole aperture in the pupil is 0.1 mm. Thus, most of the light reaching the retina can be directed through a relatively clear area of a cataractous lens. Hence, a normal acuity task is presented to the patient instead of the recognition of gratings, which may give an optimistic result as already described or possibly underestimate the acuity through unfamiliarity. Surveys were conducted by Fish *et al.* (1986) on patients with macular degeneration but clear media. Their results showed that the PAM results correlated better with Snellen acuities than those obtained with laser interferometry, suggesting a better prediction in cataract patients. In order to find a reasonably clear part of the lens, the pupil should be dilated. An allowance may be necessary for the Campbell effect, whereby the visual acuity is less for light entering the eye through a peripheral part of the pupil than through the centre. In practice, diffraction at the slide of the Snellen chart means that light will enter the eye around the imaged pinhole, exactly as in the Abbe theory of the microscope, where light enters the objective at angles outside that of the illuminating beam. It is left to the reader to calculate the theoretical limit of resolution if the real pupil diameter were 0.1 mm.

The standard pinhole disc (page 94) provides a simpler and much cheaper approach. While the patient views the letter chart, he/she is encouraged to move the head slightly, in order to try to align the pinhole with a clear zone in the lens, in which case a significant improvement may occur. If the cataract is uniform in haze, then no clear zone can be found through which to view, so only a small improvement in acuity from the reduction in scattered light may result. An objective test is to project an acuity grating on to the retina using a direct ophthalmoscope* (*see* Chapter 16). Allowance for the double passage of light through the media having been made in the calibration of the grating, the smallest size of detail that can be resolved by the observer should correspond to the patient's present visual acuity if the retina is functioning normally – Brown *et al.* (1987a). With experience, the clarity of view with the small stop of the ophthalmoscope also gives a similar indication.

The hyperacuity tests (*see* page 26) have also been used in laboratory investigations (for example, Enoch *et al.*, 1985; Hurst *et al.*, 1995), but have not yet found clinical acceptance.

Reviews of methods for verifying retinal function in the presence of cataract are given by Charman (1987), Whitaker and Buckingham (1987), Hurst and Douthwaite (1993), Hurst *et al.* (1993) and McGraw *et al.* (1996). Recent papers questioning the ability of such tests to predict the postoperative acuity from the preoperative value include Barrett *et al.* (1994, 1995) and Bueno and Hurst (1995). To a certain extent, the present author feels that, since surgery for cataract is now undertaken at a much earlier stage when both the patient's visual acuity is not severely impaired (around 6/12) and the retina can be inspected visually (*see* Chapter 16), there may not be such a need for these tests, though the presence of minor changes in the macular region can still lead to uncertainty.

Blindness and partial sight

The British statutory definition for the purpose of registration as a blind person under the National Assistance Act 1948 is that the person is 'so blind as to be unable to perform any work for which eyesight is essential'.

As a working basis, people have been considered legally blind if:

(1) the binocular acuity is poorer than 3/60, or
(2) the binocular acuity is between 3/60 and 6/60 and there is also considerable contraction of the visual field, or
(3) there are gross field defects, even if the acuity is better than 6/60.

In England and Wales, about 0.2% of the population are on the Blind Register, but it is estimated that two to three times as many are eligible for registration. About 15% of those registering have no perception of light or perception of light only; the acuity of about 55% varies from hand movements to 3/60 (20/400), while 30% have an acuity better than 3/60. Blindness is a problem of age in that only 15% of those registered are younger than 50, whereas 25% are between 50 and 69 and 60% are 70 or over. Unfortunately, the younger person has much longer to live with his or her disability. New registrations show an even greater proportion in the 70-plus age group.

Patients whose near acuity is N12 or lower and wish to become members of the Talking Book Service of the Royal National Institute for the Blind can have their application form signed by an optometrist. They may have to pay the annual subscription themselves.

In the UK, registered blind people are eligible for various concessions including an increased tax allowance and, if necessary, higher rates of supplementary benefit. Braille and Moon embossed-type books and tape-recorded books are available on loan, while local authorities can provide welfare services.

In one of a series of official reports on blindness (Department of Health and Social Security, 1979), the incidence, degree and causes of blindness in England were shown to be broadly similar in the two sexes. Among children, the major causes are congenital anomalies, optic nerve atrophy and cataract. The last two conditions, together with choroidal atrophy, glaucoma, diabetes, retinitis pigmentosa and other retinal conditions, are the main causes of blindness in adults.

A further report by the Department was published in 1988, presenting statistics for 1976/77 and 1980/81. Though there has been little change in the annual number of new registrations, the increasing life span is reflected in the fact that the age group 75 and over constitutes a growing percentage of the total of the registered blind. In the four years separating the two periods studied, the percentage rose from 54.1 to 58.6. In this most elderly group, retinal degenerative conditions are the largest single cause of blindness.

Among adults up to 64 years old, diabetic retinopathy is the largest single cause. A point of particular interest is the marked increase in the proportion of women to men who become blind for this reason within the age group 55–64.

A more detailed study of this report has been made by Giltrow-Tyler (1988).

In the USA, a typical definition of blindness is that 'a person shall be considered blind who has a visual acuity of 20/200 or less in the better eye with proper correction, or limitation in the field of vision such that the widest diameter of the visual field subtends an angular distance no greater than 20°'. This definition may vary in different States. According to the amended AMA visual efficiency ratings published in 1955, a person would be considered blind if his binocular visual efficiency was below 10%.

Statistics and clinical data on blindness in the USA are compiled by a Model Reporting Area on Blindness Statistics. This is a voluntary association of States having uniform definitions and procedures for that purpose.

---

* The Acuity Scope, available from Keeler Ltd, Clewer Hill Road, Windsor, Berks SL4 4AA.

Publication of reports is undertaken by the US Department of Health, Education and Welfare.

There is no British legal definition of partial sight, but registration is normally open to those whose visual acuity is:

(1) from 3/60 to 6/60 with full visual field,
(2) up to 6/24 with moderate contraction of the field, opacities in the media or aphakia,
(3) 6/18 or better if there is a gross field defect.

Children with acuities between 3/60 and 6/24 may be taught in special schools for the partially sighted, but a child with acuity better than 6/24 will usually be taught in a normal school.

In England, about 0.1% of the population are registered as partially sighted, but the number eligible for registration is thought to be considerably more than this. The main reason is that registration carries no entitlement to the tax and certain other of the concessions available to the blind. The age distribution of the registered partially sighted in England is similar to that of the registered blind. New registrations account for about one-fifth of the total annually.

Modulation transfer function and the eye

The sinusoidal grating

Conventional clinical assessments of visual acuity are related to the eye's resolving power. Another method of

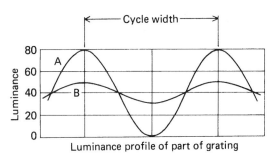

Figure 3.24.   Sinusoidal grating: luminance profile. Curve A has greater modulation than curve B.

assessment is based on the eye's sensitivity to luminance contrast. Although 'square wave' or Foucault gratings could be used for this purpose, sinusoidal gratings (*Figure 3.23*) are preferred. The name arises from the fact that a continuous plot of the luminance along a perpendicular to the bars would represent the function

$$y = a \sin (bx) + c$$

An important advantage of this type of grating is that even when defocused or affected by aberrations, its image generally retains the sinusoidal luminance pattern.

Basic definitions may be understood by reference to *Figure 3.24* which shows the luminance curves of two sinusoidal gratings having the same mean luminance and cycle width.

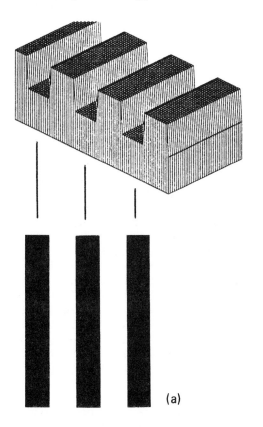

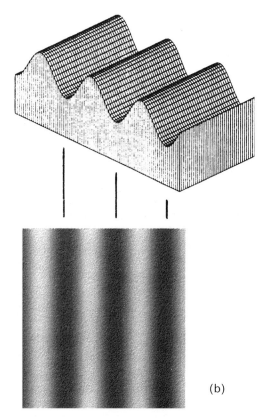

Figure 3.23.   (a) A square-wave or Foucault grating. (b) A sinusoidal grating of the same frequency. The upper drawings show corresponding three-dimensional representations of the spatial luminance profile (material for this illustration kindly provided by Professor J. Barbur).

Table 3.4 Values for luminance curves A and B in *Figure 3.24*

Curve	L_{min}	L_{max}	Mean luminance	Modulation
A	0	80	40	1
B	30	50	40	0.25

If L_{min} is the minimum and L_{max} the maximum luminance, then

$$\text{Modulation} = \frac{L_{max} - L_{min}}{L_{max} + L_{min}} \qquad (3.16)$$

Table 3.4 gives the values of L_{max}, L_{min} and the modulation for the two curves illustrated in *Figure 3.24*.

The modulation can be regarded as the maximum change in luminance from its mean value, expressed as a ratio of this value. When the minimum luminance is zero, as in curve A, the modulation is equal to unity.

In the literature of contrast sensitivity, the term 'contrast' has come into general use to denote a numerical value of modulation as defined by equation (3.16). This is sometimes termed Michaelson contrast, and is usually expressed as a percentage. For purposes of comparison, this same definition of contrast is sometimes applied to test charts of both high and low contrast. In other contexts including standardization, the contrast of a test chart is defined differently as noted earlier (*see* page 34 and Exercise 3.16 which derives relationships between the two expressions). Occasionally, contrast sensitivity is expressed in decibels – Verbaken (1987) recommends that for this purpose the dB scale should be equated to $10 \times \log$ Contrast Sensitivity.

The cycle width of a sinusoidal grating corresponds to the 'grating interval' of a square grating, but is usually expressed as a spatial frequency. Thus, if the cycle width subtends an angle of $\theta°$ at the observer's eye,

Spatial frequency $v = 1/\theta$ cycles/degree

For example, 60 cycles/degree corresponds to a cycle width subtending 1 minute of arc. Gratings used as test objects do not necessarily have a uniform spatial frequency. For some purposes it may vary in a definable manner, such as logarithmically.

If a sinusoidal grating is presented to the eye, its threshold of recognition as a grating is affected both by its spatial frequency and its luminance contrast.[*] As the contrast is reduced, recognition becomes harder as with other test objects. Moreover, with high spatial frequencies the loss of contrast in the retinal image is greater than with low frequencies, again making recognition more difficult.

In numerical terms, contrast sensitivity at a given spatial frequency is the reciprocal of the threshold value of the modulation as defined by equation (3.16). It is a measure of the eye's ability to detect small differences in luminance.

For example, if a grating can just be resolved when the modulation has been reduced to 0.08, the contrast sensitivity is 12.5. If the threshold modulation had

been at the lower figure of 0.02, the contrast sensitivity would have risen to 50. This higher value indicates a superior performance.

The modulation transfer function

When a sinusoidal grating is imaged by an optical system, the contrast of the image is reduced by the effects of aberrations and diffraction. Nevertheless, it retains the sinusoidal luminance pattern, though with a lowered modulation. In general, the ratio of the modulation of the image of a grating of given spatial frequency to that of the object is called the modulation transfer factor. A plot of this transfer factor against spatial frequency depicts the modulation transfer function (MTF). It provides a good indication of the performance of the image-forming system at varying frequencies, not just the finest.

Modulation transfer functions for the optical system of the human eye were obtained from a two-stage experimental process by Campbell and Green (1965a). In brief, their method was to form sinusoidal interference fringes on the retina by an adaptation of Young's double-slit system (*see also* page 44). In this arrangement, the angular separation θ between successive bright fringes is given by

$$\theta \, (\text{rad}) = (\lambda/a) \times 10^{-6} \qquad (3.17)$$

where λ is the wavelength (in nm) of the monochromatic light source used (632.8 nm in this experiment) and a (in mm) the separation of the slits. To vary the contrast of the interference pattern, the source producing it was dimmed. At the same time, the mean retinal illuminance was kept constant by the addition of a uniform field of light of the same wavelength. Since the interference fringes are not affected by the eye's optics, measurement of the threshold modulation as a function of spatial frequency gives the contrast sensitivity of the retina and neural system alone.

To provide a comparable test object viewed directly by the entire visual system, including the degrading effects of the ocular dioptrics, a sinusoidal grating was generated by means of an oscilloscope with a spectral luminance peak at 530 nm. The performance of the eye was considered not to vary significantly between wavelengths of 530 and 632.8 nm if the luminance were the same. The contrast sensitivity was determined over the same range of variables as before. For the same observer with a 2 mm pupil, the results are shown by the lower curve in *Figure 3.25*. Since the actual contrast in the retinal image at the threshold of recognition can be assumed to be the same in both cases, the reduced contrast sensitivity for the grating imaged by the eye can only be due to the defects and limitations of the eye's optical system with a pupil diameter of 2 mm. The oscilloscope observations can be repeated with other pupil diameters.

For a spatial frequency of 1 cycle/degree, a sinusoidal grating viewed at 40 cm would need to have a cycle width of 7.0 mm. As suggested by *Figures 3.25* and *3.26* and confirmed by other results, the spatial frequency for which the contrast sensitivity is greatest is

---

[*] In this context, the term 'luminance contrast' has come to be used as a synonym for modulation in its quantitative sense.

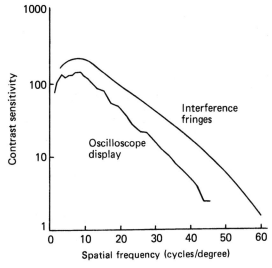

Figure 3.25. Contrast sensitivity of the human eye. Upper curve: measurements obtained from interference fringes, assessing retinal/neural function; lower curve: measurements obtained from an oscilloscope display, assessing optical as well as retinal/neural factors. (Redrawn from Campbell and Green, 1965a, by kind permission of the publishers of *J. Physiol.*)

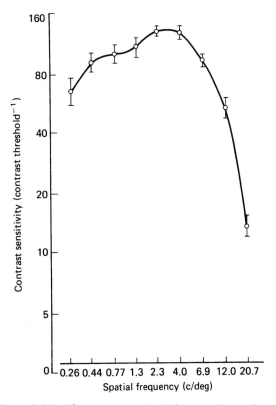

Figure 3.26. The contrast sensitivity function (mean of measurements on ten normal subjects aged between 18 and 27 years). The bar lines represent ±1 standard error. Note that both scales are logarithmic. (Reproduced from Wright and Drasdo, 1985, by kind permission of the publishers of *Documenta Ophthalmologica* and reprinted by permission of Kluwer Academic Publishers.)

about 3 cycles/degree for a typical observer. A limiting frequency of 30 cycles/degree, corresponding to a cycle width of 2 minutes, would conventionally be equated to an acuity of 6/6 (20/20), at least for a square-wave grating.

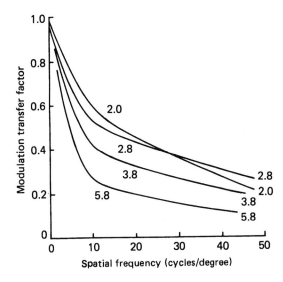

Figure 3.27. Modulation transfer function for a human eye at various pupil diameters. (Reproduced from Campbell and Green, 1965a, by kind permission of the publishers of *J. Physiol.*)

A modulation transfer function can be plotted from the data of *Figure 3.25*. Because contrast sensitivity is the reciprocal of modulation, it follows that the modulation transfer factor is the inverse ratio of the sensitivity for the interference fringes to that for the oscilloscope display. For example, at a spatial frequency of 10 cycles/degree the two values are approximately 206 and 128, giving a transfer factor of 128/206 or 0.62. At 40 cycles/degree the values are approximately 17.5 and 4.9, the transfer factor being 0.28.

The complete graph of the modulation transfer function for this pupil diameter is shown in *Figure 3.27*, together with the curves for pupil diameters of 2.8, 3.8 and 5.8 mm, all for the same subject. It can be seen that the curves for 2 and 2.8 mm pupils are not only very close together, but actually cross over at about 27 cycles/degree. On this evidence, the eye's performance changes little within this range of pupil diameters – a result confirmed by the lightly curved top of the acuity/pupil diameter graph of *Figure 3.6*.

Campbell and Green (1965b) showed that the contrast sensitivity measured binocularly was approximately 40% better than that found under monocular conditions over a wide range of frequencies. They attributed this to the summation of signals from the two eyes.

Normalized spatial frequency

If an eye of pupil diameter g had a perfect optical system limited only by diffraction, the minimum angle of resolution $\theta_{\min}$ for two point sources would be

$$\theta_{\min} \text{ (rad)} = 1.22\lambda/g \tag{3.2}$$

For a sinusoidal grating, with $\theta_{\min}$ the smallest angular cycle width which can be resolved, the corresponding relationship is

$$\theta_{\min} = \lambda/g \text{ (rad)}$$
$$= 57.3\lambda/g \text{ (degrees)} \tag{3.18}$$

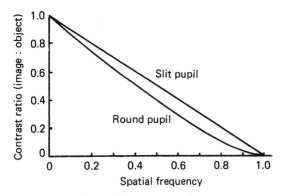

Figure 3.28. The modulation transfer function for a diffraction-limited eye or system with a slit and a round pupil. (Reproduced from Westheimer, 1972a, by kind permission of the publishers, Springer, Berlin and New York.)

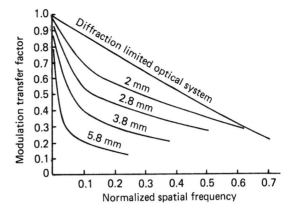

Figure 3.29. The modulation transfer function of a human eye plotted for a normalized spatial frequency. (Reproduced from Campbell and Green, 1965a, by kind permission of the publishers of *J. Physiol.*)

The maximum spatial frequency (ν_{max}) which can be discerned – the 'cut-off point' – is thus

$$\nu_{max} = 1/\theta_{min} = g/57.3\lambda \text{ (cycles/degree)} \qquad (3.19)$$

For example, given $g = 3$ mm and $\lambda = 560$ nm

$$\nu_{max} = 3 \times 10^{-3}/(57.3 \times 560 \times 10^{-9})$$

$$= 93.5 \text{ cycles/degree}$$

To facilitate comparison between the MTF of an actual eye and that of a diffraction-limited eye, the concept of normalized spatial frequency is used. Irrespective of pupil diameter and wavelength, the cut-off frequency ν_{max} for the diffraction limited eye is fixed at unity. On this normalized scale, any actual value of ν is replaced by the normalized value ν_n such that

$$\nu_n = \nu/\nu_{max}$$

From equation (3.19) it follows that

$$\nu_n = (57.3\lambda/g)\,\nu \qquad (3.20)$$

with ν_n and ν both in cycles/degree.

In this way a single MTF curve can be used to represent any diffraction-limited optical system, irrespective of particular values of g and λ.

The complete MTF for a diffraction-limited eye or optical system can be calculated by standard mathematical procedures (Westheimer, 1972a). If the pupil were rectangular in shape, with its narrower width g perpendicular to the grating bars, the MTF graph would be a straight line as shown in *Figure 3.28*. For a circular pupil, the graph assumes the shape indicated in the diagram. The cut-off point is the same for both.

In *Figure 3.29*, the MTF curves of *Figure 3.27* are shown re-plotted on a normalized frequency scale. This process could have been carried out by using equation (3.20). For example, the end-point of the graph for 5.8 mm pupil size in *Figure 3.27* occurs at an actual frequency of about 45 cycles/degree, the wavelength being 530 nm. Accordingly,

$$\nu_n = \frac{57.3 \times 530 \times 10^{-9}}{5.8 \times 10^{-3}} \times 45 = 0.24$$

which agrees with *Figure 3.29*. If continued, the graph representing the diffraction-limited system would meet the *x*-axis at the cut-off point where $\nu_n = 1$.

The curves in *Figure 3.29* for various pupil diameters of the same eye should not be compared with each other, but only with the theoretical comparison curve. The diffraction-limited eye performs better as its pupil diameter increases and so becomes a harder standard of comparison.

The double-pass technique

The double-pass technique requires only one set of experimental results from which to compute the MTF of an eye. It has been used in many investigations. In the arrangement described by Campbell and Gubisch (1966), the image of a narrow illuminated slit is formed on the fundus. Acting as a diffusing surface, the fundus reflects a portion of the incident light back through the pupil. It then passes through a beam-splitter and a converging lens which forms an aerial image of the fundus streak. This can be examined either photographically or photoelectrically, allowance being made for the effects of the reverse passage through the optical media. Analysis of the light distribution in the streak image enables the line-spread function of the eye's optical system to be determined. Its graph resembles a Gaussian normal distribution curve. By a mathematical process known as Fourier analysis, the modulation transfer function can be computed from the line-spread function. In this context, Fourier's more general theorem shows that the light distribution across a narrow slit or its image can be resolved into an infinite series of sine waves of increasing frequency.

The conventional index of the narrowness of a Gaussian-type curve is its 'half-width' – the width at half the peak value. Graphs of the image line-spread for one of Campbell and Gubisch's subjects showed the half-width to decrease with pupil size: from 6.2 minutes of arc at 6.6 mm pupil diameter to 2.2 minutes at 2.4 mm pupil diameter. For smaller pupil sizes, the half-width increased, reaching 3.2 minutes with a 1.0 mm pupil. Over this range, the reduction in the eye's aberrations becomes increasingly outweighed by the effects of diffraction.

The MTF graphs obtained by Campbell and Gubisch

Table 3.5 Frequency and amplitude of odd-numbered harmonics

Harmonic	Frequency	Amplitude
First	v	$4a/\pi$
Third	$3v$	$4a/3\pi$
Fifth	$5v$	$4a/5\pi$
.	.	.
.	.	.
.	.	.

for their three subjects are broadly similar to the results of Campbell and Green (1965a). For two of their subjects the curves for 2.0 and 3.0 mm pupils cross over as in *Figure 3.27*.

Square-wave (Foucault) gratings

Unlike sinusoidal ones, square-wave gratings are easily produced without special equipment, making them useful experimentally. According to Fourier analysis, a square wave of frequency v and amplitude a, denoting $\frac{1}{2}(L_{max} - L_{min})$ is equivalent to a sine wave of the same frequency v but of amplitude $4a/\pi$ plus a series of sine waves of increasing frequency and decreasing amplitude. Each wave, including the first, is called a harmonic. The nth harmonic has the frequency nv and amplitude $4a/\pi n$, but in this series only the odd-numbered values of n are included, as shown in *Table 3.5*.

The bold lines in *Figure 3.30* show one half of a square wave of amplitude a and the corresponding half of the first harmonic of the equivalent sine-wave series. The lower part of the diagram shows the third and fifth harmonics. Curves representing the sum of the first and third, and the sum of the first, third and fifth harmonics are also displayed. It can be seen that even though these curves still oscillate, they steadily approach the outline of the square wave.

If the third and subsequent harmonics are ignored, a square-wave grating can be regarded as a sinusoidal grating of the same spatial frequency but of $\pi/4$ times the amplitude. It then follows that the contrast sensitivity thresholds for square-wave and sinusoidal gratings of the same frequency and amplitude should in theory be in the ratio of $4/\pi$.

Since the frequencies of the subsequent harmonics are multiples of the basic frequency (of the first harmonic), they could all be situated beyond the cut-off point. For this reason alone it is evident that they can become significant only when the basic frequency lies within a restricted range. The limits of this range were explored by Campbell and Robson (1968) by determining the contrast sensitivity thresholds for square and sinusoidal gratings of the same frequency and amplitude. The expected ratio of $4/\pi$ was found to hold good for gratings of spatial frequency exceeding 0.8 cycles/degree. At lower frequencies, the ratio increased rapidly, probably due to selective response by individual neural elements in the visual system to particular frequencies.

Effects of defocus and spurious resolution

All the MTF results described above have assumed the eye to be in focus for the grating. When it is out of focus, the theory of both geometrical and physical optics predicts that modulation transfer suffers appreciably, even for very small errors. This is shown in *Figure 3.31* (Charman and Jennings, 1976), which refers to the theoretical diffraction-limited eye with a 5 mm pupil. Even with an error as small as 0.12 D, the modulation falls much more rapidly with increasing spatial frequency than in the perfect eye. As the image modulation in the defocused eye drops to zero, it falls below the threshold for detection. The grating can no longer be resolved but assumes a uniform grey appearance.

At spatial frequencies greater than this threshold value, a phenomenon known as spurious resolution may occur. A simple explanation in general terms can

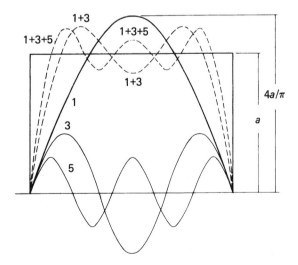

Figure 3.30. Partial generation of a square wave by compounding sine waves of frequencies of the first, third and fifth harmonics.

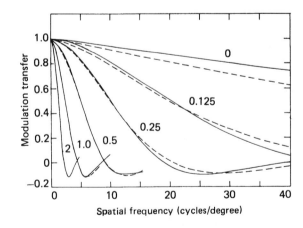

Figure 3.31. Variation in the modulation transfer function with defocus for an aberration-free eye with a 5 mm diameter entrance pupil, according to physical optics. The solid curves show the MTFs at 450 nm, the broken curves the MTFs at 650 nm, for both positive and negative errors of focus of the amounts indicated in dioptres. There is very little difference between the MTFs at the two wavelengths when the errors of focus are large. (Reproduced from Charman and Jennings, 1976, by kind permission of the publishers of *Br. J. Physiol. Optics.*)

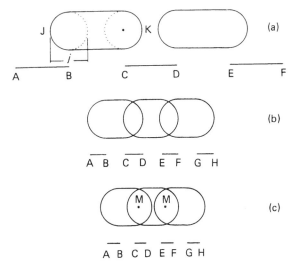

Figure 3.32. Spurious resolution: an explanation based on geometrical optics.

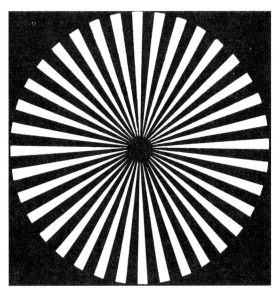

Figure 3.33. Radial square-wave grating to demonstrate unresolved annuli and zones of spurious resolution when held close to the eye and viewed out of focus.

be given with reference to a Foucault grating of relatively low spatial frequency. The effects of diffraction can then be ignored, being negligible in relation to those of geometrical out-of-focus blurring.

In *Figure 3.32*, the lines AB, CD, etc. represent the dark bars of a Foucault grating, equal in width to the white bars. If BC is taken to be a luminous line, the cross-section of a white bar, its blurred image consists of a succession of overlapping blur circles of diameter *j* and its overall length JK is equal to (BC + *j*). When the bar width is greater than *j*, as in *Figure 3.32(a)*, the blurred images of the white bars are well separated and in register with the actual white bars.

An essential part of this explanation is that the luminance of the blurred image of any white bar such as BC is not uniform along its centre line JK but tapers off identically at each end.

As the bar width decreases with *j* remaining constant, the successive blurred images begin to overlap as in *Figure 3.32(b)*. For one particular bar width, the overlap of the two end portions of diminishing relative luminance is such that their combined luminance visually matches that of the surrounding areas. This condition occurs when the bar width is approximately equal to *j*/2.

At first sight this would appear to indicate the cut-off spatial frequency of the grating for the given degree of blurring. If, however, the bar width is further decreased beyond this point, as in *Figure 3.32(c)*, the areas of overlap become larger. The sum of the two separate luminances then reaches a peak at the midpoint M of the overlap area, higher than that in the area surrounding the overlap. A periodic pattern thus re-emerges visually, giving rise to 'spurious resolution'. However, since the luminous peaks at M are situated at the centre of the black bars of the grating, a black/white reversal has occurred.

As the bar width continues to be reduced, a second point is reached where the luminance across the grating is apparently uniform. This occurs when the bar width is approximately *j*/4. Spurious resolution also recurs as

the bar width continues to decrease and further similar sequences are possible, though not necessarily discernible .

These appearances can best be observed in a radial grating, such as *Figure 3.33*, which gives increasing spatial frequency towards its centre. Grey annuli separating zones of successive contrast reversal or discontinuity can be seen if the grating is held close to the eye with the accommodation relaxed.

In *Figure 3.31*, contrast reversal of spurious resolution occurs when the modulation transfer factor assumes a negative value. These graphs, calculated on the basis of physical optics, give a more reliable picture than computations based on geometrical optics. Nevertheless, as shown by Charman and Jennings, the differences are negligible when the defocus error exceeds 0.50 D.

A detailed theoretical analysis of spurious resolution has been given by Smith (1982a). One of his conclusions is that spurious resolution is unlikely to be visible when the spatial frequency exceeds about 35 cycles/degree.

Contrast sensitivity

Clinical considerations

Contrast sensitivity testing is normally undertaken at photopic luminances. The results of Van Nes and Bouman (1967), *Figure 3.34*, show a steady decline in the contrast sensitivity of the eye with decreasing luminance, together with a shift in the peak response towards lower frequencies. Similar results have been found by Sloane *et al.* (1988).

Figure 3.31 predicts that high-frequency gratings must be focused accurately before they can be resolved, whereas coarse gratings allow a much greater tolerance to defocus. For example, with a grating of spatial fre-

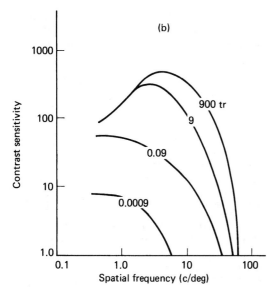

Figure 3.34. Typical changes in contrast sensitivity function with retinal illuminance. The curves are marked with the corresponding retinal illuminance in trolands. In the original study, the gratings were illuminated with green light (525 nm) and viewed through a 2 mm artificial pupil. (The original data are from Van Nes and Bouman, 1967, as replotted by Tucker and Charman, 1986). (Reproduced by kind permission of the publishers of *Am. J. Optom.*)

quency 2 cycles/degree, the modulation transfer would be reduced to about 0.1 by a focusing error of 2.0 D, whereas with a frequency of 8 cycles/degree the same reduction to 0.1 would result from a focusing error of only 0.5 D.

The contrast sensitivity function (CSF) of the eye is represented by a graph in which contrast sensitivity – the reciprocal of the grating modulation at threshold – is plotted against spatial frequency. Charman (1979) has investigated this function experimentally for various levels of defocus and pupil diameters. His results confirm the greater tolerance of low spatial frequencies to focusing errors. In fact, with normal pupil sizes, extremely accurate focusing was required when the spatial frequency exceeded about 10 cycles/degree. However, by using an artificial pupil of 1mm diameter it should be possible to make reliable measurements for frequencies up to about 25 cycles/degree, given adequate illumination.

Whereas clinical tests for contrast sensitivity examine the performance of the eye at the lower end of the spatial frequency spectrum at low contrasts, conventional test charts for visual acuity examine it at the high frequency end and at high contrast. Indeed, the intercept of the contrast sensitivity curve in *Figure 3.26* with the spatial frequency axis should indicate the visual acuity at 100% contrast. Investigation suggests that the visual system has separate channels devoted to interpreting specific data, for example, from ranges of different frequencies and orientations. The curve in *Figure 3.26* could possibly be regarded as the envelope of certain of these channels. It is also to be noted that the coarser frequencies require functional integration over a much larger retinal area than the fovea. For these reasons, reduced contrast sensitivity at low frequencies can still be

accompanied by a normal Snellen acuity – hence measurement of low-frequency contrast sensitivity may give additional information on a patient's ocular condition. A review of the role of contrast sensitivity measurements is given by Woods and Wood (1995).

In normal observers, optically corrected if necessary for the distance of the grating, the difference in contrast sensitivity between the two eyes is usually less than 25%. The variation between individuals, however, can be much greater (Weatherill and Yap, 1986). As shown by several studies, age is an important factor (Owsley *et al.*, 1983; Ross *et al.*, 1985; Wright and Drasdo, 1985; Elliott, 1987; and others). Contrast sensitivity declines with increasing age, particularly in the higher frequencies in the range investigated, 0.5–19 cycles/degree. Both Owsley and colleagues and Wright and Drasdo concluded that the main causes were the reduction in pupil diameter and increasing absorption by the ocular media with advancing age, thus reducing the retinal illumination. Owsley and colleagues found that the fall in contrast sensitivity in the 60 year old could be partly reproduced in a younger patient viewing through a neutral filter of 0.5 density,[*] which transmits about one-third of the incident light. They also found that the peak of the contrast sensitivity curve shifted from 4 to 2 cycles/degree. Elliott, however, who used interference fringes to measure the function, concluded that decline in neural capability was the principal factor. A similar conclusion was reached by Sloane *et al.* (1988) who considered that increased light scatter and absorption by the ageing crystalline lens were important subsidiary factors.

Contrast sensitivity is also impaired by pathological conditions and ocular abnormalities. While its loss from such causes has been well documented, no typical pattern has yet been found in amblyopia. Some amblyopes show a loss only at high frequencies, others over the whole range. This topic will be further discussed on page 55.

Clinical tests

For experimental purposes, the contrast sensitivity of the eye is usually determined by generating a sinusoidal pattern electronically on a TV-type monitor. Simpler techniques are required for clinical purposes. Those known to the authors will now be briefly described.

Arden Test Gratings†

The Arden test comprises a set of seven printed plates covering frequencies from 0.2 to 6.4 cycles/degree when viewed at the stipulated distance of 57 cm. On each plate the contrast increases from top to bottom, and the patient has to state when he first detects the pattern as the higher contrast part of the plate is gradually uncovered. The results are compared with the values

---

[*] Optical density is the logarithm to base 10 of the reciprocal of transmittance (expressed as a ratio, not a percentage).

† American Optical Co. Renamed AO Contrast Sensitivity Test Plates.

obtained for normal observers as listed in the instruction manual. In a clinical study of this test, Reeves *et al.* (1988) found that the significant variation in the results by different examiners was largely accounted for by differences in the technique employed. A similar tendency had been noted by Yap *et al.* (1985), who also suggested that because optometrists' patients, being mostly ametropic, are not typical population samples, it would be better for practitioners to compile their own norms for each age group, than to rely on those in the instruction manual. This advice applies generally to contrast sensitivity tests. Elliott and Whitaker (1992) give data for the Cambridge gratings and the Pelli–Robson chart, described below.

The Vistech system*

To utilize the more positive end-point of a forced-choice response, Ginsburg (1984, 1986) introduced his Vistech system. A single chart presents five rows of photographed gratings, each contained within a circle and with the lines randomly set from a choice of three orientations which the patient is required to identify. The nine gratings in each row decrease progressively in contrast by a factor of $1/\sqrt{2}$, while retaining the same spatial frequency. This increases from row to row, covering a range from 1.5 to 18 cycles/degree. Distance and near versions of the chart are available, to be used at 10 ft and 18 in, respectively. A suitable spectacle correction needs to be worn. As with the Arden test, the results can be compared with given norms.

Reeves and Hill (1987) and Reeves *et al.* (1991) have presented critical reviews of the test. In particular, they consider that the large range in contrast covered in only eight steps means that small changes in sensitivity cannot be identified.

Square-wave gratings

It was pointed out in an earlier section (*see* page 50) that for spatial frequencies greater than 0.8 cycles/degree, a square-wave grating should give results for contrast sensitivity consistently 1.27 times as high as those given by a sinusoidal grating of the same frequency and amplitude. Provided this is borne in mind, square-wave gratings offer an attractive alternative to sinusoidal ones, which are very difficult to produce.

The decrease in the modulation transfer function of the eye with increasing spatial frequency reduces the contrast in the image of a sine-wave grating but does not change its form. Drasdo and Cox (1987) have calculated the image contrast for square-wave gratings of different frequencies. Their results, illustrated in *Figure 3.35*, show an increasing departure from the square-wave form, together with decreasing amplitude, as the frequency increases.

In 1970, the present writer (AGB) was impressed by a

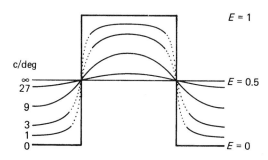

Figure 3.35. Cross-sectional profile of the retinal illuminance (E) of the image of a square-wave grating of 100% object contrast. Gratings of various frequencies have been superimposed by normalizing, i.e. adjusting the horizontal scale for each frequency so that one complete cycle is shown for all. (Reproduced, with new lettering, from Drasdo and Cox, 1987, by kind permission of the publishers of *Clin. Vision Sci.*)

test chart of square-wave gratings of varying frequency and contrast, shown to him by Dr J. K. Davis. Although not intended as a test of contrast sensitivity, it could be a useful point of departure for such a design. The chart was subsequently described and illustrated in a joint paper by Davis and Ward (1972).

Cambridge Low-contrast Gratings*

This test was designed by Dr A. J. Wilkins and Dr J. G. Robson and uses square-wave gratings in which the bars are of dot matrix construction. At the testing distance of 6 m, the appearance is that of a bar because the individual dots cannot be discerned. All the gratings have the same spatial frequency of 4 cycles/degree but with a different contrast in each of the ten plates in the set, varying from 5% to 0.14%.

The test is relatively inexpensive, simple and quickly conducted, and the plates can be placed in any orientation, thus allowing the accuracy of the results to be checked (Wilkins, 1986). Because most pathological conditions have been shown to cause losses in sensitivity at 4 cycles/degree, or also at this frequency even if others are more strongly affected, it is claimed that the test is effective in detecting such conditions.

A City University test

Photographically produced square-wave grating plates, each of a fixed contrast, are used in this uncomplicated apparatus designed at City University (London) and described by Barbur *et al.* (1986). The test and its method of use incorporate several novel features including a continuously variable spatial frequency scale. With eight different plates it is possible to determine a complete contrast sensitivity curve over a frequency range of 1.4–36 cycles/degree. The testing distance is 2 m but can be reduced to 1 m so as to extend the low end of the frequency range to 0.7 cycles/degree.

With this system it is possible to produce absolute sensitivity curves comparable to those obtained from elec-

* Obtainable from Keeler Ltd, Clewer Hill Road, Windsor, Berks SL4 4AA.

* Obtainable from Clement Clarke International Ltd, Edinburgh Way, Harlow, Essex CM20 2TT.

tronically generated gratings. The apparatus is not at present commercially available but is in use at City University for research purposes.

The Melbourne Edge Test

Described by Verbaken and Johnston (1986), the Melbourne Edge Test is a chart of 20 circular patches of 25 mm diameter, spread over four rows. Each is divided into two semicircular halves by a straight line 'edge' forming a boundary between a darker and a lighter shade of grey. In this respect, the test has similarities with a square-wave grating. The contrast diminishes with each successive patch. To incorporate the principle of forced-choice response, the edge is set in one of four orientations (0, 45, 90, and 135° in standard axis notation) which the patient has to identify. The test is based on the principle that the contrast sensitivity measured for a single edge is a reliable indicator of its value at the peak of the contrast sensitivity function.

Low-contrast test charts

Contrast sensitivity testing requires the patient to learn a new and rather difficult end point criterion. This is avoided by using a conventional test chart but at much lower contrast levels than the normal.

A notable study of the effects of decreasing luminance and contrast on Snellen letter acuity was undertaken by Oscar Richards (1977).[*] Eight special test charts were prepared, with contrasts ranging from approximately 90% to 6%. Each was presented at four levels of luminance from about 34 to 0.0034 cd/m^2 in equal logarithmic steps. The 149 subjects were chosen to represent a typical sample of the general population.

With each drop in luminance there was not only the expected reduction of visual acuity at peak contrast but also a marked increase in the rate of decline with decreasing levels of contrast. This was especially pronounced in the older age groups. At all luminance levels and in all age groups the fall in acuity became precipitous at contrasts below 20%. Similar results were also obtained by Johnson and Casson (1995), whose findings in the presence of blur are discussed on page 72.

Using three different test charts with contrasts of 88%, 21% and 14%, and a similar range for near, Ho and Bilton (1986) found that the reduction in visual acuity with induced refractive blur up to 2.50 D was substantially the same at all three contrast levels. On the other hand, 'diffusive' blur artificially simulated at four different levels reduced the acuity at a faster rate with each drop in contrast. For this reason they advocated the use of charts with two different contrast levels to help differentiate between causes of visual degradation.

Low-contrast letter charts designed for clinical use were described by Regan and Neima (1983, 1984), a de-

velopment from previous work by Regan *et al.* (1977). Five specially prepared charts were used, one resembling a standard Snellen chart with the same high contrast and the other four with decreasing contrasts covering a wide range. Clinical trials were made with these and also with a sine-wave grating test. From the results, it was concluded that low-contrast letter charts are equally capable of detecting visual loss in patients with diabetic retinopathy and Parkinson's disease, even when the visual acuity was normal.

A similar study was made by Greeves *et al.* (1988) using specially prepared letter charts of the Bailey–Lovie design, but at contrasts from 95% to 0.1%. Clinical trials on the control group of 15 normal subjects showed the letter charts to give results comparable with CRT generated square-wave gratings and edge tests. Their patients with age-related maculopathy (or senile macular degeneration) showed good agreement in the mid-frequency range. The use of 10% contrast charts was recommended to differentiate between normal patients and those with macular disease.

The utility of low-contrast letter charts in the field of contact lens practice has been studied by Guillon *et al.* (1988) and Guillon and Sayer (1988). They recommend the use of high- and low-contrast charts, the latter at 10% possibly supplemented by one at 20% contrast. To test at scotopic luminances they suggest the use of welding goggles fitted with neutral filters of density 2, transmitting 1% of the incident light. Specific luminance ranges are indicated. As the result of this procedure, differences in the performance of various types of contact lenses on the eye can be demonstrated, even if the acuity is similar at high contrast in high illumination.

The limb width of a test chart letter can be notionally equated to a spatial frequency by regarding the limb as half of one complete cycle of a square-wave grating. Thus, a limb width of angular subtense 6 minutes of arc is notionally equivalent to 5 cycles/degree. Consequently, a low-contrast letter chart is testing sensitivity over a wide range of spatial frequencies. The view was taken by Pelli *et al.* (1988) that the main purpose of a clinical test is to discover whether subjects with normal visual acuity (i.e. at high frequencies) show abnormally poor contrast sensitivity at lower spatial frequencies. It would therefore be preferable to use only one letter size, notionally equivalent to a spatial frequency in the neighbourhood of 5 cycles/degree. This is near the peak of the normal contrast sensitivity curve.

A similar view has since been expressed by Tunnacliffe (1989). In the chart which he designed for use in his own practice, the letters all have a notional spatial frequency of 5 cycles/degree. The drop in contrast between each of the five lines of the chart covers a total range of 0.9 log units, the successive intervals having been determined by trial to give good repeatability of results on successive days.

The Pelli–Robson chart

Despite their comments on spatial frequency quoted above, the Pelli–Robson chart, introduced in 1988, shows 5 × 5 Sloan letters, of height 49 mm to be

---

[*] His figures have been converted here into cd/m^2 and (percentage) contrast as now understood in this field.

viewed at 1 m. This gives a limb width subtense of 0.57°, corresponding to about 0.9 cycle/degree. The individual limbs of the letters are effectively square-wave gratings, and so, however, their third and fifth harmonics lie close to the peak of the contrast sensitivity function. Zhang *et al.* (1989) demonstrated that the end-point for young observers remained constant despite varying the viewing distance from 0.3 m to 3 m. The chart shows 16 groups of three letters; the contrast of each group decreases from log contrast sensitivity of 0.00 (i.e. contrast, not modulation, of 100%) in 0.15 log unit steps to 2.25 – *see* Exercise 3.17. The subject reads down the chart; the faintest group of three letters for which two letters are correctly identified is generally taken as the end-point, though Elliott *et al.* (1991) suggested giving each letter read correctly a score of 0.05, the first three 100% contrast letters being ignored. Elliott *et al.* (1990b) found that the letter C was often misread as the letter O, and recommended that this mis-identification should be accepted as being correct. On this basis, Elliott *et al.* (1990a) with young subjects and Reeves *et al.* (1993) with eye hospital patients selected for VAs not worse than 6/18, both found a test–retest reliability score around ±0.3 or two groups of letters. This indicates the change in test score needed to indicate a change in performance. Because the letters at threshold may take some time to appear, the patient must be encouraged to continue looking at the chart for 20 seconds or so to try to see letters in the next faintest group.

Rabin and Wicks (1996) report on a similar chart, in which each successive line of 10 letters decreases in contrast in 0.1 log steps. The 5 m letter size is viewed at 4 m, and so is testing at the high frequency end of the CSF. The chart was shown to be very sensitive to small amounts (+0.50 DS or +1.00 DC) of blur, early cataract and amblyopia. This is attributed to the shape of the CSF curve. As shown in *Figure 3.26*, a small drop in VA from the equivalent of 20.7 cycles/degree to 17 cycles/degree would correspond to a drop in contrast sensitivity from about 16 to 35, a factor of more than double.

Use of computer displays

While the use of computer displays for laboratory sine-wave contrast sensitivity testing has already been described, the power of modern computers and improvements in the display screen equipment enable them to provide many charts for subjective examination. The UMIST Eye Systems and TVA[*] provide both grating and low-contrast test charts for contrast sensitivity testing.

Colour Contrast Sensitivity

One of the earliest functions to suffer in retinal disease is

---

[*] Available from Department of Optometry and Vision Sciences, UMIST, PO Box 88, Manchester M60 1QD and Innomed Corporation, Brea, CA 92621, USA respectively.

discrimination in the blue–yellow colour axis. Thus Arden *et al.* (1988) developed a computer system for investigating the loss of contrast sensitivity in ophthalmologists working with the blue–green light from an argon laser. Arden (pers. comm.) has suggested the use of a studio-quality TV monitor to present blue gratings of frequency 0.6 cycles/degree very briefly exposed on a yellow background (or vice versa). Loss in colour contrast sensitivity has also been found in ocular hypertensives and diabetics.

Amblyopia

The ability of the above-described clinical tests to screen successfully for amblyopia is uncertain. Glover *et al.* (1987) concluded that neither the Arden nor the Vistech tests were satisfactory in this respect because too many false results were given. On the other hand, Brown *et al.* (1987b) concluded that the Arden gratings performed well in revealing interocular differences. They thought that if the plates were presented at twice the prescribed distance so as to double the spatial frequency at the high end, the test would become a useful technique for monitoring amblyopia treatment.

Cataract

See the last section in Chapter 15.

Vision through optical instruments

Optical instruments are used as an aid to vision when the angular subtense of the image is too small for resolution by the naked or corrected eye, and in astronomy when the luminance is too low.

The minimum angle of resolution of a perfect or aberration-free eye is limited by two factors: one is the size of the Airy discs formed by diffraction and the other is the sensitivity of the retinal/neural system. The latter must ultimately set the limit. For example, a perfect eye with a pupil diameter of 6 mm could have a minimum angle of resolution as small as 25 seconds of arc, if diffraction were the only factor. It does not follow, however, that the retinal/neural system could distinguish detail as fine as this.

Vision with telescopes and prism binoculars

Consider an instrument whose objective (object glass) is of aperture *d*. Its limit of resolution θ for two neighbouring points is given by the standard formula

$$\theta \text{ (rad)} = 1.22\lambda/d \qquad (3.21)$$

which represents half the angular subtense of the Airy disc. If the instrument magnification is *m*, the angular separation θ_i of the two points in the image presented to the eye is

$$\theta_i = m\theta = 1.22m\lambda/d$$
$$= 1.22\lambda/d' \qquad (3.22)$$

since d', the diameter of the exit pupil, is equal to d/m.

The minimum angle of resolution θ_e of a hypothetical diffraction-limited eye of entrance pupil diameter g is given by

$$\theta_e = 1.22\lambda/g \tag{3.23}$$

so that

$$\theta_i/\theta_e = g/d' \tag{3.24}$$

If g is smaller than d', θ_i is smaller than θ_e. This means that the magnification of the instrument is insufficient for full advantage to be taken of the objective's aperture. It should be such that θ_i is equal to or greater than θ_e, the exit pupil then being no larger than the eye's pupil.

Equation (3.24) refers to an optically perfect eye. If we now turn to a typical human eye, *Figure 3.6* shows that its performance approximates to the ideal only at pupil diameters less than about 2.5 mm. Consequently, for maximum resolution, the human eye requires the magnification to be such that the exit pupil is less than 2.5 mm.

Consider a 10×50 prism binocular, the first number denoting the magnification and the second the effective diameter of the objective in millimetres. If the user's daytime pupil diameter is 2 mm, the magnification needed to maximize resolution is $25\times$. However, even if such a specification as 25×50 were manufactured, the instrument could not be held steadily in the hands. Indeed, for this reason binoculars for general use are seldom manufactured with magnifications greater than $12\times$ unless intended for tripod mounting.

If the exit pupil is larger than the eye's pupil, the effective aperture of the objective is reduced proportionately. Thus, given a 10×50 binocular with its 5 mm exit pupil but a real pupil of only 2 mm diameter, the objective's useful aperture would be reduced to $m \times 2$ or 20 mm. The user would be carrying much excess weight in daytime. The large exit pupil does, however, allow more latitude in positioning the binocular in relation to the eye. Also, at night, the large objectives give a brighter image because of their greater area, provided of course that the pupil dilates sufficiently.

If aberrations are ignored, a distant source such as a small star is imaged as an Airy disc. According to the Rayleigh criterion, its angular subtense is twice the minimum angle of resolution as given by equations (3.22) and (3.23). Thus, when using a telescope, the apparent angular subtense of the retinal image is $2.44\lambda/d'$, whereas with the naked eye it is $2.44\lambda/g$. Provided that the exit pupil diameter d' and the eye's entrance pupil g are approximately the same, there is little change in the retinal image size, whether the instrument is used or not. The brightness, however, is increased by the factor $(d/g)^2$, which is the ratio of the respective areas of the telescope objective and the eye's pupil. For the particular case in which the exit pupil and the eye's pupil are equal in size, the increase in brightness is the square of the magnification. In any event, the illuminance of the retinal image may be raised above the threshold, enabling dimmer and dimmer stars to be seen by using instruments of increasing objective diameter.

The image of an extended object is, however, magnified by the instrument. Thus, a 10×50 binocular will collect 100 times as much light as an unaided eye with a 5 mm pupil, but will spread it over an area 100 times as large. The image brightness will thus remain the same, apart from the loss of light by reflection and scattering.[*]

An accepted basis for assessing the performance of a binocular in night vision is the 'twilight efficiency factor' proposed by Kuhl (cited by Haase, 1952). It takes the general form $(md)^{\frac{1}{2}}$, where m is the magnification and d is the diameter of the objective. This criterion strikes a balance between the two main factors improving the performance of the eye, magnification and light-gathering power.

Vision with microscopes

As explained in more detail on pages 247–250, the magnification of visual instruments for use with near objects is conventionally based on the assumption that the unaided eye would view the object from a distance of 250 mm. If the observer's minimum angle of resolution is θ_e in radians, the corresponding separation h_e in millimetres between two object points just resolved is $250\theta_e$. To express θ_e in minutes of arc, the conversion factor from radians of $1/3437.7$ must be applied. Accordingly,

$$h_e \text{ (mm)} = 0.0727\theta_e \tag{3.25}$$

For a microscope objective of numerical aperture NA,[†] the corresponding standard expression is

$$h \text{ (mm)} = 1.22\lambda/2\text{NA}$$

Hence, for $\lambda = 560$ nm or 5.6×10^{-4} mm,

$$h \text{ (mm)} = 3.416 \times 10^{-4}/\text{NA} \tag{3.26}$$

For the eye to take full advantage of the instrument's superior resolution, its magnification m should equalize h and h_e. From equations (3.25) and (3.26) it follows that this condition is satisfied if

$$m = h_e/h \approx 215(\text{NA})\theta_e \tag{3.27}$$

The exit pupil diameter d' of a microscope is given by the formula

$$d' = 500\text{NA}/m \tag{3.28}$$

It is usually smaller than the eye's pupil. In this event, diffraction takes place only at the objective of the instrument. The size of the eye's pupil then becomes irrelevant and the value to be assigned to θ_e problematical. In general, the conventional value of 1 minute of arc is too low. Values up to 4 minutes of arc have been generally recognized as more realistic. There is certainly a point beyond which further magnification becomes 'empty'.

---

[*] It is extremely dangerous to look through a binocular at very bright objects such as the sun, since the total energy delivered to the retina is greatly increased and can easily cause a serious retinal burn.

[†] $NA = n \sin U$, where n is the refractive index of the medium in front of the objective and U is the angle subtended by the semi-aperture of the objective at the object point on the optical axis. For well-designed objectives, the NA increases with the power from about 0.1 for a $3\times$ lens to 1.4 for $100\times$.

No further detail can then be resolved and a poorer image may result. A similar effect occurs when a newspaper photograph is viewed under magnification.

As Westheimer (1972b), Charman (1974) and others have shown, optimum magnification varies with the nature of the object studied. For non-periodic structures of low contrast, Westheimer found that the image of the Airy disc should subtend at least 5 minutes of arc at the eye. The corresponding value of θ_e is 2.5 minutes, for which equation (3.22) gives the appropriate magnification as about 550NA.

Using opaque discs and clear holes in an opaque field, Charman found that measurement of the diameters of the discs and holes – requiring precise detection of the change in illuminance at the boundary – increased in accuracy with increasing magnification until it exceeded 1500NA for green light ($\lambda = 530$ nm). A high level of retinal illuminance was maintained throughout.

For gratings or periodic structures, the contrast sensitivity of the retina was maximal for spatial frequencies within the range 5–10 cycles/degree. Charman pointed out that optimum magnification for low-contrast objects must vary with the spatial frequency. The appropriate value is that which makes the period or cycle width of the image subtend 6–12 minutes of arc at the eye. Since ϑ_e then has the same range of values, equation (3.27) shows that the optimum magnification may be as high as 2000NA or more.

At these high magnifications, it will be seen from equation (3.28) that the exit pupil becomes very small. Although the effects of ocular aberrations are then minimal, very small exit pupils can be disturbing. In particular, specks of dust on the instrument lenses and opacities in the ocular media are rendered visible.

Exercises

3.1 Construct a graph showing the variation of the eye's theoretical limit of resolution (in seconds of arc) over the range of pupil diameters from 1 to 8 mm. Take the wavelength of light as 555 nm. Using these results, comment on the possibility of an acuity better than 6/6 with a 1 mm pupil.

3.2 (a) A motorist in the UK is supposed to be able to read a number plate, the characters of which are $3\frac{1}{8}$ in high, at a distance of 67 ft. To what Snellen acuity does this correspond?
(b) The experiments of Drasdo and Haggerty (*Ophthal. Physiol. Opt.*, **1**, 39–54, 1981) suggested that a VA of $6/9 - 2$ was needed to be reasonably certain of passing the number-plate test. From your own observation of number plates, suggest reasons for the discrepancy between the answer to (a) and the experimental findings.

3.3 British Standard BS 4274: 1968 *Test charts for clinically determining distance visual acuity* specifies letters of 5×4 format, the dimensions of which must be accurate within plus or minus 5% or 0.25 mm, whichever is the less. This tolerance is increased to 10%, in respect of line thickness only, for the 4-metre and 3-metre letters. On this basis, determine the minimum and maximum permissible dimensions for: (a) the overall height, (b) the overall width, and (c) the line thickness of the 6-metre and 4-metre letters.

3.4 British Standard BS 4274: 1968 stipulates that the 12-metre line in the chart should have 5 letters of 5×4 construction and that the length of the line of letters should lie between 110 and 140 mm. Taking a length of 130 mm, calculate the space between each letter and its ratio to the width of an individual letter. Compare this ratio with that found in the printing of this question.

3.5 A patient claims to be able to discern cars on the skyline of a hill 5 km away. Is this possible, assuming a minimum angle of 30 seconds of arc for perception of an isolated object?

3.6 At what distance would you expect an observer with a visual acuity of 6/9 to be able to read a notice with letters 150 mm high?

3.7 In the printing of this question how many letters occupy a print width of 50 mm? Use this result to determine the number of letters imaged within: (a) the fovea centralis, and (b) the macula lutea, taking their horizontal dimensions as 0.3 and 1.5 mm respectively. Assume an eye of normal length ($+60$ D image distance) in a suitably accommodated state, the reading distance being one-third of a metre from the eye's principal point.

3.8 Using *Figure 3.17*, construct a double-sided scale showing the relationship between Snellen acuity and Times New Roman test letters viewed at 450 mm.

3.9 From first principles calculate the Sloan and Brown M number for a letter of x-height 2.2 mm.

3.10 Using equation (3.8), calculate the AMA visual efficiency rating equivalent to 6/12 (20/40).

3.11 Find the linear misalignment corresponding to 10 seconds of arc vernier acuity at: (a) 250 mm, (b) 400 mm, (c) 1 m.

3.12 Express the visual acuities 6/9 (20/30), 6/4.5 (20/15) and 6/36 (20/120) in decimal notation.

3.13 Non-standard testing distances are often necessary in domiciliary examinations. Convert the following to their approximate 6 m or 20 ft equivalents: 3/6, 5/18, 4/12, 2/9.

3.14 Draw to size the following 18-metre letters in 5×4 non-serif and 5×5 serif format: F, R, U.

3.15 Show that the relationship between the original AMA visual efficiency rating ($E\%$) and the corresponding angular detail size (A) as given by equation (3.8) can also be expressed as

$$E\% = 100(0.83625^{A-1})$$

3.16 Show that, if contrast, C, is defined as $(L_1 - L_2)/L_1$ (*see* page 34) and modulation, M, by equation (3.16), M can be expressed as $C/(2 - C)$ and C as $2M/(1 + M)$. Hence, draw up a table of M for $C = 1.0$ (i.e. 100%) to $C = 0$ in 0.1 steps.

3.17 Draw up a table of actual contrasts for the Pelli–Robson chart, $C = 1/10^S$, where S is the log contrast sensitivity.

3.18 From first principles, derive the relationship Decimal $V = v/30$, where v is the grating frequency in cycles/degree.

References

ADOH, T.O., WOODHOUSE, J.M. and ODUWAIYE, K.A. (1992) The Cardiff Test: a new visual acuity test for toddlers and children with intellectual impairment. A preliminary report. *Optom. Vis. Sci.*, **69**, 427–431

ALLEN, H.F. (1957) A new picture series for preschool vision testing. *Am. J. Ophthalmol.*, **44**, 38–41

AMERICAN MEDICAL ASSOCIATION: COUNCIL ON INDUSTRIAL HEALTH (1955) Special report: Estimation of loss of visual efficiency. *AMA Archs. Ophthal.*, **54**, 462–468

AMOS, J.F. (1977) Refractive amblyopia: its classification, aetiology and epidemiology. *J. Am. Optom. Ass.*, **48**, 489–497 (Reprinted in 1978 in *Optician*, **176**(4562), 13–19)

AMOS, J.F. (1978) Refractive amblyopia: a differential diagnosis. *J. Am. Optom. Ass.*, **49**, 361–366 (Reprinted in 1978 in *Optician*, **176**(4563), 16–24)

ARDEN, G.B. (1978) The importance of measuring contrast sensitivity in cases of visual disturbance. *Br. J. Ophthal.*, **62**, 198–209

ARDEN, G.B., BARNARD, W.M. and MUSHIN, A.S. (1974) Visually evoked responses in amblyopia. *Br. J. Ophthal.*, **58**, 183–192

ARDEN, G., GÜNDÜZ, K. and PERRY, S. (1988) Color vision testing with a computer graphics system: preliminary results. *Doc. Ophthalmol.*, **69**, 167–174

BAILEY, I.L. and LOVIE, J.E. (1976) New design principles for visual acuity letter charts. *Am. J. Optom.*, **53**, 740–745

BAILEY, I.L. and LOVIE, J.E. (1980) The design and use of a new near-vision chart. *Am. J. Optom.*, **57**, 378–387

BARBUR, J.I., HOBAN, B. and THOMSON, D. (1986) A new photographic-based system for the measurement of contrast sensitivity. *Ophthal. Physiol. Opt.*, **6**, 407–414

BARRETT, B.T., DAVISON, P.A. and EUSTACE, P.E. (1994) Effects of posterior segment disorders on oscillatory displacement thresholds, and on acuities as measured using the Potential Acuity Meter and laser inteferometer. *Ophthal. Physiol. Opt.*, **14**, 132–138

BARRETT, B.T., DAVISON, P.A. and EUSTACE, P.E. (1995) Clinical comparison of three techniques for evaluating visual function behind cataract. *Eye*, **9**, 722–727

BENNETT, A.G. (1965) Ophthalmic test types. *Br. J. Physiol. Optics*, **22**, 238–271

BLASKOVICS, I. (1923) Ueber Verwendbarkeit von Buchstaben und Zahlen bei Sehschärfe-untersuchungen. *Klin. Mbl. Augenheilk.*, **71**, 440

BLASKOVICS, I. (1924) The new unit of visual acuity and its practical use. *Archs Ophthal, N.Y.*, **53**, 476

BOYD, B.F. and GUYTON, D.I. (1983) What is the Potential Visual Acuity Meter (PAM)? What are its significant contributions and indications for use? How does it work? What are its limitations? *Highlights Ophthalmol.*, **11**(4), 1–8

BROWN, B. (1972a) Dynamic visual acuity, eye movements and peripheral acuity for moving targets. *Vision Res.*, **12**, 305–321

BROWN, B. (1972b) The effect of target contrast variation on dynamic visual acuity and eye movements. *Vision Res.*, **12**, 1213–1224

BROWN, B. and YAP, M.K.H. (1995) Differences in visual acuity between the eyes: determination of normal limits in a clinical population. *Ophthal. Physiol. Opt.*, **15**, 163–169

BROWN, N.A.P., BRON, A.J., AYCLIFFE, W., SPARROW, J. and HILL, A.R. (1987a) The objective assessment of cataract. *Eye*, **1**, 234–246

BROWN, V.A., DORAN, R.M.I. and WOODHOUSE, J.M. (1987b) The use of computerized contrast sensitivity, Arden gratings and low contrast letter charts in the assessment of amblyopia. *Ophthal. Physiol. Opt.*, **7**, 43–51

BUENO, G. and HURST, M.A. (1995) Displacement threshold hyperacuity as a predictor of postsurgical visual performance in patients with cataract. *Invest. Ophthalmol. Vis. Sci.*, **36**, 686–691

CAMPBELL, F.W. (1958) A retinal acuity direction effect. *J. Physiol.*, **143**, 25–26

CAMPBELL, F.W. and GREEN, D.G. (1965a) Optical and retinal factors affecting visual resolution. *J. Physiol.*, **181**, 576–593

CAMPBELL, F.W. and GREEN, D.G. (1965b) Monocular versus binocular visual acuity. *Nature Lond.*, **208**, 191–192

CAMPBELL, F.W. and GREGORY, A.H. (1960) Effect of pupil size on visual acuity. *Nature Lond.*, **187**, 1121–1123

CAMPBELL, F.W. and GUBISCH, R.W. (1966) Optical quality of the human eye. *J. Physiol.*, **186**, 558–578

CAMPBELL, F.W., KULIKOWSKI, J.J. and LEVINSON, J. (1966) The effect of orientation on the visual resolution of gratings. *J. Physiol.*, **187**, 427–436

CAMPBELL, F.W. and ROBSON, J.C. (1968) Application of Fourier analysis to the visibility of gratings. *J. Physiol.*, **197**, 551–566

CARTER, D.B. (1958) Studies of fixation disparity. *Am. J. Optom.*, **35**, 590–598

CHANDNA, A. (1991) Natural history of the development of visual acuity in infants. *Eye*, **5**, 20–26

CHARMAN, W.N. (1974) Optimal magnification for visual microscopy. *J. Opt. Soc. Am.*, **64**, 102–104

CHARMAN, W. N. (1979) Effect of refractive error in visual tests with sinusoidal gratings. *Br. J. Physiol. Optics*, **33**, 10–20

CHARMAN, W.N. (1987) Vision behind the cataract. *Ophthal. Physiol. Opt.*, **7**, 207–209

CHARMAN, W.N. and JENNINGS, J.A.M. (1976) The optical quality of the retinal image as a function of focus. *Br. J. Physiol. Optics*, **31**, 119–134

CHARMAN, W.N. and VOISIN, L. (1993) Astigmatism, accommodation, the oblique effect and meridional ambyopia. *Ophthal. Physiol. Opt.*, **13**, 73–81

CHAVASSE, F.B. (1939) *Worth's Squint*, 7th edn. London: Baillière, Tindall & Cox

COATES, W.R. (1935) Visual acuity and test letters. *Trans. Inst. Ophthal. Optns*, **III**, 1–24

CRAWFORD, H.B. (1936) *Proc. R. Soc. B.*, **121**, 376. Cited by Campbell and Gregory (1960)

DAVIS, J.K. and WARD, B. (1972) The modulation transfer function as a performance specification for ophthalmic lenses and protective devices. *Am. J. Optom.*, **49**, 234–259

DAWES, W.R. (1867) Catalogue of micrometrical measurements of double stars. *Mem. R. Astron. Soc.*, **35**, 137–502

DEPARTMENT OF HEALTH AND SOCIAL SECURITY (1979) *Blindness and Partial Sight in England 1969–1976*. London: HMSO

DEPARTMENT OF HEALTH AND SOCIAL SECURITY (1988) *Causes of Blindness and Partial Sight among Adults in 1976/77 and 1980/81*. London: HMSO

DOBSON, V., MCDONALD, M.A., KOHL, P., STERN, N., SAMEK, M. and PRESTON, K. (1986) Visual acuity screening of infants and young children with the acuity card procedure. *J. Am. Optom. Ass.*, **57**, 284–289

DOBSON, V. and TELLER, D. (1978) Visual acuity in human infants: a review and comparison of behavioural and electrophysiological studies. *Vision Res.*, **18**, 1469–1483

DOUTHWAITE, W.A. and JENKINS, T.C.A. (1987) Visual acuity prediction using the visual evoked response. *Ophthal. Physiol. Opt.*, **7**, 421–424

DRASDO, N. and COX, W. (1987) Local luminance effects of degraded pattern stimulation. *Clin. Vision Sci.*, **1**, 317–325

DUKE-ELDER, W.S. (ed.) (1958) *System of Ophthalmology*, Vol. 1, pp. 658–659. London: Kimpton

ELLIOTT, D.B. (1987) Contrast sensitivity decline with ageing: a neural or optical phenomenon? *Ophthal. Physiol. Opt.*, **7**, 415–419

ELLIOTT, D.B., BULLIMORE, M.A. and BAILEY, J. (1991) Improving the reliability of the Pelli–Robson contrast sensitivity chart. *Clin. Vision Sci.*, **6**, 471–475

ELLIOTT, D.B., SANDERSON, K. and CONKEY, A. (1990a) The reliability of the Pelli–Robson contrast sensitivity chart. *Ophthal. Physiol. Opt.*, **10**, 21–24 (*See also Matters Arising*, **12**, 111–115)

ELLIOTT, D.B., WHITAKER, D. and BONETTE, L. (1990b) Differences in legibility of letters at contrast threshold using the Pelli–Robson Chart. *Ophthal. Physiol. Opt.*, **10**, 323–326

ELLIOT, D. B. and WHITAKER, D. (1992) How useful are contrast sensitivity charts in optometric practice? Case Reports. *Optom. Vision Sci.*, **69**, 378–385.

EMSLEY, H.H. (1946) *Visual Optics*, 4th edn, pp. 499–500. London: Hatton Press

ENOCH, J.M., BIRCH, D.G., BIRCH, E.E. and BENEDETTO, M.D. (1980) Alteration in directional sensitivity of the retina by monocular occlusion. *Vision Res.*, **20**, 1185–1189

ENOCH, J.M., WILLIAMS, R.A., ESSOCK, E.A. and FENDICK, M. (1985) Hyperacuity: a promising means of evaluating vision through cataract. In *Progress in Retinal Research* (N.N. Osborne and G.J.O. Chader, eds), Vol. 4. Oxford: Pergamon

FABRY, C. (1936) Vision in optical instruments. *Proc. Phys. Soc.*, **48**, 747–762

FERRIS, F.L., KASSOFF, A., BRESNICK, G.H. and BAILEY, I.L. (1982) New visual acuity charts for clinical research. *Am. J. Ophthal.*, **94**, 91–96

FERRIS, F.L. and SPERDUTO, R.D. (1982) Standardized illumination for visual acuity testing in clinical research. *Am. J. Ophthal.*, **94**, 97–98

FFOOKS, O.O.F. (1965) The symbol test. *Br. Orthop. J.*, **22**, 98–100

FISH, G.E., BIRCH, D.G., FULLER, D.G. and STRAACH, R. (1986) A comparison of visual function tests in eyes with maculopathy. *Ophthalmology*, **93**, 1177–1182

FISHMAN, R.S. and COPENHAVER, R.M. (1967) Macular disease and amblyopia. *Archs Ophthal.*, **77**, 718–725

FOXELL, C.A.P. and STEVENS, W.R. (1955) Measurements of visual acuity. *Br. J. Ophthal.*, **39**, 513–533

FRENCH, J.Y. (1920) The unaided eye: Part III. *Trans. Opt. Soc. Lond.*, **21**, 127–156

FRIENDLY, D.S., JAAFAR, M.S. and MORILLO, D.L. (1990) A comparative study of grating and recognition visual acuity testing in children with anisometropic amblyopia without strabismus. *Am. J. Ophthalmol.*, **110**, 293–299

FRY, G.A. (1970) The optical performance of the human eye. In *Progress in Optics* (E. Wolf, ed), Vol. 8, pp. 51–131. Amsterdam and London: North-Holland Publishing Co.

GEER, I. and WESTALL, C.A. (1996) A comparison of tests to determine acuity deficits in children with amblyopia. *Ophthal. Physiol. Opt.*, **16**, 367–374

GILTROW-TYLER, J.F. (1988) Causes of blindness and partial sight. *Optician*, **196**(5159), 3

GINSBURG, A.P. (1984) A new contrast sensitivity vision test chart. *Am. J. Optom.*, **61**, 403–407

GINSBURG, A.P. (1986) The practical use of contrast sensitivity. *Optician*, **192**(5067), 17, 19–22

GLOVER, H., BIRD, S. and YAP, M. (1987) Performance of amblyopic children on printed contrast sensitivity charts. *Am. J. Optom.*, **64**, 361–366

GORMAN, J.J., COGAN, D.G. and GELLIS, S.S. (1957) An apparatus for grading the visual acuity of infants on the basis of opticokinetic nystagmus. *Pediatrics, Springfield*, **19**, 1088–1092

GORMAN, J.J., COGAN, D.G. and GELLIS, S.S. (1959) A device for testing visual acuity in infants. *Sight-Saving Rev.*, **29**, 80–84

GREEN, D.G. (1967) Visual resolution when light enters the eye through different parts of the pupil. *J. Physiol.*, **190**, 583–593

GREEN, J. (1868) On a new series of test letters for determining the acuteness of vision. *Trans. Am. Ophthal. Soc.*, **1**, pt. 3, 68

GREEVES, A.L., COLE, B.L. and JACOBS, R.J. (1988) Assessment of contrast sensitivity of patients with macular disease using reduced contrast near vision acuity charts. *Ophthal. Physiol. Opt.*, **8**, 371–377

GRIMM, W., RASSOW, B., WESEMANN, W., SAUR, K. and HILZ, R. (1994) Correlation of optotypes with the Landolt ring – a fresh look at the comparability of optotypes. *Optom. Vison Sci.*, **71**, 6–13

GROUNDS, A. (1996) Amblyopia. In *Pediatric Eye Care* (S. Barnard and D. Edgar, eds), pp. 75–101. Oxford: Blackwell Science

GUILLON, M., LYDON, D.P.M. and SOLMAN, R.T. (1988) Effect of target contrast and luminance on soft contact lens and spectacle visual performance. *Curr. Eye Res.*, **7**, 635–648

GUILLON, M. and SAYER, G. (1988) Critical assessment of visual performance in contact lens practice. *Contax*, May, 8–13

GWIAZDA, J.W., WOLF, J.M., BRILL, S., MOHINDRA, I. and HELD, R. (1980) Quick assessment of preferential looking acuity in infants. *Am. J. Optom.*, **57**, 428–432

HAASE, M. (1952) *Optiker-Taschenbuch*, 2nd edn. Stuttgart: Wissenschaftliche Verlagsgesellschaft

HALLIDAY, B.I. and ROSS, J.E. (1983) Comparison of two interferometers for predicting visual acuity in patients with cataract. *Br. J. Ophthal.*, **67**, 273–277

HARTRIDGE, H. and OWEN, H.B. (1922) Test types. *Br. J. Ophthal.*, **6**, 543–549

HO, A. and BILTON, S.M. (1986) Low contrast charts effectively differentiate between types of blur. *Am. J. Optom.*, **63**, 202–208

HOFSTETTER, H.W. (1950) The AMA method of appraisal of visual efficiency. *Am. J. Optom.*, **27**, 55–63

HOLLADAY, J.T. (1986) Brightness Acuity Tester measures functional vision. *Ocular Surgery News*, August 1, pp. 1, 20

HOOKE, R. (1705) In R. Waller (ed.), *Posthumous Works*. Section 3 of Lectures of Light, p. 96. London: The Royal Society

HOOVER, H.L. (1987) Sunglasses, pupil dilation, and solar ultraviolet irradiation of the human lens and retina. *Appl. Optics*, **26**, 689–695

HURST, M.A. and DOUTHWAITE, W.A. (1993) Assessing vision behind cataract – a review of methods. *Optom. Vis. Sci.*, **70**, 903–913

HURST, M.A., DOUTHWAITE, W.A. and ELLIOTT, D.B. (1993) Assessment of retinal and neural function behind a cataract. In *Cataract Detection, Measurement and Management in Optometric Practice* (W.A. Douthwaite and M.A. Hurst, eds), pp. 46–65. Oxford: Butterworth-Heinemann

HURST, M., WATKINS, R. and BUCKINGHAM, T. (1995) Optimal temporal frequencies in oscillatory movement hyperacuity measurements of visual function in cataract patients. *Ophthal. Physiol. Opt.*, **15**, 49–52.

IKEDA, H. (1976) Electrophysiology of the retina and visual pathway. In *Medical Ophthalmology* (F.C. Rose, ed.). London: Chapman and Hall

JACOBSON, S.G., MOHINDRA, I. and HELD, R. (1981) Development of visual acuity in infants with congenital cataracts. *Br. J. Ophthal.*, **65**, 727–735

JENKINS, T.C.A., ABD-MANAN, F. and PARDHAN, S. (1995) Fixation disparity and near visual acuity. *Ophthal. Physiol. Opt.*, **15**, 53–58

JENNINGS, J.A.M. (1993) Amblyopia. In *Visual Problems in Childhood* (T. Buckingham, ed.), pp. 124–151. Oxford: Butterworth-Heinemann

JOHNSON, C.A. and CASSON, E.J. (1995) Effects of luminance, contrast and blur on visual acuity. *Optom. Vis. Sci.*, **72**, 864–869

KAY, H. (1983) New method of assessing visual acuity with pictures. *Br. J. Ophthalmol.*, **67**, 131–133

KEELER, C.H. (1956) In Symposium on visual aids for the pathological eye. *Trans. Ophthal. Soc. UK*, **76**, 605–614

KETTESY, A. (1948) Preliminary proposal to standardise the examination of visual acuity. *Revta Oftal.*, **1**, 125

KITCHIN, J.E. (née Lovie) and BAILEY, I.L. (1981) Task complexity and visual acuity in senile macular degeneration. *Aust. J. Optom.*, **64**, 235–242

LAUGHLIN, S.B. (1992) Retinal information capacity and the function of the pupil. *Ophthal. Physiol. Opt.*, **12**, 161–164

LAW, F.W. (1952) Reading types. *Br. J. Ophthal.*, **36**, 689–690

LE GRAND, Y. (1948) *Optique Physiologique*, Vol. 2: *Lumière et Couleurs*. Paris: Editions de la Revue d'Optique (English translation by Hunt, R.W.G. (1968) *Light and Colour*, 2nd edn. London: Chapman and Hall)

LENNE, R.C., VINGRYS, A.J. and SMITH, G. (1995) Using computers to test visual acuity. *J. Am. Optom. Assoc.*, **66**, 766–774

LONG, G.M. and MAY, P. (1992) Dynamic visual acuity and contrast sensitivity for static and flickered gratings in a college sample. *Optom. Vis. Sci.*, **69**, 915–922

LOTMAR, W. (1980) Apparatus for the measurement of retinal visual acuity by moiré fringes. *Invest. Ophthalmol. Vis. Sci.*, **19**, 393–400

LOVIE-KITCHEN, J.E. (1988) Validity and reliability of visual acuity measurement. *Ophthal. Physiol. Opt.*, **8**, 363–370.

LOVIE-KITCHEN, J.E. (1989) Matters arising, authors reply. *Opthal. Physiol. Opt.*, **9**, 458

LOW, F.N. (1951) Peripheral visual acuity. *AMA Archs Ophthal.*, **45**, 80–99

LOWE, J. (1977) Prescribing closed circuit television. *Optician*, **174**(4503), 29–30, 35

LUCKIESH, M. (1945) *Light, Vision and Seeing*. New York: Van Nostrand

LUDVIGH, E.J. and MILLER, J. (1958) Study of visual acuity during the ocular pursuit of moving test objects. *J. Opt. Soc. Am.*, **48**, 799–802

MCDONALD, M.A., DOBSON, V., SEBRIS, S.L., BAITCH, L., VARNER, D. and TELLER, D.Y. (1985) The acuity card procedure: a rapid test of infant acuity. *Invest. Ophthalmol. Vis. Sci.*, **26**, 1158–1162

MCGRAW, P.V., BARRETT, B.T. and WHITAKER, D. (1996) Assessment of vision behind cataracts. *Ophthal. Physiol. Opt.*, **16**, Suppl. 2, S26–S32

MCGRAW, P.V. and WINN, B. (1993) Glasgow Acuity Cards: a new test for the measurement of letter acuity in children. *Ophthal. Physiol. Opt.*, **13**, 400–404

MCGRAW, P.V. and WINN, B. (1995) Measurement of letter acuity in preschool children. *Ophthal. Physiol. Opt.*, **15**, Suppl. 1, S11–S17.

MCKEE, S.P., WELCH, L., TAYLOR, D.G. and BOWNE, S.F. (1990) Finding the common bond: stereoacuity and the other hyperacuities. *Vision Res.*, **30**, 879–891

MALLETT, R. (1988) The management of binocular vision anomalies. In *Optometry* (K. Edwards and R. Llewellyn, eds), pp. 270–284. London: Butterworths

MALLETT, R.F.J. (1969) Investigation and management of amblyopia. *Ophthal. Optn.*, **9**, 768–780

MARG, E., FREEMAN, D.N., PELTZMAN, P. and GOLDSTEN, P.J. (1976) Visual acuity development in human infants: evoked potential measurements. *Invest. Ophthalmol. Vis. Sci.*, **15**, 150–153

MAYER, D.L. and GROSS, R.D. (1990) Modified Allen pictures to assess amblyopia in young children. *Ophthalmology*, **97**, 827–832

MAYER, D.L., BEISER, A.S., WARNER, A.F., PRATT, E.M., RAYE, K.N. and LANG, J.M. (1995) Monocular acuity norms for the Teller acuity cards between ages one month and four years. *Invest. Ophthalmol. Vis. Sci.*, **36**, 671–685

MILLER, J.W. and LUDVIGH, E.J. (1962) The effect of relative motion on visual acuity. *Surv. Ophthal.*, **7**, 83–116

MILLER, S.J. and REEDER, C.E. (1965) Kinetic visual acuity. *Br. J. Physiol. Optics*, **22**, 46–52

MILLODOT, M. (1966) Foveal and extra-foveal acuity with and without stabilised retinal images. *Br. J. Physiol. Optics*, **23**, 75–106

MILLODOT, M. and RIGGS, I.A. (1970) Refraction determined electrophysiologically. *Archs Ophthal. N.Y.*, **84**, 272–278

MITCHELL, D.E., FREEMAN, R.D., MILLODOT, M. and HAEGER-STROM, G. (1973) Meridional amblyopia: evidence for modification of the human visual system by early visual experience. *Vision Res.*, **13**, 535–558

MONOYER, F. (1875) Echelle typographique décimale pour mesurer l'acuité de la vue. *C. r. hebd. Séanc. Acad. Sci., Paris*, **80**, 1137–1138

NACHMIAS, J. (1960) Meridional variations in visual acuity and eye movements during fixation. *J. Op. Soc. Am.*, **50**, 569–571

NAWRATZKI, I., AUERBACH, E. and ROWE, H. (1966) Amblyopia ex anopsia: the electrical response in the retina and occipital cortex following photic stimulation of normal and amblyopic eyes. *Am. J. Ophthal.*, **61**, 430–435

NELSON, J. (1988) Amblyopia: the cortical basis of binocularity and vision loss in strabismus. In *Optometry* (K. Edwards and R. Llewellyn, eds), pp. 189–216. London, Butterworths,

OGLE, K.N. (1951) On the resolving power of the human eye. *J. Opt. Soc. Am.*, **41**, 517–520

OWSLEY, C., SEKULER, R. and SIEMSEN, D. (1983) Contrast sensitivity throughout adulthood. *Vision Res.*, **23**, 689–699

PALMER, D.A. (1966) The size of the human pupil in viewing through optical instruments. *Vision Res.*, **6**, 471–477

PEARSON, R.M. (1966) The objective determination of vision and visual acuity. *Br. J. Physiol. Optics*, **23**, 107–128

PEARSON, R.M. (1970) An evaluation of Wagner's method of objective determination of visual acuity. *Ophthal. Optn*, **10**, 1229–1233

PELLI, D.G., ROBSON, J.G. and WILKINS, A.J. (1988) The design of a new letter chart for measuring contrast sensitivity. *Clin. Vision Sci.*, **2**, 187–199

POINTER, J.S. and HESS, R.F. (1989) The contrast sensitivity gradient across the human visual field. With emphasis on the low spatial frequency range. *Vision Res.*, **29b**, 1131–1151

POINTER, J.S. and HESS, R.F. (1990) Contrast sensitivity gradient across the major oblique meridians of the human visual field. *Vision Res.*, **30**, 497–501

PRINCE, J.H. (1958) New reading material for sub-normal vision subjects. *Am. J. Optom.*, **35**, 629–636

PRINCE, J.H. (1959) Special print for sub-normal vision patients. *Am. J. Optom.*, **36**, 659–663

RABIN, J. and WICKS, J. (1996) Measuring resolution in the contrast domain: the small letter contrast test. *Optom. Vision Sci.*, **73**, 398–403

RASSOW, B. and RÄTZKE, P. (1978) The prognostic value of the laser interferometer – fringe test with cataract patients. *Ophthal. Optn*, **18**, 578–582

REEVES, B.C. and HILL, A.R. (1987) Practical problems in measuring contrast sensitivity. *Optician*, **193**(5085), 29, 30, 33, 34; (5086), 30, 32, 34

REEVES, B.C., HILL, A.R. and ROSS, J.E. (1988) Test–retest reliability of the Arden grating test: inter-tester reliability. *Ophthal. Physiol. Opt.*, **8**, 128–138

REEVES, B.C., WOOD, J.M. and HILL, A.R. (1991) Vistech VCTS 6500 charts: within- and between-session reliability. *Optom. Vis. Sci.*, **68**, 728–737

REEVES, B.C., WOOD, J.M. and HILL, A.R. (1993) Reliability of high- and low-contrast letter charts. *Ophthal. Physiol. Opt.*, **13**, 17–26

REEVES, P. (1918) *Psychol. Rev.*, **28**, 330. Cited by Campbell and Gregory (1960)

REGAN, D., GIASCHI, D.E. and FRESCO, B.B. (1993) Measurement of glare sensitivity in cataract patients using low-contrast letter charts. *Ophthal. Physiol. Opt.*, **13**, 115–123

REGAN, D., GIASCHI, D.E., KRAFT, S.P. and KOTHE, A.C. (1992) Method for identifying amblyopes whose reduced line acuity is caused by defective selection and/or control of gaze. *Ophthal. Physiol. Opt.*, **12**, 425–432

REGAN, D. and NEIMA, D. (1983) Low-contrast letter charts as a test of visual function. *Ophthalmology*, **90**, 1192–1200

REGAN, D. and NEIMA, D. (1984) Low-contrast letter charts in early diabetic retinopathy, ocular hypertension, glaucoma and Parkinson's disease. *Br. J. Ophthal.*, **68**, 885–889

REGAN, D., SILVER, R. and MURRAY, T.J. (1977) Visual acuity and contrast sensitivity in multiple sclerosis – hidden visual loss: an auxiliary diagnostic test. *Brain*, **100**, 563–579

RICHARDS, O.W. (1977) Effects of luminance and contrast on visual acuity, ages 16–90 years. *Am. J. Optom.*, **54**, 178–184

ROSS, H.E. (1992) Orientation anisometropy: some caveats in interpreting group differences and developmental changes. *Ophthal. Physiol. Opt.*, **12**, 215–219

ROSS, J.E., CLARK, D.D. and BRON, A.J. (1985) Effect of age on contrast sensitivity function: uniocular and binocular findings. *Br. J. Ophthal.*, **69**, 51–56

RYAN, V. (1962) The quantitative estimation of vision – historical review. *Am. J. Optom.*, **39**, 317–334

SALOMÃO, S.R. and VENTURA, D.F. (1995) Large sample population age norms for visual acuities obtained with Vistech–Teller acuity cards. *Invest. Ophthalmol. Vis. Sci.*, **36**, 657–670

SCHAPERO, M. (1971) *Amblyopia*. Philadelphia: Chilton

SHEEDY, J.E., BAILEY, I.L. and RAASCH, T.W. (1984) Visual acuity and chart luminance. *Am. J. Optom.*, **61**, 595–600

SHERIDAN, M.D. (1963) Diagnosis of visual defect in early childhood. *Br. Orthop. J.*, **20**, 29–36

SHERIDAN, M.D. (1970) Sheridan–Gardiner test for visual acuity. *Br. Med. J.*, **2**, 108–109

SHERIDAN, M.D. (1973) The Stycar graded-balls vision test. *Devel. Med. Child Neurol.*, **15**, 423–432

SHLAER, S. (1937) The relation between visual acuity and illumination. *J. Gen. Physiol.*, **21**, 165–188

SHLAER, S., SMITH, E.I. and CHASE, A.M. (1941) Visual acuity and illumination in different spectral regions. *J. Gen. Physiol.*, **25**, 553–569

SILVER, J. and FASS, V.H. (1977) Closed circuit television as a low-vision aid – development and application. *Ophthal. Optn*, **17**, 596, 598, 600–602

SIMMERS, A.A., GRAY, L.S. and WINN, B. (1996) The effect of abnormal eye movements upon visual acuity. *Ophthal. Physiol. Opt.*, **16**, 253 (abstract)

SIRETEANU, R., FRONIUS, M. and KATZ, B. (1990) A perspective on psychophysical testing in children. *Eye*, **4**, 794–801

SLOAN, L.I. (1951) Measurement of visual acuity. *AMA Archs. Ophthal.*, **45**, 704–725

SLOAN, L.I. and BROWN, D.J. (1963) Reading cards for selection of optical aids for the partially sighted. *Am. J. Ophthal.*, **55**, 1187–1199

SLOAN, L.I. and HABEL, A. (1956) Reading aids for the partially blind. *Am. J. Ophthal.*, **42**, 863–872

SLOAN, L.I., ROWLAND, W.M. and ALTMAN, A. (1952) Comparison of three types of test target for the measurement of visual acuity. *Q. Rev. Ophthal.*, **8**, 4–16

SLOANE, M.E., OWSLEY, C. and ALVAREZ, S.L. (1988) Ageing, senile miosis and spatial contrast sensitivity at low luminance. *Vision Res.*, **28**, 1235–1246

SMITH, G. (1982a) Ocular defocus, spurious resolution and contrast reversal. *Ophthal. Physiol. Opt.*, **2**, 5–23

SMITH, G. (1982b) Measurement of luminance and illuminance using photographic (luminance) light meters. *Aus. J. Optom.*, **65**, 144–146

SMITH, T.W., REMIJAN, P.W., REMIJAN, W., KOLDER, H.E. and SNYDER, J. (1979) A new test of visual acuity using a holographic phase grating and a laser. *Archs. Ophthal., N.Y.*, **97**, 752–754

SNELL, A.C. and STERLING, S. (1925) The percentage evaluation of macular vision. *Archs Ophthal., N.Y.*, **54**, 443–461

SOKOL, S. and DOBSON, V. (1976) Pattern reversal visually evoked potential in infants. *Invest. Ophthalmol. Vis. Sci.*, **15**, 58–62

SONKSEN, P.M. and MACRAE, A.J. (1987) Vision for coloured pictures at different acuities: the Sonksen Picture Guide to Visual Function. *Developmental Medicine Child Neurology*, **29**, 337–347

STANLEY, P.A. and DAVIES, A.K. (1995) The effect of field of view size on steady-state pupil diameter. *Ophthal. Physiol. Opt.*, **15**, 601–603

TELLER, D.Y., MORSE, R., BORTON, R. and REGAL, D. (1974) Visual acuity for vertical and diagonal gratings in human infants. *Vis. Res.*, **14**, 1433–1439

THIBOS, L.N., BRADLEY, A. and STILL, D.L. (1991) Interferometric measurements of visual acuity and the effect of ocular chromatic aberration. *Appl. Optics*, **30**, 2079–2087

THOMPSON, C. and DRASDO, N. (1988) Clinical experience with preferential looking tests in infants and young children. *Ophthal. Physiol. Opt.*, **8**, 309–321

THORN, F. and SCHWARTZ, F. (1990) Effects of dioptric blur on Snellen and grating acuity. *Optom. Vison Sci.*, **67**, 3–7

TOMLINSON, A. (1969) Alignment errors. *Ophthal. Optn*, **9**, 330–341

TOOTLE, J.S. and BERKLEY, M.A. (1983) Contrast sensitivity for vertically and obliquely oriented gratings as a function of grating area. *Vision Res.*, **23**, 907–910

TUCKER, J. and CHARMAN, W.N. (1986) Depth of focus and accommodation for sinusoidal gratings as a function of luminance. *Am. J. Optom.*, **63**, 58–70

TUNNACLIFFE, A. (1989) A new clinical contrast sensitivity test. *Optician*, **197**(5185), 13–15, 17–18

VANNES, F.L. and BOUMAN, M.A. (1967) Spatial modulation transfer in the human eye. *J. Op. Soc. Am.*, **57**, 401–406

VERBAKEN, J.H. (1987) Standardization of contrast sensitivity measurements. *Clin. Exp. Optom.*, **70**, 19

VERBAKEN, J.H. and JOHNSTON, A.W. (1986) Population norms for edge contrast sensitivity. *Am. J. Optom.*, **63**, 724–732

VERNON, S.A., HARDMAN-LEA, S., RUBINSTEIN, M.P. and SNEAD, M.P. (1990)Performance on three point vernier acuity targets as a function of age. *Eye*, **4**, 802–805

VILAR, E.Y.-P., GIRALDEZ-FERNANDEZ, M.J., ENOCH, J.M., LAKSHMINARAYANAN, V., KNOWLES, R. and SRINIVASAN, R. (1995) White light interferometry in amblyopic—a pilot study. *J. Opt. Soc. Amer. A*, **12**, 2293–2304

VOIPIO, H. (1961) The objective measurement of visual acuity by arresting optokinetic nystagmus without change in illumination. *Acta Ophthal.*, Suppl. 66

VOS, J.J., PADMOS, P. and BOOGARD, J. (1994) Occupational testing of near vision. *Ophthal. Physiol. Opt.*, **14**, 413–418

WAGNER, H.N. (1950) Objective testing of vision with use of the galvanic skin response. *Archs. Ophthal., N.Y.*, **43**, 529–536

WALSH, G. and CHARMAN, W.N. (1985) Measurement of the wavefront aberration of the human eye. *Ophthal. Physiol. Opt.*, **5**, 23–31

WATT, R.J., MORGAN, M.J. and WARD, R.M. (1983) Stimulus features that determine the visual location of a bright bar. *Invest. Ophthalmol. Vis. Sci.*, **24**, 66–71

WEATHERILL, J. and YAP, M. (1986) Contrast sensitivity in pseudophakia and aphakia. *Ophthal. Physiol. Opt.*, **6**, 297–301

WERTHEIM, T.H. (1894) Uber die indirekte Sehschärfe. *Z. Psychol. Physiol. Sinnesorg.*, **7**, 172–189

WESTHEIMER, G. (1954) Eye movement responses to a horizontally moving stimulus. *AMA Archs. Ophthal.*, **52**, 932–941

WESTHEIMER, G. (1972a) Optical properties of vertebrate eyes. In *Handbook of Sensory Physiology* (M.G.F., Fuortes, ed.), Vol. VII/2, pp. 449–482. Berlin and New York: Springer

WESTHEIMER, G. (1972b) Optimal magnification in visual microscopy. *J. Opt. Soc. Am.*, **62**, 1502–1504

WESTHEIMER, G. (1976) Diffraction theory and visual hyperacuity. *Am. J. Optom.*, **53**, 362–364

WESTHEIMER, G. and MCKEE, S.P. (1977) Integration regions for visual hyperacuity. *Vision Res.*, **17**, 89–93

WEYMOUTH, F.W., HINES, D.C., ACRES, I.H., RAAF, J.E. and WHEELER, M.C. (1928) Visual acuity within the area centralis and its relation to eye movements and fixation. *Am. J. Opthal.*, **11**, 947–960

WHITAKER, D. and BUCKINGHAM, T. (1987) Theory and evidence for a clinical hyperacuity test. *Ophthal. Physiol. Opt.*, **7**, 431–435

WHITAKER, D. and WALKER, H. (1988) Centroid evaluation in the Vernier alignment of random dot clusters. *Vision Res.*, **28**, 777–784

WILKINS, A. (1986) Contrast sensitivity and its measurement. *Optician*, **192**(5054), 13–14

WILLIAMS, R.A. and ESSOCK, E.A. (1986) Areas of spatial interaction for a hyperacuity stimulus. *Vision Res.*, **26**, 349–360

WILSON, H.R. (1986) Responses of spatial mechanisms can explain hyperacuity. *Vision Res.*, **26**, 453–469

WINN, B., WHITAKER, D., ELLIOTT, D.B. and PHILLIPS, N.J. (1994) Factors affecting light-adapted pupil size in normal human subjects. *Invest. Ophthalmol. Vis. Sci.*, **35**, 1132–1137

WOODHOUSE, J.M. (1975) The effect of pupil size on grating detection at various contrast levels. *Vision Res.*, **15**, 645–648

WOODHOUSE, J.M., ADOH, T.O., UDUWAIYE, K.A., BATCHELOR, B.G., MEGJI, S., UNWIN, N. and JONES, N. (1992) New acuity test for toddlers. *Ophthal. Physiol. Opt.*, **12**, 249–251

WOODS, R.L. (1991) The aging eye and contact lenses – a review of ocular characteristics. *J. Br. Contact Lens Ass.*, **14**, 115–127

WOODS, R.L. and WOOD, J.M. (1995) The role of contrast sensitivity charts and contrast letter charts in clinical practice. *Clin. Exp. Optom.*, **78**, 43–57 (Reprinted in *Optom. Today* (1996), **36**(12), 19–22; (13), 21–24 and (14),34–37.

WORTH, C. (1903) *Squint: Its Causes, Pathology and Treatment.* London: Bale and Danielsson

WRIGHT, C.E. and DRASDO, N. (1985) The influence of age on the spatial and temporal contrast sensitivity function. *Documenta Ophthal.*, **59**, 385–395

YAP, M., CREY, C., COLLINGE, A. and HURST, M. (1985) The Arden gratings in optometric practice. *Ophthal. Physiol. Opt.*, **5**, 179–184

ZHANG, L., PELLI, D. and ROBSON, J.G. (1989) The effects of luminance, distance and defocus on contrast sensitivity as measured by the Pelli–Robson Chart. *Invest. Ophthalmol. Vis. Sci.*, **30**, Suppl., 406

4

Spherical ametropia

Main classification of ametropia

An unaccommodated eye which brings parallel pencils of rays from a distant object to a sharp focus on the retina is said to be emmetropic. An eye which is not emmetropic is termed ametropic. An ametropic eye is said to have a refractive error or an error of refraction. Since the cause is an optical and not a functional defect, it is reasonable to suppose that an optical means of correcting it could be found.

Ametropia is divided into two main categories: spherical ametropia and astigmatism. In spherical ametropia, to which this chapter is devoted, the eye's refractive system is symmetrical about its optical axis. It is therefore capable of forming a sharp image, but the retina is not in the right position. In simple terms, the axial length of the eye and its focal length are out of step.

Since the image on the retina of the unaccommodated ametropic eye is, by definition, out of focus, vision is adversely affected.

Myopia

If the sharp image is formed in front of the retina (*Figure 4.1*), the resulting error of refraction is called myopia (from the Greek meaning peering, as through half-closed eyes).

The myopic eye can be regarded as having an optical system too powerful for its axial length. To be focused on the retina, light must therefore reach it in a state of divergence. In other words, the object must be at some finite distance from the eye. The higher the refractive error, the shorter this object distance must be.

The point conjugate with the fovea of the unaccommodated eye is called the far point (or *punctum remotum*). It is denoted by the symbol M_R and its distance from the eye's principal point, the far point distance, by

k. In the myopic eye, the far point is at a finite distance in front of the eye, the distance k being negative in sign (*Figure 4.2*).

By means of an effort of accommodation, a myope can focus objects at a shorter distance than the far point but not objects beyond it. Vision at such distances would, on the contrary, be worsened by accommodation. The uncorrected myope is therefore handicapped by having a very restricted range of clear vision. In extreme cases, this may extend to only a few centimetres from the eyes. The popular name for this refractive state – short-sightedness – is certainly apt.

The myope can, perhaps, console himself with the thought that since he can focus objects at shorter distances than is usual, he can obtain larger retinal images and should hence be able to distinguish more detail. We may, in fact, be indebted to myopic craftsmen for some of the intricate and beautiful works of art which have survived from epochs long before the appearance of optical aids.

Hypermetropia

If the pencils within the eye are intercepted by the retina before reaching their focus (*Figure 4.3*) the resulting error of refraction is hypermetropia. This term is due to Donders, and means 'beyond the measure of the eye', referring to the position of the eye's focus relative to the

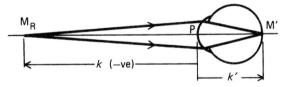

Figure 4.2. The far point of the unaccommodated myopic eye.

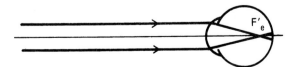

Figure 4.1. The myopic eye and rays from a distant axial object point.

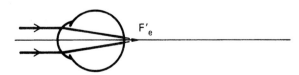

Figure 4.3. The unaccommodated hypermetropic eye and rays from a distant axial object point.

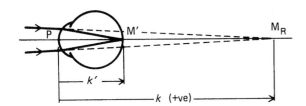

Figure 4.4. The far point of the unaccommodated hypermetropic eye.

retina. Similarly, the term emmetropia means that the focus is at the retina and ametropia that it is not. The former term is sometimes shortened to hyperopia, and in lay-person's language, is the so-called long-sightedness.

The unaccommodated hypermetropic eye is relatively too weak to suit its axial length. As a result, light must reach it in a state of convergence in order to be focused on the retina. The far point is thus a virtual one, situated behind the eye (*Figure 4.4*). Without some form of correction, no real object, whatever its distance, can be sharply focused on the retina. However, if the deficiency in the eye's dioptric power can be made up by an effort of accommodation, distant objects can then be seen clearly. The young hypermetrope does this quite unconsciously, and since he is then able to obtain a normal standard of vision he may not even suspect the presence of a refractive error.

Ocular refraction

The ocular refraction (or principal point refraction), denoted by the symbol K, is the reciprocal of the distance k in metres. In words it can be defined as the dioptric distance to the eye's far point. For example, if a myope's far point is 200 mm from the eye's principal point, then

$$k = -200 \text{ mm}$$

$$K = 1/k = 1000/-200 = -5.00 \text{ D}$$

Since K is a measure of the eye's ametropia, the term 'ocular refraction' is not well chosen but is too entrenched in the literature and in professional parlance to be easily displaced.

The axial length of the reduced eye is denoted by the symbol k'. If k' is regarded as an image distance, the corresponding image vergence K' is given by

$$K' = n'/k' \quad (k' \text{ in metres})$$

K' may be called the 'dioptric length of the eye'. It is the image vergence needed for sharp retinal imagery.

For the reduced eye

$$L' = L + F_e \tag{4.1}$$

in which L' and L are image and object vergences respectively. For a sharp retinal image we must have $L' = K'$ and the object must be situated at the eye's far point, so that $\ell = k$ and $L = K$. When these special values of L' and L are substituted in expression (4.1), it becomes

$$K' = K + F_e \tag{4.2}$$

or

$$K = K' - F_e \tag{4.3}$$

The ocular refraction is thus the eye's dioptric length minus its power. For emmetropia we must have $K' = F_e$ so that $K = 0$.

Example (1)

A reduced eye has an axial length of 21 mm and a power of +62.00 D. What is the ocular refraction and where is the far point situated?

$$K' = n'/k' = 1336/21 = +63.62 \text{ D}$$

and

$$F_e = +62.00 \text{ D}$$

Thus

$$K = K' - F_e = +1.62 \text{ D (hypermetropia)}$$

and

$$k = 1/K = 1000/1.62 = +618 \text{ mm}$$

'Axial' and 'refractive' ametropia

It is usual to make a distinction between 'axial' and 'refractive' ametropia. In the former, the eye is assumed to have its 'standard' power +60 D, so that any refractive error can be attributed to an 'error' in the axial length. In 'refractive' ametropia, the axial length of the reduced eye is assumed to have its standard value of 22.27 mm, the defect being attributed to an 'error' in the power.

In the higher degrees of myopia, there is undoubtedly a tendency for the globe to become elongated, giving rise in extreme cases to an abnormal protrusion (proptosis). On the other hand, investigations by Stenstrom, Tron, Sorsby and others have shown that the important ocular dimensions, like other bodily measurements, follow a normal distribution law. Sorsby, in particular, has demonstrated that the growth of the eye is organized in such a way that its focal length tends to keep in step with its axial length. Moreover, as far as the lower degrees of ametropia are concerned, the correlation between ametropia and axial length is not marked.

In short, the distinction between 'axial' and 'refractive' ametropia seems devoid of statistical foundation and in the opinion of the authors should now be abandoned.

Nevertheless, it is not without point to consider what change in ametropia would result from a given change in axial length, the power of the eye remaining the same. Since $K = K' - F_e$, any change $\Delta K'$ in the value K' would produce an identical change ΔK in the refractive error if F_e remained constant. We have

$$K' = n'/k' = n'k'^{-1}$$

Differentiating gives

$$\frac{dK'}{dk'} = -n'k'^{-2} = \frac{-n'K'^2}{n'^2} = \frac{-K'^2}{n'}$$

Thus

$$\Delta K' = \frac{-K'^2}{n'} \Delta k' \quad (k' \text{ in metres}) \tag{4.4}$$

If $+60$ D is taken as a mean value for K', this expression becomes

$$\Delta K' = \frac{-3.6}{n'} \Delta k' \quad (k' \text{ in millimetres})$$

$$= -2.7 \Delta k' \tag{4.5}$$

Thus, an increase of 1 mm in the axial length would produce a change in ametropia of -2.7 D, that is, in the direction of myopia. Conversely

$$\Delta k' = -\Delta K'/2.7 = -0.37 \Delta K' \tag{4.6}$$

This relationship is often expressed as 'a variation of three-eighths of a millimetre in axial length alters the refractive state by one dioptre'.

Thus, if $\Delta K'$ is 0.25 D, $\Delta k'$ is approximately 0.09 mm, which is only slightly greater than the combined length of the inner and outer segments of a foveal cone (about 0.07 mm).

The correcting lens

Principle of distance correction

The unaccommodated eye is in focus for objects in the plane of its far point. A lens forms images of distant objects in the plane of its second principal focus. Thus an eye is corrected for distance vision by a lens with its second principal focus coinciding with the eye's far point.

If the correction takes the form of a contact lens, represented schematically in *Figures 4.5* and *4.6*, its focal length f'_c must be the same as the far point distance k, and so its power* F_c must be equal to K.

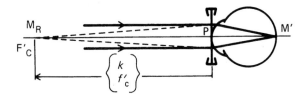

Figure 4.5. Optical principle of the correction of the myopic eye by a contact lens for distance vision.

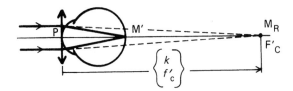

Figure 4.6. Optical principle of the correction of the hypermetropic eye by a contact lens for distance vision.

The ocular refraction therefore indicates the power of the distance correction needed at the eye's principal point.

Spectacle refraction

The power of a spectacle lens is universally understood to mean its back vertex power. This is defined as the reciprocal of the distance in metres from the back vertex of the lens to its second principal focus.

From the point of view of ophthalmic prescribing and dispensing, the numbering of lenses in terms of their back vertex power has important practical advantages. For example, if fitted at the same distance from the cornea, any two lenses of the same back vertex power would have the same effect in distance vision, even if they differed considerably in form and thickness.

As far as distance vision is concerned, and until magnification properties are considered, we can regard the actual lens as being replaced by a thin lens of power F_{sp}† equal to the back vertex power F'_v of the actual lens and situated at its back vertex A_2 (*Figure 4.7*). The position at which A_2 is placed in relation to the eye may be termed the spectacle point, denoted by S.

The positive distance d from the back vertex of the lens to the eye (*Figure 4.7*) is known as the vertex distance. Measured to the true cornea, the vertex distance usually falls within the range 10–14 mm, so it can be taken as 12–16 mm to the principal point of the reduced eye.

The power of the spectacle lens needed to correct a given ametropia is called the spectacle refraction and presupposes a known value of the vertex distance. *Figure 4.8* represents a myopic eye corrected for distance by a thin lens of power F_{sp} and focal length f'_{sp}, its second principal focus F' coinciding with the eye's far point M_R. A similar diagram for the corrected hypermetropic eye is provided by *Figure 4.9*. In each case it is evident that

$$k = PM_R = PS + SF' = -d + f'_{sp}$$

$$= f'_{sp} - d \tag{4.7}$$

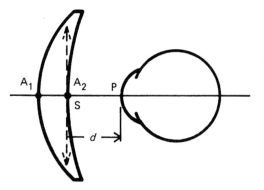

Figure 4.7. A thick lens of back vertex power F' replaced by a thin lens of the same power F_{sp}.

---

* In this context, the 'power' of a contact lens denotes its power when on the eye and includes the effect of the liquid-filled space between the contact lens and the eye.

† The symbol F_{sp} has been used in preference to F_s because the latter is the standard symbol for sagittal power (in oblique astigmatism).

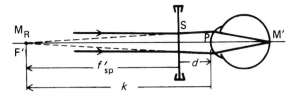

Figure 4.8. A myopic eye corrected for distance by a thin spectacle lens.

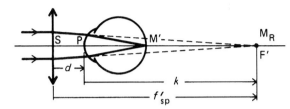

Figure 4.9. A hypermetropic eye corrected for distance by a thin spectacle lens.

so that

$$K = \frac{1}{k} = \frac{1}{f'_{sp} - d} = \frac{F_{sp}}{1 - dF_{sp}} \qquad (4.8)$$

Equation (4.7) can be rewritten as

$$f'_{sp} = k + d \qquad (4.9)$$

which gives

$$F'_{sp} = \frac{K}{1 + dK} \qquad (4.10)$$

Equations (4.8) and (4.10) are useful for analysis, but numerical calculations are most simply carried out as in the following examples.

Example (2)

An eye with an ocular refraction of $+5.00\,D$ is to be corrected by a spectacle lens placed at a vertex distance of 13 mm. What should be its power?

$$k = 1000 / +5.00 = +200\,mm$$

$$f'_{sp} = k + d = +200 + 13 = +213\,mm$$

$$F_{sp} = 1000 / +213 = +4.70\,D$$

Example (3)

An eye is corrected for distance vision by a lens of power $-15.00\,D$ placed 14 mm from its principal point. What is the ocular refraction?

$$f'_{sp} = 1000 / -15.00 = -66.67\,mm$$

$$k = f'_{sp} - d = -66.67 - 14 = -80.67\,mm$$

$$K = 1000 / -80.67 = -12.40\,D$$

Change in vertex distance

It should be clear from the above that an ophthalmic prescription is not strictly complete if it specifies only the spectacle refraction F_{sp}. The vertex distance d at

which the refraction was determined may also need to be measured and recorded. This is well understood in contact-lens practice, where a knowledge of the ocular refraction K is required.

Where spectacles are concerned, it is not considered essential to record the vertex distance, provided that the prescription is of fairly low power, say, 5.00 D or less. If the prescription is of higher power and especially if close liaison between prescriber and dispenser cannot be assumed, the vertex distance used in testing should be recorded in millimetres as in Example (4) below.* In these circumstances the centration distance should also be specified.

The report of a Ministry of Health Committee, published in 1956, states quite clearly that 'the onus is on the dispenser to determine whether there will be any change in the vertex distance, and if so, to modify the prescribed power accordingly'.

Since the second principal focus of the correcting lens should coincide with the eye's far point (*Figures 4.8* and *4.9*), the modified prescription can be deduced from the following rule, namely, if the lens is to be moved x mm nearer to the eye's far point, reduce its focal length by x mm. The converse is also true.

Example (4)

A prescription reads

R −8.00 at 16

What lens power would be needed if the vertex distance were reduced to 13 mm?

The lens is to be moved 3 mm nearer to the eye, hence, in this case, 3 mm away from the eye's far point. The focal length of the lens must be increased accordingly.

$$\text{Original } f'_{sp} = 1000 / -8.00 = -125\,mm$$

$$\text{New } f'_{sp} = -(125 + 3) = -128\,mm$$

$$\text{New } F_{sp} = 1000 / -128 = -7.81\,D$$

Rounded off to the nearest regular interval, the modified prescription would read

R −7.75 at 13

A useful approximation can be obtained as follows. Let F_o be the power of the original lens and let F_{sp} be the modified power needed when the vertex distance is changed by x mm. Then

$$F_{sp} = \frac{1}{f'_o \pm x} = \frac{F_o}{1 \pm xF_o}$$

$$= F_o \pm xF_o^2 \pm \ldots$$

The necessary change in power is $(F_{sp} - F_o)$, found from

$$F_{sp} - F_o \approx \pm xF_o^2 / 1000 \quad (x \text{ in millimetres}) \qquad (4.11)$$

---

* The method recommended in BS 2738 Part 3: *Specification for the presentation of prescriptions and prescription orders for ophthalmic lenses.*

The question whether the original power is to be increased or decreased by this amount follows from the rule already given on this page.

Applied to Example (4), the above approximation gives

$$F_{sp} - F_o = \pm 0.19\,D$$

which agrees with the answer already obtained.

Equation (4.11) may also be used to calculate those powers where a change in vertex distance is important. On the basis that lens powers are manufactured in 0.25 D steps, a change of 0.13 D may be regarded as the threshold where a correction for effectivity is necessary. Thus

$$F_{sp} - F_o = \pm 0.13 \approx \pm x F_o^2 / 1000$$

For contact lens calculations, x will equal the vertex distance, say 15 mm, giving F_o a value around 3 D, while for high-power spectacle lenses, x represents the change in vertex distance requiring a power modification. For a $+10.00\,D$ lens, x is only 1.3 mm.

Hypermetropia and accommodation

There is clearly an intimate link between hypermetropia and accommodation. The emmetrope needs to accommodate only when viewing objects at relatively near distances and the uncorrected myope only to see objects nearer than his far point. On the other hand, the uncorrected hypermetrope has to exert a sustained effort of accommodation to see clearly at all and a correspondingly greater effort in near vision.

Because of this excessive activity, the ciliary muscle of the young hypermetrope acquires some degree of physiological 'tone', which means that a certain amount of accommodation remains permanently in play and cannot be relaxed at will. Hypermetropia may therefore be regarded as consisting of two parts: manifest and latent. The manifest error is measured by the strongest plus lens 'accepted' in distance vision, that is, the strongest lens with which the visual acuity remains at its maximum level. The latent error is the residue masked by involuntary accommodation due to physiological tone.

Experience has shown that after a first correction for hypermetropia has been worn for some time, a stronger correction may be accepted, part of the latent error having become manifest.

As we shall see in more detail in Chapter 7, the amplitude of accommodation (the maximum amount that can be exerted) decreases with age at a predictable rate. As the amplitude of accommodation declines, so does the proportion of latent to the total hypermetropia. In subjects of primary-school age as much as two-thirds to three-quarters of the total hypermetropia may be latent, but this proportion will have dwindled to zero by the middle forties, when only about 4 D of accommodation are left.

Hypermetropia, or that part of it which can be corrected by accommodation, is termed facultative. Because of the gradual loss of accommodation with age, hypermetropia of a degree which is unnoticed in youth eventually asserts itself. Any hypermetropia in excess of the amplitude of accommodation is termed absolute, since it is not correctable by natural means.

The relationship between the various components of hypermetropia is shown schematically in *Figure 4.10*.

Aphakia

Aphakia (from the Greek meaning without a lens) is the condition in which the crystalline lens is either absent, or, in very rare cases, displaced from the pupillary area so that it plays no part in the eye's optical system. The former condition may be congenital, but is usually the result of surgery. With advancing age the crystalline lens tends to develop opacities – a condition known as cataract – which would eventually lead to blindness. In the absence of other pathology, or degenerative changes, removal of the crystalline restores the possibility of good vision, but a strong plus lens is generally needed to make good the deficiency in the eye's power.

Removal of the crystalline lens entails the loss of ability to accommodate, so additional positive power is needed for near vision.

Depending upon the operative technique, the after-effects of surgery on the cornea may leave the aphakic eye needing a correction for astigmatism as well, but since the major element of the prescription is normally

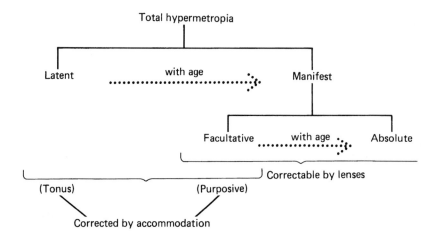

Figure 4.10. Classification of hypermetropia and its change with age.

a high spherical power it is reasonable to consider aphakia as primarily a type of spherical ametropia.

The aphakic eye presents a number of distinctive features. In the absence of the lens, the iris tends to recede, giving the anterior chamber an unusually deep and conical appearance. The iris also shows a tremulous movement (iridodonesis) when the eye is turned. Another indication is the absence of the third and fourth Purkinje images (*see* Chapter 12) formed by reflection from the lens surfaces.

If an operation for cataract is performed on one eye only, the resulting condition is termed 'unilateral aphakia'. This refractive state presents a number of optical problems in an acute form (*see* pages 262–263).

To study the optics of aphakia one must start with a schematic eye in which the crystalline lens is represented. In the Bennett–Rabbetts schematic eye, treated in detail in Chapter 12, the cornea is represented by a single spherical surface of radius of curvature +7.8 mm, the refractive index of the humours is taken as 1.336 and the overall axial length in emmetropia is 24.09 mm. After removal of the crystalline lens, this eye has the same construction as a reduced eye although its dimensions are different. Thus we have

$$F_e = \frac{n'-1}{r} = \frac{336}{7.8} = +43.08\ \text{D}$$

and

$$K' = \frac{n'}{k'} = \frac{1336}{24.09} = +55.46\ \text{D}$$

which gives $K = K' - F_e = +12.38\ \text{D}$.

This indicates the necessary power of a contact lens *in situ* when used as a distance correction for this aphakic eye.

If a spectacle correction were to be fitted at a vertex distance d of 12 mm, its second focal length f'_{sp} would need to be

$$f'_{sp} = k + d$$
$$= (1000/+12.38) + 12 = +80.78 + 12$$
$$= +92.78\ \text{mm}$$

from which

$$F_{sp} = 1000/+92.78 = +10.78\ \text{D}$$

In this example the eye was previously emmetropic. The aphakic correction needed by any given eye would, of course, be affected by any previous error of refraction and by any significant departure in optical dimensions from the values assumed in the schematic eye. A comprehensive survey of the range of possibilities has been made by Bennett (1968).

The retinal image in corrected ametropia

In studying the formation of retinal images when the eye is corrected or assisted by a lens, two separate stages should be distinguished. First, the lens forms a real or virtual image, independently of the eye, in accordance with the laws of conjugate foci. Secondly, this image becomes an object for the eye. As far as the eye is concerned, the first image becomes a real object if formed in front of the eye and a virtual object if formed behind it.

Figure 4.11 represents an unaccommodated hypermetropic eye corrected for distance by a lens of power F_{sp} at a vertex distance d. Parallel rays from the extremity Q of a distant object make an angle u_o with the optical axis and are converged by the lens to form a real image Q'_1 in the plane of its second principal focus F'. The position of Q'_1 in this plane is determined by the undeviated ray through the optical centre of the lens, which coincides with the spectacle point S. The distance $F'Q'_1$, denoted by h'_1, represents the image height after the first refraction and becomes the object height for the second refraction, by the eye.

If a line is drawn from Q'_1 through the eye's principal point P and continued until it meets the lens at T, then TQ'_1 represents the path of the ray from Q after refraction by the lens. This ray is incident on the lens at T. We can therefore take TP as a ray incident on the eye at P, making an angle u with the optical axis. After refraction by the eye, this ray makes a reduced angle u' with the axis such that $u' = u/n'$. The intersection of this refracted ray with the retina determines the second image point Q'_2 and its distance h'_2 from the optical axis.

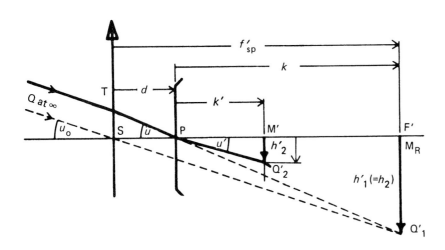

Figure 4.11. Formation of the retinal image in the corrected hypermetropic eye.

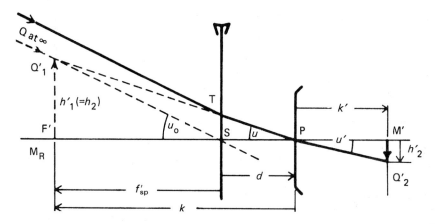

Figure 4.12. Formation of the retinal image in the corrected myopic eye.

Figure 4.12 shows essentially the same construction applied to a myopic eye corrected by a minus lens.

The retinal image size, h'_2, can be determined as follows. First, if u_o is considered positive, then

$$h'_1 = h_2 = -u_o f'_{sp} \quad (u_o \text{ in radians}) \quad (4.12)$$

$$= \frac{-u_o f'_{sp}}{100} \quad (u_o \text{ in prism dioptres, } \Delta) \quad (4.13)$$

This gives the height of the first image, acting as an object for the eye.

Next, since this object must lie in the eye's far point plane in order to be conjugate with the retina, the object and image vergences for the second refraction, L_2 and L'_2, must be equal to K and K' respectively. Thus

$$h'_2 = \frac{h_2 L_2}{L'_2} = \frac{h_2 K}{K'} \quad (4.14)$$

Example (5)

An eye of axial length 24.80 mm is corrected for distance by a -5.00 D lens placed 12 mm from its principal point. Find the size of the retinal image of a distant object subtending an angle of 15Δ. (Assume $n' = 1.336$)

First refraction

$$f'_{sp} = 1000/-5.00 = -200 \text{ mm}$$

$$u_o = 15\Delta$$

$$h'_1 = h_2 = \frac{-15 \times -200}{100}$$

$$= +30 \text{ mm}$$

Second refraction: Method 1

$$k = f'_{sp} - d = -200 - 12 = -212 \text{ mm}$$

$$K = 1000/-212 = -4.72 \text{ D}$$

$$K' = \frac{n'}{k'} = \frac{1336}{24.80} = +53.87 \text{ D}$$

$$h'_2 = \frac{h_2 K}{K'} = \frac{30 \times -4.72}{53.87} = -2.63 \text{ mm}$$

Second refraction: Method 2

$$k = f'_{sp} - d = -200 - 12 = -212 \text{ mm}$$

$$u = -h'_1/\text{PM}_\text{R} = h'_1/k = \frac{-30}{-212} \text{ (rad)}$$

$$u' = u/n' = \frac{30}{212} \times \frac{1}{1.336} = 0.106 \text{ (rad)}$$

$$h'_2 = -0.106 \times 24.80 = -2.63 \text{ mm}$$

Blurred retinal imagery

Blur-circle diameter

The requirements for a sharp retinal image are that after refraction by the eye, the image-forming pencils are homocentric (i.e. free from astigmatism) and the image vergence L' is equal to K' (the dioptric length of the eye). In this chapter, the study of blurred imagery is restricted to eyes with axial symmetry, that is, either emmetropic or with spherical ametropia. There is thus no defect in the optical image and blurring results only if this image does not lie on the retina. In this event, the retinal image is composed of overlapping blur circles each corresponding to a point on the sharp optical image.

The size of each individual blur circle is related to the degree of focusing error, but is also affected by the pupil size. In *Figure 4.13* the refracting surface of a reduced eye and the retina are each represented by a straight line perpendicular to the optical axis, the extremities of the pupil being denoted by H and J. A pencil of rays filling the pupil HJ from an axial object point B is converged towards the image point B', shown in the diagram as lying behind the retina. If g is the pupil diam-

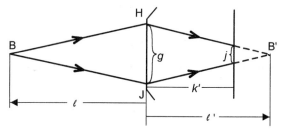

Figure 4.13. Blur-circle formation in the ametropic eye.

eter and j the diameter of the blur circle on the retina, then, from similar triangles

$$\frac{j}{g} = \frac{\ell' - k'}{\ell'}$$

so that

$$j = g\left(\frac{\ell' - k'}{\ell'}\right) \qquad (4.15)$$

Since, in most real situations, ℓ' and k' would differ only by a small amount, each would have to be worked out to several decimal places to obtain a value of j in millimetres correct to two decimal places. If, however, ℓ' and k' are replaced by the corresponding vergences, the expression assumes a much more convenient form. Thus

$$j = g\left(\frac{n'/L' - n'/K'}{n'/L'}\right)$$

$$= g\left(\frac{K' - L'}{K'}\right) \qquad (4.16)$$

Since $K' = K + F_e$ and $L' = L + F_e$, equation (4.16) could be rewritten as

$$j = g\left(\frac{K - L}{K'}\right) \qquad (4.16a)$$

If the image point B' lies in front of the retina, expressions (4.16) and (4.16a) still apply, but the result gives a negative j. This has no real significance apart from indicating a crossing over of the refracted rays before reaching the retina.

The quantity $(K' - L')$ may be regarded as the focusing error E in dioptres. In distance vision, $L' = F_e$ so that

$$E = K' - F_e = K$$

in which case

$$j = gK/K' \qquad (4.17)$$

Example (6)

An unaccommodated eye which has a power of $+62.00\,D$, an ocular refraction of $-6.00\,D$, and a pupil diameter of 4 mm views a point object at a distance of 250 mm. Find the diameter of the retinal blur circle.

$$L = 1000/-250 = -4.00\,D$$

$$L' = L + F_e = -4.00 + 62.00 = +58.00\,D$$

$$K' = K + F_e = -6.00 + 62.00 = +56.00\,D$$

$$j = g\left(\frac{K' - L'}{K'}\right) = 4\left(\frac{56.00 - 58.00}{56.00}\right)$$

$$= -8/56 = -1/7 = -0.14\,mm$$

It will be recalled that due to the wave nature of light the best image of a point source is an Airy disc of finite size. The Airy disc should not be confused with the blur circle due to out-of-focus conditions and its effect on the distribution of light in the retinal image should not be overlooked, especially when the blur circle is relatively small. A more detailed treatment is offered by Fry (1955, 1970).

Blurred image of an extended object

Figure 4.14 shows an object BQ situated on the axis of a myopic reduced eye. A pencil of rays from Q fills the pupil HJ, its centre being assumed to coincide with the principal point P. The ray directed toward P is the chief or central ray of the incident pencil, any cross-section of the refracted pencil having its centre on the conjugate refracted ray from P. Consequently, this is the most important ray path for the study of blurred imagery. In this context, the nodal point has no relevance. For example, in reality a ray aimed at the nodal point N at an angle of $30°$ from the axis could not even enter a 4 mm pupil.

The intersection with the retina of the refracted ray through P determines the centre of the retinal blur circle. Moreover, this ray path is not affected by accommodation or by a change in pupil size. Consequently, even if the size of the blur circle were altered by either or both of these causes, its centre would not shift. We may therefore define the basic height h'_b of an extended out-of-focus retinal image as the distance between the centres of the limiting blur circles.

Consider the blurred image of a line of negligible thickness (*Figure 4.15*). Its basic height is h'_b. Every point on the sharp optical image is represented by a blur circle of diameter j, only a few of which are shown.

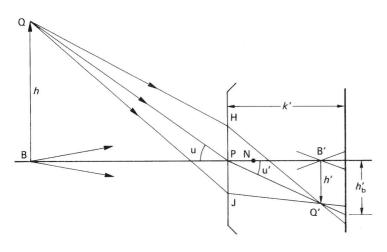

Figure 4.14. Basic image height h'_b of an out-of-focus extended object.

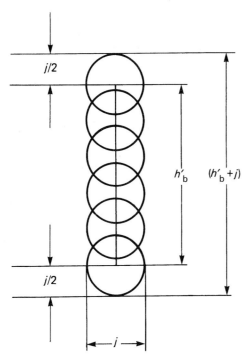

Figure 4.15. Blurred image of a line object.

The total length of the blurred image is clearly $(h'_b + j)$, while its width is j.

From *Figure 4.14*, we can see that

$$h'_b = -u'k' = \frac{-uk'}{n'} = -u/K' \qquad (4.18)$$

If the object is of height h at a distance ℓ,

$$u = -h/\ell = -hL$$

which gives

$$h'_b = hL/K' \qquad (4.18a)$$

The height h' of the sharp optical image is given by the familiar expression

$$h' = hL/L'$$

It can be seen that h'_b is greater than h' if the optical image lies in front of the retina. The reverse applies if it lies behind the retina.

When the summation of the overlapping blur circles is closely examined, it is evident that at the extremities of the image the effect of blurring tapers off. Thus, if the image is of a luminous line, the illumination at the ends falls away. Similarly, if the image is of a black line on a lighter ground, the contrast is reduced. To some extent, the effect of blurring on vision is thereby mitigated. As with visual acuity in general, a high level of illumination could be another mitigating factor.

Blur ratio

Since recognition of the blurred image of a letter depends on the relative size of the component blur circles, we may conveniently introduce the concept of 'blur ratio' defined as

$$\text{Blur ratio (BR)} = \frac{\text{blur-circle diameter}}{\text{basic height of retinal image}}$$

$$= j/h'_b$$

Experiments by Swaine (1925) showed that some test letters could be recognized when the blur ratio was as high as 0.5.

A theoretical expression for blur ratio in terms of the unaided vision in various degrees of spherical ametropia may be derived as follows. From equations (4.17) and (4.18) we obtain

$$\text{BR} = \frac{gK/K'}{-u/K'} = \frac{-gK}{u} \qquad (4.19)$$

in which u is in milliradians (mrad) if g is in millimetres.

A test letter of size D (denominator of the Snellen fraction) subtends an angle u given by

$$u = 5D/6 \text{ minutes of arc} \approx 0.24D \text{ mrad}$$

Hence

$$\text{BR} \approx gK/0.24D \approx 4gK/D \qquad (4.20)$$

in which g is in millimetres. The minus sign has been omitted as irrelevant in this context.

In *Figure 4.16*, this approximation is represented graphically for pupil diameters of 3 and 4 mm. For example, with a 3 mm pupil, the blur ratio of a 12 m (40 ft) letter viewed by a subject with 0.75 D of uncorrected ametropia would be 0.8. The small black circles indicate mean corresponding values of letter size D and K as found in

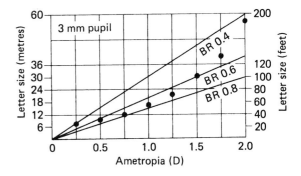

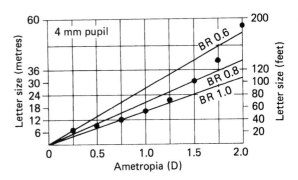

Figure 4.16. Relationship between unaided vision spherical ametropia. The ordinates represent the denominator D of the Snellen fraction at 6 m and 20 ft. Black circles: mean of experimental results from *Figure 4.18*; straight lines: theoretical relationships for stated blur ratios.

clinical practice and shown by the dotted line in *Figure 4.18*. It can be seen from *Figure 4.16* that Swaine's criterion – a limiting blur ratio of 0.5 – is well on the conservative side. If the clinical findings are generally valid for a 4 mm as well as a 3 mm pupil size, recognition of test letters is possible with blur ratios up to 1.0.

In near vision by the *unaccommodated* eye at a dioptric distance L, the blur ratio for an object of height h can be found by dividing equation (4.16a) by equation (4.18a), which yields

$$BR = \frac{g(K - L)}{hL} \qquad (4.21)$$

If, however, the subject exerts A dioptres of accommodation while viewing at this distance, the term $(K - L)$ must be replaced by $(K - L - A)$.

Projected blurs

In *Figure 4.17* the blurred image of an object point has a diameter j and subtends an angle θ' at P, considered as the pupil centre. Corresponding to this angle θ' is an angle θ in object space such that

$$\theta = n'\theta'$$

This is the angle which the perceived blur could be expected to subtend at the eye. Its apparent size y when projected to a distance x can be calculated from the relationship $y = x\theta$. An experimental determination can be made by placing a screen at the given distance x and attaching two vertical markers to it so as to straddle the perceived blur. Their positions are then adjusted so that they appear simultaneously tangential to it.

For a distant object point, the diameter of the retinal blur circle has been shown to be given by

$$j = gK/K' \qquad (4.17)$$

Since

$$\theta' = \frac{j}{k'} = \frac{jK'}{n'}$$

then

$$\theta = n'\theta' = jK' = gK \qquad (4.22)$$

in which θ is in radians and g in metres. Alternatively,

$$\theta \text{ (in prism dioptres)} = gK \text{ (g in centimetres)} \qquad (4.22a)$$

The perceived blur of a point source in real or simulated spherical ametropia differs in several respects from the over-simplified geometrical construction suggested by ray diagrams. The boundary is often ill-defined

and the blurred patch, instead of being uniformly bright, has a streaky or structured appearance, no doubt the result of diffraction by the fibres of the crystalline lens.

Vision in spherical ametropia

If uncorrected by accommodation, 1 D of hypermetropia would produce the same degree of blurring in distance vision as 1 D of myopia.

The effect on vision of uncorrected spherical ametropia can be studied by placing a series of plus lenses of known power in front of the emmetropic or corrected eye. By this means the eye is rendered artificially myopic and vision cannot be improved by accommodation.

The results of such experiments are in reasonable agreement with those of similar studies conducted on uncorrected myopes. There is some evidence to suggest, however, that myopes may, as a result of experience, acquire some ability to interpret blurred images that may not be developed in other refractive states.

The mean results of Hirsch (1945), Crawford *et al.* (1945) and Rubin *et al.* (1951) are plotted in *Figure 4.18*. In the diagram the abscissa represents dioptres of spherical ametropia S (the minus sign omitted), while the ordinate represents the denominator D of the corresponding Snellen acuity, graduated in a logarithmic scale. The graduations on the right-hand side of the graph show the value of D in metres when the testing distance d is 6 m, those on the left-hand side being the values of D in feet when d is 20 ft.

When plotted on this basis the relationship is approximately linear, in which case it would be expressed by an equation of the form

$$\log D = mS + c$$

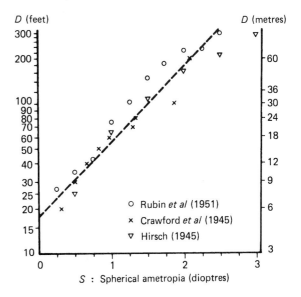

Figure 4.18. Relationship between unaided vision and spherical ametropia as determined by various investigators. The ordinates are the denominator D of the Snellen fraction at 6 m and 20 ft.

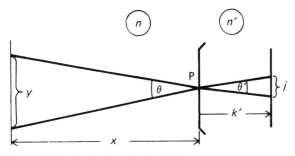

Figure 4.17. Projection of retinal blur.

The dotted line in *Figure 4.18*, representing a reasonable approximation to the mean of all the results plotted, is in fact the graph of the equation

$$\log D \text{ (in metres)} = 0.5S + 0.73 \qquad (4.23)$$

or

$$\log D \text{ (in feet)} = 0.5S + 1.25 \qquad (4.23a)$$

A similar expression can be obtained in terms of decimal V instead of D. Since $V = d/D$,

$$\log V = \log d - \log D$$

in which d is 6 (metres) or 20 (feet). With the appropriate substitution, equations (4.23) and (4.23a) both become

$$\log V = 0.05 - 0.5S \qquad (4.24)$$

In general, this gives V a negative value, which needs to be converted to the standard logarithmic form with a positive mantissa. For example, if $S = 1.00 \text{ D}$,

$$\log V = 0.05 - 0.5 = -0.45$$

$$= \bar{1}.55$$

which gives

$$V = 0.36$$

These expressions should be recognized as approximations to a mean about which a certain spread is to be expected in practice. Moreover, if myopia of much higher degree than two or three dioptres is taken into consideration, the expression relating D and S may take a different form from equations (4.23) and (4.23a). Thus Smith (1991, 1996), arguing from an equation similar to (4.22a), suggested that vision should be linearly proportional to gS, giving

$$D = pgS \qquad (4.25)$$

where p is a constant of proportionality. This might depend on the criterion for vision. For example, a clinician might expect a cut-off of 80% correct answers, whereas a person undertaking physiological research might accept a lower proportion of correct answers. From a clinical point of view, the deterioration in vision caused by small errors of refraction is more important than for very large errors. Very few people have large uncorrected focusing errors, while objective refraction (*see* Chapters 17 and 18) allows the practitioner to estimate the required lens power. Depending upon the aberrations in any particular eye, the drop in vision for any given small amount of blur may vary.

The results of Smith *et al.* (1989) can be expressed in a slightly different form as:

$$D \text{ (in metres)} = 5.46gS - 19.14 \qquad (4.26)$$

where g is in millimetres.

The relationship between D and S is sometimes expressed in the form

$$\log D = m \log S + c$$

Smith (1991, 1996) suggests that this equation was used to give a more uniform distribution to data where most has been collected for low to medium values of S. Because of aberrations and diffraction, he suggests that

the expression relating vision to S for small focusing errors should take the form

$$D = d\sqrt{(MAR)^2 + (pgS)^2} \qquad (4.27)$$

where MAR is the minimum angle of resolution, i.e. the best acuity expressed for the limb width of the test chart letter. Substituting $MAR = 1$, $p = 0.66$ as detailed in the second work cited, and $g = 5$ mm gives similar results to those shown in *Figure 4.18* for ametropias up to about 2 D, but predicts better resolution for blurs between 2 D and 3 D.

Because this equation has been derived from a simple reduced eye, Smith points out that there are very small errors arising from ignoring the separation between the principal points and the entrance pupil of the eye, and also of the small changes in their positions with accommodation.

Johnson and Casson's (1995) four observers also showed a slightly lower drop in acuity than the line in *Figure 4.18*, with the rate of deterioration slowing with increasing blur up to the 8 D investigated. They also measured the effects of blur over the range of photopic and mesopic luminances from 75 to 0.075 cd/m^2 and over Michaelson contrasts from 97% to 6%. Roughly similar shaped plots of vision against dioptric blur were obtained in all cases, the vision deteriorating with both reduced luminance and contrast, particularly when the latter fell below 12%. Low-contrast stimuli appeared more sensitive to blur than high-contrast letters. The vision dropped by approximately 1 logMAR unit for a reduction to 1/10 of the previous luminance, and by about 0.5 logMAR if the contrast was halved. They concluded that the effects of low luminance and contrast on blur were additive.

The pinhole and Scheiner discs

The pinhole disc

The pinhole disc is a useful trial case accessory, its function being to reduce the effective pupil size. This affects vision in three different ways. First, if the retinal image is in sharp focus and resolution is limited by diffraction, a small pinhole may impair the vision by increasing the size of the Airy discs. For this reason, the diameter of the pinhole should not be less than 1.0 mm. Secondly, a pinhole reduces the illumination of the retinal image, which again may impair the vision. Thirdly, if the retinal image is out of focus, resulting in poor vision, a pinhole will reduce the size of the retinal blur circles and may bring about a noticeable improvement.

If poor vision is not improved by a pinhole disc, the indication is that it is not due to a blurred retinal image but to some deeper underlying cause.

The Scheiner disc

Every point on a retinal blur circle corresponds to a unique ray path from a given object point and hence to a unique point of incidence at the refracting surface. This is illustrated in *Figure 4.19*, which shows a pencil

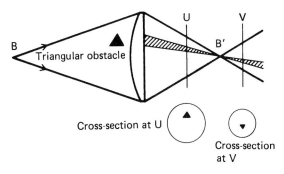

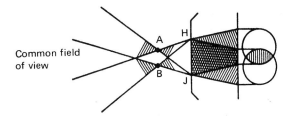

Figure 4.21. Blurred retinal images and fields of view of the Scheiner disc pinholes.

Figure 4.19. Point-to-point relationship between an obstacle and its shadow in the ray bundle.

of rays from an object point B filling the aperture of a converging lens and brought to a focus at B′. If a small area of the aperture is occluded, say by an opaque triangle, every cross-section of the refracted pencil will show a triangular shadow varying in position and possibly in orientation as shown in the diagram.

This basic fact has given rise to a number of different ways of determining ametropia. For example, if a fine wire is moved across the pupil and the retinal image of a small distant source is out of focus, the apparent direction in which the shadow moves across the blur indicates whether the eye is myopic or hypermetropic.

A particularly simple application of the general principle is the disc devised by and named after Scheiner (b.1573). It consists of an opaque disc pierced with two holes, each of about 1.0 mm diameter with their centres 2–4 mm apart. This separation must always be less than the pupil diameter. The disc is placed close to the eye, carefully centred with respect to the pupil, and the subject looks at a small distant spotlight. The disc occludes the pencil that would otherwise fill the pupil and admits only two narrow separated pencils, as shown in *Figure 4.20*. If the eye is hypermetropic, these pencils are intercepted by the retina before they unite at their common focus B′. As a result, the subject perceives two separated images – an effect known as 'doubling'. In hypermetropia, the illuminated retinal patches are uncrossed in relation to their respective pinholes, but because the retinal image is inverted perceptually, the doubled images as seen will be crossed. That is, if the

pinholes were set vertically and the upper one occluded, it is the lower image that would seem to disappear.

In myopia, the doubling is crossed on the retina but uncrossed by mental projection. Only the emmetropic eye, where the common focus of the two pencils lies on the retina, receives an image free from doubling. To distinguish between myopia and hypermetropia it is merely necessary to occlude one pinhole and discover which of the two images has disappeared.

Irrespective of any object viewed through them, the appearance of the pinholes themselves deserves study. For this purpose they can be regarded as luminous points sources, A and B in *Figure 4.21*. Since they are close to the eye's anterior focal plane, they will each give rise to an approximately parallel pencil within the eye, of the same diameter as the pupil HJ. Provided that AB is less than HJ, these pencils will illuminate two overlapping circular areas of the retina, and this is how the pinholes will appear to the subject. The area of overlap on the retina, shown shaded in the diagram, corresponds to the common field of view in object space.

The sensitivity of the device is probably improved by replacing the distant spotlight with a narrow illuminated slit. If the holes in the Scheiner disc were set horizontally, the slit would need to be vertical. The effect of such an arrangement is illustrated in *Figure 4.22*, in which L and R denote, respectively, the left-hand and right-hand pinholes as seen by the subject; *ℓ* denotes the perceived slit image seen through the left-hand pinhole and *r* the image seen through the right-hand pinhole. To a myopic subject, the appearance would then be as shown in the upper part of the figure in which

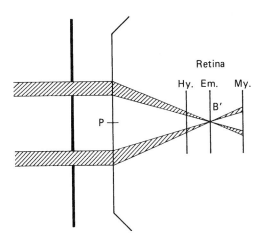

Figure 4.20. Principle of the Scheiner disc test for ametropia.

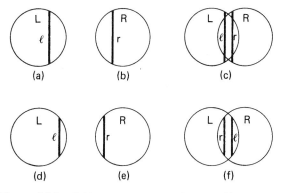

Figure 4.22. Subjective appearance of a vertical line seen through a horizontally orientated Scheiner disc. Upper row: view seen by a myopic patient; lower row: view seen by a hypermetropic patient. L indicates the view through the left pinhole, R the view through the right pinhole; (c) and (f) the combined view.

(a) represents the slit as seen through the left pinhole and (b) as seen through the right. The combined effect is illustrated in (c). It could be inferred from *Figure 4.22(c)* that the doubling is perceived as uncrossed because it is the left-hand one of the two slit images that is bounded by the left-hand pinhole. The lower half of *Figure 4.22* represents the corresponding appearances to a hypermetropic subject. In this case the doubling is perceived as crossed, the slit image seen on the left at (f) being bounded by the right-hand pinhole.

Subjective optometers

Optometers in general

Methods of estimating errors of refraction are divided into two categories: subjective and objective. In the former, reliance is placed on the subject's co-operation during the test. In objective methods, the examiner relies on his own observations and judgement.

Although the term optometer could be applied to any apparatus for measuring errors of refraction, it is generally confined to devices which obviate or restrict the need for a set of trial lenses.

The term was introduced in 1737 by William Porterfield, a Scottish surgeon (Porterfield, 1737, 1759). He gave few details of the construction beyond making it clear that a Scheiner double-slit aperture was an essential feature; there was no mention of a lens.

During the latter part of the nineteenth century, a great number of subjective optometers of different types were devised, but they have since been superseded in everyday practice by more reliable methods of refraction. Objective optometers, discussed in Chapter 18, have long been in demand both for clinical use and for research.

The subjective optometers described below are limited to those of historical or particular technical interest.

The simple optometer

The simple optometer consists essentially of a plus lens of power about +8 or +10 D, mounted at the end of a graduated bar along which a test object can be freely moved. The device is usually held by hand such that the lens is close to the eye. The test object, initially placed at the remote end of the bar, is moved towards the eye until it is seen clearly. If the subject has succeeded in relaxing his accommodation completely, the test object will then be at such a distance from the lens that its image is formed at the eye's far point where it is conjugate with the fovea.

Unfortunately, the subject's knowledge that he is looking at a physically near test object – no matter where its image may be – is bound to stimulate an involuntary effort of accommodation, especially so in young subjects. Because of this 'proximal' accommodation, the test object is brought too close to the eye. In consequence, the results recorded err in the direction of myopia. This is a major disadvantage of all such devices employing a palpably near test object.

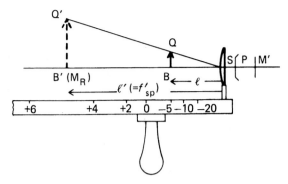

Figure 4.23.   Principle of the simple optometer.

The calibration of the simple optometer can be deduced from *Figure 4.23*. It is assumed that the optometer lens, of power F_o is thin and placed at the spectacle point S. To correct the unaccommodated eye, the test object must be placed at a dioptric distance L from the lens such that the image vergence L' is equal to the power F_{sp} of the distance correcting lens required. Hence

$$L' = L + F_o = F_{sp}$$

or

$$L = F_{sp} - F_o$$

and

$$\ell(\text{mm}) = \frac{1000}{F_{sp} - F_o} \qquad (4.28)$$

This equation gives the theoretical distance ℓ of the test object from the lens, enabling the bar of the optometer to be graduated directly in terms of F_{sp}.

As indicated in *Figure 4.23*, which has been drawn to scale, the interval of graduation is far from uniform.

Another disadvantage of this simple form of optometer is that the apparent size of the image varies considerably as the test object is moved along the bar. If Q is a point on the test object (*Figure 4.24*), its locus as the object is moved is the straight line QT parallel to the optical axis of the optometer lens. If QT is taken as an incident ray path, the refracted ray path is TF'_o, F'_o being the second principal focus of the optometer lens. Consequently, TF'_o or TF'_o produced backwards is the image locus on which Q', the image of Q, is bound to lie. If Q'_1 and Q'_2 are two different positions of Q', it is evident from the diagram that Q'_1 subtends a greater angle at the eye than Q'_2. The closer Q' lies to the lens, i.e. the greater the myopic correction required, the larger the apparent size of the test object becomes.

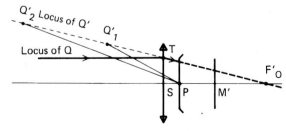

Figure 4.24.   Varying magnification of the simple optometer.

In his Bakerian lecture to the Royal Society, delivered in 1800 and published in 1801, Thomas Young described an improved Porterfield optometer for clinical use. In Young's model, a straight line was engraved along the centre of the bar, appearing as an elongated X when viewed through a Scheiner double-slit aperture. The apparent point of intersection of the two lines, being free from doubling, must be conjugate with the fovea and thus mark the position of the eye's far point. Another innovation was the addition of a +4.00 D lens placed close to the eye to enable the instrument to be used in cases of hypermetropia. It is characteristic of Young's genius that he noted a general tendency to accommodate on the part of the subject and advised that the glasses prescribed (for myopia) should be 'two or three degrees [power intervals] lower than that which is thus ascertained'.

The Badal optometer

The improved form of optometer introduced in 1876 by the French ophthalmologist Badal has two important advantages: its power scale is uniform and the apparent size of the test object is not greatly affected by the state of adjustment.

Only one lens is used, but it is moved forward so that its second principal focus F_o lies either at the spectacle point S or at the eye's principal point P, according to whether the spectacle refraction or the ocular refraction is the result desired.

In *Figure 4.25*, the instrument is positioned to determine the ocular refraction, F'_o coinciding with P.

If x is the distance of the test object BQ from the first principal focus F_o of the optometer lens, x' the distance of the image B'Q' from the second principal focus F'_o of the optometer lens and f'_o the second focal length of the optometer lens, then, from a general relationship discovered by Newton and named after him,

$$xx' = -f'^2_o \qquad (4.29)$$

so that

$$x = \frac{-f'^2_o}{x'}$$

To be seen distinctly without accommodation, the test object must be positioned so that its image lies in the eye's far-point plane. In this setting of the instrument

$$x' = PM_R = k$$

and

$$x = \frac{-f'^2_o}{k} = \frac{-1000\,K}{F^2_o}\,\text{mm} \qquad (4.30)$$

Since the image of Q must invariably lie on the ray path TF'_o or TP produced, the image of the test object subtends a constant angle u at the eye's principal point. It can also be seen from equation (4.30) that the distance through which the test object must be moved from its zero position at F_o is directly proportional to the refractive error.

To determine the spectacle refraction, the optometer must be moved slightly forward from the position shown in *Figure 4.25* so that F'_o coincides with the spectacle point S. The distance x' now becomes SM_R which is equal to the focal length f'_{sp} of the correcting spectacle lens (*Figure 4.11*). Consequently, the calibration equation becomes

$$x = \frac{-1000\,F_{sp}}{F^2_o}\,\text{mm} \qquad (4.31)$$

Although the image of the test object continues to subtend a constant angle u at F'_o, its angular subtense at P will now vary with the state of adjustment. The variation will nevertheless be small compared with that of the simple Porterfield–Young construction because of the much greater proximity of F'_o and P.

The Badal principle is embodied in Schober's subjective optometer (Rodenstock) designed for domiciliary use and is also used in a number of more elaborate objective optometers.

Telescopic optometers

The optometers described so far have used a fixed lens or lens system in conjunction with an adjustable test object which can be moved through a range of near distances. An alternative arrangement is to use a fixed test object at a normal testing distance together with an adjustable lens system. By this means, the stimulus to proximal accommodation is reduced.

One possibility, described by Von Graefe in 1863, is to use a Galilean telescope and to vary the separation between object glass and eye lens to alter the vergence of the emergent light. Racking the eyepiece towards the eye produces a convergent (plus) effect, away from the eye a divergent (minus) effect. The telescope tube can thus be graduated to show the effective power in dioptres as the eyepiece is moved back and forth. A binocular version was introduced by Von Graefe in 1865.

Two drawbacks of this type of optometer should be noted: the dioptric scale is not a uniform one and the apparent size of the test object varies with the state of adjustment. These drawbacks are removed in an ingenious telescopic optometer described in 1951 by Dudragne. A +20 D lens, fixed in position, is placed so that its second principal focus lies in the spectacle plane. In front of this lens is a −20 D lens that is axially movable. When in contact with the +20 D lens the combined power is zero, but as the minus lens is moved forward, the combination produces variable plus power.

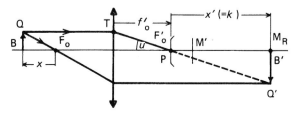

Figure 4.25. Principle of the Badal optometer.

Measured at the spectacle point, this power is directly proportional to the movement of the −20 D lens at a uniform rate of 1D per 2.5 mm of movement.

To cope with myopia, a second −20 D lens is placed in the spectacle plane, its power being effectively reduced as the first minus lens is moved forward from the zero position.

The optometer is used in conjunction with a distant test object. It was shown by Dudragne that the lens system used produced an image of very nearly the same size as that which would be given by a single correcting lens placed at the spectacle point.

The cobalt disc

A simple form of subjective test based on the chromatic aberration of the eye was introduced many years ago. It made use of a plane filter of cobalt blue glass – the 'cobalt disc' – which absorbs most of the middle region of the visible spectrum while transmitting a sufficient proportion at each end, red and blue. Since the eye is a strong positive system exhibiting marked chromatic aberration, its focal length for the longer (red) wavelengths is appreciably greater than for the shorter (blue) wavelengths. In general, the retinal image of a small white source will be formed by overlapping red and blue diffusion circles. If both foci are in front of the retina, as in myopia, the red blur circle will be smaller than the blue because the red is more nearly in focus. The subject should thus perceive a small reddish spot surrounded by a blue ring. The reverse applies in hypermetropia. It is commonly assumed that the 'best focus' would normally correspond to the middle of the visible spectrum.

The object of the test is therefore to find the spherical correction which causes the red and blue foci to straddle the retina, such that the two blur circles are equal in size.

The cobalt disc, though once a standard trial case accessory, is now obsolete. However it is worthy of mention because of the current widespread use of 'bichromatic' tests based on a similar principle. A more detailed examination of the rationale of such tests will be found in Chapters 6 and 15.

Exercises

4.1 Find the position of the far point for each of the following ocular refractive errors: (a) ±2.50 D, (b) ±5.00 D, (c) ±7.50 D, (d) ±10.00 D.

Make a graph of the results, choosing suitable scales for each variable.

4.2 Calculate the static refractive error (if any) of each of the following reduced eyes, taking n' as 1.336:

	corneal radius	*axial length*
(a)	5.58 mm	21.42 mm
(b)	5.30 mm	21.20 mm
(c)	5.42 mm	25.89 mm
(d)	5.86 mm	22.22 mm

4.3 Assuming a reduced eye of power +60 D and $n' = 1.336$, calculate the axial length for values of spherical ametropia at 2.50 D intervals from −10.00 D to +5.00 D. Draw a graph of your results. On the basis of this graph, what variation in axial length corresponds to one dioptre of ametropia? Verify your result algebraically.

4.4 If, in the standard reduced eye of power +60 D and $n' = 1.336$, the refractive index were increased by 5%, what would its refractive condition be?

4.5 Calculate the ocular refraction corresponding to a spectacle refraction of: (a) +8.00 DS, (b) −8.00 DS. Assume the spectacle point to be 14 mm from the eye's principal point.

4.6 A reduced eye ($n' = 1.336$) has a corneal radius of 5.75 mm and an axial length of 21.6 mm. What lens placed 15 mm from the principal point of this eye will correct it for distance?

4.7 (a) A myope is found to require −12.00 D, the spectacle point being 13 mm from the reduced surface. Determine the distance correction required if this vertex distance were altered to (i) 11 mm, (ii) 15 mm. (b) Repeat (a) for an original correction of +15.00 D, all other values being unchanged.

4.8 (a) An eye of axial length 25 mm sees clearly an object which is distant 500 mm. What is the power of the eye, assuming $n' = 1.336$? (b) If the object is 2 mm high, what is the size of the retinal image?

4.9 Calculate the position and size of an object which forms a sharp image 0.1 mm high on the retina of an uncorrected and unaccommodated hypermetrope of +5.00 D, assuming the static power of the eye to be +60 D and n' to be 1.336. What is the nature of this object?

4.10 An eye with axial myopia is corrected for distance by a −8.00 D sphere placed 14 mm from the reduced surface. Find the size of the retinal image, in this corrected eye, of an object 15 m high at a distance of 1.056 km. Also find the size of the image that would be formed in the standard emmetropic reduced eye and hence determine the relative spectacle magnification (first answer divided by second).

4.11 In general, an ametropic eye is corrected for distance by a lens of power F_{sp} at a distance d from the reduced surface of the eye, which has a power F_e and a refractive index n'. Find an expression for the size of the retinal image of a distant object subtending an angle w.

4.12 An object 50 mm high is situated on the optical axis of the standard emmetropic reduced eye at a distance of 200 mm from its principal point. Calculate: (a) the basic size of the blurred retinal image (that is the distance between the centres of the limiting blur circles) and (b) the total extent of retina stimulated, assuming a pupil diameter of 4 mm.

4.13 A −2.00 D myope of reduced eye power of +60 D views a test chart at a distance of 6 m. Find the diameter of the retinal blur circle corresponding to each object point, assuming a pupil diameter of 5 mm and also the basic size of the retinal image of the 6-metre and 60-metre letters.

Comment on the legibility of these two letter sizes on the basis of the figures obtained.

4.14 An eye of standard power and −10.00 D of myopia looks through a Scheiner disc at a bright point of light 6 m away. The pinholes are each of 1 mm diameter and their centres are 3 mm apart on a vertical line. The upper pinhole is covered with a red filter. Giving dimensions, describe what the subject will see, projected on a plane at the same distance as the luminous point.

4.15 When the eye is under water ($n = 1.334$), the power of the cornea is almost abolished and the eye could reasonably be regarded as a (thin) crystalline lens of power +20 D situated 18 mm from the retina. Assuming a pupil diameter of 4 mm, investigate (on paper) the possibility of distinguishing under water a 60-metre letter at half a metre from the crystalline lens of the naked eye.

4.16 A simple optometer has a thin lens of power +8.00 D, the test object being 2 mm high. Find the size of the retinal image when the instrument is focused: (a) for an axial hypermetrope of +5.00 D *spectacle* refraction, (b) for an axial myope of −5.00 D spectacle refraction. Assume the optometer lens to be situated in the spectacle plane, 15 mm from the principal point of the reduced eye.

4.17 (a) A Badal-type optometer has a thin lens of power +8.00 D arranged so that its second principal focus coincides with the principal point of the eye under test. Show that the scale can be uniformly calibrated to record the ocular refraction and find the interval of graduation per dioptre of ametropia.

(b) Assuming a test object 2 mm in height, find the size of the retinal image when the instrument is focused: (i) for an axial hypermetrope of +5.00 D ocular refraction, (ii) for an axial myope of −5.00 D ocular refraction. (c) Where would the second focal plane of the optometer lens need to be placed to give constant retinal image height irrespective of axial length?

4.18 An unaccommodated eye views a point source at a finite distance for which it is not in focus. Rays drawn from opposite extremities of the pupil through the eye's far point intersect a vertical plane through the source at P and Q. Show that PQ is the apparent size of the blurred image of the source when projected to this plane.

4.19 A +1.00 D absolute hypermetrope with a 2 mm pupil and a −3.00 D myope with a 4 mm pupil each view a Bjerrum screen (for testing visual fields) at a distance of 1 m. Both patients are uncorrected. Find the blur ratio for a target stimulus of 1 mm diameter and comment qualitatively on the effect of the blur on the fields plotted, taking into account the intensity of retinal illumination, summation areas and visual thresholds.

4.20 Equation (4.21) shows the blur ratio for an uncorrected and unaccommodated eye viewing a near object to be proportional to $\{(K/L) - 1\}$ for given values of g and h. Plot graphs of $\{(K/L) - 1\}$ for values of K from −8.00 to +8.00 D: (a) when $L = -2.00$ D, (b) when $L = -4.00$ D. From these results, discuss the change in the blur ratio on bringing an object closer.

4.21 A Dudragne optometer is constructed from plus and minus 16.00 D lenses. Show that the scale for the −16.00 D lens movement is linear and calculate its travel for each dioptre of the subject's ametropia.

4.22 A myopic reduced eye with a 3 mm pupil views a car at 100 m. If the rear lights are 1.5 m apart and the retinal blur circles just touch, what is the ametropia?

4.23 Use equation (4.11) to evaluate the lens power that gives rise to an effectivity difference ±0.13 D for a vertex distance change of (a) 12 mm, and (b) 2 mm. What is the relevance of this to (a) contact lens practice and, for (b), the dispensing of high-power lenses?

References

BADAL, J. (1876) Optomètre métrique international. *Annls Oculist.*, **75**, 101–117

BENNETT, A.G. (1968) The corrected aphakic eye: a study of retinal image sizes. *Optician*, **155**, 106–111, 132–135

CRAWFORD, J.S., SHAGASS, C. and PASHBY, T.J. (1945) Relationship between visual acuity and refractive error in myopia. *Am. J. Ophthal.*, **28**, 1220–1225

DUDRAGNE, R.A. (1951) Optomètre à variation continue de puissance. *International Optical Congress 1951*, pp. 286–298. London: British Optical Association

FRY, G.A. (1955) *Blur of the Retinal Image*. Columbus: Ohio State University Press

FRY, G.A. (1970) The optical performance of the human eye. In *Progress in Optics* (Wolf, E., ed.), Vol. 8, pp. 51–131. Amsterdam and London: North-Holland Publishing Co.

GRAEFE, A. VON (1863) Optométrie. *Annls Oculist.*, **49**, 200–208

HIRSCH, M.J. (1945) Relation of visual acuity to myopia. *Archs Ophthal. N.Y.*, **34**, 418–421

JOHNSON, C.A. and CASSON, E.J. (1995) Effects of luminance, contrast and blur on visual acuity. *Optom. Vis. Sci.*, **72**, 864–869

PORTERFIELD, W. (1737) Essay concerning the motions of our eyes. In *Medical Essays and Observations*, Vols 3, 4. Edinburgh: 'A Society in Edinburgh'

PORTERFIELD, W. (1759) *Treatise on the Eye*. Edinburgh: Hamilton and Balfour

RUBIN, L., SILVERSTEIN, H. and SILVERSTEIN, I. (1951) The significance of Snellen acuity in uncorrected myopia. *Am. J. Optom.*, **28**, 484–488

SMITH, G. (1991) Relation between spherical refractive error and visual acuity. *Optom. Vis. Sci.*, **68**, 591–598

SMITH, G. (1996) Visual acuity and refractive error. Is there a mathematical relationship? *Optom. Today*, **36**(17), 22–27

SMITH, G., JACOBS, R.J. and CHAN, C.D.C. (1989) Effects of defocus on visual acuity as measured by source and observer methods. *Optom. Vis. Sci.*, **66**, 430–435

SWAINE, W. (1925) The relation of visual acuity and accommodation to ametropia. *Trans. Opt. Soc.*, **27**, 9–27

YOUNG, T. (1801) On the mechanism of the eye. *Phil. Trans. R. Soc. 1800*, **92**, 23–88 + plates

5

Astigmatism

Astigmatism in general

Spherical lenses and systems of coaxial spherical surfaces possess symmetry about an optical axis. Subject to
paraxial limitations, rays diverging from a point on the
axis are converged to (or made to diverge from) a conjugate axial image point. Pencils of rays having this type
of symmetry are termed stigmatic (from the Greek
stigma, denoting the mark made by a pointed object).

There is another class of reflecting and refracting surfaces termed astigmatic which possess a lower order of
symmetry and which do not form point images of axial
object points. A property common to all astigmatic surfaces is that they have two mutually perpendicular principal meridians, the curvature of the surface varying
from a minimum in one of these meridians to a maximum in the other. Corresponding to the curvature in
each of the two principal meridians is a different 'principal power' as given by equation (2.3) on page 8. The astigmatism of the surface may be expressed in dioptres
as the difference between the two principal powers.

The simplest astigmatic surface is the cylindrical,
shown in *Figure 5.1*. It can be regarded as generated by
the rotation of a straight line LL about an axis of revolution YY parallel to it. Only a small part of the surface,
such as the circular area shown in the diagram, would
be used. The meridian of minimum curvature, zero in
this case, is AA which is parallel to the axis of revolution
and thus called the 'axis meridian' or simply the 'axis'.
The meridian of maximum curvature is PP, which is
perpendicular to AA and known as the 'power meridian'. The radius of curvature in this meridian (r_c) is
that of the circular cross-section of the complete cylinder.

Another form of astigmatic surface, commonly used
in spectacle lenses, is the toroidal, one form of which is
illustrated in *Figure 5.2*. This surface forms part of the
complete figure known as a 'torus', which is generated
by the revolution of a circular arc GH about an axis YY

in the same plane as the arc but not passing through its
centre of curvature C_t. In spectacle lens terminology,
the meridian of minimum curvature is known as the
'base meridian',[*] BB in the diagram. It corresponds to
the axis meridian of a cylindrical surface. The meridian
of maximum curvature, CC in the diagram, is perpendicular to the base meridian and is called the 'cross
curve'. In the type of torus illustrated (known as 'barrel
formation'), the base meridian has the same curvature
as the generating arc GH, while the curvature in the
cross-curve meridian is that of the equator MM of the
complete torus.

An astigmatic lens or system is one which has at least
one astigmatic surface. The simplest lens of this type,
having one plane and one cylindrical surface, is called
a 'plano-cylinder' or 'plano-cylindrical lens'. Such a
lens may be as, for example,

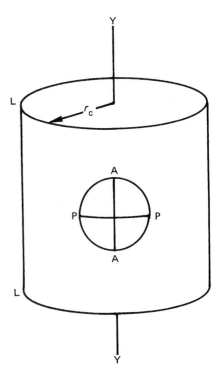

Figure 5.1. The cylindrical astigmatic surface. The circular
area denotes the part used: AA its axis meridian and PP its
power meridian. Principal powers: zero along AA, +4.00 D
along PP, equivalent to plano/+4.00 DC axis AA.

---

[*] For many years, the term 'base curve' has meant both the
surface power of the flattest meridian of a toroidal surface and
an identification of the power of the front surface of the lens.
This was sensible when almost all lenses had toroidal front surfaces, but these are now rare. Hence, the author has adopted
the term 'base meridian' rather than 'base curve meridian' in
the present text.

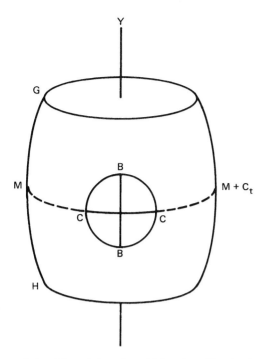

Figure 5.2. A barrel-shaped toroidal surface. The circular area denotes the part used, BB the base meridian (of shallowest curvature), CC the cross-curve meridian (of steepest curvature). Principal powers: +3.00 D along BB, +7.00 D along CC, equivalent to +3.00 DS/+4.00 DC axis BB. C_t is the centre of curvature of the arc GH.

Plano/ +2.00 DC

in which +2.00 DC denotes a plus or convex cylindrical surface of power +2.00 D. A lens bounded by one spherical and one cylindrical surface is termed a 'spherocylinder' or 'sphero-cylindrical lens'. It is specified as in

+1.50 DS/ +2.00 DC

denoting a +1.50 D spherical surface combined with a +2.00 D cylindrical surface.

In general, any astigmatic surface can be regarded as combining an element of spherical power with an element of cylindrical power. It is optically equivalent to a sphero-cylindrical lens. The cylindrical surface is a limiting case in which the spherical element is of zero power.

The cylindrical element of power is invariably the difference between the two principal powers. In the case of toroidal surfaces, the following rules can be applied:

(1) spherical power, that of weaker principal meridian,
(2) cylindrical power, power in stronger principal meridian minus power in weaker.

For example, if the principal powers of the toroidal surface illustrated in *Figure 5.2* were +3.00 D (base meridian) and +7.00 D (cross-curve meridian), the surface would be optically equivalent to the sphero-cylinder

+3.00 DS/ +4.00 DC

In the same way that a +5.00 D spherical lens, for example, could be 'neutralized' or reduced to zero by a −5.00 D spherical lens placed in contact with it, it is possible to neutralize the cylindrical element of an astigmatic lens or system by a correcting cylinder. For example, a convex plano-cylinder could be neutralized by a concave plano-cylinder of equal (and opposite) power. The two lenses would fit together to form a parallel plate of zero power. It is not necessary for the correcting lens to be in contact with the given astigmatic lens or system. Like a correcting lens for spherical ametropia, its power can be adjusted to suit the separation between the two. It is on this basis that the astigmatism of an eye can be neutralized by a correcting cylinder, the spherical power of the lens simultaneously correcting any accompanying spherical ametropia.

For a fuller treatment of astigmatic lenses, the reader is referred to any modern textbook on ophthalmic lenses.

Even spherical refracting and reflecting surfaces give rise to what is termed 'oblique astigmatism', unless the incident pencil is normal to the surface. If the incidence is oblique, symmetry is lost and the refracted pencil (if narrow) exhibits characteristics very similar to those of the axial pencils formed by astigmatic lenses or systems. Oblique astigmatism is an important geometrical aberration affecting lenses and optical systems in general.

Refraction by astigmatic systems can be studied by considering each of the two principal meridians separately.

Ocular astigmatism

Most human eyes show at least a slight degree of astigmatism. There are two contributory factors. First, the cornea is seldom truly spherical, even in the immediate vicinity of the eye's optical axis. By means of an instrument called a keratometer (*see* Chapter 20), the curvature of the front surface of the cornea can readily be measured to a sufficient degree of accuracy. The evidence of several large-scale investigations has proved beyond doubt that in early life the cornea tends to be slightly astigmatic with the meridian of maximum curvature in or near the vertical – *see*, for example, *Figure 21.4*. Corneal astigmatism of this type is called 'with the rule'. If the meridian of maximum curvature lies in or near the horizontal, the astigmatism is said to be 'against the rule'.

The curvature of the back surface of the cornea is far more difficult to measure, but there is evidence to suggest that at least in cases of marked corneal astigmatism both surfaces have the same general configuration. This would mean that a small fraction – about one-tenth – of the corneal astigmatism due to the front surface is neutralized by the back surface. As we shall see in Chapter 20, the calibration of the keratometer makes an arbitrary allowance for the effects of the back surface of the cornea.

The second possible source of ocular astigmatism is the crystalline lens. Either or both of its surfaces may be astigmatic, though accurate measurements of their curvature are difficult to make. Even if both surfaces could be regarded as spherical, any decentration or tilting of the crystalline lens with respect to the cornea would give rise to oblique astigmatism. Whatever the

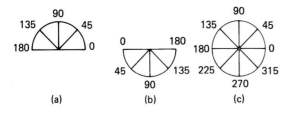

Figure 5.3.   Standard axis notation (ISO, Tabo, Axint). Observer's view. (a) Preferred upper semi-circle notation, (b) alternative lower semi-circle notation, (c) complete 360° protractor.

cause, any astigmatism due to the crystalline lens is simply known as 'lenticular astigmatism'. This component can conveniently be supposed to account for any difference between the corneal astigmatism as given by the keratometer and the total ocular astigmatism as indicated by the spectacle lens found necessary to correct it, due allowance having been made for the vertex distance.

Axis notation

Numerous different systems have been in use for specifying a particular meridian of the eye, the axis direction of a correcting cylinder and the base setting of a prescribed prism. Although there are alternative methods for expressing the prism base setting, the International Standards Organization has adopted the scheme known variously as Standard Notation, Tabo* or Axint† in its 1986 standard: ISO 8429 *Graduated dial scale*, republished as BS 6903: 1987 *Graduated dial scales for ophthalmic instruments*. According to this method, a meridian is specified by the anticlockwise angle which it makes with the horizontal. The viewpoint is that of an observer looking at the eye or at the lens as worn, and the same system is used for the right and left eyes or lenses.

The notation may be represented graphically on prescription forms by either *Figure 5.3(a)* or *(b)*, but the former is preferred because it is consistent with the '360° protractor' shown in *Figure 5.3*. This protractor is used in some countries for specifying the base setting of prescribed prisms. It has the advantage of being a more concise notation for this purpose than any other. In view of the ISO standard, the protractor is no longer recommended in BS 2738 Part 3: 1991 *Specification for the presentation of prescriptions and prescription orders for ophthalmic lenses*.

In writing prescriptions, the degree sign is deliberately omitted so that, for example, 15° cannot be mistaken for 150 or vice versa. By convention, the horizontal setting is denoted by 180 and not by 0.

* From the initial letters of Technisher Ausschuss für Brillenoptik.

† As adopted in 1950 by the International Federation of Ophthalmological Societies.

Image formation in the astigmatic eye

For most purposes, ocular astigmatism can be studied on the basis of the reduced eye. The single refracting surface is then supposed to be toroidal in form with different curvatures and different powers in two mutually perpendicular principal meridians. To distinguish between them we will denote the meridian of greater curvature by α and the meridian of the lesser curvature by β. The subscript letters α and β will be used in the same way. Thus

$$F_\alpha = \text{power of eye in stronger principal meridian}$$

and

$$F_\beta = \text{power of eye in weaker principal meridian}$$

Given an object at a dioptric distance L, the respective image vergences after refraction by the eye are

$$L'_\alpha = L + F_\alpha \tag{5.1}$$

and

$$L'_\beta = L + F_\beta \tag{5.2}$$

Strictly, the ocular astigmatism, Ast, is merely the difference between F_α and F_β, and no plus or minus sign need be given to it, but since it is sometimes convenient to do so, we may write

$$\text{Ast} = F_\alpha - F_\beta \text{ or } F_\beta - F_\alpha \tag{5.3}$$

Figure 5.4 is an isometric drawing (though not to scale) showing the main features of the refracted pencil within an astigmatic eye. Purely for convenience, the principal meridians have been taken as horizontal and vertical, the latter being the more powerful one as in astigmatism 'with the rule'.

Consider an incident pencil of rays from an object point B on the axis. The rays incident at points on the vertical meridian α will be converged to a focus B'_α on the optical axis. Incident rays contained in other vertical sections of the pencil will be brought to a focus in the same plane as B'_α but at different distances from the axis, thus forming a horizontal focal line of which B'_α is the mid-point. Similarly, rays incident at points on the horizontal meridian β will be focused at an axial point B'_β lying at a greater distance from the surface than B'_α because of the lower power in this meridian. As in the previous case, the axial focus B'_β will be extended into a focal line – this time vertical – by the refracted rays passing through other horizontal sections of the lens. The rear focal line is always parallel to the more powerful meridian. Assuming that the limiting aperture (in this case, the pupil) is circular, the cross-section of the refracted pencil is, in general, elliptical, its dimensions and shape varying with the distance from the lens. As we have seen already, the ellipse degenerated into a line in each of the two principal image planes. Dioptrically – *not* geometrically – mid-way between these planes, the cross-section of the pencil is circular. This 'circle of least confusion' is shown in *Figure 5.4*, its centre being denoted by B'_z. It is customary for the dis-

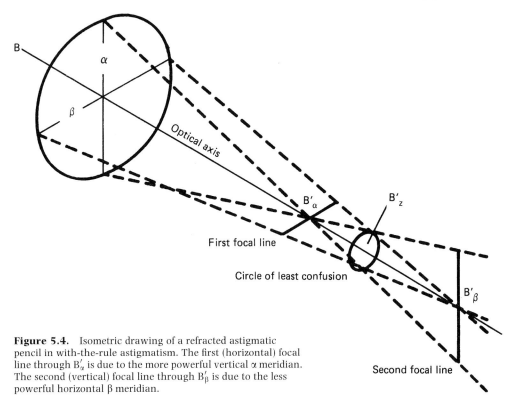

Figure 5.4. Isometric drawing of a refracted astigmatic pencil in with-the-rule astigmatism. The first (horizontal) focal line through B'_α is due to the more powerful vertical α meridian. The second (vertical) focal line through B'_β is due to the less powerful horizontal β meridian.

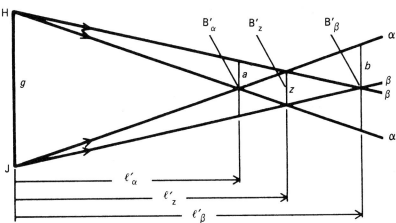

Figure 5.5. Analysis of the refracted astigmatic pencil by superimposing the cross-sections in the two principal meridians.

tance between the two focal lines to be called the 'interval of Sturm', but Thomas Young was undoubtedly the first to describe the geometrical structure of an astigmatic pencil.

The lengths of the focal lines and the diameter of the circle of least confusion can readily be found with the aid of a diagram such as *Figure 5.5*, in which cross-sections of the astigmatic pencil in the two principal meridians are superimposed. The rays in the more powerful meridian converge to the first focal line through B'_α, while the second focal line passes through B'_β. The lengths of these two lines, denoted by a and b respectively, are each determined by the cross-section of the pencil in the other meridian. It is evident that the circle of least confusion must have its centre at B'_z where the two cross-sections of the pencil have the same width, z. Let the distances of B'_α, B'_β, and B'_z from the eye's principal point P be denoted by $\ell'_\alpha, \ell'_\beta$ and ℓ'_z respectively, and let g denote the pupil diameter.

Then, from the similar triangles in the diagram, the following expressions are readily deducible:

Length (a) of first focal line

$$a = g\left\{\frac{\ell'_\beta - \ell'_\alpha}{\ell'_\beta}\right\} = g\left\{\frac{L'_\alpha - L'_\beta}{L'_\alpha}\right\}$$

$$= \frac{g\,\mathrm{Ast}}{L'_\alpha} \tag{5.4}$$

Length (b) of second focal line

$$b = g\left\{\frac{\ell'_\beta - \ell'_\alpha}{\ell'_\alpha}\right\} = g\left\{\frac{L'_\alpha - L'_\beta}{L'_\alpha}\right\}$$

$$= \frac{g\,\mathrm{Ast}}{L'_\beta} \tag{5.5}$$

Diameter (z) of circle of least confusion

$$z = g\left\{\frac{\ell'_\beta - \ell'_z}{\ell'_\beta}\right\} = g\left\{\frac{\ell'_z - \ell'_\alpha}{\ell'_\alpha}\right\} \qquad (5.6)$$

from which

$$L'_z = \frac{L'_\alpha + L'_\beta}{2} \qquad (5.7)$$

and

$$z = g\left\{\frac{L'_\alpha - L'_\beta}{L'_\alpha + L'_\beta}\right\} = \frac{g \, \text{Ast}}{L'_\alpha + L'_\beta} \qquad (5.8)$$

Example (1)

An astigmatic reduced eye ($n' = 1.336$) with a pupil diameter of 5 mm has a power of $+62.00$ D in the $30°$ meridian and $+64.00$ D in the $120°$ meridian.

Determine the main features of the image of an axial object point at a distance of 1 m from the eye's principal point.

The numerical work can be conveniently set out in parallel columns.

	120° Meridian (α)	30° Meridian (β)
L	-1.00 D	-1.00 D
F_c	$+64.00$ D	$+62.00$ D
L'	$+63.00$ D	$+61.00$ D
ℓ'	$\dfrac{1336}{63} = +21.21$ mm	$\dfrac{1336}{61} = +21.90$ mm
Length of focal lines	$a = 5\left\{\dfrac{63-61}{63}\right\}$	$b = 5\left\{\dfrac{63-61}{61}\right\}$
	$= 0.159$ mm	$= 0.164$ mm

Circle of least confusion
$$L'_z = \tfrac{1}{2}\{63 + 61\} = +62.00 \text{ D}$$
$$\ell'_z = \frac{1336}{62} = +21.55 \text{ mm}$$
$$z = 5\left\{\frac{63-61}{63+61}\right\} = 0.081 \text{ mm}$$

These calculations assume that the presence of the retina may be ignored.

It should be noted that the first focal line, associated in this case with the $120°$ meridian, will be perpendicular to this, i.e. at $30°$. The second focal line will be at $120°$.

This example illustrates a general proposition that can be inferred from a study of equations (5.4)–(5.8). Since L'_α and L'_β differ only by the amount of the ocular astigmatism, which is relatively small, the two focal lines must be of very nearly the same length, about twice the diameter of the circle of least confusion.

Classification of astigmatism

A self-explanatory method of classifying astigmatism in the unaccommodated eye is based on the position of the retina in relation to the focal lines of the refracted pencil (*Figure 5.6*). Given a distant object point, each of

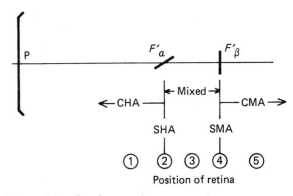

Figure 5.6. Classification of astigmatic refractive errors according to position of retina in relation to focal lines. CHA, compound hypermetropic astigmatism; SHA, simple hypermetropic astigmatism; Mixed, mixed astigmatism; SMA, simple myopic astigmatism; CMA, compound myopic astigmatism.

the two focal lines is situated at the principal focus of the corresponding meridian, F'_α and F'_β. There are five different possibilities:

(1) *Compound hypermetropic astigmatism (CHA)*
  The retina is situated in front of the first focal line.
(2) *Simple hypermetropic astigmatism (SHA)*
  The retina is situated at the first focal line.
(3) *Mixed astigmatism*
  The retina lies between the focal lines.
(4) *Simple myopic astigmatism (SMA)*
  The retina is situated at the second focal line.
(5) *Compound myopic astigmatism (CMA)*
  The retina lies behind the second focal line.

The distance correcting lens

Corresponding to each of the two principal meridians of an unaccommodated astigmatic eye is a separate far point. The correcting lens must be astigmatic, its principal meridians aligned with those of the eye and its principal powers such that the second principal focus coincides in each case with the eye's far point.

As with spherical ametropia, the ocular refraction K of an unaccommodated astigmatic eye represents the power of the correcting lens placed in contact with the eye.

Example (2)

An astigmatic eye has principal powers of $+64.00$ D along $60°$ and $+68.00$ D along $150°$. Its dioptric length K' is $+61.00$ D. What is the ocular refraction?

	Along 60°	Along 150°
K'	$+61.00$ D	$+61.00$ D
F_e	$+64.00$ D	$+68.00$ D
$K = K' - F_e$	-3.00 D	-7.00 D

This result could be expressed in sphero-cylindrical form as

$$K = -3.00 \text{ DS}/-4.00 \text{ DC axis } 60$$

To find the spectacle correction needed at a given vertex distance, for example, 14 mm, the procedure is exactly as for spherical ametropia. Thus:

	Along 60°	Along 150°
K	−3.00 D	−7.00 D
k	−333.3 mm	−142.9 mm
d	14 mm	14 mm
$k + d = f_{sp}$	−319.3 mm	−128.9 mm
F_{sp}	−3.13 D	−7.76 D

The power of the correcting spectacle lens would thus be

−3.13 DS/−4.63 DC axis 60

or, in the abbreviated form commonly used in practice,

−3.13/−4.63 × 60

This procedure could be reversed in a self-evident manner (*see* Example (3) on page 65) to determine the ocular refraction, given the spectacle refraction and the vertex distance.

To compensate for a change in the vertex distance, the method on page 65 should be applied to each principal meridian of the lens in turn .

Example (3)

A prescription reads

+12.50/+3.50 × 170 at 14

What modified power would be needed at 12 mm?

In this case, the spectacle plane is being moved 2 mm nearer to the eye's far points, so the focal lengths of the lens must be reduced by this amount. Accordingly:

	Along 170°	Along 80°
Original power F_{sp}	+12.50 D	+16.00 D
f_{sp}	+80.00 mm	+62.50 mm
−2 mm	−2.00 mm	−2.00 mm
New f'_{sp}	+78.00 mm	+60.50 mm
Modified power	+12.82 D	+16.53 D

These principal powers are given by the lens

+12.82/+3.71 × 170

Rounded off to the nearest 0.25 D, the modified prescription would be

+12.75/+3.75 × 170 at 12

Astigmatic blurring

Images of straight lines

The intersection of an astigmatic refracted pencil with the retina may form an ellipse, a circle or a line. In general, there is some degree of elongation as a result of which lines in or close to one particular orientation will be seen more clearly than any other. This is one of the main characteristic features of vision in the astigmatic eye.

Suppose, for example, that with a given eye every object point at a certain distance gives rise to an ellipti-

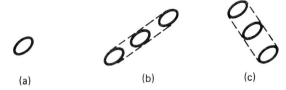

Figure 5.7. The retinal image in uncorrected astigmatism: (a) the blur ellipse due to a point object, (b) the blurred image of a line parallel to the major axis of the blur ellipse, (c) the blurred image of a line perpendicular to the major axis of the blur ellipse.

cal blur on the retina with its long axis at 30°, as shown in *Figure 5.7(a)*.

The image of a line of negligible thickness could be constructed simply by considering the line as a number of points, each separately imaged as an elliptical blur. If the line were at 30°, that is, parallel to the long axis of the individual blur ellipses, the image would be formed as indicated in *Figure 5.7(b)*. This is clearly the most favourable orientation, in which the blurring is least apparent. It is equally evident that the blurring would be worst in the meridian perpendicular to this, as indicated in *Figure 5.7(c)*.

Images of extended objects

In the case of astigmatism, the blurred retinal image of an extended object can be constructed by the method previously described in relation to spherical ametropia (*see* pages 69–70). There are two main steps: one is to determine the basic size of the retinal image, the other to calculate the dimensions of the blurred patch on the retina corresponding to any point on the given object.

Example (4)

An unaccommodated astigmatic eye of axial length 23.00 mm, pupil diameter 4 mm, and ocular refraction

−1.00 DS/−3.00 DC axis 60

views, at a distance of 6 m, an 18-metre test letter V of 5 × 4 format. Find the principal dimensions of the blurred retinal image.

The basic size of the retinal image is found by ignoring the effects of out-of-focus blurring, that is, by imagining the pupil to be indefinitely small. In *Figure 5.8*, the test letter is represented by the object BQ lying on the eye's visual axis and subtending an angle u at the eye's principal point P, which is also taken to be the centre of the

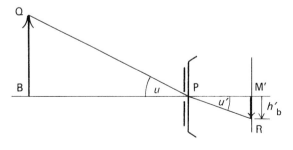

Figure 5.8. Basic retinal image height h'_b of object BQ.

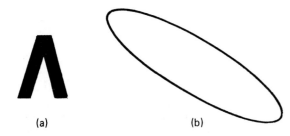

(a)   (b)

Figure 5.9.   (a) The basic inverted retinal image of test letter V. (b) The blur ellipse corresponding to a single point of the object, drawn to the same scale.

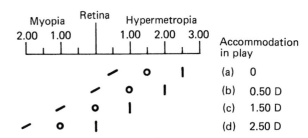

Figure 5.10.   Effect of accommodation on the position of the astigmatic focal lines in relation to the retina.

pupil. The upper extremity of the basic retinal image lies at the centre of the fovea, at M'. Its lower extremity R is determined by the refracted ray PR, conjugate with QP, making an angle u' with the visual axis such that

$$u' = u/n' = 0.75u$$

Since the axial length of the eye is 23 mm, the basic height h'_b of the retinal image is given by

$$h'_b = M'R = -23u' = -23 \times 0.75u$$

Viewed at 6 m, an 18-metre test letter subtends an angle three times as large as the 6-metre letter, that is, 15 minutes of arc or $\pi/720$ rad. Hence,

$$u = \pi/720$$

and

$$h'_b = \frac{-23 \times 0.75 \times \pi}{720} = -0.075 \, \text{mm}$$

Since the letter is of 5×4 construction, the width of the basic image will be four-fifths of h'_b or 0.060 mm and the line thickness 0.015 mm.

To determine the dimensions of the individual retinal blurs of which the image is composed, we need only apply equation (4.16) or (4.17), whichever is appropriate, to each principal meridian in turn. In this case we may use equation (4.17) since it is customary to regard an object at 6 m as lying at infinity. Thus

	Along 60°	Along 150°
k'	23.00 mm	23.00 mm
$K' = 1336/k$	+58.09 D	58.09 D
K	−1.00 D	−4.00 D
g	4 mm	4 mm
$j = gK/K'$	−0.069 mm	−0.275 mm

This shows that each point on the object gives rise to a retinal blur ellipse measuring approximately 0.28×0.07 mm, the long axis parallel to the 150° meridian. In *Figure 5.9*, which has been drawn to scale, the basic (inverted) retinal image is shown at (a) and the blur ellipse at (b). The retinal image of the test letter can be visualized by imagining every point on the basic image (a) to be replaced by an ellipse of the relative size and shape indicated at (b). In this instance it is fairly evident that the letter could not then be recognized.

Effect of accommodation

When studying an astigmatic pencil, it is often helpful to think of the position of the two focal lines and the circle

of least confusion in terms of their ametropic distance from the retina. For example, 1.00 D in front of the retina represents the image position corresponding to 1.00 D of myopia and so on. The scale in *Figure 5.10* has been numbered on this basis.

Consider a case of compound hypermetropic astigmatism in which the ocular refraction is

$$+0.50 \, \text{DS}/+2.00 \, \text{DC axis} \, 90$$

with the accommodation fully relaxed. A distant object point would give rise to a horizontal focal line 0.50 D behind the retina, a circle of least confusion 1.50 D behind the retina, and a vertical focal line 2.50 D behind it, as in *Figure 5.10(a)*. In general, the effect of exerting A dioptres of ocular accommodation is to move all the features of the refracted pencil towards the eye's principal point by this same dioptric amount. Consequently, the exertion of first 0.50 D, then 1.50 D and finally 2.50 D of accommodation would place, in turn, the horizontal focal line, the circle of least confusion, and the vertical focal line on the retina, as shown respectively in *Figure 5.10(b)*, *(c)* and *(d)*. It should be noted that the dioptric separations between these various features of the refracted pencil remain unchanged by accommodation.

The best position of focus of an astigmatic pencil evidently lies within the region bounded by the two focal lines. The exact position depends on the nature of the object viewed. For example, the plane of the circles of least confusion would not be the best position of focus for an object consisting mainly of fine lines parallel to one of the eye's principal meridians.

Vision in uncorrected astigmatism

Unaided vision in the astigmatic eye is affected by a number of different factors: the amount of astigmatism, the type of astigmatism, and the axis direction.

Amount of astigmatism

It follows from equations (5.4)–(5.8) that, all other factors being equal, the dimensions of the focal lines and of the circle of least confusion of an astigmatic pencil are directly proportional to the amount of astigmatism in dioptres. This has a direct bearing on the unaided vision, subject to the other factors involved.

Type of astigmatism; mean ocular refraction

Consider a single pencil of rays from a distant object point. Given the pupil diameter, the retinal blur depends on which cross-section of the astigmatic pencil lies on the retina and on whether any improvement can be brought about by accommodation.

To simplify the discussion, we shall introduce the term 'mean ocular refraction' to denote the mean of the refractive errors in the two principal meridians of an astigmatic eye. For example, given an ocular refraction of $-1.00\,DS/-2.00\,DC$, indicating myopia of $-1.00\,D$ in one principal meridian and $-3.00\,D$ in the other, the mean ocular refraction would be $-2.00\,D$. It is evident that the mean ocular refraction gives the position of the circle of least confusion in terms of ametropia. In terms of the powers needed in the spectacle plane, this is often termed the mean refractive error, the mean sphere or the equivalent sphere.

In simple and compound myopic astigmatism, the distance vision cannot be improved by accommodation. In such cases the vision would be expected to be approximately the same as in spherical ametropia equal to the mean ocular refraction.

In cases of simple and compound hypermetropic astigmatism, the subject can place the most favourable cross-section of the astigmatic pencil on his retina, provided that sufficient accommodation is available. Suppose that the circle of least confusion is brought into focus. Equation (5.8) shows its diameter z to be given by

$$z = \frac{g\,Ast}{L'_\alpha + L'_\beta}$$

but the mean of the two image vergences L'_α and L'_β, must in this case be equal to the dioptric length K' of the eye and so

$$z = \frac{g\,Ast}{2K'} \tag{5.9}$$

In the case of spherical ametropia, however, we found the diameter j of the blur circle in the unaccommodated eye to be given by

$$j = \frac{gK}{K'} \tag{4.17}$$

Thus, for the same pupil diameter, the circle of least confusion given by x dioptres of astigmatism is only half the size of the blur circle given by the same amount of spherical ametropia.

This can be a useful pointer to the amount of astigmatism: the estimate for a case of spherical ametropia is simply doubled. For example, a vision of 6/18 would indicate spherical ametropia in the neighbourhood of 1.00 D or astigmatism of about 2.00 D if it could be assumed that the most favourable part of the pencil was focused on the retina.

In the unaccommodated eye with mixed astigmatism, only one focal line is behind the retina. There is thus, in general, a more limited scope for the improvement of vision by accommodation. Much depends on the position of the circle of least confusion, which may be in front of or behind the retina according to whether the mean ocular refraction is on the side of myopia or hypermetropia.

Axis direction

Since vertical and horizontal lines predominate in test letters as well as in most of the objects in our environment, vision is poorest when the ocular astigmatism is at an oblique axis, all other factors being equal. In printed matter, where lower-case letters predominate, there is no doubt that the vertical strokes are collectively the most important. One reason is that the ascending strokes of letters such as b, d, h and t are important clues to their recognition, as are the tails of letters such as p and y. Another important factor is that in printed matter there is usually less space between the letters on a line than between the lines themselves. Consequently, if horizontal focal lines or ellipses are being formed on the retina, the letters will appear to 'run together' and become indistinct or illegible.

Although the analogy should not be pushed too far, a reasonably good idea of the effect of astigmatic blurring can be given by photography. *Figure 5.11* shows a portion of a test chart of 5×5 test letters photographed normally and through a $+1.00\,DC$ plano-cylinder in four different axis settings. The effect of this lens is to simulate the condition of simple myopic astigmatism. Though there is little to choose between the 90° and 180° directions, the legibility is markedly inferior in the oblique directions. For comparison, a photograph with a blur from a $+0.50\,D$ spherical lens is included.

Figure 5.12 presents a similar set of photographs of part of a reading test card in Times Roman lettering. In this case there is a marked difference between the vertical and horizontal axis setting, the print being quite legible when the vertical lines are in focus but nearly illegible when they are blurred.

Perhaps the best way for the student to study the effects of uncorrected astigmatism on vision is by simulating various astigmatic refractive states with the aid of trial lenses. They should be held close to one eye while the other is occluded. An illuminated pinhole, an illuminated narrow slit and a Snellen letter chart provide excellent test objects for this purpose.

The stenopaeic slit

This simple device was once in fairly common use as a means of testing for astigmatism, sometimes as an adjunct to an optometer. Greatly superior methods have now taken its place, but there is a certain historical interest attached to the device, and the principle on which it is based may still find occasional applications.

The stenopaeic slit is a trial case accessory consisting of an opaque disc having a central slit aperture about 1 mm in width. Correctly centred, it has the effect of reducing the effective pupil diameter in the meridian perpendicular to the slit.

The first use of the device is to locate the principal meridians of the astigmatic eye. Provided that the individual blurs (focal lines or ellipses) composing the ret-

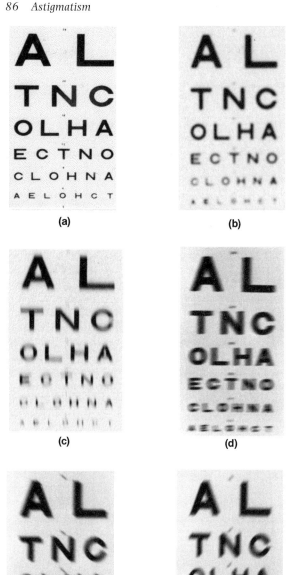

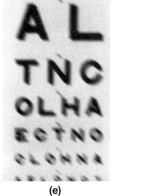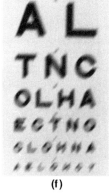

Figure 5.11. Portion of test chart photographed: (a) in focus, (b) through a +0.50 DS lens, (c) through a +1.00 DC lens at axis 180, (d) axis 90, (e) axis 135, (f) axis 45. A 5.7 mm aperture and the supplementary lenses were placed near the principal planes of a 135 mm telephoto lens, the 1 D error giving a blur ratio for the 18 m line of approximately 0.54 for the object distance of −2.5 m.

inal image are sufficiently elongated, rotation of the slit will enable a 'best position' to be found. This will clearly occur when the slit is perpendicular to the major axis of these blur ellipses or focal lines.

The next step is to carry out a subjective refraction, using spherical lenses only, first with the slit in the best position and then turned through 90°. In each case the best sphere should approximate to the spectacle refraction in the meridian of the slit. For example, if the best sphere is −1.50 D with the slit along 90° and −0.50 D

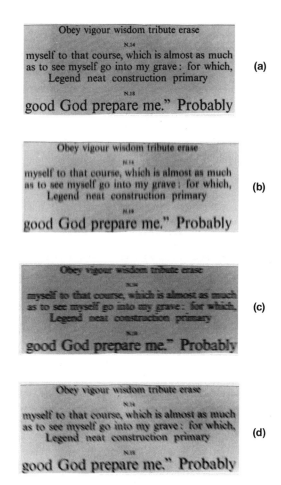

Figure 5.12. Portion of a near test chart photographed (a) in focus, (b) through a +0.50 DC lens at axis 180, (c) axis 90, (d) axis 45. Blur ratio for the N14 letters approximately, 0.67 ($\ell = -540$ mm, other details as for *Figure 5.11*).

with the slit at 180°, the refractive error is approximately −0.50 DS/−1.00 DC × 180.

The diagram in *Figure 5.13* will help to explain this rule. The upper part (a) of the diagram shows a typical astigmatic pencil when the entrance pupil is circular, the principal meridians being horizontal and vertical and the astigmatism with the rule. The lower part (b) of the diagram illustrates the action of the stenopaeic slit when it is vertical. The waist of the pencil is accentuated and is displaced such that the focal plane of the vertical rays is in the middle of the region of best focus. It will be seen that there are two different positions, denoted by Z_1 and Z_2 where the cross-section of the pencil is approximately circular, having the same width in both principal meridians. A similar diagram would show that when the slit is turned to the horizontal, the region of best focus then straddles the focal plane of the horizontal rays.

Residual errors: obliquely crossed cylinders

Suppose that an eye needs a cylinder correction of −1.50 DC × 20 but is given −1.00 DC × 10. There will

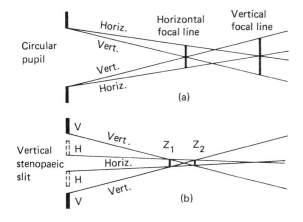

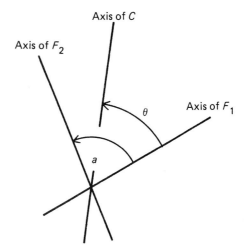

Figure 5.13. (a) The refracted astigmatic pencil with its two principal meridians superimposed. (b) The reduction in width of the pencil in the horizontal meridian, caused by a stenopaeic slit with its length vertical.

Figure 5.14. Compounding obliquely crossed cylinders: the positive sign convention for anticlockwise acute angles.

be remaining a 'residual error', meaning the power of the *additional* lens needed to put matters right. First, the incorrect lens must be neutralized, in this example by $+1.00$ DC $\times$ 10 and then the correct lens added, -1.50 DC $\times$ 20. The residual error is the sum of these two. To resolve this combination we must resort to the theory of obliquely crossed cylinders.

There are two basic theorems. The first is that a combination of any two or more cylinders placed in contact with their axes at random has the same fundamental properties as a single sphero-cylinder. This statement may easily be verified with two trial case cylinders and a focimeter. Two different power readings in mutually perpendicular meridians will invariably be obtained.

The second proposition is that the sum of the two given cylinder powers, F_1 and F_2, is equal to the sum of the two principal powers of the equivalent sphero-cylinder. Let the spherical power of this latter be denoted by S and its cylindrical power by C. Then its principal powers are S and $(S + C)$ and

$$F_1 + F_2 = S + (S + C)$$

which gives

$$S = \tfrac{1}{2}(F_1 + F_2 - C) \qquad (5.10)$$

This expression enables us to find the spherical power of the equivalent sphero-cylinder as soon as its cylindrical power has been determined.

A graphical solution

The complete resolution of two obliquely crossed cylinders can be carried out by a well-known graphical construction. The first step is to set out the given data. To avoid mistakes at this stage, an angle convention must be followed. As shown in *Figure 5.14*, the positive (anticlockwise) angle a between the given cylinder axes is the *acute* angle measured *from* the axis of the F_1 cylinder *to* the axis of the F_2 cylinder. It is wise to draw or visualize these axes before deciding which of the cylinders should be labelled F_1. For example, if the two axes are 20° and 140°, F_1 is the cylinder at axis 140 and the angle a is 60°. The axis direction of the resultant

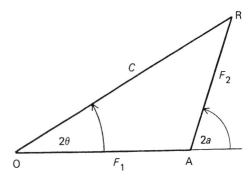

Figure 5.15. Graphical construction for compounding two obliquely crossed cylinders of like sign.

cylinder C is expressed by the angle θ measured *from* the F_1 cylinder. When the obliquely crossed cylinders are of like sign, the relationship illustrated in *Figure 5.14* will invariably hold good. The equivalent spherocylinder having the same sign as F_1 and F_2 will have its axis *within* the angle a and nearer to the axis of the stronger given cylinder.

A distinctive feature of the conventional graphical method is that the angles a and θ are doubled. *Figure 5.15* shows the construction when the two given cylinders are of like sign. On a chosen scale, OA is drawn proportional to F_1 and AR proportional to F_2 making an angle $2a$ with OA. The resultant cylinder power C, of the same sign as F_1 and F_2, is proportional to OR and makes a positive angle 2θ with OA.

If the cylinders are of opposite sign, the construction is modified as in *Figure 5.16*. The line AR is drawn below OA, and the resultant cylinder is of the same sign as F_1. In this construction, the angle 2θ becomes clockwise and therefore negative in sign. Consequently, the axis of the resultant cylinder is that of F_1 minus θ.

Mathematical solutions

Mathematical solutions for the resultant of two obliquely crossed cylinders have been devised in the form

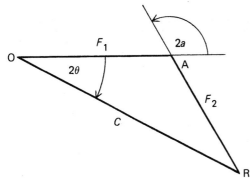

Figure 5.16. Graphical construction for compounding two obliquely crossed cylinders of opposite sign.

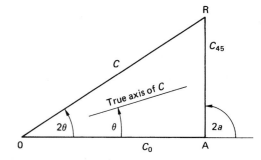

Figure 5.17. Graphical construction based on *Figure 5.15* for the combination of two cylinders C_0 and C_{45} at axes $0°$ and $45°$ respectively to produce an oblique cylinder of power C at axis θ.

of various sequences of equations. The most convenient of them seems to be the following. First, the resultant cylinder C is found from

$$C = \sqrt{(F_1 + F_2)^2 - 4F_1 F_2 \sin^2 a} \qquad (5.11)$$

Next,

$$\theta = \arctan \frac{-F_1 + F_2 + C}{F_1 + F_2 + C} \tan a \qquad (5.12)$$

Finally, the resultant spherical power S is found from equation (5.10).

There is, however, a much simpler solution which needs no preliminary arrangement of data, dispenses with the angle a altogether, and can cope with *any* number of astigmatic lens or surface powers with the axes at random. It is described in the section immediately following.

Astigmatic decomposition

The theory of obliquely crossed cylinders, first propounded by Stokes (1883), shows that any combination of plano-cylinders in contact with their axes at random is equivalent, in general, to a single sphero-cylinder. A corollary to this theorem is that any given cylinder is replaceable by a combination of two separate cylinders with their axes in any specified meridians. On this basis, Dr W. E. Humphrey was able to incorporate a new method of refraction in the Humphrey Vision Analyser which he designed (Chapter 19). In effect, the correcting cylinder of power C is the resultant of two components, C_0 at axis $0°$ and C_{45} at axis $45°$. As explained in Chapter 19, the preliminary step of locating the eye's principal meridians is thereby made unnecessary.

Humphrey's principle of 'astigmatic decomposition' can further be utilized to produce the simplest of all methods of performing calculations involving obliquely crossed cylinders. As a first step, each of the given cylinders is decomposed into its C_0 and C_{45} components, which need not be of like sign. When expressed in such a form, cylinders become additive if due regard is paid to their signs and to resultant spherical components.

The construction illustrated in *Figures 5.15* and *5.16* is followed in *Figure 5.17* in which OA represents C_0 and AR represents C_{45}. Since all angles have to be doubled, AR is at right-angles to OA. The length OR

represents the cylindrical element of C_0 and C_{45} in combination. Conversely, C_0 and C_{45} are components into which a given cylinder of power C can be resolved, its axis direction (θ in standard notation) being half the angle AOR. From *Figure 5.17* it is evident that

$$C_0 = C \cos 2\theta \qquad (5.13)$$
$$C_{45} = C \sin 2\theta \qquad (5.14)$$

and

$$C = \sqrt{C_0^2 + C_{45}^2} \qquad (5.15)$$

To deal with the spherical element of power we can take advantage of another additive property, the mean power M of an astigmatic lens, often termed the 'mean sphere'. This is the algebraic mean of the two principal powers, which are S and $(S + C)$. Hence,

$$M = S + C/2 \qquad (5.16)$$

The new method of calculation is to express each of the given lens or surface powers in terms of C_0, C_{45} and M, to find their respective algebraic sums, ΣC_0, ΣC_{45}, and ΣM, and then to re-convert these totals into orthodox sphero-cylinder notation.

In the following numerical example there are only two astigmatic lens or surface powers to be summed. This is the usual form in which the problem arises.

Example (5)

Find the resultant of the combination of

$$-2.75\,\mathrm{DS}/ + 1.00\,\mathrm{DC} \times 10$$

and

$$+4.25\,\mathrm{DS}/ - 1.50\,\mathrm{DC} \times 20$$

Table 5.1 Worked example of a method of calculating the resultant of any number of astigmatic lens or surface powers

Given prescription			Required components		
Sphere S	Cylinder C	Axis θ	C_0 $C \cos 2\theta$	C_{45} $C \sin 2\theta$	M $S + C/2$
−2.75	+1.00	10	+0.940	+0.342	−2.25
+4.25	−1.50	20	−1.149	−0.964	+3.50
			ΣC_0	ΣC_{45}	ΣM
	Summation		−0.209	−0.622	+1.25

Since equations (5.13) and (5.14) represent additive quantities, the resultant cylinder C_R can be found from

$$C_R = \sqrt{(\Sigma C_0)^2 + (\Sigma C_{45})^2} \qquad (5.17)$$

The sign taken must be the same as that for ΣC_0. In this case,

$$C_R = -\sqrt{0.0437 + 0.3869}$$
$$= -0.656\,\text{D}$$

Next, the axis θ_R of the resultant cylinder C_R of the sign specified above is given by

$$\theta_R = \tfrac{1}{2}\arctan\left(\Sigma C_{45}/\Sigma C_0\right) \qquad (5.18)$$
$$= 35.7°$$

Alternatively, C_R may be given either sign and θ_R evaluated from

$$\theta_R = \arctan\left\{(C_R - \Sigma C_0)/\Sigma C_{45}\right\} \qquad (5.18a)$$

If θ_R emerges from either routine with a minus sign, $180°$ should be added to it.

Finally, the spherical power S_R of the combination can be found by transposing equation (5.16) into

$$S_R = \Sigma M - C_R/2 \qquad (5.19)$$
$$= +1.25 + 0.328 = +1.578\,\text{D}$$

Rounded off, the resultant is

$$+1.58\,\text{DS}/-0.66\,\text{DC} \times 36°$$

It is left as an exercise for the student to compare this result with that obtained from the graphical construction of *Figure 5.16*.

Astigmatic analysis

Mean of many values

The technique of astigmatic decomposition may be extended to find the mean of any number of astigmatic values. As shown by Bennett (1984), each astigmatic power is expressed as its Humphrey components (C_0, C_{45} and M), and the individual components summed. Proceeding exactly as for the resultant of two obliquely crossed cylinders, the subsequent totals may be used to find the resultant. If, for example, the sum of six astigmatic values is: $\Sigma C_0 = -13.28$, $\Sigma C_{45} = -4.13$ and $\Sigma M = -11.50$, the resultant sphero-cylinder is $-4.55\,\text{DS}/-13.91\,\text{DC} \times 8.6$. If, however, the mean value is needed, the subtotals should be divided by the number of values before calculating the conventional power. *Table 21.6* gives a further example.

Subtraction of cylinders

The difference between two values may also be determined by the Humphrey method. For example, suppose an estimate of a patient's refractive error was $+3.25\,\text{DS}/-2.25\,\text{DC} \times 10$ and the final prescription given was $+3.75\,\text{DS}/-3.00\,\text{DC} \times 12$, then the difference between the two may be given either by subtracting the components as shown in *Table 5.2*, or by adding the power that neutralizes the second value to that of the

Table 5.2 Worked example of a method of calculating the difference between a pair of astigmatic lenses or values

Sphere S	Cylinder C	Axis θ	C_0 $C\cos 2\theta$	C_{45} $C\sin 2\theta$	M $S + C/2$
+3.75	−3.00	12	−2.74	−1.22	+2.25
+3.25	−2.25	10	−2.11	−0.77	+2.125
			ΔC_0	ΔC_{45}	ΔM
	Difference		−0.63	−0.45	+0.125

giving, in conventional form, $+0.51\,\text{DS}/-0.77\,\text{DC} \times 18$

first, i.e. reversing the signs of both sphere and cylinder of the first value.

Scalar representation of astigmatism

Three values are required to specify a sphero-cylindrical power, namely either the spherical and cylindrical powers and cylinder axis, or the two principal meridional powers and the orientation of one of these. Although $+2.00\,\text{DS}/-1.00\,\text{DC} \times 20$ and $+2.00\,\text{DS}/-1.00\,\text{DC} \times 50$ have the same principal powers, their orientation is different. For some purposes, it is useful to be able to represent such powers by a single scalar quantity, u. The Humphrey components may again be used, as in equation (5.20):

$$u = \sqrt{C_0^2 + C_{45}^2 + M^2} \qquad (5.20)$$

the positive root, in general, being taken irrespective of the sign of the components. The value of u for both these two powers is $+1.80$. Thus the difference between two powers cannot be represented by the difference in their scalar values, but a scalar value can be found for the difference. Thus in this example, the difference between the two powers is $+0.50\,\text{DS}/-1.00\,\text{DC} \times 170$, giving a scalar difference of 1.00.

Comparison between a series of retinoscopy (Chapter 17) or autorefractor (Chapter 18) results and subjective refraction (Chapter 6) values can thus easily be evaluated – Rabbetts (1996). As pointed out by McCaghrey and Matthews (1993), the disadvantage of always taking the positive root for a scalar quantity such as u is that it is impossible to differentiate between findings where, say, the retinoscopy result is always more positive than the subjective from results where the findings may be more or less positive. A suggestion here would be to give u the same sign as that of the mean sphere M of the difference.

An alternative method for deriving a similar scalar value was presented in the series of papers by Harris and co-workers; for example, Harris (1988, 1994), Harris and Malan (1992). The two methods were brought together by Harris (1996). The properties of the oblique cylinder components of the Humphrey decomposition method have been further amplified by Thibos, Wheeler and Horner (1996). They also point out that this method of analysis was first developed by Gartner (1965).

The Stokes lens

The Stokes lens is a variable cylinder named after its inventor and described by him in 1849. Sometimes used as an ophthalmic trial case accessory, it consists of two plano-cylinders of equal and opposite power ($\pm F$) mounted in a cell and geared to rotate equally in opposite directions from a zero setting. In this setting, the two cylinder axes coincide, resulting in neutralization. When the lenses have been rotated so as to make an angle a between their axes, the resultant cylinder power is equal to $2F \sin a$ with its axis always at $45°$ to the zero setting. There is also a resultant spherical power of $-F \sin a$. The mean power of the combination is invariably zero. A Stokes lens has been used in a number of ophthalmic instruments. Mounted on a suitable handle, it would serve as a cross cylinder (Chapter 6) of variable power.

Irregular astigmatism

Astigmatism of the type discussed so far is termed 'regular' because it possesses a certain symmetry and is correctable by suitable lenses.

Irregular astigmatism – a better term for which would be irregular refraction – denotes a condition in which poor focusing results from asymmetrical or local variations in the curvature of one or more of the eye's refracting surfaces, notably the cornea. In severe cases only a contact lens will give satisfactory results. Irregular refraction may also be caused by local variations in the refractive index of the crystalline lens.

In reality, no sharp dividing line can be drawn between regular and irregular astigmatism. No eye is free from some irregularities and some degree of asymmetry and it would be a mistake to imagine that the refracted pencils in a typical astigmatic eye bear more than a general resemblance to the neat geometrical structure illustrated in *Figure 5.4*.

In 1924, Tscherning suggested that irregular astigmatism is most conveniently studied by observing, at various distances or through various lenses, an illuminated pinhole of about 0.2 or 0.3 mm diameter (Tscherning, 1924). From the varying size and shape of the blurred image, and by occluding different parts of the pupil in turn, it is possible to make certain deductions about the nature of the refracted pencils. Tscherning stated some useful rules relevant to this interpretation.

Figure 5.18, reproduced from Chapter 10 of Tscherning's book, illustrates the appearance of a luminous point as seen at different distances by his right eye. Row A refers to vision through the whole pupil, row B to vision when the lower half of the pupil was occluded and row C to the upper half occluded. The columns (a) to (d) relate respectively to viewing distances of 60 cm, 1 m, 1.5 m and 'infinity'. Tscherning remarks that 'these figures are, up to a certain point, analogous to those which are obtained with a lens placed obliquely'. It will be noted that all the figures show marked symmetry about a nearly vertical axis. The streaky appearance of some of the figures is produced by the fibrous structure of the crystalline lens.

In cases of marked irregular refraction, a pinhole disc will generally improve the best visual acuity otherwise obtainable, by isolating a relatively homogeneous portion of the eye's optical system.

Historical notes

The concept of astigmatism originated with Newton, who was the first to pay attention to rays in the plane now called sagittal, perpendicular to the (tangential) plane of the diagram. Newton discovered that rays in these two planes are focused at different distances if the

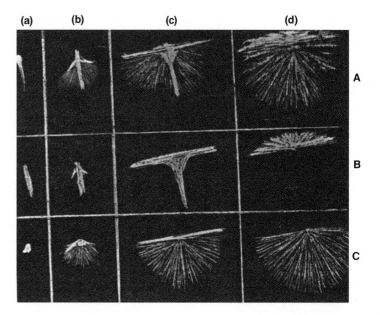

Figure 5.18. Self-drawn appearances of a luminous point to Tscherning's right eye. Columns (a) to (d): viewing distances of 60 cm, 1 m, 1.5 m and infinity respectively. Row A: view with full pupil; row B: with lower half of pupil covered; row C with upper half covered. (Reproduced from Tscherning, 1924.)

incident pencil is oblique and he devised elegant graphical methods of constructing both foci.

There is nothing in Newton's *Opticks* or in his *Optical Lectures* devoted to either axial or ocular astigmatism, but he did make some interesting speculations as to which section of an astigmatic pencil would be selected by an eye for focusing on the retina. As pointed out by Bennett (1961), the section which he suggested as the most probable can be shown to be that containing the circle of least confusion.

After Newton, the subject seemed to arouse little interest until Young turned his attention to it towards the end of the eighteenth century. In his famous Bakerian Lecture to the Royal Society, delivered in 1800, Young presented the results of a brilliant series of experiments and theoretical calculations on the dioptric system of the eye.

Incidentally to his main purpose, which was to identify the mechanism of accommodation, Young determined the refraction of one of his own eyes, finding it to be (in our notation) about 4.00 D myopic in the vertical meridian and 5.75 D myopic in the horizontal. This is the first recorded astigmatic refraction. Since Young also discovered that the same amount of astigmatism remained when his cornea was immersed in water, he concluded that his own astigmatism must be due to an obliquity of the crystalline lens. He remarked that it had never troubled him and that he had been unaware of it before he started his experiments.

In the same lecture Young expounded his own contribution to the study of oblique astigmatism, and one of his diagrams showed various cross-sections of the astigmatic pencil formed by oblique refraction. Another diagram showed what we would now term the tangential and sagittal image shells formed by the successive refracting surfaces of the eye, from which Young concluded that the curvature of the retina has the required value for optimum focusing over a wide field.

It was in 1825 that Airy read his famous paper to the Cambridge Philosophical Society describing how he had measured the refraction of his own astigmatic eye and had had a sphero-cylindrical lens specially made to correct it. This and subsequent papers by Airy on the same subject evoked a world-wide interest.

After Airy's discourse had been given, but before it appeared in print in 1827, hints on the use of Young's optometer for determining the ocular refraction in two mutually perpendicular meridians had been published by a remarkable English engineer, J. I. Hawkins (1826). A printed music stave was suggested as a suitable test object. Hawkins described not only how he worked out a sphero-cylindrical correction for himself, but also how he had it made up in trifocal form, each separate portion being correctly centred and angled. His paper is an astonishing *tour de force* for a layman.

Another English contribution to the study of astigmatism is the term itself, attributed to Dr Whewell who became Master of Trinity College Cambridge in 1841 and Vice-Chancellor of the University in 1855.

A detailed account of progress in the study and correction of astigmatism from 1800 onwards can be found in the work by Levene (1977).

Exercises

5.1 The principal powers of a reduced astigmatic eye are +62.00 D in the horizontal and +64.00 D in the vertical meridian. The eye has the normal emmetropic length, a pupil of 6 mm, and it views a distant point source. Calculate: (a) the position of the two focal lines and the circle of least confusion, (b) the lengths of the two focal lines and the diameter of the circle of least confusion, (c) the dimensions of the blurred patch on the retina.

5.2 A 60-metre Landolt ring is viewed at 6 m by an unaccommodated uncorrected eye of ocular refraction −1.00 DS/ −4.00 DC axis 90 and of pupil diameter 6 mm. Calculate the apparent size of the blur ellipse corresponding to a point on the object when projected to a distance of 6 m. On a scale one-half actual size, draw the projected blur patch alongside the 60-metre ring and discuss the apparent blurred appearance of the latter. Assume the eye to be of normal length.

5.3 An astigmatic chart consisting of four thin lines each 100 mm long intersecting centrally at 45° intervals is viewed at 1 m by an uncorrected eye whose ocular refraction is −3.00 DS/−3.00 DC axis 45. Draw a careful enlarged diagram of the blurred retinal image, indicating the scale. Assume that the eye has the normal length and a pupil diameter of 6 mm.

5.4 An unaccommodated uncorrected eye with pupil diameter 10 mm has an ocular refraction of +2.00 DS/−4.00 DC axis 180. The eye views a distant point source of light through a centred pinhole disc in which there are two pinholes, A and B, each of diameter 2 mm and with centres 5 mm apart symmetrically disposed about the disc centre. From simple geometrical considerations describe the illumination on the retina when the line of the pinhole centres is: (a) horizontal with A lying outwards, (b) vertical with A lying upwards, (c) in meridian 45° with A lying up and out. If pinhole A is occluded in each case, describe how the observer looking through the disc would see its apparent eclipse.

5.5 An eye provided with a centred pinhole disc views a cross-line with its limbs, each 100 mm long, horizontal and vertical. The cross-line chart is 1 m from the eye and mid-way between them is a circular lens of diameter 50 mm and power +2.00 DS/+2.00 DC axis 90. How will the cross-line appear to the eye viewing through the lens? Give an explanation with diagrams.

5.6 An uncorrected and unaccommodated eye sees clearly a vertical line at a distance of 850 mm and a horizontal line at a distance of 270 mm from its principal point. What lens fitted at 14 mm from the reduced surface would correct this eye for distance? What is the ocular refraction?

5.7 An astigmatic reduced eye has an axial length of 26 mm and principal powers of +62.00 D along 30° and +59.50 D along 120°. What is the power of the distance correcting lens needed if placed at 13 mm from the reduced surface?

5.8 A patient has a spectacle correction of +10.00/ −4.00 × 90 at 15 mm. Calculate: (a) the ocular refraction and (b) the spectacle correction required at 12 mm (suitably rounded off).

5.9 A patient has a spectacle correction of −6.00/ −4.00 × 180 at 15 mm. Calculate: (a) the ocular refraction and (b) the spectacle correction required at 12 mm (suitably rounded off).

5.10 From the results of Exercises 5.8 and 5.9, formulate a qualitative relationship between ocular astigmatism and the necessary spectacle cylinder correction in compound hypermetropia and compound myopia.

5.11 A patient with an uncorrected refractive error of +1.00/−5.00 × 180 views a distant spotlight without accommodating. Draw to scale the blur ellipse when viewed through: (a) the natural 4 mm pupil and (b) through a stenopaeic slit 1 mm wide orientated (i) along 180°, (ii) along 90° and (iii) along 135° (Hint: draw an isometric diagram for this last orientation.)

5.12 Find the resultant of three +1.00 D plano-cylinders placed in contact with their respective axes at 10°, 40°, and 70°.

References

AIRY, G.B. (1827) On a peculiar defect in the eye and a mode of correcting it. *Trans. Camb. Phil. Soc. 1825*, **2**, 267–271

BENNETT, A.G. (1961) Some unfamiliar British contributions to geometrical optics. *International Optical Congress 1961*, pp. 274–291. London: British Optical Association

BENNETT, A.G. (1984) A new approach to the statistical analysis of ocular astigmatism and astigmatic prescriptions. In Trans. First International Congress, *The Frontiers of Optometry* (W. N. Charman, ed.), Vol 2, pp.35–42, British College of Ophthalmic Opticians (Optometrists)

GARTNER, W.F. (1965) Astigmatism and optometric vectors. *Am. J. Optom.*, **53**, 459–463

HARRIS, W.F. (1988) Algebra of sphero-cylinders and refractive errors, and their means, variance and standard deviation. *Am. J. Optom.*, **65**, 794–802

HARRIS, W.F. (1994) Dioptric strength: a scalar representation of dioptric power. *Ophthal. Physiol. Opt.*, **14**, 216–218

HARRIS, W.F. (1996) Author's reply to Rabbetts (1996). *Ophthal. Physiol. Opt.*, **16**, 261–262

HARRIS, W.F. and MALAN, D.J. (1992) Meridional profiles of variance–covariance of dioptric power. Part 2. Profiles representing variation in one or more of sphere, cylinder and axis. *Ophthal. Physiol. Opt.*, **12**, 471–477

HAWKINS, J.I. (1826) On the means of ascertaining the true state of the eye, and of enabling persons to supply themselves with spectacles, the best adapted to their sight. *Repertory of Patent Inventions*, **3**, 347–353, 385–392 + plate VIII

LEVENE, J.R. (1977) *Clinical Refraction and Visual Science*, pp. 203–285. London: Butterworths

MCCAGHREY, G.E. and MATTHEWS, F.E. (1993) Matters arising – residual refraction. *Ophthal. Physiol. Opt.*, **13**, 432–433

RABBETTS, R.B. (1996) Scalar representation of astigmatism. *Ophthal. Physiol. Opt.*, **16**, 257–260

STOKES, G.G. (1883) *Mathematical and Physical Papers*, Vol. 2, pp. 172–175. Cambridge: Cambridge University Press

THIBOS, L.N., WHEELER, W. and HORNER, D. (1996) Power vectors, an application of Fourier analysis to the description and statistical analysis of refractive error. *Optom. Vision Sci.*, **74**, 367–380

TSCHERNING, M. (1898) *Optique Physiologique*. Paris: Carré et Naud

TSCHERNING, M. (1924) *Physiologic Optics*, 4th edn (English translation by C. Weiland). Philadelphia: Keystone Publishing Co.

YOUNG, T. (1801) On the mechanism of the eye. *Phil. Trans. R. Soc. 1800*, **92**, 23–88 + plates

6

Subjective refraction

Introduction

A patient may wish to have an eye examination for one of many reasons such as poor vision either at distance or in close work, asthenopic symptoms such as head or eye aches or for a general check on the state of his eyes. An eye examination consists of four main parts: checking the health of the eyes, measuring any optical errors of focusing, evaluating the efficiency with which the two eyes work together and deciding whether to prescribe some form of optical correction or treatment (such as orthoptic training) to improve the binocular functioning of the eyes.

The patient's refractive error, or refraction as it is often called, may be estimated by two broad methods: objective and subjective. The former requires no help from the patient except to look in a certain direction or into an instrument, the adjustments being made by the examiner (*see* Chapters 17 and 18). Subjective refraction requires the co-operation of the subject and many of the specific techniques will be discussed in this chapter. Although it is based on scientific principles, the experienced refractionist realizes that subjective work is partly an art; the ability to know which method to use for a particular patient and the ease with which understanding is established with patients can come only with experience.

In general, a patient's refractive error is first estimated objectively. There may be errors involved in an objective measurement, so the refraction is usually checked subjectively in order to refine it. There are patients, for example, young children, with whom it is not possible to make a satisfactory subjective examination, in which case the prescriber relies on the objective results alone. In order to impart a thorough understanding of the methods of subjective work, it is better, however, to describe subjective refraction without assuming an initial objective assessment. The later parts of this chapter will describe how the various subjective techniques are normally linked with a prior objective refraction. Some of the more sophisticated methods of balancing the monocular findings will then be discussed.

Unaided vision and refractive error

The first step in measuring a refractive error is to determine the patient's unaided vision with each eye separately and then binocularly. As shown in Chapter 4, myopia will cause a reduction in distance vision from a standard which is usually taken as 6/6 or better. A hypermetropic error may also cause a reduction in vision, depending on the ability of the eye to increase its refractive power by accommodation. In a young person there is usually ample accommodation and such a patient with a small or medium hypermetropic error will be able to read the small lines on the test chart. Even so, prolonged use of the eyes for detailed vision may cause discomfort since more than the usual amount of accommodation is required. The maximum power of accommodation declines with age (*see* Chapter 7), therefore an older person with even a small hypermetropic error of one or two dioptres will have reduced vision.

An astigmatic error may be combined with either myopia or hypermetropia. With myopia or high hypermetropia, both the astigmatic and spherical components of the error reduce the unaided vision. When astigmatism is combined with a low hypermetropic error in a young patient, accommodation can be brought into action so as to place either of the focal lines or the circle of least confusion on to the retina. Even so, vision is usually reduced. With a small astigmatic error, the vision may be almost normal, but if either focal line may be brought on to the retina, accommodation is unstable and asthenopic symptoms often result. Paradoxically, a larger astigmatic error may cause less asthenopia, because the vision is too poor to stimulate alternations of the level of accommodation between the two astigmatic foci. Moreover, the change in accommodation required may be too great for easy adjustment. If the axes of the error are approximately horizontal or vertical, unaided vision is often reduced less than with an oblique error; this is because most letters are composed of vertical and horizontal strokes.

Table 6.1, which is based on the studies plotted in *Figure 4.18*, gives the approximate relationship between unaided vision and spherical and astigmatic ametropia. With modern apparatus using non-serif letters and higher luminances, the predicted ametropia may be slightly higher than the figures tabulated. For example, a score of 6/12 (20/40) is often possible with ametropia of 1.00 D.

The predicted vision in astigmatism is tabulated on the assumption that the circles of least confusion lie on or close to the retina, either naturally or with the aid of accommodation or trial lenses. The vision with a given

Table 6.1 Expected vision in various ametropic states

Vision	Refractive error (D)	
	Spherical*	Astigmatic
6/6 (20/20)	small	small
6/9 (20/30)	0.50	1.00
6/12 (20/40)	0.75	1.50
6/18 (20/60)	1.00	2.00
6/24 (20/80)	1.50	3.00
6/36 (20/120)	2.00	4.00
6/60 (20/200)	2.00 to 3.00	high

* Myopia or absolute hypermetropia.

Note: The predicted vision in astigmatism is on the assumption that the circles of least confusion lie on or close to the retina.

dioptric value of astigmatism is better than for the same amount of spherical ametropia (compare equations (4.17) and (5.9)). For a patient already wearing spectacles, or halfway through a subjective routine, *Table 6.1* can be used to predict the remaining error.

This table is reasonably accurate for a pupil size of about 4 mm. With much larger pupils, which can occur in young patients or in low illumination, the same deterioration in vision will be caused by a smaller error. Conversely, a patient with small pupils, about 2 mm, will be able to see better than predicted for the refractive error. A patient who is used to being undercorrected may see far better than expected from the size of the error, because he or she is used to interpreting blurred images, whereas a person who has recently broken his spectacles will be more greatly handicapped and may accordingly be led to the erroneous conclusion that the spectacles have made the sight worse.

Some people habitually squeeze their eyelids together in order to see clearer: reducing the effective pupil size decreases the retinal blurs. This habit or manoeuvre is sometimes erroneously called 'squinting'.

The practitioner can make use of the pinhole disc to test whether reduced vision is due to poor focusing or to a retinal defect such as amblyopia or macular degeneration. If the pinhole – about 1 or 1.5 mm diameter – improves the vision, then in general there is ametropia to be corrected. An exception to this rule occurs when opacities in the ocular media produce an irregular focusing effect. In this case the pinhole may give a better acuity than a lens alone if it isolates a small region which is sufficiently homogeneous to give a good focus.

Basic equipment for refraction

The distance test chart has already been discussed in Chapter 3. By convention, the normal testing distance is 6 m or 20 ft but is sometimes varied slightly to suit the size of the consulting room. To enable the patient to adopt a comfortable posture, the chart should be placed at an average eye-level. Frequently, a reversed or indirect chart is used, viewed by the patient in a mirror. In this case, the mirror and image of the chart should be at the patient's eye level, the mirror being angled if necessary to enable the test chart or cabinet to be

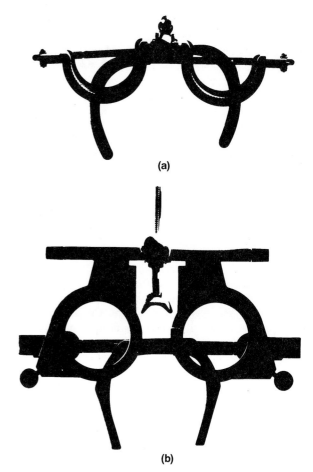

(a)

(b)

Figure 6.1. (a) Oculus drop cell and (b) rotating cell trial frames. Photographs reproduced by kind permission of Oculus Optikgeräte GmbH.

placed at a greater height convenient for the practitioner.

It is important that the mirror should be large enough so that the test-chart surroundings are visible even to patients not of average height or tending to sit to one side. If the mirror is framed, the colour of the frame should merge with the surrounding wall. This reduces any tendency on the patient's part to accommodate for the distance of the mirror instead of attempting to relax his accommodation as fully as possible.

The room illumination should be at a comfortable indoor level: pupils dilate in the dark and a refraction under these conditions will be influenced by the aberrations due to the peripheral parts of the eye's optical system. The correction found under these conditions may not be the best for use in daylight out of doors with a normal size pupil. A trial case of separate lenses is a necessity, even if a refracting unit (or phoropter) is normally in use. Trial case lenses are placed in a trial frame (*Figure 6.1*) worn by the patient, or, less frequently, supported by a wall bracket. They may either be full aperture, about 38 mm diameter, or of a reduced aperture of 20 mm or so in a full-size mount. The larger lenses enable the practitioner to obtain a better view of the patient's eyes and similarly give the patient a larger field of view. On the other hand, reduced-aperture lenses are lighter and thinner. They are better protected by the wide rim and less likely to break if dropped. The wide rim also tends to prevent finger marks on the lenses and permits clearer power markings. A further advantage is that the trial sets are available in a more extensive range of fractional powers than full-aperture trial sets.

In a refracting unit, discs of reduced-aperture lenses are so mounted that any sphero-cylinder combination can quickly and easily be placed before the patient's eye.

Such units are large and must be mounted mechanically. As a result, the patient's head has to be kept pressed against the unit, which can be uncomfortable. Also, in some designs the unit cannot be tilted, which means that near vision testing has to be undertaken in a horizontal plane. Nevertheless, refracting units have many practical advantages.

The designs of trial lenses, whether for use with a trial frame or in a refracting unit, raises several problems arising from effectivity, that is, the effect of lens form, thicknesses and separations on the vergence of the emergent pencils of light. As far as distance vision is concerned, these problems can be overcome by designs based on the principle of additive vertex powers, but in near vision the full-aperture symmetrical and reduced-aperture curved forms are generally superior (*see also* Report of a Ministry of Health Committee, 1956; Bennett, 1968).

The trial frame or refracting unit should carefully be centred to the patient's inter-pupillary distance (abbreviated to PD). There are specialized instruments for measuring the PD (*see* page 221), but reasonable accuracy may be obtained with a simple ruler or, better still, a rule with a fixed cursor at the zero of the scale and a movable cursor. The rule is held in the spectacle plane and the patient is directed to look at the examiner's right eye. Using this eye, the examiner lines up the zero cursor with the centre of the patient's left pupil. With the rule still held in this position, the patient's attention is redirected to the examiner's left eye, and using this eye the second cursor is lined up with the centre of the patient's right pupil. This gives the distance PD. The near PD is measured by asking the patient to look at one of the examiner's eyes, the examiner leaning forward so that the distance from patient to practitioner is the same as the usual working distance. The cursors are lined up with this eye alone, the rule again being held in the spectacle plane.

Available trial case accessories include centring discs, which can be used in a similar manner to adjust the trial frame directly to the patient's PD. They also facilitate the vertical adjustment* which is no less important than the horizontal centration. Another necessary adjustment, made by angling the sides, is to set the plane of the lenses at right-angles to the line of sight.

---

* Trial frames and many refractor heads cannot be adjusted to compensate for a marked vertical difference in eye and pupil positions. With some patients, the final spectacles may best be fitted off the horizontal so as to match the brow line, in which case the trial frame may be similarly tilted. In other cases, the spectacles and trial frame or refractor head should remain horizontal. An allowance for induced prism, such as discussed on pages 263–265, may then be needed.

Finally, the projection of the trial frame should be adjusted so that the vertex distance, as far as can be judged, will be little changed if spectacles are subsequently worn. Because of effectivity considerations, the strongest spherical lens needed should be placed in the rear cell, with any weaker auxiliary lenses in front of it. When the lens power exceeds about 5 D, the vertex distance should be measured and recorded as part of the prescription. At the dispensing stage, when the frame and lens type have both been chosen, the vertex distance with these spectacles can then be estimated. If it differs from that recorded in the prescription, calculation as in Chapters 4 and 5 or reference to tables will show what alteration, if any, to the original prescription should be made to reproduce the same effect at the eyes.

The vertex distance may be measured with special calipers, by placing a stenopaeic slit in the rear cell of the trial frame and pushing a thin card scale through it to meet the patient's closed eyelid, or, less accurately, by viewing from the side with a rule held against the side of the head.

Since trial frames are relatively heavy, it is more comfortable for the patient if the frames are removed occasionally during the refraction, for example, when writing down the objective findings and later the subjective results for distance.

The many other items of equipment in general use will be described in the relevant places.

Measurement of a spherical ametropia

A standard routine

Although the possibility of astigmatism should never be excluded, it is simpler initially to assume that any ametropia present is purely spherical. The first stages in the routine apply in either case. The unaided vision will give some guide as to the possible size of any error. If the vision is good, for example 6/9 or better, it indicates a small amount of myopia, emmetropia or hypermetropia. If hypermetropia, there could be a small absolute error in a middle-aged person or a medium or large error in a young patient. While the patient is still observing the distant test chart, with the other eye occluded, add +1.00 DS. If the vision is made worse, try +0.50 DS; if the vision again deteriorates, the patient is emmetropic or myopic. Then try −0.50 DS; if the vision improves, the patient is myopic. From *Table 6.1*, −0.50 DS should improve the vision from 6/9 to 6/6, but some patients with 6/9 vision may need slightly more negative power.

If the initial +1.00 DS made a slight improvement or no difference to the vision, hypermetropia is confirmed. Since accommodation can overcome all or part of a hypermetropic error, positive sphere should continue to be added until the vision no longer continues to improve. Initially, the plus power should be increased in whole dioptre steps until the next addition of +1.00 DS causes a reduction in vision. At this stage, half- and quarter-dioptre steps should then be used.

Now suppose the patient's unaided vision to be 6/24. *Table 6.1* predicts an error of about 1.50 D, so a

+1.50 DS lens should be tried initially. If this improves vision, continue adding positive spherical power as in the previous example until no more is accepted, that is, further addition causes blurring. On the other hand, if the initial positive lens made the vision even worse, then a minus lens, say −1.00 DS, should be tried next. This should improve the vision to about 6/9, and a little more negative sphere should then give the best VA. The change in minus sphere should be consistent with the improvement in acuity; for example, it should not require −4.00 DS to improve the vision from 6/24 to 6/6. Over-minusing an eye merely stimulates accommodation without improving vision and makes the eye effectively hypermetropic.

It is, however, a familiar fact that if a myopic eye is slightly over-corrected (too much minus power) or a hypermetropic eye is slightly under-corrected, the test letters or symbols generally appear smaller and blacker. The accepted rule is that the highest positive or lowest negative power that gives the best acuity should be regarded as the ametropic error. Other factors have to be taken into consideration, and we shall discuss this rule later in greater detail.

In order to verify the refractive findings so far determined, check tests must be applied. The simplest test is to add positive power to the correction, whether the patient is hypermetropic or myopic. If the patient's acuity is 6/6, then addition of +0.25 DS should blur the line fractionally, but without rendering it illegible. An addition of +0.50 DS should blur the vision back to 6/9, and a +1.00 DS to 6/18, as predicted by *Table 6.1*. If the patient can still read 6/9 through an extra +1.00 DS then either the first result is incorrect or the patient has either a smaller pupil or greater ability in interpreting blurred images than average. Normally, this check test is carried out only with a +1.00 DS.

A disadvantage of increasing positive power from zero when refracting a hypermetropic patient is that accommodation is then brought into play until the ametropia is fully corrected. Some patients, however, find it difficult to make the accommodation relax once it has been exerted. Accordingly, an alternative approach is to start by obtaining the best spherical lens, as described above. The +1.00 DS check test is then applied. Next, this extra lens power is reduced* by a quarter of a dioptre at a time until the best line is again read. Perhaps only half a dioptre need be removed if some relaxation has taken place. This method is called 'fogging'.

Unfortunately, some eyes will react to a 'fogged' image by accommodating, even though this makes the retinal image worse. Ward (1987) showed that this reaction does not usually occur unless the eye is fogged by more than +1.5–2.0 D. The resulting vision of about 6/30 is then too blurred to control accommodation which may then drift towards its resting state (*see* the discussion on inadequate stimulus myopias in Chapter

7). The binocular methods of refraction to be described later are greatly superior.

Bichromatic (duochrome) methods

The human eye is not corrected to focus light of different wavelengths at the same image point, that is, it suffers from both axial and transverse chromatic aberration. The axial aberration may be used to help determine the spherical component of the refractive error. If yellow light is focused exactly on the percipient layer of the retina, the blue–green focus will lie in front of the retina and the red focus behind it.

One of the earliest tests based on this principle and suitable for clinical use was designed by Clifford Brown and patented in 1927. It used carefully selected red and green glass filters and was marketed under the tradename 'duochrome'. More recently, the word 'bichromatic' has become an accepted generic term for tests of this kind, though 'dichromatic' is said to be etymologically more correct.

Although the retina is most sensitive to light of a greenish hue in photopic conditions, Ivanoff (1953) found that for distance vision the eye tends to select a yellow focus in preference to green. The choice of filters takes this into account, together with the spectral distribution of energy of the typical tungsten-filament light source and the spectral luminous efficiency curve of the eye. Thus, green filters conforming to the British Standard† have their peak luminosity at wavelength approximately 535 nm and the red at approximately 620 nm. Relative to a best focus in the yellow at 570 nm, these filters give a green focus about 0.20 D forward and a red focus at about 0.24 D behind (Bennett, 1963). Another property of these filters is that they appear of approximately equal brightness to the observer with normal colour vision (*see also* pages 289–290).

Since the red and green foci are equally spaced about the yellow, an emmetrope (or corrected ametrope) should see black test objects on the two coloured backgrounds equally clearly (*Figure 6.2a*). Bichromatic test panels may show a series of Snellen letters on each colour, a series of concentric rings (usually in the 4.5, 12 and possibly 24 m sizes) or a pattern of dots. Since the 'white' focus for a low myope falls a short distance in front of the retina, a myope will see the pattern on the red background clearer; and, conversely, a hypermetrope will prefer the green. This means that if the red is seen clearer a minus lens is required (*Figure 6.2b*) and a plus lens if the green pattern appears clearer.

The bichromatic panel may be used as another check test: the patient is asked whether the pattern appears clearer (or blacker) on the red or the green background. It sometimes has to be stressed that no attention must be paid to any apparent brightness difference. The trial lenses are adjusted to make both rings equally clear, or

---

* During these lens changes, add the new lower powered lens before removing the original lens or use the other hand as an occluder. Accommodation will be stimulated if the patient is allowed to see the chart with less than the full correction in the trial frame.

---

† BS 3668: *Red and green filters used in opthalmic dichromatic and dissociation tests.*

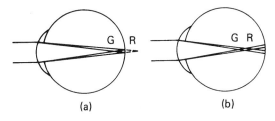

Figure 6.2. (a) Principle of the bichromatic (duochrome test). G indicates the focus for green light, R the focus for red light. When yellow light is in focus, these should lie approximately equidistant from the retina, one in front and one behind. (b) In the myopic eye, the red focus lies closer to the retina.

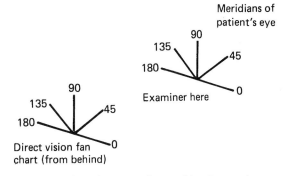

Figure 6.3. Three-dimensional view of fan chart and meridional notation of a patient's eye. Viewed from behind, the direct vision fan chart has the same meridians as the eye.

if this is not possible, clearer just on the red or just on the green, according to the purpose of the examiner.

Where the ametropia is considerable, the patterns on both colours will be grossly out of focus and the test will be unreliable. (This is probably the reason for the indecisive findings of O'Connor Davies, 1957, when recording the bichromatic preference of uncorrected subjects.) When the correction is within about 1 D of the optimum, the bichromatic test does appear to work satisfactorily. If the best acuity is poorer than the detail size of the test pattern, the contrast of the frame surrounding the test panel can sometimes be used though the test is generally omitted in these circumstances .

With older patients, the crystalline lens becomes markedly yellow, blue–green light being partially absorbed and scattered. This gives a marked red bias to the test and it sometimes becomes impossible to obtain apparent equality. Where it is obtained in such cases, too much minus lens power has usually been added and on returning to the black and white Snellen chart, an addition of about +0.50 DS may well be preferred, improving the acuity. Colour defectiveness should not upset this test too much, since the sharpness of focus is not affected, only the appearance of the colour. The protanopic or strongly protanomalous patient has a reduced sensitivity to the red end of the spectrum and this can cause difficulty, since the red background will appear much dimmer than the green.

Determination of the astigmatic error

There are two main methods of determining the astigmatic component of the refraction. The older method, using a special 'fan' chart of radial lines, will be described first since it illustrates the nature of the refractive asymmetry extremely well. The newer method, using a specially mounted cross cylinder, is now used more often because of its advantages, but not all patients respond satisfactorily and it is useful to be able to return to the older technique.

The fan and block method

In *Figure 5.4* we can see that the first focal line of an astigmatic pencil is parallel to the weaker or more hypermetropic β meridian of the eye, while the second

focal line is parallel to the more myopic α meridian. This figure illustrates diagrammatically the convergent astigmatic pencil where the principal meridians are horizontal and vertical.

They may, of course, be oblique. Suppose that an eye with simple myopic astigmatism has its more powerful principal meridian along 45° (*Figure 6.3*). The axis of the minus correcting cylinder is thus at 135°. Since the focal line on the retina lies along the 45° meridian, this must also be the direction of the clearest line seen. According to standard axis notation (*Figure 5.3*), meridians are numbered anticlockwise from the horizontal. Nevertheless, from the examiner's position between the patient and the fan chart, the line on the chart which is parallel to the patient's 45° meridian appears to be 45° clockwise from the horizontal. A reverse numbering is thus required for fan charts viewed directly (*Figure 6.4a*).

When a mirror is used, this reverse numbering is no longer required but, despite this, a different system is commonly used for convenience. The principle is to assume each line in turn to be the clearest and to number it with the axis direction of the minus correcting cylinder, which is always perpendicular to the given line. The resulting scheme is shown in outline in *Figure 6.4(b)*.

The complete fan chart is illustrated in *Figure 6.5*. Radial lines of thickness about the limb width of an 18-metre letter are spaced at 10° intervals around a central panel carrying an arrowhead and two sets of mutually perpendicular lines. The arrow or ∨ is due to Maddox and is used to refine the determination of the axis of the astigmatism. Thus, if the patient says the group of lines near the top of the chart are the clearest, the arrow is rotated to point at the clear group. Suppose that, as in *Figure 6.5*, the right-hand side of the arrowhead appears the clearer: this side is more nearly parallel to fan lines on the left of the arrow tip.[*] Thus, to find the axis of the astigmatism more accurately, the arrow is rotated away from its clearer side until equality is obtained.

The patient's attention is then directed to the two sets of lines or 'blocks' and he is asked which is the clearer: this should be the set parallel to the clearest line on the

---

[*] When the patient views the chart in a mirror, his left will be the refractionist's right for both the Maddox ∨ and the blocks.

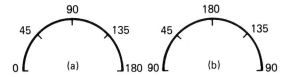

Figure 6.4. (a) Direct vision fan chart, giving a reversed protractor, being the examiner's view of the chart in *Figure 6.3*. (b) Indirect fan chart, numbered to indicate the required minus trial cylinder axis, for viewing by reflection in a mirror.

fan chart. Negative cylinder power is then brought into play, the axis being at right-angles to the lines of the clearer block, until the two sets of lines are equally clear.

Using this method, the refraction of an astigmatic eye may be undertaken as follows:

(1) Occlude the second eye and measure the unaided vision of the first eye.
(2) Determine the sphere giving the best vision obtainable with spherical lenses alone by the methods on pages 95–97. This lens is called the 'best vision sphere'. If the resulting vision is 6/12 or better, a bichromatic test may also be used. This new vision is then noted, and from *Table 6.1* the amount of astigmatism present may be estimated. It is assumed that the best vision sphere puts the circle of least confusion on the retina. Hence, in order to bring the eye into a state of simple myopic astigmatism:
(3) Add a positive sphere equal to half the estimated amount of astigmatism (since the circle of least confusion lies dioptrically mid-way between the two focal lines) or add +1.00 DS if vision at this stage is 6/9 or better.
(4) Refer the patient to the fan chart and ask which line or group of lines appear clearest and darkest. This gives the approximate direction of the astigmatic error. However, a simple check test should be made by temporarily adding an extra +0.50 DS in order to confirm that the eye is in a state of simple myopic astigmatism. The blackest lines should blur, but if not, more positive sphere should be added until they do. (In some cases the clearest lines will change through 90°, indicating that the eye had been in a

state of simple hypermetropic astigmatism, with the anterior focal line near the retina. In this case, continue adding positive sphere until this new set of lines just begins to blur.)
(5) Direct the attention to the Maddox arrow and rotate it away from its blacker limb until both limbs appear equally blurred. This gives the axis of the astigmatism, but care must be taken to ensure that the patient's head is upright.
(6) Directing attention now to the blocks, add negative cylinder at the appropriate axis until the second becomes as clear as the first. If this is not quite possible, it is better to just under-correct than over-correct the astigmatic error, that is, leaving the first group of lines the clearer or blacker of the two.
(7) Make a second check test by again adding +0.50 DS or, if the patient is a critical observer, +0.25 DS. Both blocks should blur equally, but if the blackest lines change over, the astigmatism has been over-corrected. If the originally darker block again becomes blacker, the original sphere from step (4) was wrong and must be re-checked.
(8) Return to the letter chart and determine the sphere giving best acuity, the cylindrical element remaining as just determined. As usual, a positive lens should be tried first, but a weak minus lens will most frequently be required.

If in step (4) no lines appear blacker than the others, there may be no astigmatism present, but other possibilities are that the eye is excessively fogged, has the circles of least confusion on the retina or is in a state of compound hypermetropic astigmatism. The +0.50 DS check test will show up either of these last two conditions, by making some lines darker. On the other hand, if the eye is already fogged, extra positive power will blur the lines even more, whereas the addition of minus power will make some lines blacker in the presence of astigmatism, or all equally black if there is no astigmatism.

To summarize the technique:

(1) Obtain sphere giving best vision.
(2) Estimate power of astigmatic error from the vision at this stage.

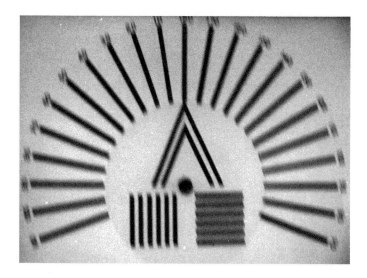

Figure 6.5. Photograph of a fan and block chart taken through a plus cylinder at axis 20°. The unequal clarity of the limbs of the Maddox ∨ shows that an anticlockwise rotation is needed to give equality and identify the axis.

(3) Assuming that the lens found in (1) was that putting the circle of least confusion on the retina, add plus spherical power equal to half the estimated minus cylinder.

(4) Find the clearest line(s) on the fan. Temporarily add an extra +0.50 DS to check that the blackest lines blur.

(5) Refine the cylinder axis using the ∨.

(6) Equalize the clarity of the blocks with minus cylinders.

(7) Ensure that the eye is not spherically under-corrected by adding +0.50 DS and checking that the blocks are equally blurred or at least not reversed in clarity from the original appearance. If necessary, adjust cylinder power.

(8) Refine sphere with Snellen or bichromatic chart.

The present writer's (RBR's) redesign of the ∨ and blocks is described on pages 104–105.

The cross cylinder

Introduction

This is an astigmatic lens in which the two principal powers are numerically equal but opposite in sign, the mean power thus being zero. According to the relevant British Standard,[*] the power of a cross cylinder should be denoted by its meridional power, but some manufacturers label their lenses with the total astigmatic power, which is twice the meridional power. Theoretically, a 0.25 D cross cylinder denotes the lens

+0.25 DC axis θ/−0.25 DC axis (θ ± 90)

but, in manufacture, an equivalent sphero-cylindrical form is preferred for practical convenience. The recommended term 'cross cylinder' is thus more appropriate than 'crossed cylinder'.

The lens is marked with the position of the axes, preferably with plus or minus signs or with coloured dots. In the UK, + is usually red and − is usually white or black, but the opposite code is generally used elsewhere.

If used in conjunction with a trial frame, the lens is mounted in a handle which is at 45° to the axes (*Figure 6.6*). By twirling the handle, the positions of the axes are rapidly interchanged. A similar principle applies to cross cylinders incorporated in refracting units.

The cross cylinder technique was introduced by Jackson, initially to determine or check the cylinder power (1887) and later (1907) the cylinder axis. Unlike the fan and block method, successful use of the cross cylinder requires the circle of least confusion to lie on the retina. Since the mean power of the lens is zero, it does not affect the position of this circle relative to the retina, but does affect its size and resultant blurring by altering the interval of Sturm. This is its basic principle when used as a check on cylinder power.

In current practice, the cross cylinder is commonly used to refine the results of an objective test, such as re-

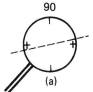 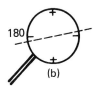

Figure 6.6. The cross cylinder and axis determination. The position of the minus cylinder axis is indicated by the two minus signs and the numerical value of the axis. In this and the next three figures, the dashed line is in the position of the required minus axis, assumed to be at 10°. Hence the minus axis of the cross cylinder lies nearer the correct axis in (b) than in (a).

tinoscopy, but in the routine to be described no such prior information is assumed.

Axis determination

To simplify the following discussion and diagrams, the refracted pencil within the eye refers to a single distant object point. This is sufficient to indicate the nature of any blurring of the complete retinal image.

The circle of least confusion is put on or slightly behind the percipient elements of the retina by obtaining the best vision with spherical lenses on the test chart, or, where the bichromatic method is reliable, equalizing the clarity of the rings. For a young patient, a further −0.25 DS may be added to allow accommodation to put the circle of least confusion on the retina.

If the patient's vision is good at this stage, such as 6/9 or better, his attention should be directed to a circular test object of size equivalent to 6/12. This next larger size is used because the cross cylinder often reduces the vision in one of its positions. Concentric circles, for example 6/12 with 6/4.5, are quite useful because if the vision is good through the cross cylinder, the patient will also be helped by the clarity of the smaller ring. If the vision is poor, a larger circle should be used.

The cross cylinder is then placed in front of the trial lens(es) already before the patient's eye with its axes vertical and horizontal (*Figure 6.6*). The lens is then twirled about its handle direction, interchanging the positions of the two axes, and the patient asked whether the circle appeared sharper (clearer or blacker) with the lens in its first or second position. If the patient preferred the position where the minus axis was horizontal, the minus axis of his astigmatism lies nearer the horizontal than the vertical. The cross cylinder is then turned so that its handle is horizontal (or vertical), thus putting its axes at 45° and 135° (*Figure 6.7*). With the patient

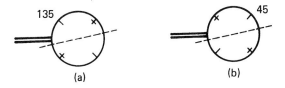

Figure 6.7. Cross cylinder handle horizontal to give 135°/45°. The minus axis of the cross cylinder lies nearer the correct axis in (b) than in (a).

---

[*] BS 3521: *Glossary of terms relating to ophthalmic lenses and spectacle frames.*

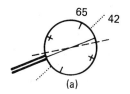
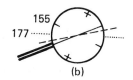

Figure 6.8. A trial cylinder of −0.50 D at axis 20° (solid line) has been added and cross cylinder handle orientated along this axis. The resultant (minus) axis of the trial and cross cylinder combination is shown as a dotted line and is nearer correct axis in (b) than in (a).

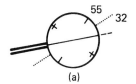
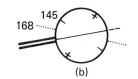

Figure 6.9. The axis of trial cylinder and cross cylinder handle adjusted to 10°. The resultant axis of trial and cross cylinder combination is equidistant from axis 10° in both positions.

still watching the test circles, the better position of the cross cylinder is determined, say, with the minus axis at 45°.

These two findings indicate that the patient's minus axis lies between 180° (or 0°) and 45°. A negative trial cylinder is then placed in position, axis about 20°, together with the addition of positive spherical power equal to half the cylinder power. This keeps the circle of least confusion near the retina. The power of the cylinder should be chosen as indicated by *Table 6.1*. (In *Figures 6.8* and *6.9* the power of the cylinder has been taken as −0.50 D to provide a numerical example. A +0.25 D sphere would have been added as well.) The cross cylinder is placed with its handle along or perpendicular to the axis of the trial cylinder, whichever is the easier position to hold. The cross cylinder axes are then at 45° to those of the trial cylinder (*Figure 6.8*). The resultant of this combination of cross and trial cylinders has its minus axis between the two individual axes. Twirling the cross cylinder may therefore, in this situation, be regarded as swinging the trial cylinder first in one direction, then, by the same amount, in the opposite one. In this example, if the preferred position of the cross cylinder was the one with the minus axis at 155° (that is, clockwise from the trial cylinder position), then the preferred resultant axis shift was also clockwise from the initial trial cylinder axis. This indicates that the trial cylinder should be rotated clockwise, say through 10°, so that its new axis is at 10°.

The cross cylinder handle is then placed along 10° and the lens twirled (*Figure 6.9*). If the ring appears equally clear in these two positions, the vision is the same whether the trial cylinder is effectively rotated by the same amount in one direction or the other. Thus the patient's astigmatic error lies at axis 10°.

The numerical values of the resultant cylinder axes given in *Figures 6.8* and *6.9* assume the cross cylinder to be of meridional power ±0.25 D.

Determination of cylinder power

The next step is to determine the cylinder power required, its axis direction having been accurately located at 10°.

To do this, the cross cylinder is now held so that its axes are respectively parallel and perpendicular to the axis of the trial cylinder. In one setting, the cross cylinder will then add minus cylinder power at the same axis as the trial cylinder, whereas after twirling, it will add plus cylinder power at this same axis. The power of the trial cylinder is thus checked by being increased and decreased to the same extent, without displacing the circles of least confusion from the retina.

Reverting to the example being considered, let us suppose that at the end of the axis check procedure there was a −0.50 D trial cylinder in position, but the patient's astigmatism was actually 1.00 D. Then, if it is assumed that the circles of least confusion had been maintained on the retina by adjustment to the spherical power as described, the residual refractive error will be

+0.25 DS/−0.50 DC axis 10

This represents hypermetropia of +0.25 D along the 10° meridian and myopia of −0.25 D along the 100° meridian, the focal lines lying as indicated in *Figure 6.10(a)*. A +0.25 D cross cylinder is now introduced with its minus axis at 10°, as shown in *Figure 6.10(b)*. This adds −0.25 D along the 100° meridian and +0.25 D along the 10° meridian, thus correcting the residual refractive error. The two focal lines would collapse to form a retinal point image of a distant object point. The second setting in which the axes of the cross cylinder are interchanged is shown in *Figure 6.10(c)*. In this position, the effect is to increase the residual myopia along the 100° meridian by −0.25 D and the residual hypermetropia along the 10° meridian by a further +0.25 D. As a result, the dioptric interval between the focal lines is doubled, together with the diameter of the circle of least confusion.

Twirling of the cross cylinder showed that better vision was obtained with its minus axis at 10°, in the same setting as the −0.50 D trial cylinder. The power of this cylinder should therefore be increased by, say −0.50 D. At the same time, +0.25 D sphere should be added so as to keep the circles of least confusion on the retina. If the astigmatic error has now been corrected, twirling the cross cylinder will give no advantage in either position since half a dioptre of astigmatism results in each case.

In some cases, the astigmatic power of the cross cylinder is greater than the residual astigmatic error of refraction. Suppose, for example, that the residual astigmatic error is −0.25 D axis 10°. With the minus axis set at 10°, an 0.25 D cross cylinder will reverse the residual astigmatic error, making it +0.25 D axis 10°. In the other setting it will be increased to −0.75 D axis 10°. Since the circles of least confusion remain on the retina, this reversal causes no problems. The first setting with the minus axis at 10° is clearly the better one since it results in a smaller residual astigmatism, and it indicates that additional minus cylinder power at axis 10° is required. If too much extra power is added, the

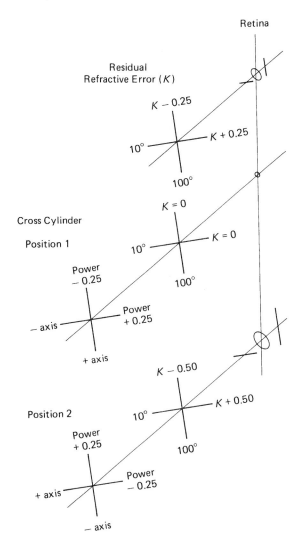

Figure 6.10. The cross cylinder and astigmatic power determination: (a) the residual refractive error of $+0.25/-0.50 \times 10$ and the position of the astigmatic pencil relative to retina, (b) a cross cylinder with its minus axis along $10°$ corrects the refractive error, as shown by $K = 0$ in the column for residual refractive error, (c) when the cross cylinder is twirled into its second position, the astigmatic refractive error is doubled.

next trial with the cross cylinder will reveal the over-correction.

To summarize the technique:

(1) Put the circle of least confusion on or behind retina, employing bichromatic test or Snellen chart.
(2) With patient observing appropriate test object, twirl cross cylinder with axes along horizontal and vertical. Note clearer direction.
(3) Twirl with axes along $45°$ and $135°$.
(4) Insert trial cylinder (and appropriate sphere) with axis as indicated by (2) and (3).
(5) Twirl cross cylinder, with handle along or at right angles to trial cylinder axis. Note clearer direction.
(6) Rotate trial cylinder in this direction.
(7) Repeat (5) and (6) until no preference, or mid-point of range obtained.
(8) To measure power, twirl cross cylinder with handle at $45°$ to trial cylinder axis.

(9) Alter cylinder (and sphere) power as indicated, and repeat until equality is obtained.

As a sequel to objective refraction, the trial cylinder is left in place and steps (2), (3) and (4) omitted.

When a high astigmatic error is found, say 3 D or more, greater accuracy may be obtained by transferring the trial frame complete with lenses to a focimeter to measure the axis direction, instead of relying on the engravings. This refinement is not possible with a refractor head, which does not permit the manufacturer's accuracy to be checked.

Relevant clinical matters

The cross cylinder test is a simple one to use, but its success depends on two factors: maintenance of the circle of least confusion on the retina and speed of rotation of the lens. The lens should be held in front of the patient's eye for two or three seconds, then rapidly twirled and again held steadily in place. This enables the patient to make a quick comparison between the two successive images. The ease of rotation is improved on some cross cylinders by having a pair of flats on the handle to be held between finger and thumb, while the smaller overall diameter of the lenses due to Freeman also helps.

If the eye is either fogged or excessively under-plussed, then the apparent clearest 'focus' might occur when one of the focal lines is nearer the retina, despite the total astigmatism being greater under these conditions. *Figure 6.11* shows an over-plussed eye with

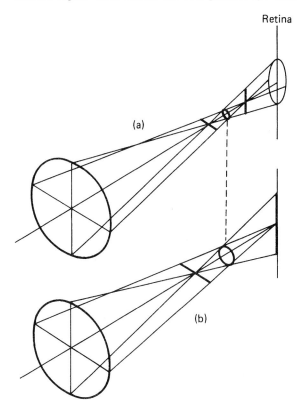

Figure 6.11. The cross cylinder and the over-plussed eye: (a) cross cylinder in its first position, reducing the total astigmatic error but giving a large blur ellipse on the retina, (b) cross cylinder in second position shows an increased astigmatic error giving a focal line on the retina, a position likely to be preferred.

both focal lines in front of the retina. Both settings of the cross cylinder leave the circles of least confusion in their original position. In setting (a), the astigmatism is reduced and the focal lines brought nearer together, but there is a large elliptical blur on the retina. In setting (b), the astigmatism is increased and the rear focal line moved backwards to the retina. Depending on the nature of the test object, the patient might find this setting the better of the two, thus giving a false indication that a stronger cylinder is needed. It is because of this paradoxical situation that the use of rectangular letters should be avoided (Williamson-Noble, 1943), especially since letters may often be read more clearly with their vertical strokes in focus than the horizontal ones. A circular test object (not a 5 × 4 letter chart O) avoids this problem and is strongly recommended. Another suitable test object is a cluster of dots, each of about 2 minutes angular subtense. The cluster pattern reduces the apparent distortion often noticed with ring test objects. An alternative test object frequently used in the USA is a Maltese cross.

The size of the test pattern to be used depends on the patient's vision, as discussed on page 99. The power of the cross cylinder used is chosen in a similar manner. Cross cylinders are commonly available in powers of ±0.12, ±0.25, ±0.37 and ±0.50 D. The ±0.25 is the most useful, provided the patient's vision with spherical lenses has reached 6/12. With poorer vision or small pupils, one might start with a ±0.50 cross cylinder but switch to ±0.25 when making the final check on cylinder power. However, since the ±0.50 cross cylinder does tend to over-blur, a ±0.37 cross cylinder is an extremely useful compromise.

If, on rotation of the cross cylinder, an increased cylinder power is indicated, it may be more convenient to do so by holding up a second cross cylinder than to change the spherical and cylindrical trial lenses. This second cross cylinder is held stationary, close to the trial lenses, and the first one twirled again. If this new total power is rejected, the extra cross cylinder is merely taken away; if accepted, the trial lenses are altered.

Since the cross cylinder is a lens of symmetrical plus and minus power and is employed with the circle of least confusion on the retina, the method may equally well be employed with plus cylinders, unlike the fan and block where only minus cylinders may be used.

When determining the axis with plus trial cylinders, the axis of the combination of cross and trial cylinders will lie between the cross cylinder's plus axis and that of the trial cylinder. Hence the trial cylinder's axis should be moved towards the preferred plus cylinder axis direction of the cross cylinder. When verifying the power, the trial cylinder should be increased or decreased, depending on whether the preferred position of the cross cylinder had the plus or minus axis respectively lying along that of the trial cylinder.

Background theory

(1) *Spherical power adjustment.* The importance of keeping the circle of least confusion on the retina when using the cross cylinder has already been stressed. For

Table 6.2   Effective cylinder axis shift by cross cylinders

Power of trial cylinder (D)	Axis shift (degrees)	
	±0.25 D cross cyl.	±0.50 D cross cyl.
0	±45	±45
0.50	22.5	31.5
1.00	13.5	22.5
1.50	9	17
2.00	7	13.5
2.50	5.5	11
3.00	4.5	9
4.00	3.5	7
5.00	3	5.5
6.00	2.5	4.5

Note: Figures rounded off to the nearest 0.5°.

this reason, if any change is made in the trial cylinder power as the test proceeds, it must be balanced by half the amount of spherical power of opposite sign.

This adjustment is carried out automatically by the Stokes' lens, named after its inventor who described it in 1849. In its modern form it consists of two plano-cylinders of equal and opposite power, mounted close together in a carrier cell to fit a standard trial frame. It is used in some optometer systems and could also be built into a refractor head. As the cylinders are made to rotate in opposite directions by the control screw, the cylinder power of the unit varies continuously, but the mean power remains zero. Hence, in any state of adjustment, there is a spherical power component of one half the cylinder power and opposite to it in sign.

The erroneous results which can occur if the circle of least confusion is not maintained on the retina were demonstrated graphically by Lindsay (1954).

(2) *Effective axis shift.* The angle through which a cross cylinder swings the resultant cylinder axis when used as an axis check can be calculated from well-known formulae relating to obliquely crossed cylinders. It can be seen from *Table 6.2* that the axis shift decreases as the power of the trial cylinder increases. Thus, the axis shift produced by a ±0.25 D cross cylinder is 22.5° when the trial cylinder power is 0.50 D but only 7° when the trial cylinder is 2.00 D. This is as it should be, because strong cylinders require more accurate orientation than weak cylinders.

(3) *Residual error of refraction.* The theory of obliquely crossed cylinders can also be applied to calculate residual errors of refraction. This term denotes the *additional* lens power needed to correct any remaining error of refraction when a spectacle lens or trial lens combination is already in position. In any such case the following rule can be applied: to find the residual error of refraction, cancel the lens(es) in place by a hypothetical lens of equal and opposite power and add to this the lens that fully corrects the given eye.

If the trial cylinder axis is of the correct power C but set at an angle ϕ from the true axis direction θ, the residual error of refraction thus arising can be shown from equations (5.10)–(5.12) to be

$$(C \sin \phi) \text{ DS}/(-2C \sin \phi) \text{ DC axis}(\theta + 45 + \phi/2)$$

$$(6.1)$$

Table 6.3 Residual errors of refraction produced by various incorrect cylinders, the eye requiring -1.00 DC axis $180°$

Trial cylinder	Residual error of refraction
-0.50×10	$+0.03/-0.56 \times 171$
-0.75×10	$+0.07/-0.39 \times 160$
-1.00×10	$+0.17/-0.35 \times 140$
-1.25×10	$+0.36/-0.46 \times 124$
-1.50×10	$+0.58/-0.66 \times 116$

The usual sign convention applies to the angle ϕ. If it is negative (clockwise from θ), $\sin \phi$ also becomes negative. As an example, if C is -1.00 D and ϕ is $-10°$, the residual refractive error is

$+0.17$ sph/-0.35 cyl axis $(\theta + 40)$

At the end of a preliminary objective examination, the trial cylinder before the eye may be incorrect as regards both power and axis direction. Suppose, for example, that the required cylinder is -1.00 D axis $180°$ but the trial cylinder in position is -0.50 D axis $10°$. The residual error of refraction is the sum of $+0.50$ DC axis $10°$ (to neutralize the incorrect lens) and -1.00 DC axis $180°$ which is the cylinder required. The resultant of this combination is

$+0.03$ sph/-0.56 cyl axis 171

A general idea of the magnitude of such errors can be seen from *Table 6.3*, which shows the effect of cylinders of different power all set at axis $10°$, placed before an eye requiring -1.00 DC axis $180°$. The figures listed refer to an off-axis error of $10°$ but, to a reasonable degree of accuracy, residual errors of refraction are proportional to the off-axis angular error, all other factors being unchanged.

Two points are of particular interest. First, the size of the residual astigmatic error, even when the trial cylinder is of the correct power should be noted. Secondly, the axis direction of the residual astigmatism is clockwise from the true axis if the angular setting error is anticlockwise and vice versa.

When a trial cylinder of the correct power is in place during a test, its axis can be moved through an angle – say ϕ degrees – before any change is subjectively discernible. Corresponding to this angle is a residual astigmatic error which can be calculated as already described. Comparative values of angle ϕ and corresponding astigmatic errors with ± 0.25 D and ± 0.50 D cross cylinders in use were determined experimentally by O'Leary *et al.* (1987). With the ± 0.25 D cross cylinder in use, the mean results from five subjects showed ϕ to vary from $4.2°$ to $1.0°$ as the trial cylinder power was increased from 0.50 to 1.50 D. The corresponding astigmatic power errors remained reasonably close to a mean value of 0.08 D. With the ± 0.50 D cross cylinder in use, the variation in was from $4.2°$ to $2.0°$, while the astigmatic errors ranged from 0.07 to 0.13 D. This confirms the general advice given on an earlier page to use the ± 0.25 D cross cylinder in the final stages of the test. Johnston (1990) confirmed theoretically and experimentally that axis determination is best with a cross cylinder power less than the trial cylinder power,

and also with the trial cylinder power less than the astigmatic error. This is not to suggest, however, that the trial cylinder should purposely be made weaker. The present writer occasionally uses a ± 0.12 D cross cylinder with 0.25 D trial cylinders when refracting observant patients, while if a much stronger cylinder is found than initially in place, it is sensible to re-confirm the axis with this.

Errors can also arise during axis location if the handle of the cross cylinder is not correctly aligned with the trial cylinder axis, but Rabbetts (1972) has shown that the comparative blurring in the two positions of the cross cylinder is scarcely affected until the angular positional error is of the order of $15°$.

Comparison of the fan and block and cross cylinder methods

The cross cylinder method has become the favoured technique because of the following advantages:

(1) It is possibly easier to use after objective refraction.
(2) It may be used with either plus or minus cylinders.
(3) It gives an average astigmatic 'focus' for the whole of the pupillary area with the position of best spherical focus on the retina.
(4) The cross cylinder is relatively unaffected by any head tilt by the patient (except when a refractor head is employed). The static eye reflex counterrotates the eyes through about one-sixth of the initial head rotation, but a $10°$ head tilt to one side will immediately give an erroneous axis result with the fan chart.
(5) It is convenient for the practitioner not to have to keep reaching to the fan chart for adjustments.

Errors and difficulties can, however, arise with the cross cylinder when:

(1) The sphere power is incorrect. It is very easy to under-plus the older patient, putting the best focus behind the retina.
(2) An unsuitable test object is used, especially if the important details are parallel to the principal meridians of the eye.
(3) The patient is confused by the apparent distortion of the test circle.

In addition, some patients do not understand the 'first' or 'second' approach. Their first answer, say 'second', biases their subsequent answers so that they repeat 'second' on the following trials since they do not wish to contradict themselves by replying 'first'. This problem may sometimes be overcome by labelling the next trials third or fourth, fifth or sixth (or heads or tails) before returning to first–second.

A useful but much less precise technique for finding the axis is to rotate the trial cylinder slowly away from the expected position and ask the patient to report when the letter chart begins to blur. This axis position is noted, and the process repeated in the opposite direction. The mean of the two end-points is taken as the axis. Although this is similar in principle to the action of the cross cylinder, it has been found helpful to some patients. It can also be a useful double check when the subjective axis has changed significantly from the present spectacle correction or from an objective finding.

The fan and block method is a well-tried and sound technique. It may be modified to give a logical continuation to objective refraction, as will be described on page 105. The blocks especially form a useful check test for cylinder power.

Cautious patients may prefer this method because the simultaneous display of both sides of the arrow or of the blocks enables them to look repeatedly from one to the other until they have decided which is better.

There are some disadvantages:

(1) It may be inconvenient to have to keep reaching to the fan chart for adjustments.
(2) The blocks occasionally appear coloured and hence confuse the patient. Also, if excess fogging is applied, spurious resolution may occur, causing the blocks perpendicular to those predicted to seem clearer.
(3) If the eye shows irregular refraction due to corneal or lenticular distortion, the symmetry of the refracted pencils will be disturbed. The astigmatic component is determined in a state of slight fog so that the retina intercepts the beam behind the best focus. The cylinder that provides the best balance under these conditions may not be the optimum lens when the spherical component is adjusted to put the best focus back on to the retina.

   Moreover, by concentrating attention on lines in two meridians only, equality of the blocks may again not give the best average refraction. This is likely to occur when the crystalline lens is divided into sectors by localized (spoke-like) cataractous changes.
(4) If the patient has had uncorrected astigmatism for years, the neurological response in the usually more blurred meridian may be poorer than that in the better meridian (*see* page 42). This might affect the blocks more than the test objects in the cross cylinder method.

Although Walsh *et al.* (1993) found a high correlation between the results of the two techniques, as would be expected, there was a consistent difference between them.

A redesigned ∨ and blocks

The traditional angle between the limbs of the ∨ has been about 45°–60°, values adopted following experimental work by Maddox (1925) and Verhoeff (1923). In low to moderate amounts of astigmatism, the blurring of the lines is such that the difference between the two when near correct alignment is readily perceptible (*Figure 6.12a*). In high astigmatism, the lines are both so blurred (*Figure 6.12b*) that there is little difference between them when slightly off-axis and hence the ∨ is then of little practical use in refraction. If the angle between the lines were reduced, the differential blur would be restored, as in *Figure 6.12(c)*.

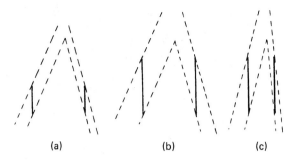

Figure 6.12.   The Maddox ∨ in low and high astigmatism. In (a) and (b) the limbs of the ∨ include an angle of 40° and in (c) 15°. The ∨ is set in all three figures at 5° from a vertical astigmatic blur. The bold vertical lines indicate the retinal focal lines determining the apparent width of the blurred limbs of the ∨, (a) in low astigmatism, (b) and (c) in high astigmatism. The narrower ∨ then permits finer discrimination.

These considerations have been incorporated in the author's (RBR's) simplification of the Raubitschek arrow or paraboline chart (*Figure 19.9*). A tapered ∨ is used with an angle of 20° between the two lines forming the apex of the arrowhead, and 50° between the extremities. The effects of various amounts of astigmatic blur with this chart are shown in *Figure 6.13*.

The patient's response to the blocks has also been improved by reducing the number of lines and increasing their separation. The original design (*Figure 6.5*), with lines and spaces of equal width, was susceptible to spurious resolution. When this occurs, the blurred block can sometimes seem clearer than the fogged reference block. In the new chart the space width is double that of the line thickness, subtending 6 and 3 minutes of arc respectively, while it is internally illuminated with yellow lamps in order to reduce the fringing from chromatic aberration.

Modification of techniques following objective refraction

If any form of objective test has been made, it is sensible to check the findings subjectively, provided that the patient is able to co-operate. The cross cylinder method can easily be adapted for this purpose.

With the objective findings (including any cylinder) in place and the other eye occluded, the patient's vision is recorded. The spherical power is then adjusted to obtain the best vision on the Snellen chart, adding perhaps −0.25 DS to ensure that the circle of least confusion can be placed on the retina. If a bichromatic test is used for this step, the rings on the green background should be left just clearer than those on the red, subject to the reservation on page 97.

The cross cylinder is now used, as described previously, to check the cylinder axis. In order to demonstrate the effect of the cross cylinder, it is useful initially to rotate the trial cylinder 5°–10° away from the objective axis so that there is a definite preference on twirling. Otherwise, if the objective axis is approximately correct, there will be little difference in sharpness, which will not help the patient to understand the procedure. The

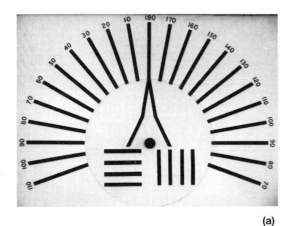

(a)

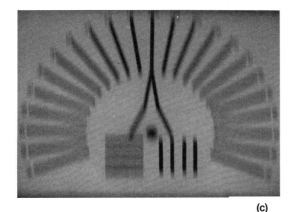

(b)

(c)

Figure 6.13. The modified design of the ∨ and blocks. (a) As seen in focus. (b) Blurred by a low plus cylinder at axis 10°. It is the wide section of the ∨ which gives the bigger blur differential. (c) Blurred by a high plus cylinder at axis 5°. It is now the narrow section of the ∨ which gives the bigger differential. (The high contrast required for photographic reproduction cannot convey exactly the appearance seen by the patient.)

astigmatic power is then confirmed and the spherical component is again checked.

If the objective test resulted in only a spherical correction, the cross cylinder should be used to make sure that an astigmatic error has not been missed, even if the vision at this stage is 6/6 (20/20).

The fan and block method may also, with some modifications, be used to check the refraction. As with the

cross cylinder method, the trial cylinder should be left in position and the best vision obtained by adjusting the spherical power. The spherical lens thus found is not the 'best vision sphere', since an astigmatic lens is also in play. If a bichromatic test is used, the preference should be just towards clarity on the red background. The eye is then fogged by the addition of a +0.50 D sphere, or stronger if the objective refraction showed high latent hypermetropia, and the trial cylinder is removed. At this stage the eye should be in a state of simple or slight compound myopic astigmatism. The astigmatic axis can then be quickly checked by using the ∨, the power by using the blocks. The spherical lens is finally checked and the visual acuity measured.

To summarize this routine:

(1) With the objective cylinder still in position, obtain red preference with the bichromatic test or find the sphere giving best vision on the Snellen chart.
(2) Add +0.50 DS (if objective refraction showed a large latent hypermetropia, use a higher power), check that vision is blurred and remove the cylinder.
(3) Set the ∨ near the objective axis and confirm. If there is a large discrepancy, use the fan chart.
(4) Using the blocks, find the cylindrical power needed.
(5) Possibly check by adding an extra +0.50 DS so that the blocks blur equally.
(6) Remove the initial +0.50 DS or other lens from step (2).

With some patients, for example those with marked lens opacities, neither an objective nor a standard subjective test can be used. No routine can be laid down for these, but various expedients may be tried. The pinhole disc or stenopaeic slit may reveal an improvement in vision. If so, a subjective test with lens changes at one or two dioptre intervals and cylinders freely rotated may result in some measure of success. If the vision is poor, 6/24 or worse, a better response often results with a standard (6 m) direct test chart placed at 3 m or even 1 m.

Balancing methods and binocular refraction

Choice of methods

When the astigmatic component of the distance refractive error has been determined, the next steps are to confirm or adjust the spherical component and, if possible, to balance the two eyes – a process sometimes known as equalizing the accommodative effort. This allows both eyes to have the retinal image simultaneously in focus. An imbalanced correction often leads to asthenopia because of unstable acccommodation, the image in first one eye and then the other being brought into sharp focus. There are many different methods of balancing, but a broad division into monocular and binocular techniques can be made.

Binocular methods of balancing can also be used to carry out a full or partial refractive test with both eyes simultaneously in use. This procedure, which goes beyond a balancing test, is best described as binocular refraction.

Since bichromatic tests can also be used in conjunction with binocular as well as monocular balancing techniques, a few general observations about them may be useful at this stage. We have already discussed the effects of poor acuity, senile crystalline lens yellowing and protanopia on the bichromatic test (*see* page 97).

Depending on whether the patient's symptoms are in distance or near vision, it may be better not to aim at equalizing the red and green but to aim at a red or green preference. For example, if the test pattern is left just clearer on the red (red preference), it means that the eye is in a slightly myopic state. This will be beneficial if the spectacles are to be worn indoors only, for example, by a young patient for close work. With the older (presbyopic) patient whose accommodation is relatively inactive, the red preference often gives better acuity on the Snellen chart and more comfortable vision, especially in the middle distance at about 2 m.

If the green is just clearer, then there is slight hypermetropia, the yellow focus lying just behind the retina. This should give the best acuity for the far distance and in the younger patient the reserves of accommodation can easily cope with the extra 0.25 D of effort. It should be remembered that a lens giving a bichromatic balance at 6 m will give −0.16 D of myopia in the far distance. Charts projected on to a screen at 3–4 m will cause even more significant errors, unless an appropriate allowance is made in the prescription.

Monocular balancing methods

Where a patient has only one working eye, the spherical component of the correction may be determined by either of the first two methods below. Where the patient has no or poor binocular co-ordination, the sphere level is again obtained under monocular conditions. The aim is to obtain the same response for each eye in turn, with the other eye occluded. Since the accommodation level may change during the time required to check the two eyes, these monocular methods should not really be called balancing techniques, but are included in this section on finishing techniques for convenience.

When a bichromatic test is used for balancing, the same preference should be obtained when each eye is alternately occluded.

Another monocular method of checking the sphere is to obtain the highest plus or lowest minus spherical power for each eye which does not impair the acuity. Assuming that 6/6 or better can be obtained, it used to be thought that the end result had been obtained when an added +0.25 DS caused a slight loss of crispness and +0.50 DS reduced the acuity by one line. Although this may be true for a good proportion of patients, it is not always so. Because of the combined effects of spherical and chromatic aberration, a paraxial pencil within the eye does not come to a geometrical focus, but converges to an ill-defined 'depth of focus', as shown in *Figure 6.14*. Within the region A to D the concentration of light produces the maximum acuity. When the pupil is

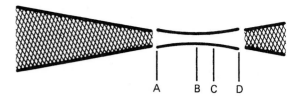

Figure 6.14. The waist or ill-defined depth of focus of the aberrated pencil within the eye.

small, the pencil is reduced in width and the depth of focus is increased. In such a case, the patient will accept more plus power before blurring becomes perceptible. As a result, it may be a cross-section at a point such as C, not at the mid-point B of the depth of focus, which lies on the retina when the next +0.25 DS just reduces the acuity.

Another monocular balancing method is the successive comparison test. An occluder is transferred from eye to eye and the patient asked to report which eye has the better vision. If there is a difference, it indicates that one eye is relatively over- or under-corrected or has inherently lower acuity. Equal plus spherical power, say +0.50 or +0.75 D, is then placed before each eye and the question repeated. The relative spherical power between the two eyes is then adjusted to give equal vision. The moderate spherical fogging reduces the effect of slight acuity differences and overcomes the uncertainty as to whether the eye is over- or under-corrected. The plus power is then reduced for the two eyes equally until the best binocular acuity is obtained.

Some drawbacks of the method should be noted. One is that the patient may accommodate while the occluder is being transferred, thus causing errors. The additional plus power should not be used in excess because it can induce accommodative spasm and very blurred images are difficult to compare. Even moderate degrees of fogging may depress the acuity of one eye more than the other (Flom and Goodwin, 1964). Unequal pupil sizes or ocular aberrations may be contributory causes. In everyday practice it is not uncommon to find patients having unequal unaided vision in the two eyes despite similar refractive errors and final corrected acuities. Hypermetropic patients with an amblyopic eye frequently prefer less positive power in front of the weaker eye monocularly than under the binocular conditions to be described.

Binocular balancing methods

For patients with good binocular vision, these methods are far superior to those just described because the fixed convergence required for viewing the test chart helps to stabilize the accommodation. They can also be used for checking the astigmatic component under binocular viewing conditions.

Turville's infinity balance test (TIB)

The infinity balance test was introduced by A.E. Turville in 1936. In its current form a mirror is used with a removable vertical septum, preferably white (though

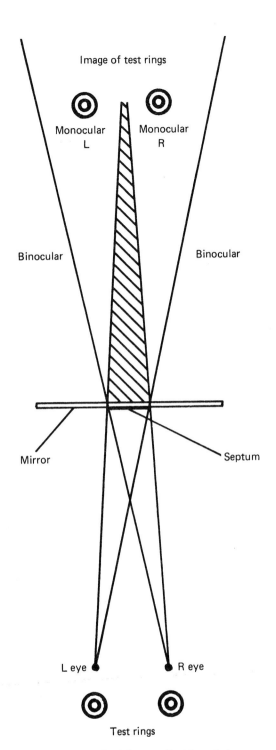

balancing, a very convenient test object often incorporated in test charts, panels or slides is two identical sets of concentric circles, one seen by the right eye and the other by the left eye only. Alternatively, a line of suitable size on a Snellen test chart can be selected.

The spherical power is adjusted to give, if possible, equal acuity to the two eyes. If there is a difference, it is generally inadvisable to fog the better eye or over-minus the poorer eye in pursuit of equality or to leave the dominant eye with an acuity lower than the poorer eye. Some practitioners prefer to use the TIB technique with a slight fog, to about 6/9, when balancing spheres. This is subject to the remarks on the previous page on unequal response to equal fogging. The method will in any case be useless if the eyes are fogged by +1.00 DS and comparison is attempted on the 24 m line: ±0.25 DS extra will then make little difference.

The bichromatic test and the TIB may be combined, but in this case the method is too sensitive to allow simultaneous comparison between right and left eyes. For each eye in turn, the clarity of the patterns on the two colours should be equalized or adjusted to a red or green preference, as appropriate. Because the two eyes have been open and the great majority of the visual field has been seen binocularly, it is unlikely that accommodative effort will alter between viewing with first one eye and then the other. It is this stability of accommodation that is the most important asset of binocular refraction.

The Humphriss fogging method

If one eye only is fogged by +0.75 or +1.00 DS, foveal vision in that eye is suspended, but paracentral and peripheral vision are maintained. This is the principle of the so-called psychologic septum, introduced as a balancing test by Humphriss (1961) and Humphriss and Woodruff (1962). Millodot's (1972) data would suggest that a central area about 2–3° diameter – about 20–30 cm at 6 m – would be suspended when vision in the fogged eye was reduced to 6/12.

Simpson (1991) showed that there was an increasing probability of suppression of detailed foveal stimuli when the monocular blur was increased from 0.50 D to 1.00 D. This confirms clinical experience that fogging by +1.00 D can generally be relied upon to ensure that the patient's attention is transferred to the other eye, but if the fogged eye is strongly dominant, transference of attention to the unfogged eye may not result.

The Humphriss fogging method may be used with the bichromatic test. Each eye observes the chart in turn while its follow eye is fogged with a +1.00 DS. The sphere before the observing eye is then adjusted to give equality, red preference or green preference as felt appropriate by the refractionist.

The Humphriss immediate contrast test (HIC)

The immediate contrast test HIC is an additional routine introduced by Humphriss. With the monocular refractive findings in place, a +1.00 DS is placed before the left eye* (Humphriss recommended a +0.75 DS, but

Figure 6.15. Principle of the Turville infinity balance or septum technique. The test rings at the bottom of the diagram are imaged by the mirror, but the septum occludes the right eye's view of the left-hand image and vice versa. The shaded area is invisible to both eyes. (The fields of view as shown vary slightly with the patient's PD.)

black is sometimes used) and of width about 30–35 mm (half the inter-pupillary distance). As shown in *Figure 6.15*, the effect of this occluding strip is to divide the central portion of the test chart image into two separate monocular fields surrounded by a binocular field of view. Originally, a special set of test cards was used with the TIB, but they are not essential. For spherical with the patient fully corrected for hypermetropia, that is, red preference on the bichromatic test. If green preference is the aim at this stage, a +1.00 D fogging lens is indicated). The patient's attention is directed to an end letter on the 9 m line and is shown this first through an extra +0.25 DS, then −0.25 DS before the right eye.† He is asked to say which lens is the more comfortable,‡ not necessarily the one which makes the letters clearer or blacker. To help relax accommodation, the plus lens should be shown first and left in place for several seconds, the minus lens for only one or two.

If the patient is already looking through a balanced correction, the +0.25 DS will blur the vision, while the −0.25 DS will tend to stimulate accommodation but still allow a reasonable view of the test object. The patient will then prefer the second (minus) lens. Accordingly, a −0.25 D lens is placed before the right eye and the +0.25/−0.25 DS choice offered again. This time the +0.25 DS will not give rise to blurring while the −0.25 DS will require 0.50 D of accommodation. The fogging produced by the +1.00 D lens before the left eye and the 0.25 D of accommodation already in play will inhibit further accommodation or make it uncomfortable. The plus lens will be preferred and so the minus trial lens is removed.

Strictly, when the −0.25 D lens was placed before the right eye, an equal lens should have been placed before the left eye. This procedure is certainly advisable when larger adjustments are required, but is of doubtful necessity when only 0.25 D is involved.

The process is repeated for the left eye, with the +1.00 D fogging lens transferred to the right eye.

To take a second example, suppose that at the end of monocular refraction the findings are

R   + 1.75 DS   L   + 2.25 DS

The steps in the HIC procedure could then be as set out in *Table 6.4*. It is strongly recommended that the reader should try this method on himself, in order to understand the appearances of the letters.

The final choice may depend on other factors: for example, the higher plus findings for the older patient (presbyope), esophore or young person who will be using the correction mostly for close work; the lower plus for a young person who will be wearing the correction for distance vision.

---

* It can be useful to have an extra lens in the trial set with the handle painted a different colour for identification and as a reminder when in the trial frame. Pinhole discs and occluders could also have painted handles.

† The use of a lens pair mounted on a single handle is recommended.

‡ Humphriss' original article suggested that the patient should be told: 'One of the two lenses put before your eyes may make the letters blacker but not clearer. Choose the clear lens, and not the lens that makes the letters blacker.' The use of the much neater phraseology in the main body of the text has been taught for many years at the Institute of Optometry, and works very well, despite the departure from the usual criterion of acuity. The practitioner must use his or her own judgement should the patient respond that the first lens is more comfortable, the second sharper.

Binocular refraction

The advantage of refracting under binocular conditions is that the eyes are in a more normal situation than when one eye is occluded. If, however, the trial cylinder before one eye is markedly incorrect in power or axis, the patient may be in an even more unnatural visual state than with one eye occluded. Therefore, unless the practitioner is very confident of the accuracy of his retinoscopy findings, it may be better to ascertain the astigmatic component in the conventional, occluded way and then verify it under binocular conditions. With experience, however, the practitioner will be able to identify those patients with whom the whole refraction may be done under binocular conditions, saving the patient repetition and himself time. Humphriss (1961) and Rabbetts (1972), for example, have shown that in unselected series of patients, slight but sometimes significant differences in astigmatic power and axis arise on changing from monocular to binocular refraction.

To determine the astigmatic correction with the Humphriss method, the +0.75 or +1.00 DS fogging lens is placed before one eye and the other eye briefly covered to check that the first eye is fogged. The sphere level for the second eye is then adjusted, using either the bichromatic or the immediate contrast method, to put the circle of least confusion on or just in front of the retina. The cross cylinder is then used in the normal way to confirm the astigmatic axis and power. The fogging lens is then transferred to the second eye and the process repeated for the first eye.

The TIB is less suitable for long processes such as the complete determination of the astigmatic correction, since the head has to be kept quite still, but it is good for the final confirmation under binocular conditions, especially where a dominant eye renders the Humphriss technique uncomfortable.

An alternative technique for binocular refraction and balancing uses polarized light and an analysing visor for the patient. In one method, test characters on duplicate panels (side by side) are mounted on polarized backgrounds. The transmission axes for the right eye's test background and analyser are parallel and perpendicular to those for the left eye. The right eye's panel thus appears black to the left eye and vice versa. This can give rise to the disconcerting effect of retinal rivalry or intermittent suppression.

In another method,* polarized characters are printed on the projector slide or near-test card. By this means, the test characters in one field appear black on a clear background to the eye with the crossed analyser, while the other sees a uniform light field. The same refracting techniques may then be used as with septum methods, for example, a bichromatic balance or the comparison of acuity between the two eyes (with black on white symbols). The printed characters for the two fields may overlap to allow tests for stereopsis.

When retinoscopy is followed immediately by binocular refraction, it is perhaps advisable to measure the

---

* Vectograph Project-O-Chart slides and Vectographic Near-Point Cards (American Optical Co.).

Table 6.4 Humphriss' immediate contrast test: example of procedure

	Right eye	Left eye
Initial spherical correction	+1.75	+2.25
L eye fogged by +1.00 D	+1.75	+3.25
+0.25 D presented to R eye	+2.00 clear	+3.25
−0.25 D presented to R eye	+1.50 effort required	+3.25
Plus lens preferred: hence add +0.25 D	+2.00	+3.25
+0.25 D presented to R eye	+2.25 blurred	+3.25
−0.25 D presented to R eye	+1.75 slight effort required	+3.25

The −0.25 D is preferred. Thus, the indicated correction for the right eye is +2.00 DS or, possibly, +1.75 DS. Repeating the process for the left eye:

	Right eye	Left eye
Initial spherical correction	+2.00	+2.25
R eye fogged by + 1.00 D	+3.00	+2.25
+0.25 D presented to L eye	+3.00	+2.50 blurred
−0.25 D presented to L eye	+3.00	+2.00 slight effort required
Minus lens preferred: hence add −0.25 D	+3.00	+2.00
+0.25 D presented to L eye	+3.00	+2.25 clear
−0.25 D presented to L eye	+3.00	+1.75 effort required

The +0.25 D is preferred. Thus, the indicated correction for the left eye is +2.25 DS or, possibly, +2.00 DS.

	Right eye	Left eye
Balanced spherical correction	+2.00	+2.25
or, possibly,	+1.75	+2.00

For purposes of record, the higher plus (or lower minus) choice may be termed the plus option and the other the minus option.

patient's vision through the objective correction with the other eye occluded. This will ensure that the correction is sufficiently exact for binocular refraction to be a help rather than a hindrance.

An alternative basis for binocular balancing and refraction originally used in the USA is to induce double vision by adding 4Δ base up before one eye and 4Δ base down before the other. The bichromatic test or comparison of acuity with or without +0.50 DS of fogging may then be made. To the present writers, the unnatural conditions of test would appear to make this method less precise than the septum, Humphriss or polarizing methods. In a comparison with vectographic methods, West and Somers (1984), however, conclude that these prism dissociation techniques do provide a valid binocular balance method.

General observations

Balancing of the sphere is a complex subject with a large choice of techniques, none of which works in all cases.

Where there is a unilateral strabismus or defective acuity in one eye, very careful balancing of the sphere levels is not required. The best lens that can be found monocularly for each eye in turn may be sufficient.

Where one eye has a slightly poorer acuity, the HIC method may work better than Turville's acuity balance, but the basic Humphriss fogging method and the TIB generally work well in conjunction with the biochromatic test. The TIB is preferable for anisometropic patients.

If transference to the non-dominant eye does not occur, it may be indicated by any of the following: indecisive results with the cross cylinder or HIC tests; red clarity from the fogged dominant eye on the biochromatic test, irrespective of the lens in front of the eye being tested; or patient discomfort shown by verbal comment or closing the dominant eye to allow refraction of the other eye.

If one eye is markedly dominant, neither of the Humphriss methods may work. Similarly, determination of the astigmatic correction under binocular conditions with the fogging method is unlikely to work for the non-dominant eye.

The binocular addition

After a subjective refraction on each eye monocularly, it is possible that when binocular vision is in play more plus power will be accepted without detriment to binocular visual acuity.

This can also happen following the use of balancing techniques, which establish the relative sphere power between the two eyes, but not necessarily the absolute level. The use of binocular refractive techniques, especially the Humphriss method, does tend to relax the patient's accommodation, making the binocular addition test less important than when following monocular refraction.

The method is straightforward: with the distance correction in place, the patient watches the lowest line of letters than he can read binocularly. A +0.25 DS lens is added simultaneously before each eye, and, if preferred, is incorporated in the correction. The process is then repeated. The practitioner should bear in mind that a test object at 6 m is dioptrically at a distance of −0.16 D, so that what is accepted in the consulting room may leave an undesirable blur outdoors. In some cases, especially where the symptoms or objective results suggest more hypermetropia than the subjective findings, the binocular addition is better determined by fogging with +1.00 DS binocularly. The resulting binocular vision is measured and the addition reduced by 0.25 DS at a time until the best acuity is again obtained.

Oculo-motor balance and previous correction

The visual axes of the two eyes may not readily intersect at the object being viewed, but may show a tendency to deviate, requiring additional adjustments by the nerves and muscles that rotate the eyes to obtain precise binocular fixation. Such a tendency to deviate is called an oculo-motor imbalance (*see* Chapter 10). Provided that binocular fixation can nevertheless be maintained, the imbalance is termed a heterophoria.

A deviation of one eye up or down relative to the other will show as an apparent relative vertical displacement of the rings on either side of the TIB septum. The rings may be levelled with plano prisms, which should then be considered for incorporation into the patient's prescription. The TIB indicates a need for prism more frequently than the fixation disparity test (*see* Chapter 10). An uncorrected vertical heterophoria will make the patient less comfortable during a binocular refraction and should be compensated by a prism before using the Humphriss methods.

In near vision, the visual axes converge to intersect at the point of regard. This convergence is normally associated with accommodation. For this reason, a hypermetrope who has to accommodate to see clearly in the distance may tend to develop esophoria (convergent heterophoria), though esophoria may be associated with any refractive error. Because balancing under binocular conditions helps to inhibit the accommodation, a higher plus correction may be found than under monocular conditions.

Conversely, a person whose eyes tend to drift apart (an exophore) may tend to accommodate more in binocular than monocular refraction, although this occurs infrequently. With the Turville septum, an exophore's visual axes may diverge enough for each axis to pass simultaneously through the appropriate circle. Fusion then occurs, giving the appearance of one ring. In this event, base-in prism will be needed to regain separate vision of the two rings before the procedure can be continued. An alternative but rarely used approach is to reduce the width of the septum to about 21 mm, as suggested by Banks (1954). It can be deduced from *Figure*

6.15 that there will then be a narrow central area which can be seen binocularly, thus providing greater binocular lock. For this purpose, an extra symbol such as a letter X or I midway between the right and left concentric rings will be needed.

The final correction obtained is not necessarily the one to be prescribed. If there is a large change in correction from that previously worn, it is often advisable to prescribe a compromise correction and give the full amount later. A previously uncorrected hypermetrope may well be very comfortable with +2.00 DS, even though the correction found was +4.00 DS. Marked changes in astigmatic power or axis can certainly cause initial discomfort with a new correction, but are usually justified by the improvement in vision obtained. An oculo-motor imbalance may also require adjustment to the refractive findings. Only experience can guide the practitioner.

With young children whose vision is in the formative stage, full astigmatic corrections, if significant, should almost always be given immediately to give the acuity the maximum chance to develop. A year's delay with a partial correction can be too long. Small refractive errors may be less significant in children than in adults, since their visual tasks are less detailed.

The repeatability of refraction

Three recent surveys on the repeatability of refractions have suggested that refraction may not be as accurate as thought. Adams *et al.* (1995) found that although the mean difference in spherical equivalent refraction between the results of two different examiners on 86 subjects aged 10–60 years was 0.12 D, there was a wide spread of results, with 95% of the differences falling between −0.90 and +0.65 DS. Perrigin *et al.* (1982) each refracted optometry students, aged 20–28 years, while McKendrick and Brennan's (1995) students were aged 19–26 years. Their results are shown in *Table 6.5*, McKendrick and Brennan's results being printed in italics.

The age of the subject or patient may have a bearing on the repeatability. Accommodation will be more active in younger patients, especially if under-corrected

Table 6.5 Percentage of subjective refraction results within the power or axis orientation limits of each other

	Power			
	The same	*Within ±0.25 D*	*Within ±0.50 D*	*Within ±0.75 D*
Spherical equivalent	27	86	98	
Spherical power	48	93	99	
		88	*97*	*97*
Cylindrical power	51	93	99	
		64	*100*	*100*
Anisometropia	44	95	100	

	Axis		
	Within 5°	*Within 10°*	*Within 20°*
	71	88	
	73	*78*	*93*

hypermetropes, while the smaller pupils and poorer media of the elderly again are likely to reduce accuracy. Conversely, the proportion of presbyopic patients who show negligible change in refraction over an interval of a year or more would suggest that the process is indeed repeatable.

Cycloplegia

Except in the mature patient, there is a normal resting state of ciliary effort and accommodation known as tonus. This accommodative tonus does not form part of the refractive error, since it will not relax even if the appropriate correcting lens is worn for a long time. In the young uncorrected or under-corrected hypermetrope, this tonus may be increased abnormally because of the habitual use of accommodation in distance as well as near vision. A normal routine examination will not reveal the full refractive error because some of the hypermetropia remains latent – masked by the accommodation. In young children a spasm of accommodation may cause excessive fluctuations in refraction, so that it is not possible to obtain a reasonable assessment of either sphere or cylinder.

Drugs known as cycloplegics, which temporarily paralyse the ciliary muscle (and also the iris sphincter) facilitate a truer determination of the refractive error. Atropine sulphate, usually as a 1% ointment, will abolish all the accommodative tonus and an allowance of about 1.00 D has usually to be made for the resting tonus regained when the effects of the drug have passed. Because it is slow both in taking effect and in wearing off, it is now rarely employed. A weaker but quicker-acting drug, 1% or 0.5% cyclopentolate hydrochloride (drops) abolishes most of the tonus and is excellent for most patients when a cycloplegic refraction is necessary.

No fixed rule can be given for the proportion of the cycloplegic refractive error to be prescribed for hypermetropes. The fullest possible correction should be given for young esotropes ('convergent' squinters, *see* Chapter 10). A partial correction leaving one or two dioptres uncorrected may be best for other young hypermetropes of over 3 D; the manifest findings and their influence on the binocular co-ordination obtained in the pre-cycloplegic examination will be a guide. If no pre-cycloplegic examination was undertaken, a post-cycloplegic refraction will be necessary to evaluate the effects of the full and partial corrections in both distance and near vision. In the absence of signs or symptoms, it may be unnecessary to correct young hypermetropes with an error of less than about +3.00 DS under cycloplegia. In myopia, cycloplegia will reveal the lowest correction giving the maximum acuity and hence the full findings should normally be prescribed.

The aberrations associated with the dilated pupil may result in an astigmatic correction that is inappropriate for the normal pupil size. It is therefore preferable to prescribe the cylinder found before cycloplegia if reliance can be placed on it. In theory, an artificial 3 mm pupil placed before the patient's eye would solve the problem, but any error of centration with respect to the visual axis could then make the refraction even less accurate. During the objective technique of retinoscopy (*see* Chapter 17), the refractionist must watch the centre of the pupil rather than the periphery, especially when dilated under cycloplegia.

A cycloplegic examination is also indicated in several other circumstances:

(1) when the symptoms appear to be of refractive origin but are not explained by the change found initially;
(2) when the accommodation measured is very low for the age;
(3) when the oculo-motor balance is markedly esophoric;
(4) when the subjective findings are considerably less hypermetropic or more myopic than the objective results.

Finally, the emmetrope or low hypermetrope with spasm of accommodation may appear to be myopic. Because of proximal accommodation myopia, this frequently occurs when children's sight is checked on a vision screener (*see* Chapter 19). This pseudo-myopia will be revealed under cycloplegia.

Exercises

6.1 Compile a third column for *Table 6.2*, relating to a ±0.37 D cross cylinder.

6.2 Calculate the effective power at the cornea of lenses of power +10.00, +11.00, +19.00 and +20.00 DS, assuming 15 mm vertex distance. What is the effective power interval between the neighbouring pairs of lenses? Repeat the calculation for negative lenses. What relevance have these figures to the choice of trial case contents and to refraction?

6.3 An objective refraction gave +2.50/−1.50 × 170. Describe the possible steps, using the modified fan and block technique, that led to the final prescription of +2.25/−1.25 × 160.

6.4 A patient's previous prescription is listed in column P, the current findings in column C. What is the lens power that has to be held over P to convert it to C, so that the change in prescription can be demonstrated to the patient? Approximate answers are adequate for (c) and (d).

	P	C
(a)	+5.00/−2.75 × 180	+3.75/−2.75 × 180
(b)	+4.00/−2.75 × 180	+4.00/−2.00 × 180
(c)	−2.25/−1.50 × 75	−3.00/−2.00 × 80
(d)	+3.00/−0.50 × 180	+3.75/−0.50 × 95

6.5 (a) A distant point source is viewed by an eye of normal length with a pupil diameter of 5 mm and principal powers of +58.00 D in the horizontal and +59.50 D in the vertical meridian. Assuming that the subject accommodates throughout so as to keep the circles of least confusion on the retina, find the diameters of this circle: (i) in the uncorrected eye, (ii) when an 0.25 D cross cylinder is placed before the eye with its minus axis vertical, (iii) when the cross cylinder is twirled to bring its minus axis horizontal. (b) Assuming that you had no knowledge of the powers of this eye, what would you deduce from your results about the cylindrical correction required?

6.6 The lens +4.75 DS/−3.25 DC axis 45 is placed before an eye having a spectacle refraction of +5.00 DS/−2.75 DC axis 35. What is the residual error of refraction, referred to the spectacle plane (that is, what additional lens is needed to correct the eye completely)?

References

ADAMS, C.W., BULLIMORE, M.A., FUSARO, R.E., COTTERAL, R.M., SARVER, J. and GRAHAM, A.D. (1995) The reliability of automated and clinician refraction. *Invest. Ophthalmol. Vis. Sci.*, **36**, S947

BANKS, R.F. (1954) A foveal lock for infinity balance. *Br. J. Physiol. Optics*, **11**, 216–225

BENNETT, A.G. (1963) The theory of bichromatic tests. *Optician*, **146**, 291–296

BENNETT, A.G. (1968) *Emsley and Swaine's Ophthalmic Lenses*, pp. 170–180. London: Hatton Press

FLOM, M. and GOODWIN, H.E. (1964) Fogging lenses: differential acuity response in the two eyes. *Am. J. Optom.*, **41**, 388–392

HUMPHRISS, D. (1961) Refraction by immediate contrast. In *International Optical Congress 1961*, pp. 501–510. London: British Optical Association

HUMPHRISS, D. and WOODRUFF, E.W. (1962) Refraction by immediate contrast. *Br. J. Physiol. Optics*, **19**, 15–20

IVANOFF, A. (1953) *Les Aberrations de l'Oeil*. Paris: Editions de la Revue d'Optique

JACKSON, E. (1887) Trial set of small lenses and a modified trial frame. *Trans. Am. Ophthal. Soc.*, **4**, 595–598

JACKSON, E. (1907) The astigmatic lens (crossed cylinder) to determine the amount and principal meridians of astigmia. *Ophthal. Rec.*, **17**, 378–383

JOHNSTON, A.W. (1990) Verification of accuracy in cross cylinder refractions – are our expectations realistic? *Frontiers of Vision – 10th Anniversary Conference*, p. 26. London: British College of Optometrists

LINDSAY, J. (1954) A theoretical investigation into the possibilities of error in the measurement of astigmatism by the crossed cylinder. *Br. J. Physiol. Optics*, **11**, 210–215

McKENDRICK, A.M. and BRENNAN, N.A. (1995) Clinical evaluation of refractive techniques. *J. Am. Optom. Ass.*, **66**, 758–765

MADDOX, E.E. (1925) The 'V' test for astigmatism. *Am. J. Physiol. Opt.*, **6**, 56–58

MILLODOT, M. (1972) Variation of visual acuity in the central region of the retina. *Br. J. Physiol. Optics*, **27**, 24–28

MINISTRY OF HEALTH (1956) *Trial Case lenses*, Report of a Committee appointed by the Minister of Health. London: HMSO

O'CONNOR DAVIES, P.H. (1957) A critical analysis of bi-chromatic tests used in clinical refraction. *Br. J. Physiol. Optics*, **14**, 170–182, 213

O'LEARY, D.J., YANG, P.H. and YEO, C.H. (1987) Effect of cross cylinder power on cylinder axis sensitivity. *Am. J. Optom.*, **64**, 367–369

PERRIGIN, J., PERRIGIN, D. and GROSVENOR, T. (1982) A comparison of clinical refractive data obtained by three examiners. *Am. J. Optom.*, **59**, 515–519

RABBETTS, R.B. (1972) A comparison of astigmatism and cyclophoria in distance and near vision. *Br. J. Physiol. Optics*, **27**, 161–190

SIMPSON, T. (1991) The suppression effect of simulated anisometropia. *Ophthal. Physiol. Opt.*, **11**, 350–358

TURVILLE, A.E. (1946) *Outline of Infinity Balance*. London: Raphaels

VERHOEFF, F.H. (1923) The 'V' test for astigmatism, and astigmatic charts in general. *Am. J. Ophthal.*, series 3, **6**, 908–910

WALSH, G., CRAWFORD, M. and DONEGAN, M. (1993) Comparison of results from common subjective methods of astigmatism determination. *Ophthal. Physiol. Opt.*, **13**, 106

WARD, P.A. (1987) The utility of fogging for relaxing accommodation. *Optician*, **194** (5119), 19–20, 22, 26

WEST, D. and SOMERS, W.W. (1984) Binocular balance validity: a comparison of five common subjective techniques. *Ophthal. Physiol. Opt.*, **4**, 155–159

WILLIAMSON-NOBLE, F.A. (1943) Possible fallacy in the use of the cross cylinder. *Br. J. Ophthal.*, **27**, 1–12

Accommodation and near vision. The inadequate-stimulus myopias

Introduction

The young eye is able to change its refractive power by alterations in curvature of the crystalline lens (*see* pages 11–12). The increase in power is known as accommodation. In the unaccommodated state, the ciliary muscle is relaxed, the suspensory zonule of Zinn is at its greatest tension, the lens takes its flattest curves and the retina is conjugate with the far point M_R. In the accommodated state, the ciliary muscle is constricted in a sphincter-like mode, relaxing the zonule of Zinn and allowing the lens to take a more convex form. In the fully accommodated state the retina is conjugate with M_P, the near point of accommodation* (in Latin, *punctum proximum*). Its linear distance from the eye is denoted by b and its dioptric distance $1/b$ by B. The maximum accommodative effort is termed the amplitude (Amp).

The above is a brief statement of the classical approach to accommodation. From this standpoint, the eye is said to be 'relaxed' when no accommodation is in play. In recent years, however, it has been demonstrated that under various conditions, including poor illumination and insufficient object detail, the accommodation tends to stabilize involuntarily at a level somewhat higher than zero. This is currently known as the 'resting state of accommodation'. The resulting ocular condition is termed (by the present authors) inadequate stimulus myopia and is discussed more fully on pages 132–138.

Although these later discoveries throw important light on the visual system, they do not invalidate the classical approach as a basis for clinical practice and the measurement of accommodation.

Figure 7.1 shows the far and near points of an emmetropic eye and *Figure 7.2* those of a myopic eye. In the general case we have the following relationships:

For the relaxed eye

$$K' = K + F_e \tag{7.1}$$

For the fully accommodated eye

$$K' = B + (F_e + \text{Amp}) \tag{7.2}$$

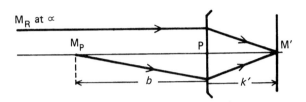

Figure 7.1. The far point M_R and near point of accommodation M_P of an emmetropic eye.

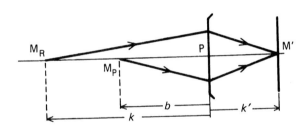

Figure 7.2. The far point M_R and near point of accommodation M_P of a myopic eye.

which gives

$$\text{Amp} = K - B \tag{7.3}$$

and

$$B = K - \text{Amp} \tag{7.4}$$

In emmetropic and myopic eyes, the near point is invariably real (b negative) but, as shown by equation (7.4), the hypermetrope's near point will be real only if his amplitude is greater than his distance refractive error.

The range of accommodation is the linear distance from the far point to the near point. Thus, for an emmetrope with 8 D of accommodation, the near point distance is $1/-8$ m or -125 mm, so the range of accommodation is from infinity to -125 mm.

Example (1)

What is the range of accommodation of an uncorrected myope of -4 D whose amplitude is 10 D?

---

* Usually abbreviated to 'near point', though in the USA this term is often used for any near point.

$k = 1/K = 1/-4 = -0.25\,\text{m} = -250\,\text{mm}$

$B = K - \text{Amp} = -4 - 10 = -14\,\text{D}$

$b = -71.4\,\text{mm}$

The range of accommodation is -250 to $-71.4\,\text{mm}$.

Example (2)

What is the range of accommodation of an uncorrected hypermetrope of $+4\,\text{D}$ whose amplitude is 6 D?

$k = 1/K = 1/4\,\text{m} = +250\,\text{mm}$

$B = K - \text{Amp} = 4 - 6 = -2\,\text{D}$

$b = -500\,\text{mm}$

Thus, in this case, the range of accommodation falls into two parts. By exerting up to 4 D of accommodation, the hypermetropia can be progressively reduced to zero, so that the point conjugate with the retina recedes from the far point to infinity. This is the virtual part of the range. This is of no use, except when using an optical instrument which can provide a virtual object for the eye. When the distance ametropia is corrected by 4 D of accommodation, the remaining 2 D of amplitude can be used to see clearly from infinity to $-500\,\text{mm}$ from the eye. This is the real part of the total range of accommodation, sometimes called the range of distinct vision.

Spectacle and ocular accommodation

Basic principles

In clinical practice most measurements are referred to the spectacle plane. Thus, in general, it is not ocular but spectacle refraction which is determined.

Consider a near object B at a distance ℓ_s from the spectacle point S (*Figure 7.3*). A paraxial pencil from B would have a vergence L_s $(= 1/\ell_s)$ at the spectacle point, but would be rendered parallel by an added lens of positive power $-L_s$. This hypothetical lens would obviate the need for accommodation and so its power is a measure of the so-called 'spectacle accommodation'. If this is denoted by A_s, then

$$A_s = -L_s \tag{7.5}$$

Because of the lens–eye separation, the required ocular accommodation A differs in general from the spectacle accommodation, often by a significant amount. If d is the vertex distance, that is, the positive distance from the spectacle point to the eye's (first) principal point, then, in the simplest case of the emmetropic eye (*Figure 7.3*), the object distance PB measured from the eye would be

$$PB = PS + SB = -d + \ell_s$$

For example, given $\ell_s = -250\,\text{mm}$ and $d = 14\,\text{mm}$ we should have $PB = -264\,\text{mm}$, which gives us

Spectacle acc $A_s = 1/0.250 = 4.00\,\text{D}$
Ocular acc $\quad A = 1/0.264 = 3.79\,\text{D}$

Thus, for the emmetrope, the ocular accommodation is less than the spectacle accommodation.

When a distance correction is worn, the relationship is complicated by the fact that the effect of the lens–eye separation varies with the vergence of the pencil emerging from the spectacle lens. In distance vision, the vergence at the eye's principal point is equal to the ocular refraction K. In near vision, pencils from the given point B reach the eye with a vergence L which is numerically less positive or more negative than K. For sharp retinal imagery, the power of the eye must therefore be increased by $(K - L)$. Hence the ocular accommodation required is

$$A = K - L \tag{7.6}$$

Figure 7.4 illustrates the case of a myopic eye corrected by a thin distance lens of power F_{sp}. The ocular accommodation required can be calculated by the 'step-along' method, as in the following examples.

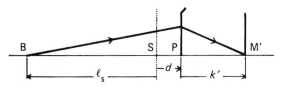

Figure 7.3. The distance ℓ_s of a near object B measured from the spectacle point S.

Example (3)

A myope is corrected by a thin $-4.00\,\text{D}$ lens at a vertex distance of 14 mm. A near object of regard is $-350\,\text{mm}$ from the eye's principal point. Compare the ocular accommodation with the spectacle accommodation and that required by an emmetrope to focus the same object.

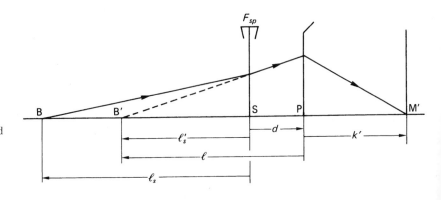

Figure 7.4. A myopic eye, corrected by a spectacle lens of power F_{sp}, viewing a near object B. The corresponding diagram for distance vision is *Figure 4.8*.

The distance $\ell_s = -336$ mm so that

Spectacle acc $A_s = 1000/336 = 2.98$ D

In distance vision

	D			mm
F_{sp}	-4.00	$\rightarrow$	f'_{sp}	-250
			$-d$	-14
K	-3.79	$\leftarrow$	k	-264

The arrow indicates the conversion from a distance in mm to the dioptric equivalent (or vice versa) by taking 1000 times the reciprocal.

In near vision

L_s	-2.98	$\leftarrow$	ℓ_s	-336
$+F_{sp}$	-4.00			
L'_s	-6.98	$\rightarrow$	ℓ'_s	-143.27
			$-d$	-14
L	-6.36	$\leftarrow$		-157.27

Ocular acc $= A = K - L = 2.57$ D

Since the near object is -350 mm from the eye, the accommodation required by an emmetrope would be $1000/350 = 2.86$ D.

The ratio of ocular accommodation to that required by an emmetrope has been termed by Pascal (1952) the 'accommodative unit'. In this case it is $2.57/2.86$ or 0.90.

Example (4)

A hypermetrope is corrected by a thin $+4.00$ D lens at a vertex distance of 14 mm. A near object of regard is -350 mm from the eye's principal point. Compare the ocular accommodation with the spectacle accommodation and that required by an emmetrope to focus the same object.

The spectacle accommodation and accommodation required by an emmetrope are as in Example 3. Figure 7.5 illustrates the calculation of ocular accommodation for the hypermetrope.

In distance vision

	D			mm
F_{sp}	$+4.00$	$\rightarrow$	f'_{sp}	$+250$
			$-d$	-14
K	$+4.24$	$\leftarrow$	k	$+236$

In near vision

	D			mm
L_s	-2.98	$\leftarrow$	ℓ_s	-336
$+F_{sp}$	$+4.00$			
L'_s	$+1.02$	$\rightarrow$	ℓ'_s	$+980.4$
			$-d$	-14
L	$+1.03$	$\leftarrow$		$+966.4$

Ocular acc $= A = K - L = +3.21$ D

In this case, the accommodative unit is $3.21/2.86$ or 1.12.

Although the above examples assume thin lenses, the principle of the method applies equally when the actual lens form and thickness are taken into account. In this case, a paraxial pencil would have to be traced through each surface of the lens. The distance ℓ_s is now measured from the front surface of the lens, while ℓ'_s becomes the image distance measured from the back surface.

Figure 7.6 shows the true ocular accommodation required over a wide range of ametropia corrected by spectacle lenses of typical form and thickness. Graphs are given for three different object distances (measured from the corneal vertex).

The circles show, for each of these distances, the value of F_{sp} at which the ocular accommodation is the same as that required by an emmetrope, that is, accommodative unit equal to unity. The squares show the value of F_{sp} at which the ocular accommodation is equal to the spectacle accommodation.

It can be seen that the demand on ocular accommodation increases rapidly as hypermetropia increases. As will be shown later, contact lenses require about the same amount of accommodation that an emmetrope would need to exert. Consequently, the advantage enjoyed by spectacle-corrected myopes disappears when they turn to contact lenses. Hypermetropes, on the other hand, may benefit substantially from the lower demand on accommodative effort.

Figure 7.6 was based on calculations in which the form and thickness of each lens were taken into account. A 14 mm vertex distance was assumed. For comparison, corresponding figures for 'thin' (zero thickness) lenses were obtained from equation (7.7) below. Over the whole range of minus lens powers, only negligible differences were found between the two sets of results. In the case of plus lenses, the thick lens values were up to about 8% greater, depending on the lens power. In the extreme case with $F_{sp} = +8.00$ D

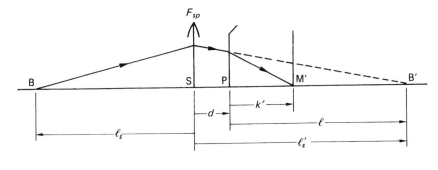

Figure 7.5. A hypermetropic eye, corrected by a spectacle lens of power F_{sp}, viewing a near object B. The corresponding diagram for distance vision is *Figure 4.9*.

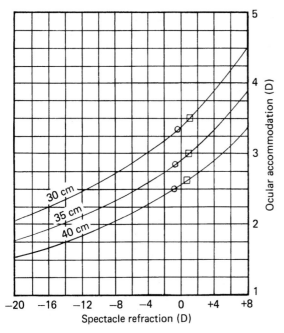

Figure 7.6. Graphs showing required ocular accommodation for stated object distances (measured from the corneal vertex) in ametropia corrected by spectacle lenses of typical form and thickness. Vertex distance taken as 14 mm. Circles: ocular accommodation equals that required by an emmetrope; squares: ocular accommodation equals spectacle accommodation.

and the object distance $-300\,\text{mm}$, the necessary ocular accommodation was found to be $4.52\,\text{D}$ for the actual lens and $4.20\,\text{D}$ for the thin lens.

Approximate expressions

By using binomial expansions it is possible to arrive at approximate expressions from which useful generalizations can be made.

Given an object distant ℓ_s from a thin lens of power F_{sp} at a distance d from the eye, the vergence L at the eye is

$$L = \frac{L_s + F_{sp}}{1 - d(L_s + F_{sp})} \quad \text{while} \quad K = \frac{F_{sp}}{1 - dF_{sp}}$$

The ocular accommodation, equal to $K - L$, is

$$A = \frac{-L_s}{(1 - dF_{sp})\{1 - d(L_s + F_{sp})\}} \tag{7.7}$$

If this is expanded by the binomial theorem and terms in d^2 and higher powers are omitted, we obtain

$$A = -L_s\{1 + d(L_s + 2F_{sp})\} \tag{7.8}$$

and

$$\frac{\text{ocular acc}}{\text{spectacle acc}} = \frac{A}{A_s} = 1 + d(L_s + 2F_{sp}). \tag{7.9}$$

Applying this approximation to Example (3) we obtain

$$A/A_s = 1 + 0.014\{-2.98 - 8.00\} = 0.85$$

The accurate figure is $2.57/2.98 = 0.86$.

For Example (4) we obtain

$$A/A_s = 1 + 0.014\{-2.98 + 8.00\} = 1.07$$

whereas the accurate figure is $3.21/2.98 = 1.08$.

From approximation (7.9) we can deduce that the ratio becomes unity when $F_{sp} = -L_s/2$, that is, when the spectacle refraction is in the vicinity of $+1.25$ to $+2.00\,\text{D}$. *Figure 7.6* gives rather lower values ranging from about $+0.50$ to $+1.00\,\text{D}$.

To obtain an approximate formula for the accommodative unit, we need an expression for A_{em}, the accommodation required by an emmetrope. The object, viewed directly, is at a distance $(\ell_s - d)$ from the eye's principal point, so that

$$A_{em} = \frac{-1}{\ell_s - d} = \frac{-L_s}{1 - dL_s} \tag{7.10}$$

Hence, from equation (7.7)

$$\text{Acc unit} = \frac{A}{A_{em}} = \frac{1 - dL_s}{(1 - dF_{sp})\{1 - d(L_s + F_{sp})\}} \tag{7.11}$$

Binomial expansion with terms in d^2 and higher powers omitted leads to the approximation

$$\text{Acc unit} = 1 + 2dF_{sp} \tag{7.12}$$

These last two expressions both show that there are two cases in which the accommodative unit becomes equal to unity:

(1) When $d = 0$. This very nearly applies to the contact lens wearer because the distance from the corneal vertex to the first principal point of the schematic eye is only about $1.5\,\text{mm}$. In terms of accommodation, the contact-lens wearer may be regarded as an emmetrope.
(2) When $F_{sp} = 0$. It also follows from equation (7.12) that the accommodative unit is greater than unity in the case of hypermetropia and less than unity in myopia. However, *Figure 7.6* shows that for lenses of average form and thickness the dividing line is not emmetropia but myopia of slightly less than $-1.00\,\text{D}$.

As a matter of theoretical interest only, equation (7.11) can also be reduced to unity when $F_{sp} = -L_s + 2/d$. This relates to the clinically impossible case in which myopia of extreme degree is corrected by a positive lens forming a real inverted image between the lens and the eye.

Equation (7.12) is a reasonably good approximation when the value of F_{sp} is not high. Applied to Example (3)

$$\text{Acc unit} = 1 + 0.028\,(-4.00) = 0.89$$

whereas the more accurate value was found to be 0.90.

For Example (4) it gives

$$\text{Acc unit} = 1 + 0.028\,(+4.00) = 1.11$$

instead of 1.12. Curiously enough, the approximation becomes increasingly inaccurate in the range of *minus* lens powers from $-8.00\,\text{D}$ upwards.

Measurement of amplitude

The distance correction must be in place before the amplitude of accommodation is measured, or else a myope would give a falsely high reading and a hypermetrope a low one. The amplitude may be ascertained both monocularly and binocularly.

In the usual clinical method, sometimes termed the push-up test, the patient observes a finely detailed test object which is brought closer to the patient's eye until the detail just begins to blur. For convenience, a near-point rule graduated in dioptric distances may be used, the reference point being approximately in the spectacle plane. Care must be taken to ensure that the test card does not fall into shade as it approaches the eye. An opposite method is to start with the card very close to the patient's eye and to move it away until the detail just becomes clear. Fitch (1971) found that except in the age group 25–40, a higher amplitude was recorded on moving the stimulus towards the patient than on sliding it away. The binocular amplitude was slightly greater than the monocular, especially on moving the test object towards the patient. Both these differences, although statistically significant, were only a fraction of a dioptre and of little clinical importance.

As with the simple subjective optometer (*see* pages 74–75) the angular subtense of the object increases as it approaches the eye, a factor which makes legibility easier. To prevent this effect, the Badal optometer can be adapted (Lindsay, 1954). Somers and Ford (1983) found the amplitude in the 32–40 age group to be only 0.6 D less when measured with a Badal optometer than the figure obtained with the push-up test.

The amplitude may also be measured with the patient observing either the distance test chart or a near chart at a fixed distance from the eye. Minus lenses are added until the acuity begins to fall, signifying that the full amplitude of accommodation has already been used to overcome the artificial hypermetropia produced by the minus lenses. Because the test object itself remains at a constant distance, there is not the same psychological stimulus to accommodate as with a genuine near object, though the fixed near object may provide a better stimulus than the distance chart because of the induced proximal accommodation (*see* page 134). For this reason, a slightly lower amplitude is often found, as by Kragha (1986) who concluded that the simpler push-up test was reliable. The method works monocularly but not binocularly, because it would then disturb the normal relationship between accommodation and convergence of the eyes.

Rosenfield and Cohen (1996) also compared these three methods for measuring the amplitude. The mean results for their five 23–29-year-old subjects were amplitudes of 11.1 D for the push-up method, 9.5 D for the slide-down and 9.1 D for the negative lens method with a test chart fixed at 0.4 m. They postulated that minification of the chart by the negative lenses may have contributed to the lower result with this method – the present writer would suggest that the minification may be caused by micropsia, described on page 119, since the angular subtense of the object does not increase in harmony with the demand on accommodation. Rosenfield and Cohen (1995) also measured the amplitude with test letters of various sizes, to find slightly greater subjective amplitude with larger letters. They attribute this to a delayed perception of blur with larger letters.

They also point out that a letter subtending, say 5 minutes, at 40 cm for an older patient will subtend a larger angle to a child with more than 10 D of accommodation. This suggests that measurements of younger people's amplitudes may be over-estimated. Exercise 7.4 also suggests another reason for the over-estimation of high values of the amplitude.

When using a near-point rule to measure the amplitude of a patient with low accommodation, a positive spherical lens should be placed in the trial frame to bring the artificial near point to a convenient distance of about 250 mm. The patient will not be able to judge an end-point if the test print is already blurred, and only large print is legible. Similarly, a minus lens may be placed before the eye of a young patient to push the near point away from the eye. Allowance must be made in each case for the supplementary lens power.

Objectively, dynamic retinoscopy (Chapter 17) may be used to measure the amplitude. A test object is mounted on the retinoscope or held just in front of it and the examiner approaches the eye while observing the movement of the reflex. When a with movement is seen, the eye is under-accommodating for the distance of the retinoscope. For research purposes an objective optometer may be used, the subject observing the test object through a beam splitter.

Accommodation and age: presbyopia

Normal amplitude

As explained on pages 11–12, the young crystalline lens is capable of being moulded into a steeper shape by its capsule when the ciliary muscle contracts and the zonule relaxes. As the crystalline ages, the alteration in curvature becomes less for the same action of the muscle, (*see* page 129). The decline in focusing ability starts in youth and continues till the age of about 60, after which the small amount that apparently remains is probably depth of field (*see* pages 288), not true accommodation.

Donders (1864) was one of the first to measure accommodation as a function of age, but his findings have been superseded by the results of Duane (1922), obtained from over 4000 eyes. Duane measured the amplitude both monocularly and binocularly, taking as the origin a point 14 mm in front of the cornea, approximately 15.5 mm from the eye's first principal point. In effect, spectacle accommodation was measured in emmetropes and fully corrected ametropes. *Figure 7.7* shows the results for monocular accommodation. The binocular results were 1–2 D higher in patients up to 15 years of age, the increase falling to below 1.0 D in the 45- to 50-year group, and usually less than 0.5 D higher in the over-50 group. These differences are far greater than those reported by Fitch (1971). Comparisons of Donders' and Duane's results have been made by Hofstetter (1944) and Turner (1958).

The shape of the curve in the 45–60 year old is debatable. As these measurements of the amplitude have been done subjectively, they include depth of field. Since the N5 print frequently employed as the stimulus

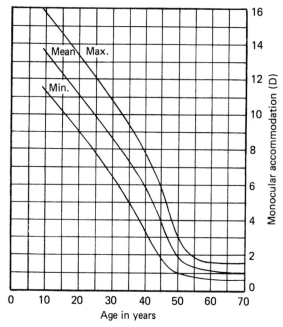

Figure 7.7. Variation of amplitude of accommodation with age. Monocular values (after Duane, 1922) related to the spectacle plane.

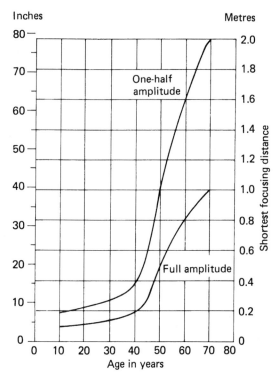

Figure 7.8. The shortest linear focusing distances corresponding to exertion of all and half the available mean amplitude of accommodation as a function of age.

corresponds to about 6/12 (*see Figure 3.17*), coupled with relatively small pupils in this age group, a high value for the depth of field or apparent amplitude is given. Thus, Millodot and Millodot (1989) measured the depth of field to be just over 2 D, a figure much greater than the 0.3 D cited on page 289.

Objective measurements of the amplitude have been made. Hofstetter (1965) made studies on two subjects, finding a linear reduction in amplitude, with it falling to zero before the age of 50, while Hamasaki *et al.* (1956) found less than 0.50 D of accommodation in their subjects who were aged over 48.

Charman (1989) argued that the gradual slowing in loss of accommodation shown in *Figure 7.7* for the 50–55 age group was a statistical consequence of taking the mean of many subjects for each age group. He postulated that for any particular individual, the amplitude was a linear function of age which declined to zero, but the spread of ages at which the zero point was reached softened the otherwise abrupt intercept between the linear decline and the horizontal line corresponding to the depth of field.

At the other end of the age scale, Sokol *et al.* (1983) used the method of visually evoked response to try to determine the accommodative response of infants. Most 2–4-month-old infants showed some response, while those 4–5 months old could accommodate up to 5–6 D. This was confirmed by Howland *et al.* (1987), who, using the method of photorefraction, found that all of their infant subjects aged 2–10 months altered their accommodation appropriately for stimuli at distances between −25 and −100 cm. In *Figure 7.8*, Duane's mean results have been re-plotted in terms of the nearest distance from the spectacle plane at which an emmetrope can see clearly when the full amplitude of accommodation has been exerted. While a child of 10 can focus at 10 cm or so, an adult of 50 can just see clearly at only

about arm's length. A separate graph shows the increased distances when only half the amplitude is in play.

Extra focusing power is therefore needed by the older eye in the form of a 'near addition' of positive power to the distance correction. A person needing such help for close work is said to be presbyopic. Presbyopia (from Greek roots meaning old eye) cannot be defined in terms of a specific amplitude of accommodation. The need for a near addition or correction depends not only on the available amplitude, but also on the habitual working distance and nature of the near visual task. Though sufficient for reading a short article, the amplitude may not serve for a day's close work.

Corrected hypermetropes have a lower spectacle accommodation than emmetropes and will tend to need a near addition at a younger age. The converse applies to myopes. In fact, myopes of less than 4 or 5 D can often cope with close work by merely removing their distance correction.

A hypermetrope's first distance correction, whether full or partial, will also be helpful to him in near vision and may postpone the need for a near addition. Even so, this is likely to be required at an earlier age than the emmetrope, because of the greater demand on ocular accommodation imposed on hypermetropes in general.

Variations from the normal

Figure 7.7 shows not only the mean value but also the normal spread of amplitude at any particular age.

Thus, approximately:

Age	Spread of amplitude
20–45	±2.00 D
50	±1.00 D
50 and over	±0.50 D

This spread was confirmed by Rosenfield and Cohen (1996) in the work already cited. The mean of their five subjects' standard deviations was 0.7 D, which suggests that a minimum change of around 1.5 D in a patient's recorded amplitude is necessary before it is meaningful, especially as usually only one measurement, not several, are made in the consulting room.

Some young patients have reserves of accommodation which are markedly subnormal (Francis *et al.* 1979), and this is why accommodation should always be measured, even in the young. Such deficiency may be due to latent hypermetropia, general poor health, Down's syndrome (Woodhouse *et al.* 1993), cerebral palsy (Leat, 1996), ocular disease, a side-effect of medical treatment or lack of normal use. This latter can occur, for example, in myopes who do not wear their spectacles for close work. Poor accommodation, sometimes associated with poor convergence, can also occur idiopathically, that is, without discoverable cause. On the other hand, some elderly patients have accommodative reserves much greater than normal, possibly because of a large depth of field due to a small pupil.

If a patient's amplitude is low, a greater than normal mental effort or neurological stimulus is needed to obtain the required amount of accommodation. The brain interprets this excessive effort as the object being closer than it really is and hence smaller because a small object at a short distance subtends the same angle at the eye as a larger object at a greater distance. The apparent reduction in size is known as micropsia: the opposite effect – macropsia – results from a spasm of accommodation. These effects occur particularly when drugs affecting the ciliary muscle are instilled into the eye.

There is a controversy over whether or not different ethnic groups or people living in hotter climates have a lower accommodation for age than Europeans. Edwards *et al.* (1993) found their sample of Hong Kong Chinese to have amplitudes of accommodation between 1 and 2 D lower than Duane's findings, with depth of field only being reached between the ages of 45 and 50. Coates (1955) found little difference in the variation in amplitude with age between South Africans of European stock who had lived in Africa for at least five years and other ethnic groups – all, however, had amplitudes below those given by Duane. Hofstetter (1968) obtained studies of typical bifocal additions from Fiji and Ghana, suggesting that the Fijians and Ghanaians needed near additions about 0.50 D stronger in the early presbyopic years than Europeans living in the same country. Weale (1981) plotted the average age at which accommodation fell below 3 D against both latitude and average ambient temperature. He found a decrease in this age with increasing temperature and attributed this to the fact that the surroundings can influence the temperature of the body to a depth of 10 mm below the sur-

face. The lens obviously lies within this region. The relationship with latitude was not significant.

The opposite view was taken by Bergman (1957) who found that the Afrikaan group (who had lived in South Africa all their life) had similar amplitudes to those given by Duane and Donders. This view is supported by Kragha (1986) in a study of Nigerians, and by Kragha and Hofstetter (1986) who found no significant difference in near additions prescribed in a survey covering the north to the south of North America.

Since there is a natural spread of amplitude within any one age group, it is not surprising if patients need a first near prescription at both earlier and later ages than normal. The amount of close work undertaken, the habitual working distance (both closer or further than average), pupil size and illumination are all obvious factors. In some countries, the availability of spectacles and their expense may also influence the age at which a correction is first sought. The patient's pride or self-consciousness may also be factors.

The near addition

There are three ways in which the initial near addition may be selected. These are based on the measurement of the amplitude of accommodation, age or the symptoms and strength of the present spectacles.

From measurement of the amplitude

The first step is to measure the available accommodation. *Table 7.1* gives approximate expected values which are easy to remember.

The third column gives an approximate addition, which may usefully be incorporated in the trial correction before the amplitude is measured, due allowance being made as already noted. It must be emphasized that the addition prescribed depends on the patient's working distance and actual amplitude and should never be based solely upon age.

To use one's full accommodative power for any length of time is not possible, but a fraction between one-half and two-thirds can be sustained. Thus, if L_s is the dioptric working distance and Amp_s the full amplitude measured from the spectacle plane,

$$\text{Add} = (-L_s) - \tfrac{1}{2}\,Amp_s \qquad (7.13)$$

$$\text{or} = (-L_s) - \tfrac{2}{3}\,Amp_s \qquad (7.14)$$

Table 7.1 Expected amplitude of accommodation and approximate near additions at various ages

Age (years)	Expected amplitude (D)	Near addition (D)
20	10	–
30	8	–
40	6	–
45	4	0–1.00
50	2	1.00–1.75
55	1	1.50–2.25
60	1	1.75–2.50

As a rule of thumb, the fraction of two-thirds seems too high to the present writers, who also demur at the common assumption that one-third of a metre ($L_s = -3.00$ D) is the normal working distance. This may apply to people engaged in very fine work, or with defective acuity, the shorter working distance making the retinal image larger. Nevertheless, the most common working distances are found to range from about 380 to 450 mm, giving a mean value of L_s in the neighbourhood of -2.50 D. Numerically, a higher value of L_s offsets a higher fraction of the amplitude. Thus, equation (7.13) with L_s taken as -2.50 D gives very similar results (for amplitudes up to 3.00 D) as equation (7.14) with $L_s = -3.00$ D. Millodot and Millodot (1989) also investigated the proportion of amplitude used, to find $(50.7 \pm 27)\%$, the mean figure agreeing with equation (7.13) above. Both these workers and Morgan (1960) found that patients adopting a shorter working distance appeared to utilize a higher proportion of their available accommodation. Woo and Yap (1995) attributed the need for a presbyopic addition in Hong Kong Chinese at an earlier age than in Caucasians to their shorter arm length.

In view of the differences between spectacle and ocular accommodation shown by *Figure 7.6*, it may be questioned whether near additions can safely be prescribed on the basis of the spectacle accommodation. In fact, no qualms need arise. The following example, which is typical, shows that an addition based on a particular fraction of the spectacle amplitude calls into play almost exactly the same fraction of the ocular amplitude.

Example (5)

An eye is corrected for distance vision by $+4.00$ DS at 14 mm from the reduced surface. The spectacle amplitude is 3.00 D and the working distance -400 mm from the spectacle plane. What is the theoretical addition needed if based on one-half of the given amplitude and what fraction of the ocular amplitude would then be in use?

Since $\ell_s = -400$ mm, $L_s = -2.50$ D and from equation (7.13)

Add $= 2.50 - (0.5 \times 3) = +1.00$ D

As in Example (4), we now need to find the ocular refraction K:

	D			mm
F_{sp}	$+4.00$	$\rightarrow$	f'_{sp}	$+250$
			$-d$	-14
K	$+4.24$	$\leftarrow$	k	$+236$

With the $+1.00$ D addition in use, the near correction F_n is $+5.00$ D. Hence, in near vision at -400 mm:

	D			mm
L_s	-2.50			
$+F_n$	$+5.00$			
L'_s	$+2.50$	$\rightarrow$	ℓ'_s	$+400$
			$-d$	-14
L	$+2.59$	$\leftarrow$	ℓ	$+386$

The ocular accommodation in use $(K - L)$ is $(4.24 - 2.59)$ or 1.65 D.

To find the full ocular amplitude, since we know that the spectacle amplitude is 3.00 D, the test object has to be at a dioptric distance of -3.00 D from the spectacle plane with the distance correction in use. Accordingly, tracing the incident pencil to the eye, where its vergence is the dioptric distance B to the eye's near point, we have

	D			mm
L_s	-3.00			
$+F_{sp}$	$+4.00$			
L'_s	$+1.00$	$\rightarrow$	ℓ'_s	$+1000$
			$-d$	-14
B	$+1.01$	$\leftarrow$	b	$+986$

Hence, from equation (7.3)

Amp $= K - B = 4.24 - 1.01 = 3.23$ D

The ocular accommodation in use with the prescribed addition is 1.65 D out of the available total of 3.23 D, the fraction being $1.65/3.23$ or 0.51. This is almost identical with the fraction of the spectacle amplitude adopted for determining the prescribed addition. Although thin lenses were used in these calculations, the end result would have been almost the same with real lenses.

Prescribing a near addition on the basis of the measured amplitude is not sufficiently reliable, because of possible inaccuracies in this measurement. Moreover, the theoretically assumed demand on accommodation may not be the amount readily exerted.

From the patient's age

The last column of *Table 7.1* gives approximate near additions which can lead directly to refinement as described below, rather than as a preliminary to measurement of the amplitude – this is the present writer's approach. Alternatively, Bussin (1990) suggests a starting point of:

(patient's age $- 35)/10$

on the assumption of a near working distance of $-\frac{1}{3}$ m, or

(patient's age $- 40)/10$

for a longer working distance (personal communication). The steady increase in addition given by such formulae (and some published tables) for patients aged over their mid-60s should be treated with caution, since many elderly patients still prefer to read at 40 cm or more, thus needing an addition no greater than $+2.50$ D.

From the present spectacles

If the patient is relatively happy with his present correction, then it would be unwise to alter the present mean sphere by more than a small amount.

Whichever approach has been taken, the final addition should be made by one or more of the methods about to be described.

Methods of checking the addition for near vision

Range of clear vision

The reading test types are used and, with the estimated addition in place, the patient is directed to observe the smallest size of type that he can read. He is then asked to bring the card closer until the print begins to blur. The same procedure is repeated with the card moved further away. These two positions should straddle the preferred position, with the greater part of the range on the far side where it is likely to be more useful. If necessary, the trial lenses are altered to give this optimum distribution.

Trial lens method

The patient looks at the test card held at his chosen distance – which at this stage may not be the clearest position – and low-powered spherical lenses are added. If these are preferred, they are incorporated in the trial correction; if rejected, lenses of opposite power are tried. Excess minus power will be rejected because of the increased accommodation required, excess plus power because it upsets the normal relationship between accommodation and convergence (*see* pages 160–164). With many patients a state may be reached where both plus and minus quarter-dioptre lenses either cause equal deterioration in vision or make no difference. No alteration need then be made. It is interesting that the dioptric equivalent of the range is frequently larger than the ±0.25 D lenses that are rejected.

Bichromatic tests

With the addition in place, the patient holds a near bichromatic test, often a pattern of dots on the two colours (*see Figure 7.16*). The addition is adjusted to give a slight clarity preference for the green background or, perhaps, equality. The detail on the red background should become clear if the device is moved 10–30 mm further away. The senile yellowing of the crystalline lens may be raised as an objection to this test because it tends to promote a red bias typical in the elderly patient. Nevertheless, unless the lenses are very yellow or hazy, the test appears to work well. Moreover, since a red bias tends to give equality with a lower positive power, the addition prescribed would err on the safe side.

Cross cylinder method

The patient observes a grid and a ±0.50 D cross cylinder is added to the trial correction, the minus axis vertical (*Figure 7.9*). If the addition is insufficient or the eye under-accommodated, the horizontal lines appear clearer. If the reverse applies, the vertical lines are clearer. The addition is adjusted to give equal blurring. This method may be used monocularly or binocularly.

Westheimer (1958) suggested a modification whereby the patient is first asked to observe the grid without the cross cylinders. These are then put in position and the

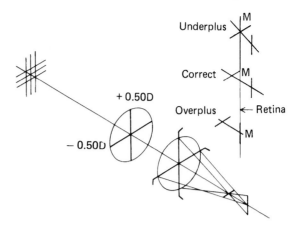

Figure 7.9. The cross cylinder technique for determining the addition. The isometric drawing shows a grid screen viewed through a cross cylinder, negative axis vertical. The rear focal line is vertical and if it appears clearer, indicates too high an addition, while clearer horizontal lines indicate too low an addition.

patient asked to report immediately whether the horizontal or vertical lines appear sharper. Because an immediate response is required, the patient has no time to adjust his accommodation so as to bring one meridian of the test object into focus. If the horizontal lines appear clearer, a low positive sphere may be added to each eye's correction and the procedure repeated until both meridians of the grid seem equally clear on introduction of the cross cylinders.

This technique may also be used as a check on the distance correction, but in this case the method of quickly introducing the cross cylinders must be used with non-presbyopic patients. If the cross cylinders are left in place for any length of time, the eye will accommodate to make the vertical lines clearer, but is unable to relax to make the horizontal lines clearer. This would suggest incorrectly that the patient needs a weaker plus correction.

The accommodative response

When considering the level of accommodative demand on the eyes, two well-established facts should be borne in mind. One is that the accommodation actually exerted is generally less than the amount theoretically needed for sharp focusing – *see Figure 7.17*. Confirmation is provided by the extremely high proportion of non-presbyopes, wearing any necessary distance correction, who see the pattern better on the green background in the bichromatic test. Reversal usually occurs with the addition of +0.50 DS. This means that a theoretical demand for, say, 2.50 D of accommodation results in an exertion of about 2.00 D. As shown on pages 288–290, the eye's depth of focus is thus used to its best advantage.

Rosenfield *et al.* (1996) compared several techniques, including an autorefractor (Chapter 18) to assess the accommodative response in a group of 25 year olds. They found that, for binocular viewing of a −2.50 D stimulus, the autorefractor and dynamic retinoscopy (Chapter

Table 7.2　Examples of demand on ocular accommodation in cases of anisometropia

Spectacle refraction	Thin lenses			Real lenses		
	R Eye	L Eye	Diff.	R Eye	L Eye	Diff.
R −1.00 DS			With no addition			
L +1.00 DS	2.43	2.57	0.14	2.47	2.65	0.18
			With +2.00 D addition			
	0.57	0.60	0.03	0.61	0.66	0.05
			With bifocal			
				0.52	0.60	0.08
R +6.00 DS			With no addition			
L +8.00 DS	2.97	3.15	0.18	3.16	3.39	0.23
			With +2.00 addition			
	0.69	0.76	0.04	0.93	1.11	0.18
			With bifocal			
				0.90	0.82	−0.08

17) measured the response to be about 2.00 D, the bichromatic test slightly more at 2.17 D, while the cross cylinder method slightly higher again. They concluded that the nature of the cross cylinder test lead to overactive accommodation. Monocularly, the autorefractor found a lag of accommodation of about 0.3 D, whereas the bichromatic test found 0.75 D. This reflects the author's experience, where monocular (including strabismic) patients usually need more plus than binocular patients to obtain reversal to seeing the stimulus on the red clearer.

On the other hand, accommodation termed 'proximal' is often stimulated by the knowledge that an object of regard is actually at a near distance, even though it is viewed through a lens or optical system intended and adjustable to place the image at infinity. For this reason, the eyepiece of instruments such as microscopes and focimeters should always be racked out towards the eye and then moved inwards until the image just comes into focus.

Proximal accommodation is quite marked in young people and would, for example, introduce serious errors in measuring their refraction with a simple type of optometer, and under-estimates of visual acuity with vision screeners.

Returning to the fact that the amplitude of accommodation has declined to just depth of focus by the age of 50, the question arises as to why the near addition continues to increase from this age. Pointer (1995), for example, found that up to the 51–55 age group, the mean near addition was given by the expression

$$0.252 + 0.0996\ (age - 40)$$

and for the group older than this, by

$$1.272 + 0.0364\ (age - 40)$$

with the two expressions meeting at around 1.8 D. This gives a rise from 1.3 to 1.8 D between ages 50 and 55, and a further 0.5 D up to the age of 70. The near bichromatic test would suggest that there is indeed a decline in accommodation, since an increasing addition is required over these periods of time to give equality. Mill-

odot and Millodot (1989) have suggested that a larger image is needed to compensate for the clarity as the ocular media deteriorates with age. They suggest that the working distance becomes shorter, possibly aided by the curving spinal posture.

Near vision and anisometropia

For a given working distance, the difference between spectacle and ocular accommodation has been shown to vary with the distance refractive error. It follows from this that in cases of anisometropia the two eyes are called upon to exert different amounts of ocular accommodation.

Table 7.2 summarizes data relating to two different refractive errors, each with 2.00 D of anisometropia. In each case the object distance was taken as −400 mm and the vertex distance as 14 mm. The ocular accommodation required for sharp focusing is shown both for 'thin' lenses and for real lenses of typical form and thickness. Figures for the latter are seen to be slightly higher.

When no reading addition is in use, the difference in the accommodative demand on the two eyes is 0.18 D in one case and 0.23 D in the other. Though these amounts may not be clinically significant, they are probably nearing the level where discomfort may result.

When a near addition is in use, less accommodation is needed and so the difference between the right and left amounts required is also reduced. For comparison, *Table 7.2* also gives the ocular accommodation needed when a +2.00 D near addition is in use, both as single vision near correction and as a front surface bifocal addition.

In the great majority of cases, the innervation to accommodate is probably the same in each eye and generally results in equal accommodative effort. Differences in flexibility of the crystalline lenses or the strength of the ciliary muscle can give unequal response between the two eyes. Innervation to one eye may also be defective. It is unlikely, however, that purposive differences in accommodation can be produced, though such a response is postulated in one of the references cited on page 125. The depth of focus of the eye and fluctuations in accommodation described on page 130 may serve to moderate the effect of any difficulties caused by anisometropia. Moreover, the depth of focus in near vision is greater than in distance vision because of the smaller pupil size.

The older ametrope requires different corrections for distance and near vision, whether in bifocal form or otherwise. In theory, the younger anisometrope – despite adequate accommodation – may also need a separate near correction designed to equalize the accommodative effort of the two eyes.

Effectivity of the astigmatic correction in near vision

The difference between spectacle and ocular accommodation is a consequence of effectivity – a concept relating to the change in vergence that occurs between two specified points on the path of a pencil of rays. Over a given distance, the change in vergence varies with its initial value, being roughly proportional to the square of this quantity.

Another consequence is that the cylindrical component of a distance correcting lens invariably has a reduced astigmatic effect in near vision.

Example (6)

The distance correction $+6.00/-3.50 \times 150$ is worn at 16 mm from the reduced surface. What is the effective cylinder power in near vision at -400 mm from the lens (assumed thin)?

The main stages in the calculation are illustrated in *Figure 7.10*.

Each principal meridian must be dealt with separately, as follows.

Distance vision

	150° meridian		60° meridian	
F_{sp}	$+6.00$		$+2.50$	
f_{sp}		$+166.67$		$+400$
$-d$		-16		-16
k		$+150.67$		$+384$
K	$+6.64$		$+2.60$	

The effective cylinder power at the eye is $(6.64-2.60)$ or 4.04 D, which can be taken as indicating the amount of ocular astigmatism.

Near vision at -400 mm

	150° meridian		60° meridian	
L_s	-2.50		-2.50	
$+F_{sp}$	$+6.00$		$+2.50$	
L'_s	$+3.50$		0	
ℓ'_s		$+285.7$		
$-d$		-16		
		$+269.71$		
L	$+3.71$		0	

The effective cylinder power at the eye is now only 3.71 D, which is 0.33 D less than in distance vision.

For a significant under-correction of 0.50 DC to occur in near vision, this result suggests that the distance astigmatism must be about 4–5 D. As in anisometropia, the normal depth of focus of the eye is capable of tolerating moderate differences. Where symptoms of asthenopia do arise in near vision, it is probably better to measure the astigmatism subjectively (*see* page 127) than to rely on theoretical allowances.

There have been many attempts to derive theoretical relationships between the correcting cylinder in distance and near vision. Fletcher (1951/52) presents a summary of these equations, while an exact expression due to Swaine is quoted by Rabbetts (1972).

The change in cylinder effectivity in near vision can also be regarded as a meridional difference in the required ocular accommodation. Numerically they are identical. Reverting to *Example (6)* it will be see that the quantity $(K-L)$ expressing the required ocular accommodation is 2.93 D in the 150° meridian and 2.60 D in the 60° meridian. The difference, 0.33 D, was the result obtained for the change in cylinder effectivity from distance to near vision. A simple approximate expression for this quantity can hence be derived.

The first step is to substitute $-L_s$ for A_s (equation 7.5) in equation (7.9) which can then be put in the form

$$A = -\{1 + d(L_s + 2F_{sp})\}L_s \qquad (7.15)$$

in which A is the ocular accommodation.

Let F_α and F_β denote the spectacle refraction in the two principal meridians of the eye and A_α and A_β the ocular accommodation theoretically required in these two meridians. Then, from equation (7.15),

$$A_\alpha = -\{1 + d(L_s + 2F_\alpha)\}L_s$$

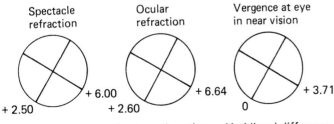

Spectacle refraction $+2.50$ $+6.00$
Ocular refraction $+2.60$ $+6.64$
Ocular astigmatism 4.04D
Vergence at eye in near vision 0 $+3.71$
Meridional difference 3.71D

Figure 7.10. Stages in the calculation of reduced cylinder effectivity in near vision.

and

$$A_\beta = -\{1 + d(L_s + 2F_\beta)\}L_s$$

which gives

$$A_\alpha - A_\beta = -2dL_s(F_\alpha - F_\beta) \tag{7.16}$$

Applied to Example (6), this approximation would give the answer 0.28 D, the correct result being 0.33 D.

A more exact expression relating the required cylinder powers in distance and near vision may be derived.

Let M denote the mean power $(S + C/2)$ of an astigmatic lens. The two principal powers of the lens are then $(M + C/2)$ and $(M - C/2)$. Also, let C be the distance-correcting cylinder, C' the effective power of C at the eye, C_n the theoretically required near-vision cylinder and C'_n the effective power of C_n at the eye. Then, by use of the exact effectivity formula, equation (2.11), the relationship in distance vision can be written as

$$C' = \frac{M + C/2}{1 - d(M + C/2)} - \frac{M - C/2}{1 - d(M - C/2)}$$

$$= \frac{C}{(1 - dM)^2 - d^2C^2/4} \tag{7.17}$$

In the general case of near vision at a dioptric distance L_s from the lens, the correction may incorporate a near addition of power N. Consequently, the quantity M in the above expressions must be replaced by $(L_s + M + N)$, leading to

$$C'_n = \frac{C_n}{\{1 - d(L_s + M + N)\}^2 - d^2C_n^2/4} \tag{7.18}$$

If C_n has the correct value, C'_n will remain the same as C' in distance vision. Little loss of accuracy will ensue if the term in d^2 in the denominators of equations (7.17) and (7.18) is omitted as being relatively small. The condition that $C' = C'_n$ is then represented by the equation

$$C_n/C = \frac{\{1 - d(L_s + M + N)\}^2}{(1 - dM)^2} \tag{7.19}$$

Expanded by the binomial theorem with terms up to d^2 retained, this becomes

$$C_n/C = 1 - 2d(L_s + N) + d^2\{(L_s + N)^2 - 2M(L_s + N)\} \tag{7.20}$$

This ratio, always greater than unity, reduces as the near addition is increased, becoming unity when $N = -L_s$. With no addition in use, the expression takes the simpler form

$$C_n/C = 1 - 2dL_s + d^2(L_s^2 - 2L_sM) \tag{7.21}$$

It will be noted that the ratio C_n/C as given by these various expressions is independent of the cylinder power. Since the term in d^2 is relatively small, especially for moderate values of M, it can be omitted if only a reasonable first approximation is sought.

Figure 7.11, plotted from equation (7.19), gives a representative range of values and also shows the effect of a +2.00 D near addition. A vertex distance of 14 mm was assumed. For a dioptric working distance of -2.50 D the cylinder power in near vision should theoretically be some 7–9% higher than the distance correct-

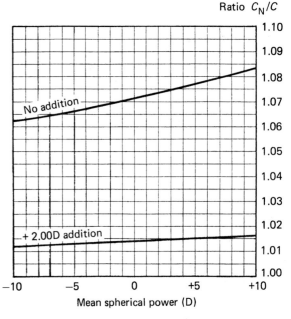

Ratio C_N/C

Figure 7.11.   The approximate ratio of required near cylinder C_N to distance cylindrical correction C as a function of mean spherical power. Vertex distance taken as 14 mm and near object vergence as -2.50 D.

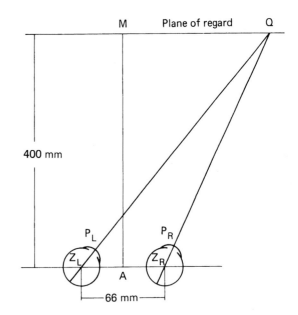

Figure 7.12.   Accommodation in asymmetrical convergence.

ing cylinder. With a +2.00 D near addition in use, the difference becomes less than 2%.

Accommodation in asymmetrical convergence

In *Figure 7.12*, Z_R and Z_L are the eyes' centres of rotation and AM is a line in the median plane, which is a vertical plane bisecting Z_RZ_L at right-angles. So far we have considered only near objects situated in the median plane, where they are equidistant from both eyes. This is not the case for any fixation point such as Q that is not in the median plane.

Referring to *Figure 7.12*, suppose the distances (taken as positive) to be as follows: $Z_R Z_L = 66$ mm, $MQ = 100$ mm, and $MA = 400$ mm. Then

$$(QZ_L)^2 = 133^2 + 400^2$$

which gives $QZ_L = 421.5$ mm.

Since the centre of rotation lies approximately 12 mm behind the eye's principal point, P_L, the object distance $P_L Q$ is -409.5 mm and the corresponding vergence -2.44 D. A similar calculation for the right eye shows the vergence to be -2.54 D, a difference of 0.10 D. If the fixation point Q were 200 mm instead of 100 mm from the median plane, the difference in vergence would become 0.16 D. Both these values are small in relation to the eye's depth of field.

The vergence difference also increases as the plane of fixation MQ approaches the eyes. For example, if MA were reduced to 200 mm, the vergence difference would reach 0.50 D with the fixation point only 70 mm from the median plane .

In general, both the head and the eyes are rotated to view objects to one side. Head movement reduces the asymmetry of the convergence. Unless the object is extremely close, the difference in object vergence at the two eyes is not significant. There have been several experimental studies of the accommodation exerted when the eyes are converged asymmetrically. Rosenberg *et al.* (1953) found that the eye nearer the object did accommodate more than its fellow eye, the difference agreeing approximately with the calculated theoretical value. Spencer and Wilson (1954) also measured small differences between the accommodation levels in the two eyes, but the eye exerting the greater amount was not always the one closer to the fixation object.

Near vision effectivity

The concept of effectivity was briefly explained on page 10. It relates to the change in the vergence of a pencil of rays from one point to another on its path. As shown by equation (2.12), the change in vergence is approxi-

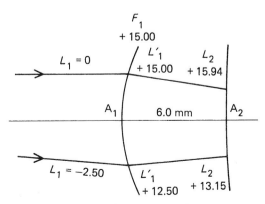

Figure 7.13. Effectivity changes arising from centre thickness of a spectacle lens in distance vision and in near vision at 40 cm.

Table 7.3 Effectivity errors of spectacle lenses in near vision ($L_1 = -2.50$ D, $n = 1.523$)

Front surface power of lens (D)	Centre thickness of lens (mm)				
	2	4	6	8	10
+10	−0.06	−0.12	−0.18	−0.25	−0.32
+15	−0.09	−0.19	−0.29	−0.40	−0.52
+20	−0.13	−0.27	−0.42	−0.58	−0.75

mately proportional to the square of its initial value. One consequence is that the change in vergence undergone between the two surfaces of a lens is not the same in both distance and near vision.

Figure 7.13 refers to a lens of front surface power +15.00 D and centre thickness 6 mm, the refractive index being 1.523. In distance vision ($L_1 = 0$), the vergence L_1' after the first refraction is +15.00 D and the vergence L_2 at the second surface is +15.94 D. The change in vergence is +0.94 D. In near vision at −400 mm ($L_1 = -2.50$ D), L_1' becomes +12.50 D and $L_2 + 13.15$ D. In this case, the change in vergence has the lower value +0.65 D. Thus, the effective power change is $(0.65 - 0.94)$ or −0.29 D, the minus sign indicating a loss of effective positive power.

A simple approximation for the effective power change can be derived from equation (2.12), with the centre thickness t replacing the distance d.

In distance vision

$$\text{Vergence change} = (t/n)F_1^2$$

In near vision

$$\text{Vergence change} = (t/n)(L_1 + F_1)^2$$

Subtracting the first of these expressions from the second we obtain

$$\text{Near effectivity error} = (t/n)(L_1^2 + 2L_1 F_1) \qquad (7.22)$$

The chief value of this approximation is the light it throws on the relationship in general. In any specific case it is just as easy to obtain an accurate value by the step-along method used on page 115. The skeleton *Table 7.3*, compiled by this accurate method, was designed to give an overall idea of the magnitude of near vision effectivity errors. Because of their small centre thickness and relatively weak front surface power, all minus lenses and plus lenses of low power can evidently be excluded from consideration.

To a good standard of approximation, the effectivity errors under discussion are proportional to the value of L_1. Thus, to find approximate values for $L_1 = -3.00$ D, the figures in *Table 7.3* should be multiplied by 1.2.

Given the same vertex distance, *any* two lenses of the same back vertex power will equally correct a static refractive error. In near vision, however, a similar equivalence may not apply to lenses of moderate and high plus powers. Ideally, trial lenses should have near effectivity errors of the same order as prescription lenses of typical form and thickness. This, unfortunately, is not the case. Lenses of the additive vertex power design have plane front surfaces giving effectivity errors in

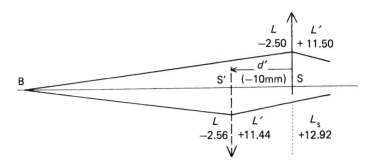

Figure 7.14.   Effect in near vision of a forward spectacle shift: thin lens power +14 D.

near vision never exceeding +0.02 D. In this respect, full-aperture bi-convex trial lenses have the advantage since their near effectivity errors (for $L_1 = -2.50$ D) range from about -0.04 D on a $+8.00$ D lens to -0.22 D on a $+20.00$ D lens.

For a fuller discussion of effective power losses in trial and prescription lenses, see Rabbetts and Bennett (1986).

Effect of forward spectacle shift

The loss of the crystalline lens in aphakia deprives the eye of its accommodative power. Nevertheless, it is well known that an effective increase in positive power can be obtained with high-powered spectacles by pushing them down the nose.

If a thin lens of power F is moved forward by a short (negative) distance d' (in metres) from the original spectacle plane, its effective power in this plane for parallel incident light is altered by approximately $-d'F^2$, which is always a positive quantity. The effect is as though the lens had been left in its original position with an additional lens of power $-d'F^2$ placed in contact with it.

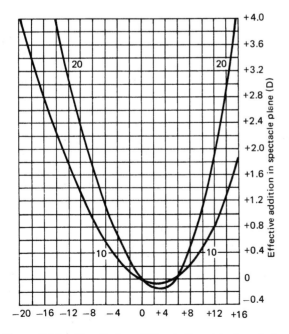

Figure 7.15.   The effective addition in the original spectacle plane when the spectacles are moved forward by 10 and 20 mm. Typical values assumed for lens form and thickness. Initial object vergence -2.50 D.

In near vision at a dioptric distance L from the lens, the effective addition in the original spectacle plane becomes approximately $-d'(L + F)^2$.

A typical case is illustrated in *Figure 7.14*. An object B is situated at a distance of -40 cm ($L = -2.50$ D) from a thin lens of power $+14.00$ D. After refraction by the lens, the vergence L' is $+11.50$ D. The lower half of the diagram represents the situation when the lens has been moved forward 10 mm from the original spectacle point S to S'. Since the object distance is now -39 cm, the vergence L becomes -2.56 D and the vergence L' after refraction is $+11.44$ D. After travelling the distance 10 mm to the original spectacle plane, the pencil has the increased vergence of $+12.92$ D. The effective addition in this plane is therefore $(+12.92 - 11.50)$ or $+1.42$ D.

When a real lens is substituted for the imaginary thin lens, the addition is reduced by a near effectivity error of the type already described. Nevertheless, there would still be a net gain with the great majority of corrections for aphakia. In the numerical example just given, the true addition would be about $+1.30$ D.

Figure 7.15, compiled by the accurate 'step-along' method used earlier in this chapter, gives an idea of the additions available by pushing spectacles down the nose. Figures have been plotted for a wide range of spectacle refractions and for forward shifts of 10 and 20 mm. Lens form and thickness were taken into account, typical values being assumed, and the initial object distance was taken as -40 cm from the front vertex of the lens. Note the loss in power with plus corrections of up to about $+6.00$ D.

The near correction

Normal routine

The relaxed or unaccommodated state of the eyes is often termed 'static' and the accommodated state 'dynamic'. In routine practice, the correction for near vision is not considered until after the static refractive error has been ascertained. One good reason is that the amplitude of accommodation cannot be measured accurately until the distance correction has been determined, and this is often required in any case. Even if the patient desires a near correction only, the practitioner has a duty to determine the corrected visual acuity. If it is subnormal, for example, 6/18 (20/60), it could be a significant pointer to some pathological or other condition requiring appropriate action to be taken.

Another reason for this procedure is that in the dynamic state, the slight pupillary contraction (miosis) and fluctuations in accommodation make it more difficult to measure astigmatism as accurately as in distance vision. This applies especially to the younger patient.

It is also routine practice to obtain the correction for near vision by giving a 'near addition' of plus power to the distance correction (*see* pages 119–121), rather than ascertaining the dynamic refraction. For the great majority of patients, this is undoubtedly a satisfactory procedure. The miosis in near vision increases the depths of field and focus, giving a slightly greater tolerance to residual errors of refraction.

When refracting in near vision it should be borne in mind that trial lenses stronger than about 4.00 D can give rise to significant amounts of oblique astigmatism, unless the visual axis is closely aligned with the optical axis of the lens (Rabbetts, 1984). From this point of view, the plano-convex form with the curved surface next to the eye is worse than others in current use. If the lens is reversed for this reason, account must be taken of its changed back vertex power. For convenience, a conversion table could be compiled with the aid of a focimeter. Careful angling and adjustment of the trial frame (if used) is a necessary precaution. For trial lenses of medium and high minus powers, the plano-concave form is particularly suitable, but careful angling is still required.

To reduce the number of lens surfaces, it is preferable to incorporate a reading addition by changing the spherical lenses, rather than by adding supplementary lenses. The trial frame generally allows the patient to reproduce the normal head and body posture better than a refractor head, hence allowing a better judgement of the patient's near vision distance.

Astigmatism in near vision

The possibility that the eye's astigmatism might show a significant change in its dynamic state should not be overlooked. From his wide-ranging investigations, Fletcher (1951/52) concluded that astigmatic accommodation does not exist as a deliberate method of compensating for ocular astigmatism, but may arise as a random by-product of the ordinary process of accommodation. He suggested it be termed 'accidental astigmatism of accommodation'. There are a number of possible causes:

(1) A tilt of the crystalline lens gives rise to astigmatism, the amount being approximately proportional to its power (pages 208–209). The astigmatism will accordingly increase with accommodation.

(2) The position and angle of tilt of the crystalline lens might also change when the suspensory zonule relaxes during accommodation.

(3) If either surface of the lens is astigmatic, the astigmatism could conceivably increase when the lens becomes more steeply curved upon accommodation.

(4) Inhomogeneities in the lens substance could give rise to an irregular change in refraction in the dynamic state.

(5) The cornea can change shape slightly upon marked eye movements from the primary position though not, perhaps, to any significant extent in normal positions of the gaze. Both Fairmaid (1959) and Lopping and Weale (1965) measured the corneal curvature before and after convergence. There was a tendency for the horizontal meridian to flatten by an amount equivalent to 0.25 D with convergence, but accommodation alone caused no appreciable change.

Despite all these possible causes for a difference in astigmatism in the eye's dynamic state, changes in astigmatic power and axis detectable by everyday clinical techniques rarely occur. Reviews on this subject have been published by (among others) Bannon (1946) and Rabbetts (1972). The latter found only nine power changes exceeding 0.25 D out of a total of 100 eyes. Significant axis changes also occurred in only a low proportion of the eyes examined.

Millodot and Thibault (1985), in a study of 122 eyes, used an objective optometer to measure changes in astigmatism as the subjects accommodated for a range of distances from 4.75 m to 30 cm. They found that those subjects who had either oblique or more than 1.0 D of with-the-rule astigmatism tended to show an increase of about 0.1 D in their astigmatism with increased accommodation. The greatest change occurred with about 2.0 D of accommodation in play. On the other hand, subjects with against-the-rule astigmatism showed a typical reduction of about 0.05 D with increased accommodation, the greatest change again occurring in the neighbourhood of 2.0 D. These results suggest that accommodation tends to produce a greater increase in power in the vertical than in the horizontal meridian.

Though these results justify the routine use of the static findings, they also indicate the occasional need to check the cylinder component in near vision. This would be necessary in cases where the patient is comfortable with his single-vision correction in distance but not in near vision. It might also be advisable if spectacles are prescribed for near vision only.

For the purpose of such a test, the cross cylinder may be used with a letter O or preferably a small circle drawn on the test card. The young subject should initially have the distance correction in place, and the presbyopic patient an adequate near addition as well. It is essential that the trial lenses be angled perpendicularly to, and centred on, the depressed line of sight, because a relative tilt will introduce oblique astigmatism.

The near refraction may be undertaken in either monocular or binocular conditions. If the former, the eye not under test should be occluded. If binocular conditions are chosen, the vision in this eye may be dimmed by a neutral filter of density 0.6–0.8 (or transmittance between 25 and 15%). Many tinted ophthalmic glasses are suitable for this purpose. An alternative method is to blur the vision with a ±1.00 D cross cylinder placed with the axes vertical and horizontal.

Polarized for R eye

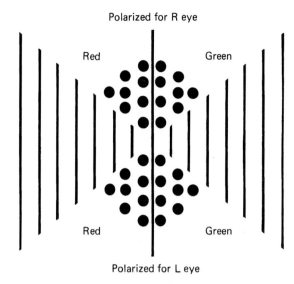

Figure 7.16. A polarized bichromatic display for near vision balancing (after Mallett), approximately three times actual size.

Critical vision is often employed in near work for much longer periods of time than in distance vision. Small uncorrected or residual astigmatic errors of the order of 0.50 D prevent sharp retinal imagery. As a result, the accommodation tends to fluctuate in search of the best focus. This may give rise to asthenopic symptoms such as tired eyes and headaches.

Balancing the spherical component

In distance vision, the spherical correction can be balanced under binocular conditions by one of the techniques described on pages 106–108. The septum technique can also be applied to near vision, as in the Esdaile–Turville equilibrium test (Turville, 1934) and the Turville near balance unit described by Giles (1960). The Humphriss method is not adaptable, because the low-powered positive lens does not fog the second eye in near vision but merely reduces the accommodative effort required. It is then not possible to tell which eye is in focus for the test object.

A technique now in common use is to combine the bichromatic method with polarization. The two halves of the bichromatic pattern are polarized in mutually perpendicular directions so that, when viewed through a similarly polarized visor, one half is visible to the right eye only and the other half to the left eye only. *Figure 7.16* shows the pattern used in the Mallett units.* To give viewing conditions as near normal as possible, the upright lines and the surround are seen binocularly. The patient's attention is directed to the upper half of the cluster of dots and the spherical correction for the appropriate eye is adjusted to give equality of contrast on the red and green backgrounds. The process is then repeated for the other eye viewing the lower cluster of dots. It is essential that this test display should have ade-

quate luminance to compensate for the light loss from the polarizing filters and analysing visor. The dots should be about 0.6–0.7 mm in diameter, subtending about 6 minutes of arc at the eye. A variant of this test uses two sets of letters instead of dots.

An objective method is to use dynamic retinoscopy (*see* Chapter 17).

The intermediate addition

The range of clear vision through a near addition decreases with increasing addition power – *see*, for example Exercises 7.5 and 7.6. Thus an early presbyope with a +1 D addition and 3 D of accommodation has a dioptric range of clear vision from −1 to −4 D, or −1000 to −250 mm if depth of field is ignored. An older patient with a +2 D addition and 1 D of accommodation can manage only from −500 to −333 mm. Consequently, an occupational need for working comfortably at distances greater than 500 mm will require a weaker addition, termed an intermediate addition. The practitioner should be careful to ascertain what is meant, however, if a patient requests help for an intermediate distance – some consider vision at 2–3 m to be intermediate.

The required intermediate addition can be determined by any of the methods described earlier in this chapter for confirming the near addition, but commencing with a power between one-half and two-thirds of the normal addition.

Depending upon the patient's needs, the prescription may be dispensed as a separate correction, a trifocal, a progressive power (progressive addition or varifocal) lens, or, rarely, an intermediate and near or distance and intermediate bifocal. The majority of trifocals have an intermediate addition fixed at 50% of the full near addition, though a few employ a 60 or 66% value. Anonymous (1980) showed that the 50% value gives a better linear overall range.

Visual display unit users

The presbyope may have difficulty working with VDUs for two reasons: first, the working distance to the screen, typically around 600 mm, is further than for conventional close work. Secondly, even when the display unit is placed in the preferred position immediately on the desk, the angle of gaze is too high for comfortable use of the bifocal's near segment, while it is too close to view through the distance portion. Burns *et al.* (1993) found that most users positioned their paperwork at a similar distance to the screen, thus suggesting that a single vision intermediate correction should perform well for most users. He also pointed out that although the keyboard is positioned closer, it has large characters and therefore does not need a near correction to view it.

European employers have a responsibility to provide special spectacles for their employees whose ordinary spectacle correction is inadequate for VDU use, for example a single vision intermediate correction supplied to a habitual bifocal wearer. The Association of Optome-

---

* Supplied by Institute of Optometry Marketing Ltd, 56–62 Newington Causeway, London SE1 6DS.

trists' recommendations on the visual standards for VDU users are given on page 370.

Specialized progressive power lenses have been developed for those users who also spend a significant amount of time working at conventional reading distances. For example, the Zeiss RD has a +0.50 D addition at the fitting cross and a slightly larger near zone than most progressives, the AO Truvision Technica has very large near and intermediate zones at the expense of a small distance zone, while the Essilor Proximal, Rodenstock Cosmolit P and Sola Access are effectively intermediate–near progressives. Although a conventional progressive power lens would allow vision with only a slight head back tilt, the width of the intermediate portion may be too narrow to allow comfortable screen work for a prolonged time. While it might be expected that the power increase down the progressive corridor might cause visual blur because of the varying power across the pupil, Burns (1995) showed that this was negligible.

Anatomy of accommodation

The fibres of the young crystalline lens form an elastic substance which is surrounded by an elastic capsule with its maximum thickness at the equator: this drives the lens into a more convex shape when the zonular tension is released by contraction of the ciliary body. Changes in the relative sizes of the lens cortex and nucleus, and their relative softness, explain the age changes in lens shape on accommodation. Thus, in the child's eye the whole lens is soft, and upon accommodation adopts a more convex spherical shape. In the young adult up to about 30 years of age, the cortex has grown to a significant thickness, but is less easily deformed than the nucleus. On accommodation, the softer nucleus thus forces the central zone of the lens to bulge more than the periphery producing an aspherical front surface with peripheral flattening. (*See* pages 281–283 for the effect of accommodation on the spherical aberration of the eye.) After the age of 30 or 40, both the nucleus and cortex stiffen, though the nucleus does so faster and eventually becomes harder than the cortex. Both the asphericity of the lens and the amplitude of accommodation continue to decrease with age. The size of the anterior portion of the ciliary muscle increases between the ages of 20 and 45, but then begins to diminish (Stieve, 1949). Thus the effort required to accommodate at the onset of presbyopia is about 50% greater than in youth. For further details, the reader is referred to the papers by Brown (1973, 1974, 1986) and Fisher (1971) and the recent reviews by Atchison (1995) and Gilmartin (1995).

Physiology of accommodation

The classical view of accommodation is that it is at rest when viewing a distant object and that the ciliary body is innervated to greater extent the nearer the object of regard. Indeed, the basis of subjective refraction is the assumption that with most patients the accommodation

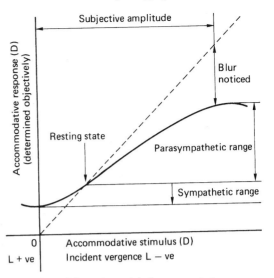

Figure 7.17. Schematic model of accommodation response in a young eye. The straight diagonal line represents coincidence of stimulus and response.

will relax when viewing the distance test chart, especially under binocular conditions.

Researches from about 1940 onwards have led to a different view. It is now thought that accommodation is exerted in both directions from an intermediate resting state. Thus, what is conventionally called over-accommodation in distance vision is an incomplete relaxation from the resting state. The accommodative function is also economical, departing from its resting state only to the extent required to give satisfactory vision. In distance vision, for example, a good Snellen acuity is consistent with slight accommodative lead (bichromatic test left clearer on the red), while the lag of accommodation in near vision has been known from the beginning of the century.

Accommodation is mediated by parasympathetic stimulation of the ciliary body under the innervation of the IIIrd cranial or oculo-motor nerve, arising in the mid-brain. In the absence of a definite visual stimulus, a low degree of neural activity gives rise to some ciliary tonus – hence an alternative description of the resting state as tonic accommodation. A reduction from the tonic level requires an inhibition of the parasympathetic effort. As it is unusual for body muscles not to be opposed, a sympathetic innervation to reduce accommodation has often been postulated. Recent evidence showing that the ciliary body contains beta-adrenergic sympathetic receptors supports this view.

The similar reaction time (latency) of about 375 ms for both reductions and increases in accommodation would suggest, however, that significant changes in either direction are mediated by the same neural system. Gilmartin (1986) gives a comprehensive review of the evidence for and against sympathetic innervation.

Experimental evidence on the performance of the accommodative system is obtained by plotting the actual accommodative response against the dioptric distance of the test object (i.e. the vergence of the incident light). If these two quantities were equal, the graph would be a straight line through the origin at 45° to both axes. As shown in *Figure 7.17*, the typical response confirms

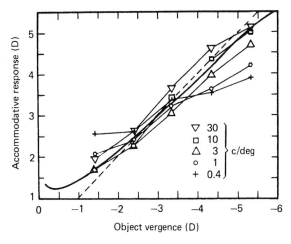

Figure 7.18. Accommodative response as a function of object vergence for a Snellen target (bold line) and for sinusoidal gratings of various spatial frequencies. (Redrawn from Charman and Tucker, 1978, by kind permission of the publishers of *Am. J. Optom.*)

the proposition that over-accommodation (or accommodative lead) is the norm in distance vision and under-accommodation (or lag) in near vision. It follows that at some intermediate distance the response curve must pass through the equality line at 45°. In a young adult, the 'cross-over point' would lie within the range 1.0–2.5 D. The portion of the curve to the right of the cross-over point is mediated by the parasympathetic system, while the portion to the left is sometimes termed the sympathetic part of the curve, despite the fact that the question is still unresolved. The cross-over point was considered to indicate the tonic accommodation at the resting state, but recent evidence discussed below finds a much lower value for the tonic accommodation.

The proposition that accommodation is exerted economically from an intermediate (resting-state) point of departure is supported by results such as those of Charman and Tucker (1978) reproduced here as *Figure 7.18*. In their experiments, the accommodative response at various viewing distances was measured for high-contrast 6 m Snellen letters and for sinusoidal gratings of five different spatial frequencies. As the gratings become coarser, the smaller the changes in accommodation become over the range of viewing distances. Comparable results had previously been obtained by Heath (1956) using distant test objects blurred by fogging lenses or ground glass plates placed immediately in front of them. The greater the blur, the greater the accommodation exerted, that is, the smaller the departure from the resting state.

The accommodative stimulus

Accommodation is a response to an out-of-focus retinal image, and thus may depend upon such factors as the duration of presentation, the contrast of the image, the size and type of detail, and its luminance.

Reaction time

Tucker and Charman (1979) showed by high-speed infra-red recording that in addition to a reaction time of about one-third of a second (0.29 ± 0.07 s from far to near, 0.34 ± 0.14 from near to far), there is a response time of about a second (0.75 ± 0.31 s from far to near, 1.19 ± 0.57 s from near to far) to reach the 'steady' state. Thus a stimulus needs to be present for at least a second for full response to occur. Moreover, even when the eye is observing a static target, infra-red optometers show that the power of the eye is fluctuating. Thus Campbell and Robson (1959) found a focusing tremor of amplitude 0.2–0.3 D at two superimposed frequencies in young subjects viewing a test object at 1 m. The low-frequency component of frequency < 0.6 Hz is probably due to the neurological control, while the high-frequency component has been shown to be related to the arterial pulse (Winn and Gilmartin, 1992). van der Heijde *et al.* (1996), using ultrasonography, confirmed variations in crystalline lens thickness (and also anterior and vitreous chamber depths) as being associated with the low-frequency component.

It is not known whether these fluctuations help in determining the direction of accommodative response to an out-of-focus image (e.g. Campbell *et al.*, 1958). With their subjects' accommodation paralysed, Walsh and Charman (1988) showed that the visual system could detect changes in focus as small as 0.1 D for a target simulating the micro-fluctuations of accommodation by oscillating to and from the eye. Maximal sensitivity occurred when the retinal image was slightly out of focus. They felt this supported Charman and Tucker's (1978) hypothesis that the fluctuations were an aid in maintaining the final level of accommodation.

Dependence on detail size

Figure 7.18 showed that the accommodative response for detailed objects in the form of fine gratings or Snellen charts was more accurate than that for coarser gratings. This might be expected since the fine target offers greater stimulus for accommodation, whereas the coarser gratings will still be visible even when out of focus – *Figure 3.31* shows a cut-off frequency of 10 cycles/degree for 0.5 D error in focus, while a 3 cycle/degree grating is still visible when 1.0 D out of focus.

The converse argument is that a grating of frequency around 5 cycles/degree at the peak of the contrast sensitivity curve is most readily perceived, and therefore most likely to stimulate accurate accommodation, whereas a fine grating must be positioned dioptrically close to the eye's present focus to make it perceptible and thus able to control accommodation. This was shown by Ward (1987b), who measured the accommodative response with an infra-red autorefractor (*see* Chapter 18) while his subjects viewed sinusoidal gratings of 25–26% modulation (contrast) at an object vergence of −5.00 D. The results plotted in *Figure 7.19* (Ward, 1987b) show the most consistent accommodation for the 5.0 cycles/degree grating, and a reasonably consistent result for the 1.67 cycles/degree grating. In

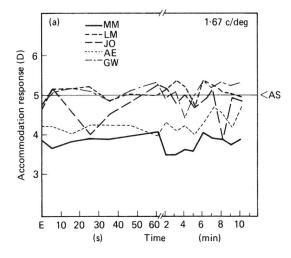

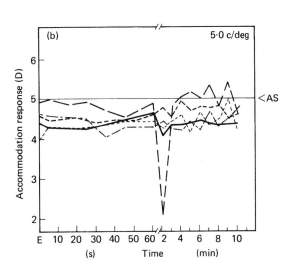

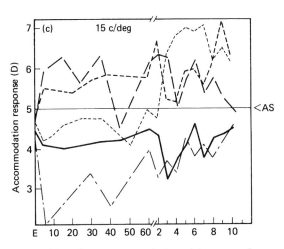

Figure 7.19. The variation with time of the monocular accommodation response of five subjects viewing gratings of contrast 25–26%. The accommodative stimulus, indicated by AS, was −5.0 D. Note the change in the time scale at 60 s. (a) 1.67 c/deg, (b) 5.0 c/deg, (c) 15 c/deg. (Reproduced from Ward, 1987b, by kind permission of Pergamon Press.)

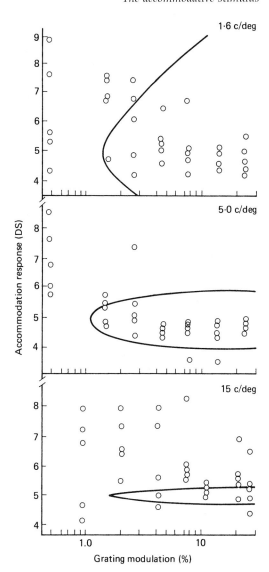

Figure 7.20. The monocular accommodation response to gratings of 1.6, 5.0 and 15 c/deg with a stimulus vergence of −5.0 D, as a function of object contrast. The individual data points of all observers are represented by circles. The region to the left of the solid lines is where the defocus produced by the accommodative error results in a sub-threshold image. (Reproduced from Ward, 1987a, by kind permission of Pergamon Press.)

both cases, the contrast of the image on the retina was above the contrast sensitivity threshold. The greater tolerance to defocus of the coarser grating was due to the larger depth of focus. The 15 cycles/degree stimulus gave widely variable accommodative results. Ward's calculations showed that the retinal image was then at the contrast sensitivity threshold and thus gave poor control over the accommodation.

This supported his suggestion (1987a) of an accommodation response contrast threshold (ARCT), below which the eye does not maintain focus. With the same three frequencies, but at modulation down to 0.5%, Ward found that accommodation was again maintained more accurately after 1 minute's observation for the 5.0 cycles/degree stimulus than for the 1.6 cycles/ degree grating, while the response to the 15 cycles/degree stimulus was poor even at 8% modulation. *Figure 7.20* shows that whereas accommodation maintained the two coarser stimuli in sufficient focus for the retinal image to be above the contrast sensitivity threshold, the fine grating's image fell below threshold, allowing accommodation to drift towards that of the field surround (at a dioptric distance of -9.0 D).

Tucker and Charman (1986) postulated that for stimuli containing a broad range of spatial frequencies, the eye's accommodation response from a very out-of-focus level may be governed in turn by increasingly finer detail. Thus, as the response becomes more accurate, relatively coarse detail drives the accommodation to a slightly more accurate level, sufficient for finer detail to surmount the accommodation response threshold. The apparent disagreement between Ward's results and those of Charman and Tucker (1978) in *Figure 7.18* could be explained by the 80% contrast used in the latter study whereas in Ward's study it was 25–26%.

Stone *et al.* (1993) investigated the accuracy of focus of subjects observing a stimulus oscillating towards and away from the eye. They found the best response for gratings between 3 and 5 cycles/degree. The effects of ocular longitudinal chromatic aberration on accommodation were examined by Kruger *et al.* (1993). Compared with the response in white light, they found the response fell when the aberration was neutralized by an achromatizing lens (*see* Chapter 15), while it was less again in monochromatic light and even less when the aberration was reversed, while the reaction time increased. Stone and colleagues also tried doubling the longitudinal chromatic aberration of the eye, but found little improvement in accommodative accuracy. They found that about 10% of subjects appeared to be relatively unaffected by changes in chromatic aberration, suggesting that their accommodation was controlled by an achromatic directional clue. Conversely, they concluded, like Edgar Fincham, that longitudinal chromatic aberration was a component in the reflex control for most people.

Voluntary control of accommodation

In both the studies last mentioned, the subject was asked to maintain the best possible focus. Some subjects are able to exert voluntary control over their accommodation, so that instructions during an investigation can make significant differences to the results. Ciuffreda and Hokoda (1985) demonstrated a 5 D response to a -6 D stimulus when the subject was instructed to keep the object looking as contrasty as possible, yet the response was only about 2.5 D after an instruction to relax when viewing the grating. (Cornsweet and Crane, 1973, showed that subjects could even learn to control their accommodation in response to an auditory stimulus.) This can be demonstrated during the push-up test for accommodation, when encouragement (the 'mental effort' of orthoptists) may result in a higher amplitude.

Square-wave gratings

Tucker and Charman (1987) measured the accommodative response to square- and sine-wave gratings. Their findings of better response for the square-wave gratings below 6 cycles/degree were explained by the help given by the higher frequency harmonics of these gratings. A similar result was found by Dul *et al.* (1988); their subjects gave the most accurate accommodative response when third and fifth harmonics were added to an 84% contrast sinusoidal grating of 1 cycle/degree. Tucker and Charman suggested that the lower amplitude of accommodation found in amblyopes, for example, by Hokoda and Ciuffreda (1982), could be caused by the lower contrast sensitivity of the amblyopic eye to higher frequency gratings.

Importance of luminance

As shown by *Figure 3.34*, the contrast sensitivity of the eye reduces with decreasing luminance, only lower and lower frequencies at higher and higher contrast being visible. Tucker and Charman (1986) investigated the depth of focus and accommodative response of the eye to sinusoidal grating stimuli as the luminance was lowered. Under these conditions, the eye's focus tends towards that of the resting state. They concluded that the reduced ability of the eye to perceive fine detail, combined with the large depth of focus of the eye to coarse detail, resulted in a very inaccurate accommodative response. The relatively myopic state thus caused in scotopic conditions has been termed night myopia.

The inadequate-stimulus myopias – tonic accommodation

Introduction

Whenever the visual stimulus is insufficient to control the accommodation accurately, it drifts towards a tonic level, governed by a low degree of parasympathetic stimulation. This has often been assumed to be equal to that of the resting state, though Rosenfield *et al.* (1993) argue that they may differ. The relatively myopic refractive state found under the various conditions indicated has been described as night (or twilight) myopia, dark field myopia, empty space (or empty field) myopia and instrument myopia.

In the recent literature, the various collective terms used for these myopias include resting state, anomalous, and accommodative myopias. The terms inadequate-stimulus myopia and tonic accommodation are used here as they give a more accurate description of their common basic cause, the drift of accommodation to its tonic value. Additional subsidiary factors may also contribute, as later described.

Rosenfield *et al.* (1993, 1994) give a comprehensive review of the subject to which the interested reader is referred. The next few pages give an introduction to the subject.

Night myopia

In low illumination the refractive state of the eye tends to change in the direction of myopia, irrespective of any ametropia at photopic luminances. As Levene (1965) has shown, this 'night myopia' was discovered independently by several astronomers, the first mention of it having been made in 1789 by Nevil Maskelyne, the Astronomer Royal at Greenwich. The discovery had hitherto been attributed to Lord Rayleigh, whose announcement on the subject in 1883 created a lasting interest in it.

Night myopia, also called twilight myopia, was studied during and after World War II because of its possible effects on visual performance, both unaided and when using telescopes or binoculars. Investigations followed two main lines.

In the first, the subject adjusted one eyepiece of the binoculars to give the best subjective quality of vision both in daylight and at scotopic luminances, the other objective being occluded. The difference between the two settings was taken to indicate the amount of night myopia. Thus, Wald and Griffin (1947) found night myopia to average −0.59 D, in 21 inexperienced observers, the spread being from +1.4 to −3.4 D. The results for 8 experienced observers out of doors ranged from +1.4 to −1.9 D, with a mean myopic shift of −0.31 D – not a particularly dramatic result. In a similar study with 28 observers viewing binocularly through field glasses, Schober (1947, cited by Knoll, 1952) found a range from −0.50 to −4.00 D, with a mean of −2.00 D.

In the second technique used by Wald and Griffin, the threshold or minimum illumination required by the subject to resolve a coarse acuity test object was measured as a function of induced ametropia. The subject viewed the chart through one half of a prism binocular, the eyepiece focusing being adjusted in turn for each of a range of dioptric values. Dark adaptation was required for mesopic and scotopic determinations. At low luminances a plot of the threshold against induced ametropia resulted in a U-shaped curve, the lowest point of which was regarded as indicating the optimum focus. When this was compared with the optimum focus at photopic luminances, a myopic shift was again found. For the five subjects concerned it averaged −1.4 D, with a range from approximately −0.75 to −2.25 D. *Figure 7.21* shows Wald and Griffin's experimental results for two observers, redrawn from the original graphs with the luminance additionally re-scaled in cd/m², the appropriate SI unit. The dotted curve gives the result after instillation of homatropine to paralyse the accommodation, while the arrows indicate the subject's own settings.

With themselves as observers, Koomen *et al.* (1951) determined the limits of resolution of a square-wave grating as a function of ametropia introduced by phoropter lenses at a series of different luminance levels. U-shaped curves (of angular resolution threshold against

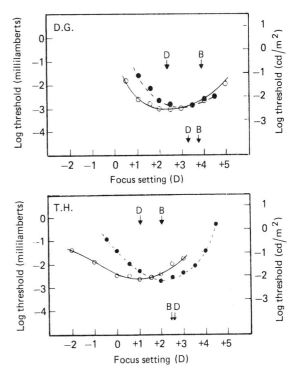

Figure 7.21. The luminance threshold for recognition of a target as a function of binocular eyepiece setting for two subjects. Solid line: normal, dark-adapted eye; broken line: with cycloplegia. The two pairs of arrows give the subjects' own preferred eyepiece setting for dim D and bright B light. Upper: normal eye, lower: with cycloplegia. Note the logarithmic luminance scales. (Redrawn from Wald and Griffin, 1947, by kind permission of the publishers of *J. Opt. Soc. Am.*)

lens power) were again obtained, with values of night myopia in the neighbourhood of −1.50 D.

Causes of night myopia

The relative weight to be attached to the various factors contributing to night myopia has been the subject of much previous speculation and discussion. Reviews of the literature at different stages have been given among others by Ball (1951), Knoll (1952) and Borish (1970). Though tonic accommodation is now accepted as the basic cause, the eye's chromatic aberration makes a fairly constant and spherical aberration a variable contribution.

Involuntary accommodation

As shown by Campbell (1954), the minimum quantity of light required to elicit the accommodative reflex is just greater than the threshold for foveal vision. It is therefore concluded that the stimulus to accommodate in the interests of visual acuity is mediated by the foveal cones. As luminance decreases and rod vision becomes more and more predominant, the accuracy of accommodation decreases and a small amount of involuntary accommodation becomes manifest. Moreover, the U-shaped curves of *Figure 7.21* indicate that the eye tends towards a fixed focus in low illumination. A markedly skewed plot would result if the eyes were able to accommodate normally to overcome hypermetropia induced by minus lenses or equivalent eyepiece settings. Thus the eye can be regarded as showing 'nocturnal presbyopia', in which the available amplitude reduces towards a relatively fixed level remaining in play as illumination falls (Durán, 1943, cited by Otero, 1951).

Chromatic aberration

At photopic luminances the eye is most sensitive to light of wavelength 555 nm, as shown by the graph of the $V(\lambda)$ function (*Figure 15.1*). In scotopic vision, however, the entire curve is displaced towards the shorter end of the spectrum, its peak occurring at about 510 nm. This is called the Purkinje shift. Because of chromatic aberration, the eye's focus for blue light is relatively more myopic than for green or yellow light. *Figure 15.5* shows the Purkinje shift to make the ocular refraction more myopic by about −0.30 D.

It should be noted, however, that the standard $V(\lambda)$ curves refer to the hypothetical equi-energy spectrum and are affected by the spectral distribution of energy of the light source. For CIE Standard Illuminant D_{65} representative of noon sunlight the peak is at 548 nm, but for Standard Illuminant A representative of tungsten-filament lamps it is at 570 nm, as shown in *Figure 15.1*. This wavelength is much closer than 555 nm to that which tends to be focused on the retina in distance vision (*see* pages 288–289). In scotopic vision the peak of the $V(\lambda)$ curve shifts only slightly with the nature of the source. With all these minor complications borne in mind, the contribution made to night myopia by the Purkinje shift can reasonably be taken as −0.35 ± 0.05 D.

Spherical aberration

The positive spherical aberration of the relaxed eye causes a refracted axial pencil of rays to take the form shown in *Figure 7.22*. At photopic luminances, the reduced pupil diameter and the Stiles–Crawford effect combine to place the effective focus close to the paraxial

focus P where the tip of the refracted ray caustic is situated.

At scotopic luminances, vision is dependent on the rod receptors, which do not exhibit the Stiles–Crawford effect. Consequently, the rays through the peripheral zone of the dilated pupil exert their full effect and shift the best focus position to W, the waist or circle of least aberration of the refracted beam. As a result, the eye becomes effectively myopic by an amount possibly up to −0.75 D in a typical eye. However, since spherical aberration shows considerable variation between individuals, its contribution to night myopia may also vary.

Having found similar values for marginal spherical aberration and night myopia with themselves as subjects, Koomen *et al.* (1951) were inclined to regard spherical aberration as the main cause of night myopia. This view was strengthened by the fact that a 3 mm artificial pupil reduced the myopia to between −0.50 and −0.75 D, about twice the amount which can be attributed to the Purkinje shift.

It can be seen from *Figure 7.22* that spherical aberration with a dilated pupil has an unequal effect on the size of the retinal blur circles in uncorrected ametropia. Because of the additional deviation of the marginal rays, the increase in the blur size as the pupil dilates is less than it would otherwise have been in hypermetropia, while the converse applies to myopia. This is an additional reason why myopes in particular are likely to complain of poorer acuity at night.

Measurement errors: proximal and cognitive myopia

There are several techniques employed to evaluate the refractive state of the eye. The laser speckle technique (*see* pages 375–376) may be used in conjunction with an optometer of the Badal type to make a subjective measurement of ametropia in, for example, total darkness. Infra-red optometers, especially the Canon Auto Ref R1 (*see* page 354) which allows the subject to view external fixation stimuli, and retinoscopy (*see* Chapter 17) allow objective measurements.

As pointed out below, results obtained with the laser speckle system show greater amounts of inadequate-stimulus myopia than the infra-red optometers. This has been attributed to various factors affecting the laser results:

(1) Proximal accommodation is induced by the knowledge that the object of regard is close to the eyes, so the laser's Badal optometer lens and drum could trigger this. A related effect produced by the awareness of, for example, the size of the room in which the experiments are conducted has been termed 'surround propinquity' (Rosenfield and Ciuffreda, 1991).

(2) Jaschinski-Kruza and Toenies (1988) and others have shown that mental effort as opposed to passive observation increases the accommodative response. It is thought that the effort of judging the direction of speckle motion might also give a falsely myopic refraction. This has been termed 'cognitive accommodation'.

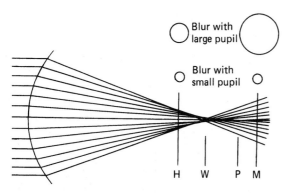

Figure 7.22.   The aberrated ray bundle: paraxial focus P, waist W. H and M indicate the positions of the retina in uncorrected hypermetropia and myopia, while the circles above indicate the diameters of the blur circles with small and large pupils.

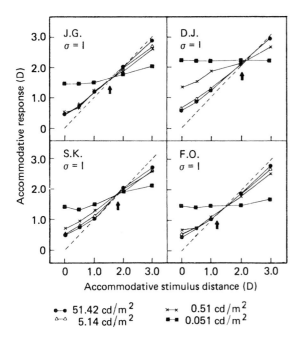

Figure 7.23. Accommodative response as a function of object vergence for a graticule target viewed at four luminance levels. Individual values of dark focus refraction are given by the arrows. The flat response at the lowest light level demonstrates nocturnal presbyopia. (Reproduced from Johnson, 1976, by kind permission of the publishers of *J. Opt. Soc. Am.*)

Dark-field myopia

To prevent confusion, the refractive error measured in darkness should be referred to as the dark-field refraction and the term dark-field myopia reserved for the shift towards myopia. For example, if the eye is hypermetropic $+2.00$ D in photopic conditions but $+0.50$ D hypermetropic in total darkness, the latter is the dark-field refraction but the dark-field myopia is -1.50 D.

Using 120 college students as subjects, Leibowitz and Owens (1975) found their dark-field myopia to range from 0 to -4.00 D, with a mean value of -1.72 D. Their results also showed dark-field myopia to be strongly correlated to night myopia, both in magnitude and individual variations. In fact, it can be regarded as a limiting form of night myopia.

The effect of night myopia on the accommodative response is shown in *Figure 7.23*, which plots the results of Johnson (1976) for 4 observers aged 22–24 at four different illumination levels decreasing by a constant factor of 10. As the luminance falls, the response curve is seen to become flatter. At the lowest level of approximately 0.05 cd/m^2, the response for all observers is never less than about 1.50 D or more than 2.25 D over the entire range of object distances from 0 to -3 D.

Levels of dark-field myopia measured with the Canon Auto Ref R1 appear significantly lower. Thus, Rosenfield (1989a) found 1.28 ± 0.48 D with the infrared instrument, as opposed to 2.01 ± 1.02 D with the laser speckle. The results for each of their 10 subjects showed little correlation between the two methods. The article by Rosenfield *et al.* (1993) gives the even lower

figure of between 0.50 and 0.75 D as the typical value for tonic accommodation.

Empty-field or Ganzfeld myopia

Though vision continues to operate in an illuminated but empty-field (or empty-space or Ganzfeld) myopia, the absence of all visual detail removes the normal stimulus to accommodation. For this reason, as in night myopia, the accommodation becomes fixed at or near to its resting state. Typical real conditions can occur in daylight fog or in high-level flight well above the clouds where little detail is visible from the aircraft.

In early investigations, Luckiesh and Moss (1937) used their 'sensitometric' technique of refraction in which the accommodation is not stimulated. In effect, the contrast threshold is measured with a range of lens powers before the eye, the luminance contrast being raised from below threshold so as to present initially an empty visual field. The 'best' refraction is indicated by the lens power giving the lowest threshold. Measurements were made on 100 subjects, from which a mean value of about -0.75 D was found for empty-space myopia, the range being -0.37 to -1.37 D. Two years later, Reese (cited by Knoll, 1952) found a mean value of about -1.00 D with a somewhat larger spread from a study of 25 subjects.

Whiteside (1952, 1957) found involuntary accommodation to fluctuate considerably in an empty visual field, both in time with a single observer and from one subject to another. These observations were confirmed by Westheimer (1957) and by Heath (1962, cited by Heron *et al.*, 1981) who found them to apply to night myopia as well.

Because of the relatively constant photopic illumination levels in empty-space situations, neither chromatic nor spherical aberration contribute to this type of myopia, which can most simply be explained by an inadequate-stimulus theory.

Instrument myopia – use of a pinhole to 'open-loop' accommodation

Instrument myopia is the well-known tendency to overaccommodate when using instruments such as microscopes. It was originally thought to be a form of proximal accommodation. This is certainly a principal factor because instrument myopia can be reduced by training and by adjusting the eyepiece from the fully racked-out (hypermetropic) side so that accommodation during this adjustment does not improve the focus. Nevertheless, it is now the opinion that instrument myopia has a contribution from tonic accommodation.

Measurements have generally been made with subjects viewing monocularly through a microscope having an exit pupil not greater than 2 mm. Results show the same spread of individual values typical of the other myopias under discussion. For example, Hennessy (1975) using as subjects 15 emmetropes aged 18–25, found a mean of -1.91 D, with a range from -0.96 to -2.78 D. The results of Leibowitz and Owens for instrument myopia, in the study mentioned previously, are

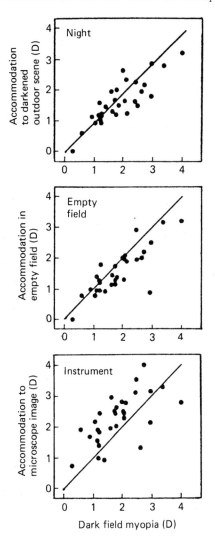

Figure 7.24.   Scatter plots for 30 subjects comparing night, empty-field, and instrument myopia with dark-field myopia. (Reproduced from Leibowitz and Owens, 1975, by kind permission of the publishers of *Science* © by the AAAS.)

shown in one of the scattergraphs included in *Figure 7.24*. The mean value, determined from this graph, is about −2.3 D, with a range from −0.7 to −4.0 D. Schober *et al.* (1970) found a similarly extensive range but a somewhat higher mean value, about −3.0 D. They reported that variables such as image configuration and contrast, magnification and luminance had only a minor influence. Their subjects were aged 25–30, but all had an amplitude of accommodation of 8 ± 1 D.

Another possible factor investigated by Hennessy was that the field stop in the microscope might bias the accommodation by virtue of the Mandelbaum effect (*see* below). He found, however, that it had no such effect, unless its normally black surface was covered with a distinctive checkerboard pattern.

Hennessy concluded that because the small exit pupil of the microscope increases the depth of field, small errors of focusing provide little stimulus to accommodation. On the other hand, if the instrument is markedly out of focus, the image is badly blurred and the accom-

modation again unstimulated. Then, as the focus is adjusted, the point where the image becomes sufficiently in focus to stimulate the accommodation is reached too suddenly for the accommodation to respond and so it remains at its tonic value.

A key point in this explanation is the assumption of a small exit pupil. For this reason, the accepted term 'instrument myopia' could be misleadingly too general. It would be interesting to have data on other monocular instruments having larger exit pupils, such as focimeters and prismatic monocular telescopes.

Because they greatly increase the eye's depth of focus, small artificial pupils are used in research into the relationship between convergence and accommodation (Chapter 9). Their effect is to remove blurring of the retinal image as a stimulus to accommodation; the blur stimulus reflex is then said to be 'open-looped', leaving the control of accommodation to other factors, for example, convergence. Ward and Charman (1987) showed that an artificial pupil used for this purpose should have a diameter not greater than 0.5 mm.

Correlations and variability of the inadequate-stimulus myopias

To investigate relative magnitudes and correlations, Leibowitz and Owens (1975, 1978) determined the night, dark-field, empty-space and instrument myopia of 30 students aged between 17 and 26, all with vision not less than 20/25 (6/7.5) and wearing their normal distance correction (if any). Their results are shown in *Figure 7.24*, in which each point on the various scattergraphs records the value of the particular myopia for one subject, plotted against his dark-field myopia. The line at 45° represents the condition for equality of these two quantities.

In these experiments, night myopia was measured in daylight, but a neutral density filter was used to attenuate the ambient illumination by a factor of 16 000. It nevertheless remained within the range of photopic vision and so the Purkinje effect component was eliminated.

Statistical analysis of the results of this study reveals a high degree of correlation between the various forms of myopia considered. There is, however, a wide range of inter-subject variation. One of the principal reasons for this may well be variations in the amplitude of accommodation within the same age group. Another reason may be variations in the level of parasympathetic activity, an excess of which would tend to reduce pupil size and raise the level of accommodation at the resting state.

There is evidence both for and against a relationship between the tonic level of accommodation and refractive error. The natural accommodative tonus would be expected to vary in low hypermetropes and myopes, depending on whether and how much a refractive correction is worn. Myopes whose error develops after the age of about 15 years appear to show tonic accommodation about 0.4 D less than emmetropes (B. Gilmartin, 1989, pers. comm.). McBrien and Millodot (1986a) found that hypermetropes had a lower ocular amplitude of accommodation than emmetropes, who in turn had a lower amplitude than myopes, especially those who became myopic after the age of 14. These effects might be explained as follows. If in *Figure 7.17*, the 'cross-over point' moved to the left in myopes as a result of reduced sympathetic tonus, a lower resting state would result. Also, the parasympathetic part of the curve would be longer, giving a larger amplitude. A similar effect was found by McBrien and Millodot (1986b), in that the gradient of the ocular accommodative response to changes in object vergence (i.e. the slope in *Figure 7.17*) was greater for hypermetropes than myopes. Current research has investigated the differences in tonic accommodation in myopes who have been recently discovered and those with long-standing corrections, in an effort to ascertain the causes of the progression of the condition.

For practical purposes, the tonic value of accommodation may be taken as its level in the dark-focus situation. Despite the wide inter-person variations, the dark-focus accommodative level is relatively stable (apart from micro-fluctuations), as several different researchers have shown. The same conclusion was reached by Heron *et al.* (1981), who also reported on the slightly different values given by different methods of measurement.

Post *et al.* (1984) investigated the stability of the resting focus when measured on several occasions. A high correlation of 0.98 was found between measurements taken a few minutes apart, falling to about 0.75 when the measurements were separated by periods of one day to two weeks. Bullimore *et al.* (1986) found that the variation in results for any individual tended to be proportional to the subject's tonic accommodation.

The Mandelbaum effect

The Mandelbaum effect refers to the response of the eyes when there are two superimposed but conflicting stimuli to accommodation: for example, when viewing a distant object through a wire fence or dirty window at some intermediate distance (Mandelbaum, 1960). The hypothesis is that the near stimulus will tend to increase the accommodative response when viewing the distant object, especially if the near stimulus is positioned close to the eye's dark focus. Conversely, if the object of regard is closer than the dark focus, then the presence of a more distant conflicting stimulus might lower the accommodative response. There is evidence both for and against this effect.

Thus, Owens (1979) monitored the actual accommodative level by means of a laser optometer. Results of one of the four subjects investigated by Owens are shown in *Figure 7.25*. In this diagram, the subject's dark-field refraction (approximately −2.25 D) is indicated by the arrows. The response R with a distant matrix stimulus S was found to be raised by the interposed screen and lowered for near vision. Both these effects were found to be greatest when the screen was placed at the eye's dark focus. However, when the object was positioned near the dark focus, the accommodative response was scarcely influenced by the position of the screen whether nearer or further than the stimulus. He concluded from these and other results that the eye's dark-field refraction can also be taken to indicate its resting state of accommodation. A further inference is that the accommodation is most accurate and stable when the object of regard is situated at the eye's dark focus. A better than average performance in distance vision would thus be predicted for low uncorrected hypermetropes – an idea earlier suggested by Whiteside (1957).

Rosenfield and Ciuffreda (1991), using a subjective optometer, found a wide variation in their subjects' responses to stimuli presented simultaneously at −1 and −5, −1 and −3 or −3 and −5 D, with only a small correlation with the dark focus. They concluded that when the eye views stimuli at various distances, the accommodative response is produced 'primarily from the interaction of proximal, convergent and tonic inputs'. Adams and Johnson (1991) similarly felt proximal accommodation to influence their subjects' results which were monitored with an infra-red optometer, though they found that three of their nine subjects did show a definite influence of dark focus on the accommodative response to conflicting stimuli, and two more a slight tendency.

The present writer (RBR) would also question the influence of the normal lead and lag of accommodation. Thus, in distance vision, if stimuli are presented at vergences of 0 and −3 D, with a dark focus of −1.0 D, then the accommodative response would be expected to be around 1 D when the subject concentrates on the further stimulus. Conversely, if the stimuli were presented at −2 and −4 D, then the normal lag of accommodation in near vision might predict that the response would be nearer the −2 D than the −4 D stimulus, coincidentally nearer the dark focus.

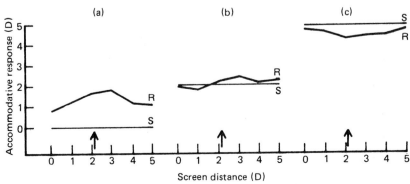

Figure 7.25. The Mandelbaum effect: accommodative response (R) as a function of the dioptric distance of the 'background' screen (plotted along the abscissa) for three different stimulus or test object distances (S). The arrow indicates the dark-focus refraction. The effective position of the letter matrix (a) at infinity, (b) at dark focus, (c) at 5 D. (Redrawn in part from Owens, 1979.)

Correction of night myopia

Night and empty-space myopia are important because they can affect the ability of the eye to perceive objects near the visual threshold. For example, empty-space myopia in an emmetrope will give a blurred retinal image. The image of a distant aircraft, whether seen in silhouette as a dark speck or relatively bright, may thus be spread over a larger region of the retina than the ganglion summation area. If so, the resultant variation in intensity may fall below the luminance contrast threshold. Whiteside (1957) found that empty-space myopia could reduce the range at which an aircraft could be perceived by one-half. He also found that a dot very close to threshold size in an otherwise empty field could suddenly disappear because it was an insufficient stimulus to prevent the accommodation assuming its resting state. This effect can be noted when watching aircraft or birds fly into the distance, especially if high in the sky. As well as affecting visual acuity, night myopia can also raise the luminance threshold (Wald and Griffin, 1947).

The luminance levels for night driving are in the range 0.35–0.7 cd/m^2 when the light is from the headlamps alone. This level could be raised to about 2 cd/m^2 or more by street lighting (Charman, 1996) and the spread of light from shop windows. It can be seen from *Figure 7.23* that for three of the four subjects the accommodative response varied very little over a luminance range from 51 down to 0.51 cd/m^2. On this basis, a separate correction for night driving may not be needed.

Richards (1968) found that only some 12% of a group of 315 subjects obtained an improvement in visual acuity from a negative addition, within the range −0.50 to −1.00 D. On the other hand, Sheard (1976) found that 17 out of the 26 subjects examined benefited from a minus addition, though never greater than −1.00 D.

As a general principle, Owens and Leibowitz (1976) suggested that the subject's dark-field myopia was the best guide to prescribing. They found that a minus addition of one-half this value gave the best acuity at low luminances. In a bright empty field Post *et al.* (1979) found detection of distant test objects to be best served by a full correction of dark-field myopia. This was confirmed for empty-space myopia by Luria (1980); for objects subtending up to 7.5 minutes of arc, correction improved their visibility, while there was no improvement for larger objects.

In clinical practice, patients reporting difficulties in night driving possibly due to night myopia should be refracted in suitably low illumination. Possible methods are either for the patient to wear very dark filters (2–3 ND) or to illuminate the distant test chart only by the ambient light from a torch. A couple of minutes should be allowed for the myopia to develop and retina to dark adapt. Bullimore *et al.* (1986) suggest that the tonic accommodation can be estimated objectively by using automated infra-red optometers in complete darkness, though the present writer would question the influence of the internal fixation scene employed in current instruments. Alternatively, the Mohindra technique of retinoscopy (*see* page 343) may be employed for each eye in turn, the other eye being occluded to prevent convergence control of the accommodation. The accommodative element of the dark-field myopia takes only a few seconds to develop, so that an adequate response may be measured after a minute. Rosenfield (1989b) felt that the Canon Auto Ref R1 provided a truer value for tonic accommodation than retinoscopy or fixation of a very low spatial frequency grating (≈ 0.1c/deg). In case of doubt, any negative addition suggested by these techniques could be fitted to a clip-over for trial.

The pupil dilation to its fullest extent and hence the spherical aberration component may take a few minutes. While a lens change might help compensate for spherical aberration, irregular refraction in the pupil periphery, for example from early crystalline lens changes, may also affect night driving. Depending on the initial state of retinal light adaptation, retinal adaptation to minimal light levels will take much longer, the Purkinje shift occurring after about 5 minutes.

Tonic accommodation theory predicts that the inadequate-stimulus myopias will become less manifest with advancing age because of presbyopia. It would also follow that any night myopia in old age must be due to chromatic and spherical aberration. The contribution of the latter will also decline with advancing age because of the smaller pupil size in low illumination. In a study of complete presbyopes and aphakics, Otero (1951) found only the amount of myopia that could be explained by aberrations, though Knoll (1952) quotes Schober as finding two septuagenarians with 1.0 and 1.5 D respectively of night myopia.

Charman (1996), in a comprehensive review, points out that under conditions of binocular viewing, any myopic shift occurring will be less that that found under monocular conditions. Moreover, an uncorrected refractive error which might give relatively insignificant blur with normal sized pupils under photopic conditions will give increased blur with dilated pupils at night. He therefore suggests that symptoms of poor vision for night driving are much more likely to be caused by uncorrected photopic refractive errors than by night myopia. Scattered light from dirty windscreens, spectacles and ocular media will also impair vision.

Adaptation of tonic accommodation

There is considerable recent experimental work on the effects of prolonged close work on the accommodative response. While this also relates to the bioengineering model of accommodation and convergence presented at the end of Chapter 9, two effects of interest here are possible changes in the level of tonic accommodation and refractive error. If an eye has been accommodating for a long time, the focus does not initially relax completely when the dioptric stimulus is reduced. Most recent work confirms that there may be a temporary shift towards a myopic refractive error and a very short-term increase in the level of the tonic accommodation of up to 0.75 D lasting 60–90 s. The latter is somewhat controversial, as, if an allowance is made for the change in the far point, there may be almost no change in tonic accommodation. There may also be different amounts of adaptation and time courses for the decay in the various types of refractive error. The interested reader is referred to Rosenfield *et al.* (1994) for a review.

Exercises

7.1 Find the distance of the near point and the range of accommodation in each of the following cases, assumed to be uncorrected:
(a) Emmetropia: amplitude of accommodation 7.50 D
(b) Hypermetropia +2.75 D: amplitude of accommodation 4.75 D
(c) Hypermetropia +3.25 D: amplitude of accommodation 2.25 D
(d) Myopia −12.00 D: amplitude of accommodation 4.00 D

7.2 (a) A myope is corrected for distance by −7.00 DS placed 14 mm from the reduced surface and the nearest point he can then see distinctly is one-third of a metre from the lens. Find the spectacle and ocular accommodation. (b) Repeat (a) for a hypermetrope corrected by +7.00 DS, all other values being unchanged.

7.3 A subject whose amplitude of (spectacle) accommodation is 2.50 D is corrected for distance by −5.00 DS fitted at 16 mm from the eye's principal point. What reading addition would be prescribed for vision at 250 mm from the plane of the lenses on the basis of leaving: (a) one-half of the available spectacle accommodation in reserve; (b) one-half of the ocular accommodation in reserve?

7.4 An emmetropic patient with PD of 64 mm observes a fine test object in the median plane of a near point rule, which is calibrated in dioptric distances from the spectacle plane. The indicated amplitude is 15 D. Allowing for the obliquity of gaze, find: (a) the true spectacle accommodation and (b) the ocular accommodation. Take the vertex distance as 16 mm, with the centre of ocular rotation 27 mm behind the spectacle plane. (c) Compare these results with the ocular accommodation for a true spectacle amplitude of 15 D.

7.5 An emmetropic patient with an available amplitude of accommodation (measured in the spectacle plane) of 2.50 D wears +1.50 DS for near vision. What is his range of clear vision: (a) ignoring depth of field, (b) assuming this to be ±0.50 D?

7.6 A mature presbyope with no accommodation has a dioptric depth of field of ±0.37 D. Tabulate: (a) the nearest position of clear vision, (b) the position of the true focus, (c) the furthest position of clear vision for additions of +2.00, +2.25, +2.50 and +2.75 DS. Compare: (d) the total range for the +2.00 and +2.50 D additions and (e) the nearer and further parts of the range for a +2.25 D addition.

7.7 A patient views a bichromatic test. If the pattern reverses clarity for a vergence change of 0.25 D, and if the green is just clearer at 400 mm, how much further away should the test be positioned to give a red preference?

7.8 An anisometrope has a spectacle plane correction of R: plano (afocal), L: +4.00 DS at 15 mm from the eye's principal point. Assuming thin lenses, calculate the demand on ocular accommodation for an object distance of −380 mm from the spectacle plane and the resultant inequality between the eyes.

7.9 The distance correction −6.00 DS/−4.00 DC axis 165° is worn at 15 mm from the eye's principal point. How much of the ocular astigmatism is uncorrected in near vision at −250 mm from the lens?

7.10 (a) A real object is situated at a dioptric distance L from a thin spectacle lens of power F_{sp}. If the lens is then moved towards the object through the negative distance δ, show that the image vergence in the original spectacle plane is given by the expression

$$\frac{L + F_{sp}(1 - \delta L)}{1 + \delta F_{sp}(1 - \delta L)}$$

(b) Show that this vergence is the same as when the lens was in

its original position, only when its power F_{sp} satisfies the equation

$$F_{sp} = \frac{-L(2 - \delta L)}{1 - \delta L}$$

(c) Determine this value of F_{sp} when $\delta = -6$ mm and $L = -3.00$ D.

7.11 The smallest size of print on a near point rule is N5, with x-height 0.95 mm. Compare its angular subtense at the 'standard' reading distance of 350 mm from the eye with that when in the position indicating 12 D of ocular accommodation. To what type size at 350 mm does the latter subtense correspond (see Exercise 3.8)?

7.12 Compile a table of decentrations for near vision for the following ranges of values: inter-ocular distances 56, 60, 64, 68 and 72 mm and working distances 25, 30, 35, 40 and 45 cm. Assume the centre of rotation distance to be 27 mm.

7.13 Owens' (1979) investigation of the Mandelbaum effect made use of a double (or consecutive) Badal optometer arrangement. If this were made of four +5.00 D lenses, positioned at −200, −600, −1000 and −1400 mm from the subject's eye, with the object and screen stimuli placed respectively between the first and second, and third and fourth lenses, show that the stimulus further from the eye would satisfy the usual linear scaling condition of the Badal optometer.

References

ADAMS, C.W. and JOHNSON, C.A. (1991) Steady-state and dynamic response properties of the Mandelbaum effect. *Vision Res.*, **31**, 752–760

ANONYMOUS (1980) Near and intermediate additions in trifocals. *Optician*, **179** (25), 18, 20 and 22

ATCHINSON, D.A. (1995) Accommodation and presbyopia. *Ophthal. Physiol. Opt.*, **15**, 255–272

BALL, G.V. (1951) Twilight myopia. *International Optical Congress 1951*, pp. 92–103. London: British Optical Association

BANNON, R.E. (1946) A study of astigmatism at the near point with special reference to astigmatic accommodation. *Am. J. Optom.*, **23**, 53–75

BERGMAN, S. (1957) Research into the amplitudes of accommodation of Afrikaans group. *Br. J. Physiol. Optics*, **14**, 59–64

BORISH, I.M. (1970) *Clinical Refraction*, 3rd edn, Vol. 1, pp. 103–109. Chicago: Professional Press

BROWN, N.A.P. (1973) The change in shape and internal form of the lens of the eye on accommodation. *Exp. Eye Res.*, **15**, 441–459

BROWN, N.A.P. (1974) The shape of the lens equator. *Exp. Eye Res.*, **19**, 571–576

BROWN, N.A.P. (1986) How the lens accommodates. *Optician*, **191**(5045), 15–16, 18

BULLIMORE, M.A., GILMARTIN, B. and HOGAN, R.E. (1986) Objective and subjective measurement of tonic accommodation. *Ophthal. Physiol. Opt.*, **6**, 57–62

BURNS, D. (1995) Blur due to pupil area when using progressive addition lenses. *Ophthal. Physiol. Opt.*, **15**, 273–279

BURNS, D., OBSTFELD, H. and SAUNDERS, J. (1993) Prescribing for presbyopes who use VDUs. *Ophthal. Physiol. Opt.*, **13**, 409–414

BUSSIN, H. (1990) Reading additions the easy way. *Optician*, **200** (2282), 12–13

CAMPBELL, F.W. (1954) The minimum quantity of light required to elicit the accommodation reflex in man. *J. Physiol.*, **123**, 357–366

CAMPBELL, F.W. and ROBSON, J.G. (1959) High-speed infrared optometer. *J. Opt. Soc. Am.*, **49**, 268–272

CAMPBELL, F.W., WESTHEIMER, G. and ROBSON, J.G. (1958) Significance of fluctuations of accommodation. *J. Opt. Soc. Am.*, **48**, 669

CHARMAN, W.N. (1989) The path to presbyopia: straight or crooked? *Ophthal. Physiol. Opt.*, **9**, 424–430

CHARMAN, W.N. (1996) Night myopia and driving. *Opthal. Physiol. Opt.*, **16**, 474–485

CHARMAN, W.N. and TUCKER, J. (1978) Accommodation as a function of object form. *Am. J. Optom.*, **55**, 84–92

CIUFFREDA, K.J. and HOKODA, S.C. (1985) Effect of instruction and higher level control on the accommodative response spatial frequency profile. *Ophthal. Physiol Opt.*, **5**, 221–223

COATES, W.R. (1955) Amplitude of accommodation in South Africa. *Br. J. Physiol. Optics*, **12**, 76–81, 86

CORNSWEET, T.N. and CRANE, H.D. (1973) Training the visual accommodation system. *Vision Res.*, **13**, 713–715

DONDERS, F.C. (1864) *Accommodation and Refraction of the Eye.* London: The New Sydenham Society

DUANE, A. (1922) Studies in monocular and binocular accommodation with their clinical applications. *Am. J. Ophthal.*, **5**, 865–877

DUL, M., CIUFFREDA, K.J. and FISHER, S.K. (1988) Accommodative accuracy to harmonically related complex grating patterns and their components. *Ophthal. Physiol. Opt.*, **8**, 146–152

EDWARDS, M.H., LAW, F., LEE, C.M., LEUNG, K.M. and LIU, W.O. (1993) Clinical norms for amplitude of accommodation in Chinese. *Ophthal. Physiol. Opt.*, **13**, 199–204 (and matters arising, 431)

FAIRMAID, J.A. (1959) The constancy of corneal curvature. *Br. J. Physiol. Optics*, **16**, 2–23

FISHER, R.F. (1971) The elastic constants of the human lens. *J. Physiol.*, **212**, 147–180

FITCH, R.C. (1971) Procedural effects on the manifest human amplitude of accommodation. *Am. J. Optom.*, **48**, 918–926

FLETCHER, R.J. (1951/52) Astigmatic accommodation. *Br. J. Physiol. Optics*, **8**, 73–94, 129–160, 193–224: **9**, 8–32

FRANCIS, J.L., RABBETTS, R.B. and STONE, J. (1979) Depressed accommodation in young people. *Ophthal. Optn.* **19**, 803–804, 807–808, 811

GILES, G.H. (1960) *Principles and Practice of Refraction.* London: Hammond, Hammond & Co. Ltd

GILMARTIN, B. (1986) A review of the role of the sympathetic innervation of the ciliary muscle in ocular accommodation. *Ophthal. Physiol. Opt.*, **6**, 23–37

GILMARTIN, B. (1995) The aetiology of presbyopia: a summary of the role of lenticular and extralenticular structures. *Ophthal. Physiol. Opt.*, **15**, 431–437

HAMASAKI, D., ONG, J. and MARG, E. (1956) The amplitude of accommodation in presbyopia. *Am. J. Optom.*, **33**, 3–14

HEATH, G.G. (1956) The influence of visual acuity on the accommodative responses of the eye. *Am. J. Optom.*, **33**, 513–524

VAN DER HEIJDE, G.L., BEERS, A.P.A. and DUBBELMAN, M. (1996) Microfluctuations of steady-state accommodation measured with ultrasonography. *Ophthal. Physiol. Opt.*, **16**, 216–221

HENNESSY, R.T. (1975) Instrument myopia. *J. Opt. Soc. Am.*, **65**, 1114–1120

HERON, G., SMITH, A.C. and WINN, B. (1981) The influence of method on the stability of dark focus position of accommodation. *Ophthal. Physiol. Opt.*, **1**, 79–90

HOFSTETTER, H.W. (1944) A comparison of Duane's and Donders' tables of the amplitude of accommodation. *Am. J. Optom.*, **21**, 345–363

HOFSTETTER, H.W. (1965) A longitudinal study of amplitude changes in presbyopia. *Am. J. Optom.*, **42**, 3–8

HOFSTETTER, H.W. (1968) Further data on presbyopia in different ethnic groups. *Am. J. Optom.*, **45**, 522–527

HOKODA, S.C. and CIUFFREDA, K.J. (1982) Measurement of accommodative amplitude in amblyopia. *Ophthal. Physiol. Opt.*, **2**, 205–212

HOWLAND, H.C., DOBSON, V. and SAYLES, N. (1987) Accommodation in infants as measured by photorefraction. *Vision Res.*, **27**, 2141–2152

JASCHINSKI-KRUZA, W. and TOENIES, U. (1988) Effect of a mental arithmetic task on dark-focus of accommodation. *Ophthal. Physiol. Opt.*, **8**, 432–437

JOHNSON, C.A. (1976) Effects of luminance and stimulus distance on accommodation and visual resolution. *J. Opt. Soc. Am.*, **66**, 138–142

KNOLL, H.A. (1952) A brief history of 'nocturnal myopia' and related phenomena. *Am. J. Optom.*, **29**, 69–81

KOOMEN, M., SCOLNIK, R. and TOUSEY, R. (1951) A study of night myopia. *J. Opt. Soc. Am.*, **41**, 80–90

KRAGHA, I.K.O.K. (1986) Amplitude of accommodation: population and methodological differences. *Ophthal. Physiol. Opt.*, **6**, 75–80

KRAGHA, I.K.O.K. and HOFSTETTER, H. (1986) Bifocal aids and environmental temperature. *Am. J. Optom.*, **63**, 372–376

KRUGER, P.B., MATHEWS, S., AGGARWALA, K.R. and SANCHEZ, N. (1993) Chromatic aberration and ocular focus: Fincham revisited. *Vision Res.*, **33**, 1391–1411

LEAT, S. (1996) Reduced accommodation in children with cerebral palsy. *Ophthal. Physiol. Opt.*, **16**, 385–390

LEIBOWITZ, H.W. and OWENS, D.A. (1975) Anomalous myopias and the intermediate dark focus of accommodation. *Science*, **189**, 646–648

LEIBOWITZ, H.W. and OWENS, D.A. (1978) New evidence for the intermediate position of relaxed accommodation. *Doc. Ophthal.*, **46**, 133–147

LEVENE, J.R. (1965) Nevill Maskelyne, F.R.S. and the discovery of night myopia. *Notes Rec. R. Soc. Lond.*, **20**, 100–108

LINDSAY, J. (1954) The Lindsay accommodation measure. *Optician*, **127**, 273–274

LÖPPING, B. and WEALE, R.A. (1965) Changes in corneal curvature following ocular convergence. *Vision Res.*, **5**, 207–215

LUCKIESH, M. and MOSS, F.K. (1937) The avoidance of dynamic accommodation through the use of brightness contrast threshold. *Am. J. Ophthal.*, **20**, 469–478

LURIA, S.M. (1980) Target size and correction for empty field myopia. *J. Opt. Soc. Am.*, **70**, 1153–1154

McBRIEN, N.A. and MILLODOT, M. (1986a) Amplitude of accommodation and refractive error. *Invest. Ophthal. Vis. Sci.*, **27**, 1187–1190

McBRIEN, N.A. and MILLODOT, M. (1986b) The effect of refractive error on the accommodation response gradient. *Ophthal. Physiol. Opt.*, **6**, 145–149

MANDELBAUM, J. (1960) An accommodative phenomenon. *AMA Arch. Ophthal.*, **63**, 923–926

MILLODOT, M. and MILLODOT, S. (1989) Presbyopia correction and the accommodation in reserve. *Ophthal. Physiol. Opt.*, **9**, 126–132

MILLODOT, M. and THIBAULT, C. (1985) Variation of astigmatism with accommodation and its relationship with dark focus. *Ophthal. Physiol. Opt.*, **5**, 297–301

MORGAN, M.W. (1960) Accommodative changes in presbyopia and their correction. In *Vision of the Aging Patient* (Hirsch, M.J. and Wick, R.E., eds), pp. 97–98. Philadelphia: Chilton Co

OTERO, J.M. (1951) Influence of the state of the accommodation on the visual performance of the human eye. *J. Opt. Soc. Am.*, **41**, 942–948

OWENS, D.A. (1979) The Mandelbaum effect: evidence for an accommodative bias toward intermediate viewing distances. *J. Opt. Soc. Am.*, **69**, 646–652

OWENS, D.A. and LEIBOWITZ, H.W. (1976) Night myopia: cause and a possible basis for amelioration. *Am. J. Optom.*, **53**, 709–717

PASCAL, J.I. (1952) Scope and significance of the accommodative unit. *Am. J. Optom.*, **29**, 113–128

POINTER, J.S. (1995) The presbyopic add. II. Age-related trend and a gender difference. *Ophthal. Physiol. Opt.*, **15**, 241–248

POST, R.B., JOHNSON, C.A. and TSEUTAKI, T.K. (1984) Comparison of laser and infrared techniques for measurement of the resting focus of accommodation: mean differences and long-term variability. *Ophthal. Physiol. Opt.*, **4**, 327–332

POST, R.B., OWENS, R.L., OWENS, D.A. and LEIBOWITZ, H.W. (1979) Correction of empty-field myopia on the basis of the dark focus of accommodation. *J. Opt. Soc. Am.*, **69**, 89–92

RABBETTS, R.B. (1972) A comparison of astigmatism and cyclophoria in distance and near vision. *Br. J. Physiol. Optics*, **27**, 161–190

RABBETTS, R.B. (1984) Oblique astigmatism of trial lenses. *Ophthal. Optn.*, **24**, 864, 866–867

RABBETTS, R.B. and BENNETT, A.G. (1986) Near vision effective power losses in trial and prescription lenses. *Optometry Today*, **26**, 14–19, 36–38

RICHARDS, O.W. (1968) Visual needs and possibilities for night driving: part 11. *Optician*, **155**, 185–190

ROSENBERG, R., FLAX, N., BRODSKY, B. and ABELMAN, I. (1953) Accommodative levels under conditions of asymmetric convergence. *Am. J. Optom.*, **30**, 244–254

ROSENFIELD, M. (1989a) Comparison of accommodative adaptation using laser and infra-red optometers. *Ophthal. Physiol. Opt.*, **9**, 431–436

ROSENFIELD, M. (1989b) Evaluation of clinical techniques to measure tonic accommodation. *Optom. Vis. Sci.*, **66**, 809–814

ROSENFIELD, M. and CIUFFREDA, K.J. (1991) Effect of surround propinquity on the open-loop accommodative response. *Invest. Ophthalmol. Vis. Sci.*, **32**, 142–147

ROSENFIELD, M., CIUFFREDA, K.J., HUNG, G.K. and GILMARTIN, B. (1993) Tonic accommodation: a review I. Basic aspects. *Ophthal. Physiol. Opt.*, **13**, 266–284

ROSENFIELD, M., CIUFFREDA, K.J., HUNG, G.K. and GILMARTIN, B. (1994) Tonic accommodation: a review II. Accommodative adaptation and clinical aspects. *Ophthal. Physiol. Opt.*, **14**, 265–277.

ROSENFIELD, M. and COHEN, A.S. (1995) Push-up amplitude of accommodation and target size. *Ophthal. Physiol. Opt.*, **15**, 231–232

ROSENFIELD, M. and COHEN, A.S. (1996) Repeatability of clinical measurements of the amplitude of accommodation. *Ophthal. Physiol. Opt.*, **16**, 247–249

ROSENFIELD, M., PORTELLO, J.K., BLUSTEIN, G.H. and JANG, C. (1996) Comparison of clinical techniques to assess the near accommodative response. *Optom. Vis. Sci.*, **73**, 382–388

SCHOBER, H.A.W., DEHLER, H. and KASSEL, R. (1970) Accommodation during observations with optical instruments. *J. Opt. Soc. Am.*, **60**, 103–107

SHEARD, D.A. (1976) The significance of night myopia for motor vehicle drivers. *Ophthal. Optn*, **16**, 151–154

SOKOL, S., MOSKOWITZ, A. and PAUL, A. (1983) Evoked potential estimates of visual accommodation in infants. *Vision Res.*, **23**, 851–860

SOMERS, W.W. and FORD, C.A. (1983) Effect of relative distance magnification on the monocular amplitude of accommodation. *Am. J. Optom.*, **60**, 920–924

SPENCER, R.W. and WILSON, K. (1954) Accommodative response in asymmetric convergence. *Am. J. Optom.*, **31**, 498–505

STIEVE, R. (1949) Uber den Bau des menschlichen Ciliarmuskels, seine Veränderungen während des Lebens und seine Bedeutung für die Akkommodation. *Anat Anz.*, **97**, 69–79

STONE, D., MATHEWS, S. and KRUGER, P.B. (1993) Accommodation and chromatic aberration: effect of spatial frequency. *Ophthal. Physiol. Opt.*, **13**, 244–252

TUCKER, J. and CHARMAN, W.N. (1979) Reaction and response times for accommodation. *Am. J. Optom.*, **56**, 490–503

TUCKER, J. and CHARMAN, W.N. (1986) Depth of focus and accommodation for sinusoidal gratings as a function of luminance. *Am. J. Optom.*, **63**, 58–70

TUCKER, J. and CHARMAN, W.N. (1987) Effect of target content at higher spatial frequencies on the accuracy of the accommodative response. *Ophthal. Physiol. Opt.*, **7**, 137–142

TURNER, M.J. (1958) Observations on the normal subjective amplitude of accommodation. *Br. J. Physiol. Optics*, **15**, 70–100

TURVILLE, A.E. (1934) New instruments. *Br. J. Physiol. Optics*, **8**, 74–189

WALD, G. and GRIFFIN, D.R. (1947) The change in refractive power of the human eye in dim and bright light. *J. Opt. Soc. Am.*, **37**, 321–336

WALSH, G. and CHARMAN, W.N. (1988) Visual sensitivity to temporal changes in focus and its relevance to the accommodative response. *Vision Res.*, **28**, 1207–1221

WARD, P.A. (1987a) The effect of stimulus contrast on the accommodation response. *Ophthal. Physiol. Opt.*, **7**, 9–15

WARD, P.A. (1987b) The effect of spatial frequency on steady-state accommodation. *Ophthal. Physiol. Opt.*, **7**, 211–217

WARD, P.A. and CHARMAN, W.N. (1987) On the use of small artificial pupils to open-loop the accommodation system. *Ophthal. Physiol. Opt.*, **7**, 191–193

WEALE, R.A. (1981) Human ocular ageing and ambient temperature. *Br. J. Ophthal.*, **65**, 869–870

WESTHEIMER, G. (1957) Accommodation measurements in empty visual fields. *J. Opt. Soc. Am.*, **47**, 714–718

WESTHEIMER, G. (1958) Accommodation levels during near crossed-cylinder test. *Am. J. Optom.*, **35**, 599–604

WHITESIDE, T.C.D. (1952) Accommodation of the human eye in a bright and empty visual field. *J. Physiol.*, **118**, 65P

WHITESIDE, T.C.D. (1957) *The Problems of Vision in Flight at High Altitudes*. London: Butterworths

WINN, B. and GILMARTIN, B. (1992) Current perspective on microfluctuations of accommodation. *Ophthal. Physiol. Opt.*, **12**, 256

WOO, G.C. and YAP, M., (1995) Is the near addition related to stature? *Optom. Vis. Sci.*, **71**, Suppl., 149

WOODHOUSE, J.M., MEADES, J.S., LEAT, S.J. and SAUNDERS, K.J. (1993) Reduced accommodation in children with Down's syndrome. *Invest. Ophthalmol. Vis. Sci.*, **34**, 2382–2387

Further reading

ALPERN, M. (1958) Variability of accommodation during steady fixation at various levels of illuminance. *J. Opt. Soc. Am.*, **48**, 193–197

CHARMAN, W.N. (1982) The accommodative resting point and refractive error. *Ophthal. Optn*, **22**, 469–473

CHARMAN, W.N. and HERON, G. (1988) Fluctuations in accommodation: a review. *Ophthal. Physiol. Opt.*, **8**, 153–164

EHRLICH, D.I. (1985) Transient myopia following sustained accommodation. *Ophthal. Physiol. Opt.*, **5**, 235

GREEN, D.G. and CAMPBELL, F.W. (1965) Effect of focus on the visual response to a sinusoidally modulated spatial stimulus. *J. Opt. Soc. Am.*, **55**, 1154–1157

HOGAN, R.E. and GILMARTIN, B.E. (1985) The effect of sustained visual tasks on tonic accommodation and tonic vergence. *Ophthal. Physiol. Opt.*, **5**, 234–235

MADDOCK, R.J., MILLODOT, M., LEAT, S. and JOHNSON, C.A. (1981) Accommodation responses and refractive error. *Invest. Ophthalmol. Vis. Sci.*, **20**, 387–391

PIGION, R.G. and MILLER, R.J. (1985) Fatigue of accommodation: changes in accommodation after visual work. *Am. J. Optom.*, **62**, 853–863

TAN, R.K.T. and O'LEARY, D.J. (1985) Steady-state accommodation response to different Snellen letter sizes. *J. Am. Optom.*, **62**, 751–754

SCHOR, C.M., JOHNSON, C.A. and POST, R.B. (1984) Adaptation of tonic accommodation. *Ophthal. Physiol. Opt.*, **4**, 133–137

WARD, P.A. (1985) A brief overview of accommodation. *Optom. Today*, **25**, 725–730

WARD, P. (1987) Parameters affecting the steady-state accommodation. *Optician*, **193**(5092), 95, 99, 102, 103, 107

8

Ocular motility and binocular vision

Introduction

In this and the following three chapters we shall be outlining the movements of the eyes, their co-ordination in binocular vision and some of the failures to achieve this co-ordination. These chapters should provide an introduction to specialized textbooks and papers on binocular vision and orthoptics or the use of eye exercises to improve co-ordination.

This chapter deals with the movements of the eyes and some of the perceptual results of well co-ordinated vision with two eyes.

Directions of ocular movements

Monocular rotations

The primary position of the eye is its position when looking straight ahead at a distant object, the head and shoulders being erect. It is from this position that the remaining positions of the eyes are defined. Rotations of a single eye are known as ductions.

The frontal or Listing's plane (*Figure 8.1*) is the vertical plane in the head passing through the centre of rotation of each eye and normal to the visual axis of the eye in its primary position. It coincides with an equatorial plane of the eye when in this position. The four secondary positions of gaze (*Figure 8.2*) result from a cardinal rotation of the eye about either a horizontal or a vertical axis in Listing's plane, as follows:

Cardinal rotation	Movement of cornea
(1) Elevation (or supraduction)	upwards
(2) Depression (or infraduction)	downwards
(3) Abduction	away from nose
(4) Adduction	towards nose

A tertiary position of regard is an oblique direction of the gaze, for example, up and to the right.

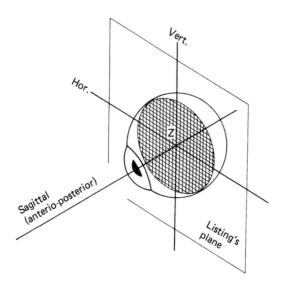

Figure 8.1. Listing's plane: a vertical section through the eye's centre of rotation Z, perpendicular to the primary line of the eye.

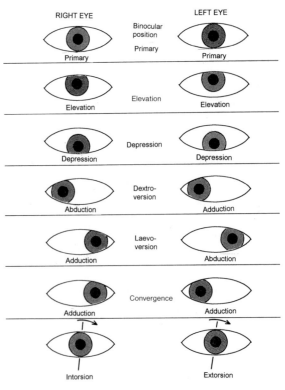

Figure 8.2. Ocular movements from the examiner's viewpoint.

Rotations of the eye about its anteroposterior axis are called torsions. They cannot be induced by voluntary effort but can result from certain reflexes, for example, in partial compensation for a tilt of the head towards one shoulder.

Extorsion occurs when the upper end of the vertical meridian of the cornea is rotated away from the median plane. Rotation in the contrary direction is known as intorsion.

Binocular movements

The secondary positions of gaze defined above apply to a single eye. If both eyes move in a similar direction, as, for example, when maintaining binocular fixation of an object moving in a fronto-parallel plane (a vertical plane parallel to the line joining the eyes' centres of rotation), the resulting binocular movement is called a version.

Elevation of both eyes is called supraversion and depression infraversion. When both eyes look to the right, the right eye abducts and the left eye adducts: the binocular movement is called dextroversion. Gaze to the left involves laevoversion.

A vergence movement occurs when the eyes rotate in opposite directions. Thus, convergence occurs when fixation is changed from a relatively distant to a nearer object, while divergence denotes the opposite.

Version movements may also be made in vertical and torsional directions under the stimulus of reflex pathways (*see* Chapter 10).

The eye's centre of rotation

Excluding the cornea, the globe of the eye is approximately spherical, and its movements resemble those of a ball and socket joint. Rotation takes places about a point approximately at the centre of curvature of the posterior sclera. Because the extra-ocular muscles alter shape during an ocular rotation, the shape and position of the orbital socket may well be changed as a result. Consequently, the centre of rotation does not remain fixed with respect to the head during a large eye movement.

Helmholtz and von Kries (Helmholtz, 1924) give a comprehensive survey of many of the early researches into the position of the eye's centre of rotation, including those of Donders and Doyer (Donders, 1864). The method they used may be simplified for use by students. First, the corneal diameter is measured with a device such as the Wessely keratometer. The subject's head is then held firmly in a rest and his eye is observed through a telescope fitted with a hair-line graticule (reticle). Two fixation objects D and E are positioned as in *Figure 8.3*, such that when the subject views D, the right-hand side of his cornea is imaged on the graticule line, and similarly for the other side when E is viewed.

If d is the corneal diameter, y_R and y_L the semi-diameters (which are not necessarily equal) and q the distance from corneal vertex A to line DE, then, from

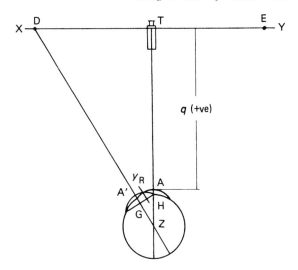

Figure 8.3. A method of determining the position of the ocular centre of rotation Z.

the similar triangles ZGH and ZTD and regarding all distances as positive,

$$\frac{GZ}{GH} = \frac{TZ}{TD} = \frac{TA + AZ}{TD} = \frac{TA + A'Z}{TD}$$

If the corneal sag A'G is neglected as being small in relation to TA, this expression may be written

$$\frac{GZ}{y_R} = \frac{TA + GZ}{TD} = \frac{q + GZ}{TD}$$

from which

$$GZ\,(TD - y_R) = y_R q$$

Similarly

$$GZ\,(TE - y_L) = y_L q$$

so that, by addition

$$GZ\,(DE - d) = dq$$

which gives

$$z = A'Z = \frac{dq}{DE - d} + \text{corneal sag A'G}$$

For emmetropic eyes, Donders and Doyer found that the mean distance z to be approximately 13.5 mm, taking the corneal sag as 2.6 mm.

Park and Park (1933) found that in the horizontal plane the motion of the eye could best be described as the rolling of a pivot of finite size near the centre of the eye on another curved surface. This is analogous to the clenched fist rolling in the gently cupped palm of the other hand. The effective centre of rotation lies on the nasal side of the visual axis, which could be predicted from *Figure 2.12* since the visual axis and the axis of symmetry of the eye do not coincide.

This was confirmed by Fry and Hill (1962), who found for 28 of their 33 subjects that the centre of rotation was at a mean distance of 0.79 mm nasalwards from the visual axis, and some 14.8 mm behind the corneal pole. For three of their subjects, however, the results suggested that they did not have a fixed centre of rotation.

Although a fixed centre of rotation situated on the visual axis is assumed for purposes such as spectacle-lens design and calculations involving convergence, the true position is more complicated as the previous discussion has shown. Experimental evidence also suggests that the centre of rotation is not the same for vertical as for horizontal movements. (For a review *see* Alpern, 1969.)

A simple technique for estimating the distance between the centres of rotation of the eyes, instead of assuming it to equal the inter-pupillary distance (PD), is described by Ryland and Lang (1913).

The extra-ocular muscles

The human orbit is approximately pyramidal in form, the square base lying open at the front. The nasal walls of the left and right orbits are roughly parallel, while the two lateral walls lie approximately at right-angles to each other. The axes of the orbits thus diverge at about 22° from the median plane (*Figure 8.4*).

The eye is rotated in its socket by six extrinsic or extra-ocular muscles. Five of these originate in a tendinous ring which surrounds the optic nerve at the apex of the orbit. Four of them, the recti muscles, pass forward and are inserted between 5 and 8 mm from the limbus. The fifth ocular muscle originating from the ring is the superior oblique, which extends forward to the superior nasal corner of the orbit. There, its tendon passes through a ring called the trochlea and turns back to its insertion in the rear portion of the sclera. Its effective axis makes an angle of 55° with the primary direction, passing behind the centre of rotation of the eye.

The sixth extra-ocular muscle, the inferior oblique, originates in the lower nasal corner of the front of the orbit and passes diagonally backwards to its insertion in the lower rear sclera. Its direction of action is at an angle of about 51° to the visual axis when the eye is in the primary position.

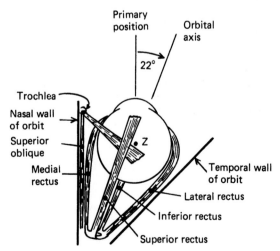

Figure 8.4. Diagrammatic representation of right orbit and extra-ocular muscles viewed from above, the inferior oblique muscle being hidden. Z denotes the ocular centre of rotation.

The levator palpebrae superioris also originates from the tendon ring at the orbital apex and controls the position of the upper lid.

This simplified picture of the attachments of the muscles is sufficient for deducing the effects of their contractions, both from the primary position and also from oblique positions of gaze. In extreme positions, the normal eye's excursions are also controlled by various check ligaments, which prevent excessive movement. Occasionally, the muscles or check ligaments are incorrectly positioned and abnormal ocular movements are produced.

The extra-ocular muscles are innervated by three of the cranial nerves. The third or oculomotor nerve innervates the superior, inferior and medial recti, and also the inferior oblique. It also innervates the levator palpebrae superioris, the ciliary muscle and the iris sphincter. The fourth nerve, the trochlear, innervates the superior oblique, while the abducens or sixth nerve innervates the lateral rectus.

The motor nerves originate in the brain stem at the base of the cerebrum. The third nerve nucleus is subdivided into parts for each muscle it controls; these and the fourth nerve nucleus lie in the tegmentum on the dorsal aspect of the mid-brain. The sixth nerve nucleus lies in the pons.

These nuclei are stimulated by supra-nuclear or intermediary nuclei, which in turn are stimulated by other pathways: for example, an involuntary pathway from the visual or occipital cortex of the cerebrum and the voluntary route from the frontal cortex. Thus, if a moving object is watched, the fixation reflex from the occipital cortex will stimulate the nerve nuclei, and hence the extra-ocular muscles, to maintain the retinal images upon the foveae. Head movements may also be produced. If the gaze is transferred to some other object, the innervation arises from the motor cortex in the frontal lobe of the cerebrum – Brodmann's area No.8.

Other stimuli, mostly reflex, arise from the sense of balance and bodily position. Thus, a head tilt to the right shoulder gives rise to a compensatory reflex tilt of the eyes in the opposite direction, as shown at the bottom of *Figure 8.2*. This compensatory tilt is, however, only about one-sixth of the head tilt. Similarly, a head rotation to the right about a vertical axis will tend to stimulate laevoversion (movement to the left). These static reflexes compensate for changes in head or body position, while stato-kinetic reflexes originate during, and allow for, accelerations and decelerations in head or body movements.

Principal and secondary muscle actions

Monocular actions

In general, co-ordinated contractions and relaxations of the extra-ocular muscles are required to produce any desired change in direction of the visual axes. Initially, it is simplest to consider the actions of the individual muscles on the eye when in its primary position. *Figures*

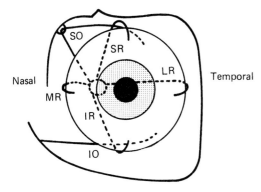

Figure 8.5. Diagrammatic representation of left orbit and extra-ocular muscles viewed from in front: SO superior oblique, SR superior rectus, MR medial rectus, LR lateral rectus, IR inferior rectus, IO inferior oblique.

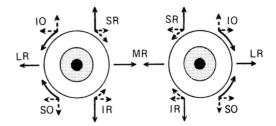

Figure 8.6. Marquez diagram: primary and secondary muscle actions in the two eyes in their primary position. Solid arrows denote primary, broken arrows secondary actions. Note that the lengths of the lines are not proportional to the effective action. Key to muscles as in *Figure 8.5.*

8.4 and 8.5 show how the effects of muscle contractions may be deduced.

Thus, contraction of the medial rectus produces only adduction, since the plane of action of the muscle is purely horizontal. Similarly, contraction of the lateral rectus abducts the eye.

The plane of action of the superior rectus is not vertical but slightly tilted. Its contraction produces elevation as the principal effect, and in addition adduction and intorsion. The direction of action of the superior oblique is defined by the line of its tendinous portion between the trochlea and its insertion into the eye. It therefore gives intorsion, abduction and depression. These results are summarized in *Table 8.1.* It will be noted that both the superior oblique and rectus muscles are intorters, while both inferior muscles are extorters. It is advisable, however, to memorize the anatomy of the orbit and deduce the muscle actions, rather than memorizing them.

These results can also be illustrated by a Marquez diagram (*Figure 8.6*) in which the arrows show the directions of action when the eye is in its primary position.

The necessity for co-ordinated action by the extra-ocular muscles arises even in cardinal rotations of the eye. Thus, in a purely horizontal movement from the primary position, muscle tone in the vertically acting muscles must be maintained because their lengths are affected by the horizontal movement of the eye. Elevation directly above the primary position requires the action of the superior rectus, but this also gives rise to intorsion and adduction. Although the inferior oblique also provides elevation, accompanied by extorsion and abduction, the latter does not counterbalance the ad-

duction produced by the superior rectus. Consequently, the lateral and medial recti also come into play to prevent horizontal movement of the eye.

Adler (1981) gives an extensive survey of muscle actions and changes in nervous stimulations when ocular movements take place. A highly detailed study of the kinematics of the extra-ocular muscles has been written by Solomons (1977).

Muscle failure and diplopia

If one of the extra-ocular muscles should cease to function efficiently because, for example, of a haemorrhage within the muscle or damage to the nerve supply, the eye will tend to deviate from its normal position. Moreover, if muscle action is suddenly and severely impaired in an adult, diplopia (double vision) will result. If the right lateral rectus were affected, then instead of both eyes looking straight ahead to view a distant object B, the right eye would adduct because the impaired action of the right lateral rectus would be outweighed by the normal muscle tone of the medial rectus (*Figure 8.7*).

In such cases, the perceived image is localized in space as though the eye were still in its primary position, as in *Figure 8.7(c).* Since, in fact, the retinal image of the distant object B lies nasally to the right fovea M'_R, the perceived image is incorrectly projected to the temporal side. The image from the left eye, however, is perceived straight ahead. In general, a diplopic image due to a malfunctioning or paretic muscle is displaced in the same direction as the rotation which contraction of that muscle normally produces.

Consider a further example: the right superior rectus. This muscle elevates, adducts and intorts the eye. If it is paretic, the eye becomes relatively depressed, abducted and extorted. Consequently, the diplopic image will be displaced in the opposite direction up and in, with the

Table 8.1 Principal and secondary actions of the extra-ocular muscles

Muscle	Principal action(s)	Secondary action(s)	
Medial rectus	Adduction		
Lateral rectus	Abduction		
Superior rectus	Elevation	Adduction	Intorsion
Inferior rectus	Depression	Adduction	Extorsion
Superior oblique	Intorsion and depression	Abduction	
Inferior oblique	Extorsion and elevation	Abduction	

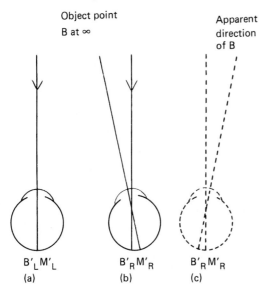

Figure 8.7. Double vision caused by loss of muscle tone in the right lateral rectus: (c) illustrates the perceptual projection of the image in the deviating eye.

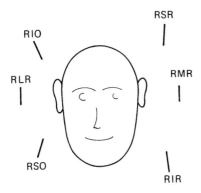

Figure 8.8. Position (from examiner's viewpoint) of the diplopic image caused by a named paretic muscle in the deviating right eye. Left eye is fixating a vertical bar light held in the median plane.

top tilted to the patient's left (*Figure 8.8*). Note that because the diplopic image lies to the patient's left, it could mistakenly be thought that the image shows extorsion.

If the paresis is only slight, the fusional reserves (*see* Chapter 9) would hold the two eyes in the correct position under normal circumstances. If the patient wears a red filter over his right eye and a green filter over the left, the retinal images will be of different colours. This dissociation technique makes fusion more difficult, so the right eye (with the paretic muscles) will deviate. If the patient now looks at a white light, the left eye's green image will be correctly projected back to the light, while the red image will be displaced. *Figure 8.8* shows the apparent position of the diplopic images, assuming that each muscle in turn of the right eye is paretic.

In order to demonstrate torsional effects, an elongated white light (bar light) is needed.

Conversely, if a muscle in the left eye becomes paretic (the right extra-ocular muscles remaining normal), the

right eye will correctly fixate the bar light. The falsely projected left eye's image will be positioned as in a mirror image of *Figure 8.8*.

This method is rarely used to diagnose faulty muscle action, since small deficiencies would be difficult to identify. The technique described on pages 147–149 is much more sensitive.

Muscle actions in binocular movements

The individual muscle actions described in the previous section are for small eye movements from the primary position, but eye movements generally require the combined actions of many of the extra-ocular muscles. Diagnosis of faulty muscle action can be simplified if it can be shown that particular directions of gaze are produced, in effect, by one muscle only in each eye.

Consider the action of the superior rectus muscle when the eye has abducted or turned out through an angle of 22° (*Figures 8.4* and *8.9*). The line of action of the muscle now passes almost exactly above the eye's centre of rotation. Its action is now purely elevation. In the primary position, the inferior oblique also has an elevating function. *Figure 8.9* shows that its elevating effect is less in the abducted position than in the primary position. Thus, when the eye is looking up and out, the muscle principally concerned is the superior rectus. By a similar analysis, a corresponding position of gaze can be found for each of the other muscles in turn.

Figure 8.10 and *Table 8.2* show these positions of gaze, which may be called the fields of action of the muscles. In the right eye, contraction of the right inferior rectus muscle is the most important when looking down and to the right. In the left eye, the most important muscle in this direction of gaze is the left superior oblique. Muscles paired in this way are known as yoke muscles or contralateral synergists.

These fields of action are also called the diagnostic positions of gaze, since they are used to check the operation of the extra-ocular muscles. Pure elevation and depression of the eyes should also be observed in order to

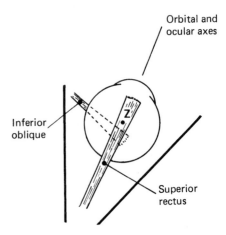

Figure 8.9. Reduction in elevating power of the right inferior oblique muscle when the eye is abducted: view of orbit from above.

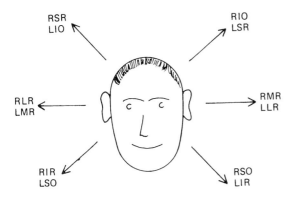

Figure 8.10. Yoke muscles: examiner's view of the field of action of each of the extra-ocular muscles.

check the operation of the lid muscles, notably the levator palpebrae superioris.

In relation to eye movements, Hering's law of equal innervation, formulated in 1868, states that the contralateral synergists receive equal stimulation. Sherrington's law of 1894 of reciprocal innervation, when interpreted for the eye, states that as the acting muscle is stimulated, so its antagonist on the same eye relaxes. The lateral and medial recti of either eye are obviously antagonists; the superior and inferior recti are also considered as antagonists since their principal actions in the primary position oppose each other, even though both are adductors. Similarly, the two obliques are antagonists.

Thus, in a binocular version movement up and to the left, the right inferior oblique and left superior rectus should receive equal innervation since they are contralateral synergists. Their antagonists, the right superior oblique and left inferior rectus, correspondingly relax.

If the left superior rectus should become paretic, the left eye will not move as far as the right eye. If the right eye maintains fixation on the test object, the left eye will lag behind. Conversely, if the paretic left eye fixates, the right eye will overshoot. Since excessive stimulus of the left muscle is required to provide sufficient movement of the eye, the overaction of the right eye will be greater than the underaction of the left eye. The primary deviation is the angle of lag when the good eye fixates, while the larger secondary deviation occurs when the eye with the paretic muscle fixates. Measurement of these deviations is discussed in the following section.

Motility testing

The clinical need for motility testing is to establish whether muscle action is normal. Faulty movement might be the result of damage to one or more of the extra-ocular muscles or their innervation. If the movement of both eyes is equally restricted in the same directions, the patient is said to have a gaze palsy. This is the effect of damage to the supra-nuclear pathways. If, however, the movement of the eyes is unequal, the malfunction is either in the nerve nuclei, their subsequent pathways or the muscle itself. Thus, motility testing is one method of investigating the functioning of various regions of the brain.

During motility tests, the patient's head must be kept still. A fixation object is initially held directly in front of the patient at about half a metre, so that the eyes are converged slightly from their primary position. The examiner then watches the relative position of the patient's eyes while he moves the fixation object first left and right and then along the four oblique diagnostic positions of gaze given in *Table 8.2*. With practice, the examiner will be able to detect small relative deviations of the eyes, while the patient will report a doubling of the fixation object if binocular fixation breaks down, unless the diplopic image from one eye is suppressed. A vertical movement should also be made to check the action of the eyelids.

A small torch or an ophthalmoscope makes a convenient fixation object, provided that the instrument is angled so that the field of illumination covers both eyes. The positions of the corneal reflexes relative to the centre of the pupil may be used to assess accuracy of fixation, particularly if the examiner moves so that his head stays behind the torch. If motility is normal, the patient's eyes should move steadily in all directions of gaze with no diplopia. If the muscle action is slightly defective in one eye, binocular fixation of the test object will probably be maintained near the central position. In the field(s) of action of the malfunctioning muscle(s), however, the paretic eye may be seen to lag behind. The diplopic image perceived by this eye will accordingly be displaced too far from the primary direction. Consequently, if this eye is covered, it is the farther image which will disappear.

Diplopia can be induced in this test more easily by dissociating the two eyes. A convenient and strongly recommended method is to use a red filter for the right eye and a green filter for the left eye. The patient can then report the relative positions of the two coloured lights in the various positions of gaze. Alternatively, the Maddox rod or the cover test may be used (*see* Chapter 10).

Observation of the patient's eyes as they follow the test object is sufficient for initial examination, but more accurate methods are needed for an assessment of complicated or long-standing cases of paresis.

Table 8.2 Yoke muscles and diagnostic positions of gaze

Muscle pair		Field of action
R medial rectus	L lateral rectus	Horizontally to the left
R lateral rectus	L medial rectus	Horizontally to the right
R superior rectus	L inferior oblique	Up and to the right
R inferior rectus	L superior oblique	Down and to the right
R inferior oblique	L superior rectus	Up and to the left
R superior oblique	L inferior rectus	Down and to the left

(a)

(b)

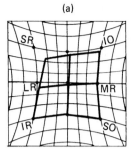
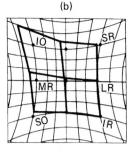

Figure 8.11. Typical plot on the Hess screen charts, indicating paresis of the left superior rectus. For clarity, only one set of fixation points is shown. (a) Plot for left eye (right-eye fixation), (b) plot for right eye (left-eye fixation).

The Lancaster and Hess screens are commonly used for this purpose. The former consists of a grid of equally spaced vertical and horizontal lines. The patient sits with his eyes level with the centre of the screen at a distance of 0.5 or 1 m, depending on the linear spacing of the lines which should subtend 4° or 7∆ at the eyes.

The Hess screen is similar, except that the lines curve inwards to the centre as in the recording chart shown in part in *Figure 8.11*. The reason for this is to overcome perspective problems: a horizontal line 20 cm above the central point of a screen used at 1 m corresponds to an elevation of 20∆ immediately above the central point, but only 18.5∆ at 40 cm to one side of it.

A light grey screen is often used, with torches projecting a red or a green streak of light. The patient wears red–green goggles to dissociate the eyes, with the red filter initially over the right eye. The examiner holds the red torch and directs its projected streak to lie horizontally at the centre of the screen. This red streak can be seen only by the patient's right eye, since the green filter over the left eye absorbs red light and vice versa. The patient holds the green torch and is asked to position its streak to lie apparently superimposed on the red streak. The actual position of the green streak indicates the projection of the left fovea.

The position of the green streak when the red streak is central is marked on the left-hand chart of *Figure 8.11*. This procedure is repeated for the six diagnostic positions of gaze and the fixation points directly above and below the centre. The positions corresponding to the inner 'square' are usually used, except when no deviation occurs between the red and green torch positions. The outer 'square' may then be brought into use.

Figure 8.11(a) shows the relative direction of the left eye when the right eye is fixing. The muscle positions shown on the chart represent the patient's (and examiner's) viewpoint and are therefore reversed left to right in comparison with *Figure 8.10* in which the examiner is facing the patient.

Either the goggles or the torches are then reversed, so it is now the patient's left eye which fixates the examiner's streak. The position of the patient's streak is now plotted on *Figure 8.11(b)*, indicating the position of the right eye and hence the action of its extra-ocular muscles.

In general, the two coloured streaks are rarely superimposed, but are separated. If the plotted figures for the two eyes are similar in size and shape, the deviation is said to be comitant or concomitant. If the plots are unequal in size and irregular in shape, the deviation is said to be incomitant and is indicative of faulty muscle action.

The chart showing the smaller figure indicates the eye with the paretic muscle, since this eye lags behind in the field of action of this muscle. Thus, *Figure 8.11* also illustrates a paresis of the left superior rectus of recent onset. The left-eye chart shows a reduced angle of movement up and out, while the right chart shows the exaggerated secondary deviation produced by overaction of the right inferior oblique – the contralateral synergist.

The Lees screen is a pair of Hess screens mounted at right-angles, the markings showing only when internally illuminated. A pair of mirrors mounted back to back bisects the angle between the screens. The patient initially faces the unilluminated left screen and views the illuminated right screen with his right eye by reflection in the mirror. The examiner indicates the various test positions to the patient's right eye and the patient uses a pointer to demonstrate the projection through the left fovea of these fixation points. These positions are marked directly on the apparently plain left screen with a glass writing pen or pencil. This left screen is then switched on, and the relative positions of the two eyes recorded on the chart. The patient then moves to view the illuminated left chart with the left eye by reflection in the mirror and the process is repeated for the right eye with the right chart switched off.

In the presence of anomalous retinal correspondence (*see* Chapter 10) the difference in position of the red and green streaks may not indicate the actual angle between the visual axes of the two eyes.

When an extra-ocular muscle paresis has been present for some time, secondary effects may occur in some of the other muscles. Thus, paresis of one muscle may be followed by permanent contraction of the antagonist of the same eye and the contralateral synergist, together with a secondary inhibition of the contralateral antagonist. For example, paralysis of the left lateral rectus may be followed by contraction of the left medial rectus and right medial rectus together with inhibition of the right lateral rectus.

A head turn to the side or up or down may reduce symptoms by avoiding the field of action of the affected muscle. Thus, from *Figure 8.10* or *Table 8.2*, a left lateral rectus palsy would give rise to a head turn to the left, while a right superior rectus palsy would give a posture of chin up and head turn to the right. The principal actions of the obliques are torsional. A slight paresis of the right superior oblique may give a head tilt or ocular torticollis to the left (to replace the intorsion – *see Table 8.1*) together with a chin-down posture. Although the muscle is an abductor, which would suggest a face turn to the right, its principal field of action or diagnostic position of gaze is down to the left. Hence there may be a face turn to the left to avoid the muscle having to move into that position. Of these three rotations, the head tilt is likely to be the greatest, but even a small head movement may be sufficient to avoid the symptoms that would otherwise be caused by a paretic muscle. It may therefore be necessary to hold the patient's head upright to achieve valid results when motility testing. Adaptations in the other extra-ocular muscles will reduce the need for an abnormal head posture, thus lessening its diagnostic value. An upwards or downwards head posture may be associated with an A or V pattern of eye movements.

A fuller explanation of the results of paresis of the extra-ocular muscles can be found in texts on strabismus.

Torsion and false torsion

True torsion

True torsion is a rotation of the eye about its anteroposterior axis, considered as a separate degree of freedom. As already noted, it is induced in both eyes as a partial compensation for a sideways tilt of the head. In the normal subject, the torsional actions of the muscles are well balanced so that little unintentional torsion occurs. This is not the case if there is a paresis of one extra-ocular muscle and over-activity by its contralateral synergist. A marked degree of torsion in the affected field of action may then result, though possibly without causing visual problems. Any torsional imbalance, however it occurs, would tend to cause perceptual disorientation of space. The same is true, though, of the aberrational distortion produced by spectacles lenses, to which most subjects eventually contrive to adapt.

Oblique eye movements

In *Figure 8.12*, Z is the eye's centre of rotation and O a point on the fixation line in the eye's primary position. Suppose that fixation is now transferred to the point Q in the vertical plane through O that is normal to ZO. Of the many routes which could be taken, the following three are of particular importance in the study of oblique movements:

(1) Elevation through the angle λ, bringing the fixation to the point S immediately above O, followed by an azimuthal rotation through the angle μ in the tilted plane ZSQ. Because of this tilt, the axis about which the second rotation takes place cannot lie in Listing's plane but is tipped backwards through the angle λ. In the diagram, the two rotations are denoted by H1 and H2 because these were the parameters used by Helmholtz.
(2) A horizontal rotation (longitude) through the angle ϕ, bringing fixation to the point T, followed by a vertical rotation (latitude) through the angle θ. They are denoted by F1 and F2, being the parameters used by Fick. Once again, it is only the first of these rotations which takes place about an axis in Listing's plane.
(3) A single rotation through the angle β in the plane OZQ, executed about the axis RR in Listing's plane making an angle α with the vertical. Since RR must be perpendicular to the plane OZQ, it follows that the angle QOT must also be equal to α – thus defining the meridian OQ in standard axis notation. This route, defined by Listing's parameters, is indicated in the diagram by the letter L.

Given that ZO = 100, OS = 50, and OT = 80, the other dimensions given in the diagram can readily be determined. The various angles can also be calculated, as

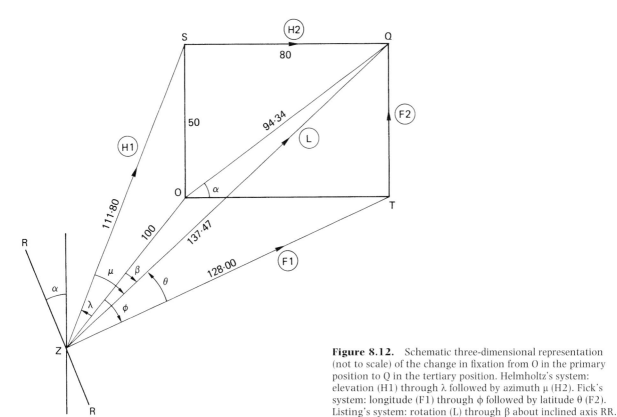

Figure 8.12. Schematic three-dimensional representation (not to scale) of the change in fixation from O in the primary position to Q in the tertiary position. Helmholtz's system: elevation (H1) through λ followed by azimuth μ (H2). Fick's system: longitude (F1) through ϕ followed by latitude θ (F2). Listing's system: rotation (L) through β about inclined axis RR.

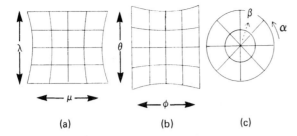

Figure 8.13. Projection of: (a) Helmholtz's, (b) Fick's, (c) Listing's system of axes on a fronto-parallel plane.

follows:

$$\lambda = \text{arc tan } 50/100 \quad\quad = 26.57° \text{ (elevation)}$$
$$\mu = \text{arc tan } 80/111.80 = 35.59° \text{ (azimuth)}$$
$$\phi = \text{arc tan } 80/100 \quad\quad = 38.66° \text{ (longitude)}$$
$$\theta = \text{arc tan } 50/128.06 = 21.33° \text{ (latitude)}$$
$$\alpha = \text{arc tan } 50/80 \quad\quad = 32.00° \text{ (meridian)}$$
$$\beta = \text{arc tan } 94.34/100 = 43.33° \text{ (eccentricity)}$$

These angles are interrelated in various ways, which may be deduced from *Figure 8.12*. For example, given λ and μ, ϕ and θ can be obtained from

$$\tan \phi = \tan \mu/\cos \lambda \quad\quad\quad\quad\quad (8.1)$$

and

$$\sin \theta = \sin \lambda \cos \mu \quad\quad\quad\quad\quad (8.2)$$

Similarly, the relationship between α and β and the other two pairs of angles is given by

$$\tan \alpha = \tan \theta/\sin \phi = \sin \lambda/\tan \mu \quad (8.3)$$

and

$$\cos \beta = \cos \phi \cos \theta = \cos \lambda \cos \mu \quad (8.4)$$

Figure 8.13 indicates the form that would be taken by flat screens or wallcharts constructed for the three different co-ordinate systems under discussion. The grid lines in each chart denote equal intervals of the two angular parameters in use.

In studies of binocular vision, Helmholtz's system offers an advantage over Fick's ϕ and θ; for a given angle of elevation λ, convergence simply becomes the algebraic difference $\Delta\mu$ between two angles of azimuth. Listing's angles α and β, sometimes called meridian and eccentricity respectively, lead to the polar chart shown at *Figure 8.13(c)*, the concentric circles representing regular intervals of the angle β.

The symmetrically curved grid of the Hess screen (*Figure 8.11*) plots regular intervals of the angles of azimuth μ and latitude θ.

Eye movements are most easily studied with the aid of an ophthalmetrope (a model eye mounted on pivots) or by using a solid rubber ball with knitting needles as the axes of rotation and fixation.

False torsion

As would be expected, horizontal and vertical ocular rotation from the primary to a secondary position are not normally accompanied by torsion. Complications arise in the case of movements to a tertiary position. Suppose that true torsion as an independent motion is not possible. Even so, it can be shown that (with one exception) the movement or series of movements by which the eye assumes a tertiary position would have to involve an incidental rotational displacement as though true torsion had occurred. A more serious complication is that the amount of incidental torsion in a given tertiary position of the eye would vary with the route by which fixation had been brought to that position. For example, in *Figure 8.12* the torsion incidental to route H would be greater than that accompanying route L, though this could not be inferred from the diagram alone. On the other hand, it can readily be visualized that route F is uniquely free from incidental torsion.

It would, of course, be highly disconcerting to the visual system if different amounts of torsion could occur in the same direction of the gaze. In fact, true torsion is used to adjust the amount of incidental torsion and so bring order into what would otherwise be an intolerable situation. Experimental studies have shown that the *actual* amount of torsion peculiar to any direction of the gaze is the same as if the eye had been brought to that position by a single rotation from the primary position about an axis in Listing's plane (route L). Paradoxically, this actual amount of torsion is termed 'false torsion'.

The observed behaviour of the eye is defined more precisely in two well-known laws:

(1) *Donders' law* states that for any given position of the line of fixation with respect to the head there exists a definite and invariable angle of false torsion, which is independent of the will of the subject and independent of the manner in which the fixation has been brought to that position.

(2) *Listing's law* states that when the line of fixation is brought from the primary to any other position, the angle of false torsion in this second position is the same as if the eye had arrived at it by rotation about an axis (in Listing's plane) perpendicular to the plane containing the initial and final positions of fixation. (In *Figure 8.12*, for example, the axis of rotation RR is perpendicular to the plane OZQ.)

Calculation of false torsion

Simple methods of demonstrating and measuring false torsion were devised by Maddox (1898). *Figure 8.14*, which is based on one of his diagrams, represents a schematic model of an eye as viewed by an observer. The point A is the corneal vertex and ZA the fixation line when the eye is in its primary position. The equatorial plane of the eye perpendicular to ZA then coincides with Listing's plane.

The eye now turns through an angle β about an axis RZ (in Listing's plane) making an angle α with the vertical VZ in this plane. As a result, A moves to A′ along a circular path in a tilted plane perpendicular to RZ, bringing the fixation line to the new position ZA′. This rotation would be upwards and to the subject's right. Simultaneously, the point in the eye's equatorial plane originally situated at V moves through the same angle β to the new position V′. Its path in this rotation lies on a circle with its centre M on RZ at the foot of the perpen-

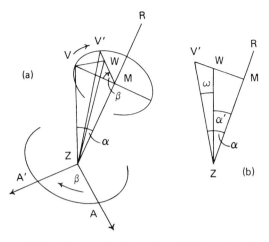

(a)

(b)

Figure 8.14. Diagram for derivation of false torsion. (After Maddox, 1898.)

dicular from V. Being the axis of rotation, RZ itself remains stationary and therefore continues to lie in the eye's equatorial plane in its new position. This is now established because it must contain the lines RZ and V′Z as well as being perpendicular to the new fixation line ZA′. Let the perpendicular from V to V′M meet this line at W. WZ is then the intersection of the eye's equatorial plane with the vertical plane containing the vertical line VZ and the fixation line ZA′. Viewed along this latter line, the appearance would be as shown in *Figure 8.14(b)*, WZ being seen in line with VZ. With respect to this true vertical the meridian V′Z, which was vertical when the eye was in its primary position, has moved through an angle ω that is clockwise from the subject's point of view. This is the angle of false torsion.

The following method of calculating its value is also derived from Maddox. Let α′ denote the angle WZR in the eye's equatorial plane. Then from *Figure 8.14* it can be seen that

$$\tan \alpha' = MW/MZ$$

and

$$\tan \alpha = MV'/MZ$$

so that

$$\tan \alpha' = (MW/MV') \tan \alpha$$

From triangle VWM it is also apparent that

$$MW/MV = MW/MV' = \cos \beta$$

Hence

$$\tan \alpha' = \tan \alpha \cos \beta$$

and

$$\omega = \alpha - \alpha'$$

$$= \alpha - \arctan (\tan \alpha \cos \beta) \qquad (8.5)$$

As shown by Helmholtz, expressions for false torsion can also be obtained in terms of the angles φ and θ, as follows:

$$\tan \omega = \frac{\sin \phi \sin \theta}{\cos \phi + \cos \theta} \qquad (8.6)$$

and

$$\tan (\omega/2) = \tan (\phi/2) \tan (\theta/2) \qquad (8.7)$$

With the help of equations (8.3) and (8.4), Helmholtz's expressions can be shown to be mathematically identical with Maddox's.

The angle of false torsion is usually quite small, with a maximum value little more than 10°. You can verify for yourself that when the relevant numerical quantities from *Figure 8.12* are inserted in any of the above expressions for false torsion, the result obtained is 7.56°.

A mathematical treatment of ocular torsion on the basis of direction cosines has been given by Solomons (1975).

Experimental verifications

The angle of false torsion implicit in Listing's law can be measured experimentally in various ways. Objective methods require a means of distinguishing one meridian of the eye as a reference line. Conjunctival sutures and a thread placed on the anaesthetized cornea are among the devices known to have been used. The iris pattern has also been used as a less drastic alternative.

Measurement of the angle of torsion requires great care because the apparent angle between two non-parallel lines in the same plane varies with the viewpoint. If photography is used, the photographic axis must be made to coincide with the fixation line in all the ocular positions investigated.

Subjective methods have used either the blind spot or an after-image as a marker. A suitable object for an after-image is an upright cross. The subject's head is constrained to ensure that his eye is in its primary position, with the centre of the cross on the fixation line. An electronic flash may be used to produce an after-image of the cross, the limbs of which correspond to the true horizontal and vertical meridians of the retina.

The orientation of the after-image when the subject now looks in various directions (with his head still fixed) is illustrated in *Figure 8.15(a)*. As predicted by Listing's law, no torsion occurs in secondary positions of the gaze, while the rotation of the after-image in tertiary positions is in the expected direction. For example, when the subject looks upwards and to his right, the rotation is clockwise as predicted by *Figure 8.14*.

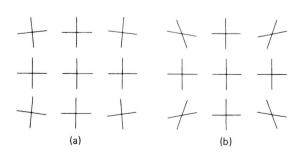

(a)   (b)

Figure 8.15. Projection of an after-image of a vertical–horizontal cross on to: (a) the inside of a sphere concentric with the eye, (b) a fronto-parallel plane.

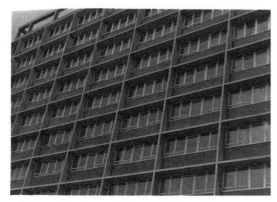

Figure 8.16. Photograph of a building, camera pointing up and to the left to show perspective distortion, opposite to that in *Figure 8.15(b)*.

A complication arises when the apparent position of the after-image is plotted on a screen which is not normal to the subject's line of sight in the particular direction studied. If plotted on a screen perpendicular to the fixation line in the eye's primary position, the after-image takes the various forms shown in *Figure 8.15(b)*. The apparent distortion of the cross which occurs in tertiary positions of the gaze arises purely from the geometry of oblique projection. A similar effect can be seen in photography, as in *Figure 8.16*, which shows a building photographed with the camera pointing obliquely upwards and to the left. In this case the distortion is of the opposite form to that shown in *Figure 8.15(b)* because the direction of projection has been reversed (backwards to the camera).

The difficulty can be overcome by plotting on the inside of a sphere concentric with the eye's centre of rotation. This was the method adopted by Quereau (1955), who used the blind spot as a marker.

In general, the truth of Listing's law has been verified by these various experimental techniques, provided that the right and left fixation lines remain substantially parallel. The angle of false torsion appears to be affected by convergence, though not in a uniform and accurately predictable manner. In the usual position of depression and convergence adopted in near vision there appears to be very little torsion.

Requirements for binocular vision

Summary of requirements

The chameleon has two eyes which are moved independently of each other. Despite its two eyes it does not have binocular vision, which may be defined as the use of two eyes in such a co-ordinated manner as to produce a single mental impression of external space. An image of partly the same scene is formed in each eye, the two images being transmitted separately to the cerebral cortex. The final mental percept is the result of the blending or fusing of the two neural representations in the higher levels of the brain – the psychological stage of the visual process. Some authors, notably Asher (1961), favour the idea of a rapid consecutive proces-

sing by the brain of the visual input from the two eyes in turn, rather than the simultaneous integration of information. This difference of opinion is not of importance for the present study.

The requirements for binocular vision can be summarized as follows:

(1) The separate visual fields must overlap in all directions of gaze.
(2) The separate fields of fixation must overlap, with co-ordinated movements of the two eyes.
(3) The neural transmission from the two eyes must reach the same area of the brain.
(4) Perceptual co-ordination must take place.

Visual fields

The visual field is that extent of space containing all points which produce perception in the stationary eye, provided that the stimulus is sufficient. For binocular vision to be possible, the two orbits and the structure of the eyes must be arranged so that the visual fields overlap. In a grazing animal, protective vision is of great importance. The rabbit has a visual field for either eye alone extending over more than a semi-circle in the horizontal plane (Duke-Elder, 1958). The two laterally placed eyes therefore provide a large area of uniocular field on each side of the head, with a small region of overlap in front and behind.

The predatory animal, however, requires a good sense of distance judgement so that it can capture its prey. This necessitates a large area of overlapping vision, resulting in a large blind area behind the head.

Man's vision is somewhat similar in its requirements to the carnivore's. The orbits are placed anteriorly, facing forwards although their axes diverge at about 45°. The eyes are nevertheless mounted so that their visual axes are approximately parallel. *Figure 8.17* shows the two uniocular visual fields, with the binocular area doubly shaded.

The uniocular field is bounded by the superior and inferior margins of the orbit, the nose, and on the temporal side by the projection of the edge of the retina (the ora serrata); this extends furthest forward in the eye on the nasal side. The field extends to about 60° nasally and 100° temporally, given a sufficient stimulus.

The visual field is measured with a perimeter. This is a hollow hemisphere or a rotatable semicircular arc, usually with radius of curvature of a half or third of a metre. The subject is positioned so that the eye under test is approximately at the centre of curvature of the perimeter surface. The second eye is covered while the first steadily fixates an object at the centre of the arc. A test stimulus, for example a 10 mm diameter white disc, is brought in from the edge of the arc until the subject is just aware of its presence in the periphery of his vision. The stimulus eccentricity is measured directly in degrees and the process repeated for other meridians.

If the fields for the right and left eyes are plotted on the same chart, the area of overlap is the binocular visual field, which is approximately pear-shaped. The monocular temporal crescents contribute significantly to our awareness of space.

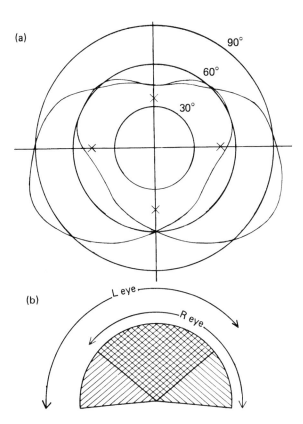

Figure 8.17. Monocular visual fields plotted on a chart. The crosses in (a) indicate the approximate limits of the field of binocular fixation. (b) Horizontal field as seen from above. The doubly shaded area represents the binocular field.

Fields of fixation

The field of fixation is that region of space containing all points which may be fixated by the mobile eye, the head remaining stationary. The eyes do not have an un-limited range of movement in their orbits, but conjugate version movements of the eyes over a range of approximately 45° from the primary position are possible. The horizontal and vertical limits are indicated by the crosses in *Figure 8.17*.

The monocular field of fixation may be determined with a perimeter by means of an after-image on the fovea produced by staring at a bright light for a few moments or at an electronic flash. The head is kept still and the eye rotated as far as the subject is able to. The position of the projected after-image on the perimeter scale gives the limit of fixation in the particular direction.

In the normal subject, the binocular field of fixation is similar to the monocular fields, but an oculo-motor paresis will reduce it in the fields of action of the affected muscle(s); compare the right and left ocular movements in *Figure 8.11*.

One method of measuring the binocular field of fixation is to ask the subject to look at a fine test object, for example, a printed word in small type. With the head stationary at the centre of the perimeter, the test object is moved out from the centre. When it appears double, binocular vision has broken down. In some cases the print may begin to blur, showing that parafoveal vision

is in use, the eyes no longer being able to follow the object movement precisely. (The monocular field may also be examined in this way, but the after-image technique is more accurate since deviation of the projected after-image from the marker which the eye is following is immediately apparent to the subject. The printed word may still be recognizable even if imaged parafoveally.)

It is important to distinguish between the fields of vision and fixation. The visual field relates to the stationary eye(s), whereas the field of fixation is the motor field – the solid angle within which the visual axes can be moved. In life, the visual field is effectively increased by both head and eye movements. An object in the peripheral field catches our attention and the eyes move so that the image falls on the fovea. Co-ordinated response of head and eye movements is required, the eye movements themselves rarely exceeding 20°.

Neural transmission

The right hemisphere of the brain is concerned with the left side of both the body and external space and vice versa. Thus the visual fibres from the two eyes might be expected to pass to the opposite side. If, however, all the fibres crossed, the neural information could not be integrated to give true binocular vision unless there were communicating tracts between the two cerebral hemispheres. Moreover, since the visual field of each eye extends over both sides of the mid-plane, some parts of the visual field would be represented in two places in the brain.

The chiasma or crossing of the two optic nerves in the cranium, behind the orbits, is only partial. Although about one-half of all the fibres (those from the nasal retina) pass to the opposite hemisphere of the brain, the temporal fibres remain on the same side. *Figure 8.18* shows schematically the path to the cortex, where the impulses from the respective parts of the two retinae are brought into proximity. Damage to one of the occipi-

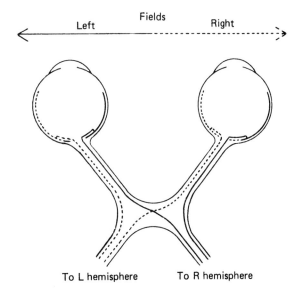

Figure 8.18. Simplified representation of nerve-fibre paths to the brain.

tal lobes therefore causes a corresponding defect in the left or the right visual field of both eyes, not to one eye alone (except for that part of the cortex corresponding to the monocular temporal crescents).

In the rabbit chiasma, the great majority of nerve fibres do cross to reach the opposite hemisphere: this arrangement is suited to the extensive uniocular fields of view but gives little binocular representation in the cortex.

Perceptual co-ordination

The partial decussation in the chiasma allows the two parts of each monocular field to be represented in the correct side of the brain. To bring these two views into association in the cortex so that there emerges out of them a single mental perception, with objects seen in their correct relative positions in space, further conditions must be satisfied.

There must be an orderly arrangement of receptors in each retina, together with their connections to the cortex. This will allow the correct monocular representation of the field of view in the brain. The terms neural and cortical image are sometimes used to describe the impulse pattern in the cortex, but this does not imply that there is a true picture in the cortex.

The two monocular representations have to be moulded into a single percept. Because the two eyes are positioned about 54–72 mm apart, they receive slightly different views of objects lying in the binocular visual field. A simple superposition of these two images would give rise to double vision and a conflicting sense of direction. The two monocular impressions must be brought into a corresponding association in the cortex and the brain must be capable of fusing or integrating them into a single binocular picture.

Monocular projection

In the normal eye the most important line of projection is that defined by the position of the centre of the fovea. For many purposes the visual axis (the line from the fovea to the centre of the exit pupil and its counterpart in object space) may be considered as the projection axis of the eye. The projection and visual axes may nevertheless differ in some anomalous conditions (*see* Chapter 10).

In the unaccommodated emmetropic eye, subject to paraxial limitations, all ray paths from the fovea emerge parallel to one another. Hence, in distance vision, any of these ray paths would lead back to the same remote object point. The simplest one to select for this purpose would be the undeviated ray through the nodal point(s) of the reduced eye. Provided that the retinal image is in sharp focus, the same simplification can be applied to near vision as well. The following discussion proceeds on this generally accepted basis, though its limitations should be borne in mind. Since the concept of nodal points is limited to paraxial rays, the construction cannot be regarded as precise.

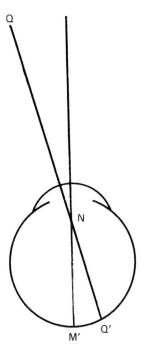

Figure 8.19.   Projection of a retinal image point Q′ into space through the nodal point of a reduced eye.

In *Figure 8.19*, the projection axis of a reduced eye is accordingly shown as the line from the fovea M′ through the nodal point N, which is taken to be the monocular centre of projection. A retinal element Q′, to the right of the fovea, would be stimulated by light from an object point Q situated anywhere on the line Q′N produced. The retinal image at Q′ is said to be projected towards Q. The direction is constant for a particular retinal element so that, when stimulated, each element always gives rise to a sensation localized in a specific direction relative to fixation. Lotze referred to this as local sign.

The monocular centre of projection should not be confused with the binocular sighting centre (*see* pages 156–157).

Corresponding points and the horopter

Whenever both foveae are stimulated simultaneously, the stimulus is invariably perceived as having a common origin in space (except in cases of anomalous retinal correspondence, *see* Chapter 10). This law applies even in artificial situations, for example, when the eyes have been made to diverge by a base-in prism or prisms.

A similar correspondence exists between a multitude of other pairs of retinal receptors, called corresponding points. When stimulated in binocular vision, they too give rise to a sensation subjectively localized at a single point. In *Figure 8.20* the eyes have converged to fixate the point B which is seen singly, and Q'_L and Q'_R are corresponding points to the left of each fovea. Since the projection lines through the respective nodal points in-

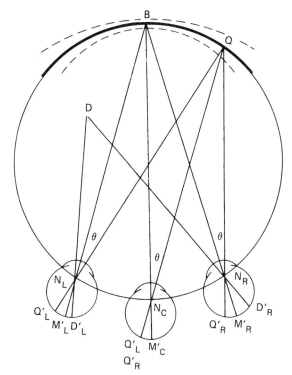

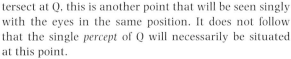

Figure 8.20. The longitudinal horopter. Subscripts L and R refer to the left and right eyes, C to the imaginary cyclopean eye.

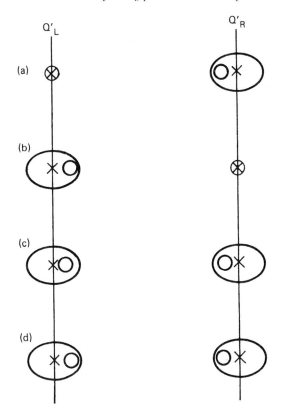

Figure 8.21. Panum's fusional areas.

tersect at Q, this is another point that will be seen singly with the eyes in the same position. It does not follow that the single *percept* of Q will necessarily be situated at this point.

For a given position of the eyes, the locus of all the object points whose images fall on corresponding points is known as a horopter, generally a curved surface. The point Q in *Figure 8.20* is said to be on the horopter of the fixation point B. The longitudinal horopter is the line formed by the intersection of the horopter with the plane containing the eyes' centres of rotation and the fixation point. In *Figure 8.20* it is indicated by the curved line through B and Q.

If perfect ocular symmetry is assumed, each point of a corresponding pair has the same angular separation from the fovea, measured from the nodal point. Thus the angles denoted by θ in *Figure 8.20* would be equal. As a result, the longitudinal horopter would form part of the circle passing through the point of fixation and the eyes' nodal points – the Vieth–Müller circle. It is a well-known property of the circle that the angle subtended by a given arc at all points on the circumference is the same. The cyclopean eye shown in *Figure 8.20* is discussed in more detail in the next section.

Despite the term 'corresponding points', the correspondence is not a precise point-to-point relationship but rather of a point to an area, named after Panum. Near the fovea, Panum's areas are approximately elliptical with the major axis horizontal and subtending about 5 minutes of arc at the nodal point. In the periphery of the retina they are larger, perhaps subtending as much as 30–40 minutes.

Figure 8.21 shows a pair of corresponding points Q'_L and Q'_R (represented by crosses), and the retinal images of the fixation object (represented by the small circles). Provided that the left image falls on Q'_L and the right within the corresponding area around Q'_R as in (a) in the figure, or vice versa as in (b), a single percept will result. Diplopia will occur if the images fall at the extremities of both corresponding areas, as in (d), though possibly not if they are only partially displaced, as in (c), which illustrates a bilateral fixation disparity (*see* Chapter 10).

Panum's areas provide not only the element of tolerance or 'slack' essential in such an arrangement, but also some latitude in the position of the horopter. The two broken lines in *Figure 8.20* enclose an area known as Panum's fusional space, within which all object points are seen singly. The increasing width of the space from the fixation point outwards arises from the increasing size of the Panum's areas towards the periphery of the retina.

Points on the two retinae which are not corresponding are said to be disparate, for example, the points D'_L and D'_R. Though corresponding points are not necessarily equidistant from the fovea, the difference in the case of D'_L and D'_R is so great that they could not be other than disparate. Consequently, the object at D which stimulates them simultaneously will be seen in diplopia.

The horopter approximates to the subjective frontoparallel plane, found by asking the subject to place a series of vertical needles so that they appear to be equidistant from him. Their position in the horizontal plane is the longitudinal horopter. Slightly differing loci will probably be plotted, depending on the instructions given to the subject and the experimental technique employed.

The shape of the horopter generally alters with the fixation distance. If this is less than about 1 m, the horopter is concave towards the subject, while for an observation distance of about 2 m or more the apparent fronto-parallel plane tends to be convex towards the subject. These departures from the theoretical Vieth–Müller circle are taken to indicate asymmetry in the location of corresponding points, though the eyes' optical aberrations may be a contributory factor. The distance at which the longitudinal horopter is approximately a straight line is called the abathic distance.

The cyclopean eye and physiological diplopia

When studying the projection of images in binocular vision, it is often helpful to use an imaginary single eye stimulated by the right and left eyes. This imaginary organ is known as the cyclopean eye or binoculus. If the longitudinal horopter is assumed to coincide with the Vieth–Müller circle, the nodal point N_C of the cyclopean eye should be placed on this circle equidistant from the real eyes' nodal points, as in *Figure 8.20*. The cyclopean fovea M'_C lies on the line from the fixation point through the nodal point N_C. Thus, when the fixation point lines in the median plane, the primary line of the cyclopean eye also lies in this plane.

When a point on the left retina is stimulated, it is conceived as stimulating a point on the cyclopean retina at the same distance and in the same direction from its fovea. The same applies to a point on the right retina. If the right and left receptors under consideration are corresponding points, they coincide when transferred to the cyclopean eye, as in *Figure 8.20*. They are then said to give rise to a single percept by projection through the cyclopean nodal point. From the geometry of *Figure 8.20*, this line is seen to pass through the point Q which stimulated the given pair of corresponding points.

If the retinal points considered are disparate, they will not coincide when transferred to the cyclopean eye. Two separate percepts in different directions then arise, resulting in physiological diplopia. This is so called because the apparent doubling is the result of the geometry of vision with two eyes and is not pathological in origin or due to a malfunction. If, when one eye is closed, the diplopic image seen on the same (right or left) side disappears, the diplopia is called homonymous or uncrossed. If the opposite occurs, the diplopia is called heteronymous or crossed.

Though physiological diplopia is seldom noticed in everyday life, it is readily perceived when attention is drawn to it. For example, if a pencil is held vertically a short distance in front of the eyes while a more distant object is steadily fixated, the pencil will appear in crossed diplopia. When the pencil is fixated, the more distant object will be seen in uncrossed diplopia. Hence the rule: uncrossed diplopia occurs when the object is

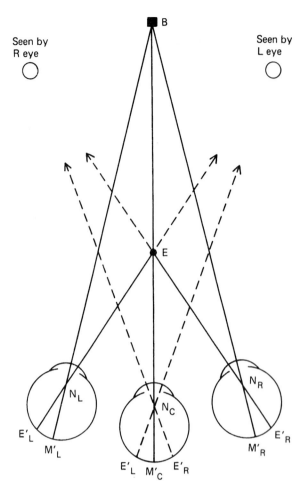

Figure 8.22. Crossed (heteronymous) physiological diplopia of the nearer point E when fixating the further point B. Projection with cyclopean eye.

farther than fixation, crossed diplopia when it is nearer than fixation.

The cyclopean eye is helpful in explaining this phenomenon. In *Figure 8.22*, the fixation object B lies in the median plane. A nearer object E in the same plane stimulates the retinal receptors E'_R and E'_L. These receptors must be disparate because they are on opposite sides of the respective foveae and hence, when transferred to the cyclopean eye, on opposite sides of its fovea, M'_C.

By monocular projection, the image of E is seen in the direction $N_L E$ by the left eye and in the direction $N_R E$ by the right eye, but the images cannot be fused into a single percept. In binocular vision, projection through the cyclopean nodal point shows that the retinal image of E in the left eye would be seen in the direction $E'_L N_C$ that is, to the right of the image due to the right eye, projected in the direction $E_R N_C$. So in this case the diplopia is crossed – true in general for objects nearer to the eyes than the plane of fixation.

The monocular and binocular projections could be reconciled by supposing the diplopic images to be subjectively located in the positions shown in *Figure 8.22*. This does *not* imply that the subject would perceive them in these locations. In general, the diplopic images are out of focus and insubstantial. Any impression of their distance from the eyes would be greatly influenced by prior knowledge of the actual positions of the objects in question, especially if the nearer one is held in the hand.

A diagram similar to *Figure 8.22* but with fixation transferred to the nearer object would show the more distant one to be seen in uncrossed diplopia.

The perfect symmetry assumed in *Figures 8.20* and *8.22* does not occur in nature. Under binocular viewing conditions, the origin of projection is seldom mid-way between the two eyes. Just as most people are definitely right- or left-handed, so one eye tends to be dominant over the other. If we wish to line up two objects accurately, we tend to close the less dominant eye (either physically or by mental suppression of that eye's image). An approximate judgement of alignment can be made binocularly, but the binocular projection centre will usually be found to lie nearer the dominant eye.

A crude way of finding the position of the cyclopean eye or the binocular projection or sighting centre is for the subject to view a pin placed in a horizontal drawing board in a plane at eye level at about half a metre from the eyes. A second pin held with both hands (to reduce the effect of hand-dominance) is pushed rapidly into the drawing board in line with the first pin, a procedure repeated several times. A line drawn backwards from the first pin through the mean position of the second pin indicates the projection axis of the cyclopean eye. Its position relative to the subject's head (which must be held rigidly in a rest) can thus be plotted. (For a more extensive treatment of this subject, *see* Francis and Harwood, 1951.)

Stereopsis

Stereopsis is the ability to perceive space as three-dimensional solely through slight differences between the right and left retinal images. It is the most highly refined attainment of binocular vision and is discussed more fully in Chapter 11.

References

ADLER, F.H. (1981) *Physiology of the Eye*, 7th edn. St. Louis: C. V. Mosby Co.

ALPERN, M. (1969) Part 1: Movements of the eyes. In *The Eye* (Davson, H., ed.), Vol. 3, 2nd edn. New York and London: Academic Press

ASHER, H. (1961). *The Seeing Eye*. London: Duckworth

DONDERS, F.C. (1864) *Accommodation and Refraction of the Eye*. London: The New Sydenham Society

DUKE-ELDER, W.S. (1958) *System of Ophthalmology*, Vol. 1, *The Eye in Evolution*, pp. 672–689. London: Henry Kimpton

FRANCIS, J.L. and HARWOOD, K.A. (1951) The variation of the projection centre with differential stimulus and its relation to ocular dominance. In *International Optical Congress 1951*, pp. 75–87. London: British Optical Association

FRY, G.A. and HILL, W.W. (1962) The center of rotation of the eye. *Am. J. Optom.*, **39**, 581–595

HELMHOLTZ, H. VON (1924) *Physiological Optics*, Vol . 3, pp. 37–154. English translation ed. by J.P.C. Southall. New York: Optical Society of America. Reprinted by Dover Publications: New York, 1962

MADDOX, E.E. (1898) *Tests and Studies of the Ocular Muscles*. Bristol: John Wright & Co.

PARK, R.S. and PARK, G.E. (1933) The centre of ocular rotation in the horizontal plane. *Am. J. Physiol.*, **104**, 545–552

QUEREAU, J.V.D. (1955) Rolling of the eye around its visual axis during normal ocular movements. *A.M.A. Archs Ophthal.*, **53**, 807–810

RYLAND, H.S. and LANG, B.T. (1913) An instrument for measuring the distance between the centres of rotation of the two eyes. *The Optician and Photographic Trade Journal*, **44**, 277–278

SOLOMONS, H. (1975) Derivation of the angle of torsion of the eye. *Br. J. Physiol. Optics*, **30**, 47–55

SOLOMONS, H. (1977) Kinematics of the extra-ocular muscles. *Ophthal. Optn*, **17**, 10–14, 46–48, 97–100, 146–156, 175–180

9

Convergence

Introduction

The term 'convergence' has two different meanings. One describes the relative position of the visual axes when they intersect at a given near point of regard, the other denotes the relative movement of the visual axes when fixation changes from a more distant point D to a nearer point N (*Figure 9.1a*). Divergence has the two corresponding opposite meanings. If fixation were to shift back from N to D or beyond, the visual axes would diverge but the final position would still be a state of convergence or parallelism. A state of divergence cannot occur with precise binocular fixation of a real object.

If the distant and near objects are both in the median plane, both eyes adduct equally in convergence and abduct in divergence. When fixating a near object placed to the right (*Figure 9.1b*), the right eye abducts and the left adducts. An interesting special case occurs when the fixation changes as shown in *Figure 9.1c*, the two object points D and N both lying on the right eye's visual axis. Only the left eye need move to change fixation from D to N but, in fact, both eyes make a small dextroversion coupled with convergence. This particular case is described by Alpern (1969) and Pickwell (1973).

Positions of rest and fixation

Position of anatomical rest

As we have already seen (page 144) the orbital axes include an angle of approximately 45°. In the absence of all innervation to the extra-ocular muscles, as in death, the eyes usually adopt a position of moderate divergence and elevation.

Position of physiological rest

This is the position assumed in the absence of all stimuli determining orientation and occurs as a result of a minimal and balanced tonus of the extra-ocular muscles, as in deep sleep or under general anaesthesia. It is again a divergent position, but less so than in the position of anatomical rest.

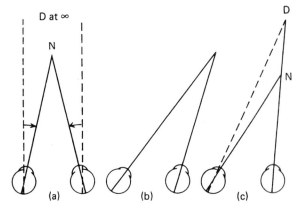

Figure 9.1. Convergence: (a) convergence from a distant object D to a near object N; (b) fixation of a point away from the median plane; (c) asymmetric convergence, the two points D and N being in line with the right eye.

When the eyes view a distant object, the visual axes are parallel, but they may not take this position in the absence of the visual stimuli.

Because the foveae in the normal individual are corresponding points, the fusion reflex directs the eyes so that the object of regard is imaged simultaneously on both foveae. If one eye is covered, it may tend to deviate from the correct position for fixation (*see* Chapter 10).

Although in clinical examination one eye maintains fixation of the test object while the second eye may deviate behind the cover or dissociating device, a theoretical position may be defined with both eyes deviating through approximately half the angle in opposite directions. Thus, the fusion-free position (passive or dissociated position) is the position adopted by the eyes when postural and fixation reflexes are active but fusion is prevented. In the particular case where the fixation object is in the distance, the fusion-free position is known as the position of functional rest.

The active or functional position of the eyes is their position when the fixation axes intersect at the point of regard and occurs when the eyes are parallel for a distant object and converged for a near object.

Figure 9.2 illustrates these various positions of the eyes, together with the angles through which the eyes move between them. Using the terms defined by Maddox (1886, 1907), the tonic convergence is that

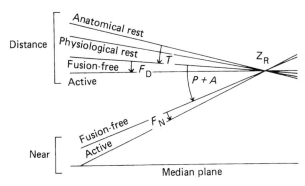

Figure 9.2. The various positions of rest and active positions of the right eye, shown looking towards the left. Z_R is the centre of rotation, T the tonic convergence, F_D the fusional convergence (distance), P the proximal convergence, A the accommodative convergence and F_N the fusional convergence (near).

bringing the eyes from the anatomical position of rest to the fusion-free position for distance.

Fusional convergence (or divergence) will bring the eyes from the fusion-free position to the active position. It is reflexly stimulated by the desire for single binocular vision. For a near object, the fusion-free position will almost certainly be converged relative to the distance fusion-free position. Two major factors contribute to this difference, proximal convergence and accommodative convergence.

Proximal convergence is that convergence induced by the knowledge that the object of regard is situated near the observer, even when viewed through a lens or optical instrument which places the image at infinity. Accommodative convergence is stimulated by the consensual linkage between accommodation and convergence (in general). Except in advanced presbyopia, accommodation and convergence are always exerted together in near vision, normal situations never demanding one without the other. The pupil also constricts when fixation is changed to a near object: the near reaction.

When proximal and accommodative convergence are in play, the eyes are in the fusion-free position in near vision. As in distance vision, fusional convergence will then be required to bring the eyes to their correct position for single binocular vision.

However, when the eyes are dissociated by being in total darkness, the fusion-free position governed by the tonic convergence is usually to an intermediate distance of about 110 cm (*see* the review in Hogan and Gilmartin, 1985, and Owens and Leibowitz, 1983). This is similar to, but not identical in value with, the tonic accommodation found in dark-field myopia (Chapter 7).

The near point of convergence

Each eye individually may be able to adduct through $40°$, but the maximum effort of convergence may correspond to an angle of much less than $80°$. This may partly be explained by different supra-nuclear innervation in the brain, even though the final nerve supply to the medial and lateral recti is by the same nerves

(cranial III and VI) for both version and vergence movements.

The closest point in the median plane to which the eyes can converge is the near point of convergence. It may be determined clinically by asking the patient to observe, for example, a vertical black line drawn on a white card. The card is then moved towards the patient's eyes and he is asked to report when the line goes double. The position of the card is then taken to mark the near point of convergence.

Disadvantages of this method are that some patients do not observe the diplopia of the test object when convergence becomes inaccurate, while others continue to converge even though single binocular vision is no longer present. It is probably better to observe the patient's eyes as the test line approaches. At a certain distance of the test line the patient's eyes will often be seen to stop adducting: they remain stationary instead of continuing to converge. Other patients continue fixating the test line with one eye – usually their preferred or dominant eye – while the second eye abducts. Sometimes this abduction is equal in amount to the continuing adduction of the fixating eye, while in other cases the visual axes become nearly parallel with the second eye turned obviously outwards.

The position of the near point of convergence varies from as close as 20 mm from the bridge of the nose to more than 500 mm. Normal values would perhaps range between 40 and 160 mm from the corneal plane. Values much greater, that is, poorer than 160 mm, may well give symptoms in near vision. Orthoptic exercises to improve the reserves of convergence and/or prismatic relief may be needed to reduce these symptoms, although patients with poor convergence often hold near work at a greater distance than normal patients.

Unlike the decline in accommodative power with age (as discussed on pages 117–119) there is no systematic decrease in amplitude of convergence with increasing age. Convergence is unlikely to be as good in age as in youth, due possibly to lack of use (since the presbyopic patient can never see very close objects clearly) and to loss of accommodative convergence. Some patients manage to maintain good powers of convergence into advanced age while others do not.

Convergence is essentially a reflex adjustment to give single binocular near vision, but it may also be produced voluntarily. With practice many people can converge (and accommodate) in the absence of a physical stimulus as if they were really viewing a near object.

Units of convergence

An ocular rotation about the eye's anteroposterior axis (torsion) is usually measured in degrees. Version movements may also be measured in prism dioptres Δ, a unit of angle explained on page 10. For convergence alone, yet another angular measure is sometimes used, the metre angle MA, devised by Nagel in 1880 before the prism dioptre had been introduced.

In *Figure 9.3* the unaided eyes have rotated to obtain binocular fixation of point B in the median plane. The

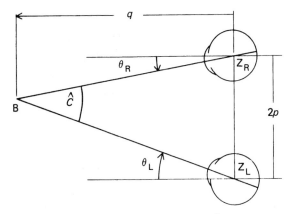

Figure 9.3.   The total angle of convergence $\hat{C}$.

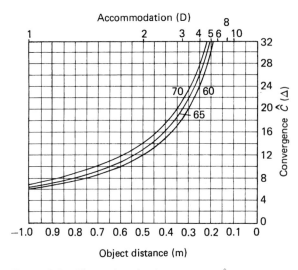

Figure 9.4.   The total angle of convergence $\hat{C}$ in prism dioptres, as a function of object distance for PDs of 60, 65 and 70 mm.

convergence of each eye is the angle through which it has rotated from its primary direction. The line joining the two rotation centres Z_L and Z_R may be called the inter-ocular base line and its length the inter-ocular distance which is approximately the same as the inter-pupillary distance PD for distance vision.

The total angle of convergence, denoted by $\hat{C}$, is the angle between the visual axes when directed towards the fixation point. It is the algebraic sum of the separate rotations θ_R and θ_L of the right and left eyes, measured in the plane containing the fixation point and the eyes' rotation centres. If $2p$ is the inter-ocular distance, q the distance of the fixation point from the base line and $Q = 1/q$ (q in metres), then to a sufficiently close approximation

$$\hat{C} = \arctan(-2p/q) \ (p, q \text{ in m})$$

$$= \arctan(-2pQ)$$

So that

$$\hat{C} \text{ (in } \Delta) = -2pQ \ (p \text{ in cm})$$

$$= -Q \times \text{PD (in cm)} \tag{9.1}$$

For example, given that $q = -250$ mm and the PD is 60 mm, $\hat{C} = 4 \times 6 = 24\Delta$.

Irrespective of the subject's PD, convergence in metre angles is simply the absolute value of the dioptric distance Q. That is, since q is negative

$$\hat{C} \text{ (in MA)} = -Q \tag{9.2}$$

and

$$\hat{C} \text{ (in } \Delta) = C \text{ (in MA)} \times \text{PD (in cm)} \tag{9.2a}$$

Convergence, accommodation and refractive error

When studying accommodation in relation to convergence, it is convenient to use the inter-ocular base line as the origin of measurement instead of the eye's principal point. The theoretical demand on accommodation in the case of emmetropia is then $-Q$. Thus, binocular fixation at a dioptric distance of -3 D would require 3 D of accommodation and 3 MA of convergence.

To simplify the treatment in the ensuing discussion, convergence will be expressed in prism dioptres. For simplicity, the fixation point will be taken as lying in the median plane and it will be assumed that the given conditions apply equally to both eyes. The total convergence $\hat{C}$ will hence be twice the inward rotation θ of the single eye considered. Marked anisometropia is not common and the expressions obtained will be sufficiently accurate for the purpose of providing a broad picture and making comparisons.

The relationship between convergence and accommodation is affected by any uncorrected ametropia and also by any correction in use. To establish a norm we shall begin with emmetropia.

Emmetropia

Figure 9.4 illustrates the theoretical demand on accommodation and convergence as the object of regard approaches the emmetropic eye. The required total convergence $\hat{C}$ is plotted in prism dioptres for three different inter-pupillary distances. A separate scale at the top of the graph, to be read directly against the object distance, gives the necessary accommodation which is numerically the same as the convergence in metre angles.

Equation (9.1) shows the total convergence required to be $-2pQ$ (p in cm), while the accommodation is $-Q$. Hence, the ratio of convergence to accommodation in emmetropia is given by

$$\hat{C}/A = 2p = \text{PD (in cm)} \tag{9.3}$$

Uncorrected ametropia

If the distance error of refraction is K, the accommodation required in near vision at a dioptric distance Q is $(K - Q)$, while the convergence is unchanged at $-2pQ$.

Hence,

$$\hat{C}/A = 2p\left(\frac{Q}{Q-K}\right) \tag{9.4}$$

This ratio has a wide range of possible values. For example, the hypermetrope will need to accommodate more than an emmetrope while converging by the same amount. If, however, the accommodation habitually needed to correct the distance refractive error is disregarded and only the additional accommodation required in near vision is considered, the $\hat{C}/A$ ratio is the same as for the emmetrope. In myopia the situation is different: a -3.00 D myope is in focus for objects at $\frac{1}{3}$ m and would not accommodate for this or any longer distance.

Emmetrope with near spectacle correction

If the spectacle lenses are optically centred for the given working distance, the convergence required is unaffected. On the other hand, the accommodative demand is reduced by the prescribed reading addition.

Spectacle-corrected ametropia

We shall assume that the spectacles are for constant wear and the lenses are optically centred for distance vision. In near vision, the ocular accommodation required has already been found to differ from the spectacle accommodation, while the convergence is affected by the prismatic effect of the lenses. The following example is typical.

Example (1)

A bilateral myope with a PD of 66 mm is corrected by lenses (assumed thin) of power -6.00 D at 14 mm from the eye's principal point. Calculate the convergence and accommodation required when viewing an object in the median plane at a distance of 400 mm from the spectacle plane. Assume the eye's centres of rotation to be 26 mm from this plane.

Using *Figure 9.5(a)*, in distance vision

	D			mm
F_{sp}	-6.00	$\rightarrow$	f'_{sp}	-166.67
			$-d$	-14
K	-5.53	$\leftarrow$	k	-180.67

In near vision

	D			mm
L_s	-2.50			
$+F_{sp}$	-6.00			
L'_s	-8.50	$\rightarrow$	ℓ_s	-117.65
			$-d$	-14
L	-7.60	$\leftarrow$	ℓ	-131.65

Occular acc $= A = K - L = +2.07$ D

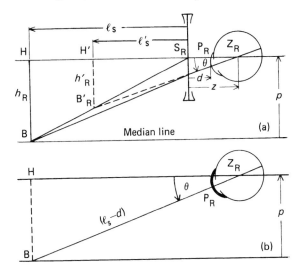

Figure 9.5. Accommodation and convergence in the myope corrected by: (a) a thin spectacle lens, (b) a contact lens.

The right eye fixates B'_R, the image of B formed by the right lens. If the distances HB and $H'B'_R$ are denoted by $h_R(=p)$ and h'_R respectively, then

$$h'_R = h_R L_s/L'_s = (33 \times -2.50)/-8.50 = 9.71 \text{ mm}$$

and the semi-convergence angle θ (in Δ) is found from

$$\theta = 100\, h'_R/H'Z_R = \frac{100\, h'_R}{H'S_R + S_R Z_R}$$

$$= \frac{100\,(9.71)}{117.65 + 26} = 6.76\, \Delta$$

so that

$$\hat{C} = 13.52\, \Delta$$

and

$$\hat{C}/A = 13.52/2.07 = 6.53$$

Contact-lens corrected ametropia

Example (2)

Retaining all the relevant data from Example (1), calculate the convergence and accommodation that would be required with a contact-lens correction in use.

Ignoring very small differences, we can take the distance of the fixation object B from the contact lens (*Figure 9.5b*) as -414 mm, the same as $P_R H$ in *Figure 9.5(a)*. The ocular accommodation is therefore $1000/414$ or 2.42 D. The convergence (in Δ) is the same as that for the emmetropic eye (equation 9.1), that is

$$\hat{C} = -2pQ \; (p \text{ in cm})$$

In this case

$$q = Z_R H = (\ell_s - z) = -426 \text{ mm}$$

so that

$$Q = -2.35 \text{ D}$$

and

$$\hat{C} = -2.35 \times 6.6 = 15.51\,\Delta$$

which gives

$$\hat{C}/A = 15.51/2.42 = 6.41$$

Thus, although the myopic contact-lens wearer in this example has to converge more and accommodate more than the spectacle wearer, the ratio of the two functions is virtually the same for both.

Summary

The generality of this last result can be demonstrated by an analysis based on binomial approximations. For the spectacle-lens wearer, this gives the ocular accommodation A as approximately

$$A = -L_s\{1 + dL_s + 2dF_{sp}\} \tag{7.15}$$

while the convergence $\hat{C}$ can be shown to be

$$\hat{C} = -2pL_s\{1 + z(L_s + F_{sp})\} \tag{9.5}$$

from which

$$\hat{C}/A = 2p\{1 + (z - d)L_s + (z - 2d)F_{sp}\} \tag{9.6}$$

For the contact-lens wearer,

$$A = -L_s(1 + dL_s) \tag{9.7}$$

and

$$\hat{C} = -2pL_s(1 + zL_s) \tag{9.8}$$

from which

$$\hat{C}/A = 2p\{1 + (z - d)L_s\} \tag{9.9}$$

Typical values of z range from 25 to 30 mm, while typical values of d range from 12 to 15 mm. Consequently, the value of $(z - 2d)$ in equation (9.6) will in general be very small. If it is ignored as relatively negligible, equations (9.6) and (9.9) become identical. Moreover, the ratio $\hat{C}/A$ now becomes independent of the power of the correcting lens.

In general, therefore, the biggest change in the convergence/accommodation ratio occurs when a first correction is worn. After this, changes in the correction make virtually no difference until the accommodation becomes depleted with the onset of presbyopia.

Accommodative convergence and the AC/A ratio

When a near object is fixated, both convergence and accommodation are normally brought into action by the non-presbyopic subject. The convergence has to be accurate to within a few minutes of arc to avoid diplopia, but the accommodation may not be exact; the eye's depth of focus still gives the observer a sharp percept.

The total angle of convergence required by the unaided eyes is the angle subtended by the inter-ocular separation $2p$ at the fixation point. For example, if $2p = 70$ mm and the fixation object is at 350 mm from the inter-ocular base line, the total convergence needed

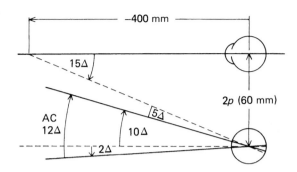

Figure 9.6.   Accommodative convergence AC from the distant to the near dissociated (fusion-free) position.

is 7000/350 or 20Δ. If the object lies on the primary line of the right eye, this total convergence would need to be made by the left eye. Suppose that, in such a situation, the left eye is now covered. Because of the habitual simultaneous use of accommodation and convergence, some convergence will remain in play, perhaps 14Δ.

If, in this same situation, the stimulus to accommodation were increased by placing a carefully centred minus lens before the right eye, the convergence of the left eye (still under cover) would probably increase, say to 18Δ. On removal of the cover, the convergence would then be increased by the amount needed to regain binocular fixation. As explained on pages 158–159, this faculty of adjustment to give accurate binocular fixation is called fusional convergence.

Convergence produced as described above by stimulating the accommodation when the eyes are dissociated was called accommodative convergence by Maddox. In clinical practice it can be utilized to modify a patient's refractive correction to provide more comfortable binocular vision. Thus, some patients tend to over-converge in near vision. If reading spectacles incorporating a plus spherical addition are prescribed, the demand on accommodation is reduced. As a result, the over-convergence may then be reduced. Conversely, a reduction in positive power may be made in order to stimulate convergence, provided that the patient has sufficient reserves of accommodation.

The ratio of accommodative convergence to accommodation, the AC/A ratio, can be used to decide how much to alter the prescription. Two clinical methods of measuring it are described below.

Direct measurement

Suppose that, in distance vision, one eye is temporarily covered and abducts through 2Δ, while in near vision with an object at -400 mm (from the inter-ocular base line) the covered eye under-converges by 5Δ. Given that the subject's PD is 60 mm, the total convergence required for binocular fixation is 6000/400 or 15Δ. As shown in *Figure 9.6*, the angle between the visual axes when the eyes are dissociated is 10Δ, being the stated 5Δ less than the amount required for binocular fixation. However, since there was 2Δ divergence from parallelism when the accommodation was relaxed, the total amount of accommodative convergence is 12Δ. If the small distance from the eye's principal point to the centre of rotation is ignored, the accommodation required in this case is 2.50 D. Hence

$$AC/A = 12/2.50 = 4.8$$

This method enables the ratio to be determined from data that are normally obtained in routine examination of the oculo-motor balance. It should be noted that the accommodative convergence measured in this way includes an element of proximal convergence.

Gradient tests

This method determines the AC/A ratio for a constant object distance: the vergence of light reaching the eyes is altered by means of lenses but since the fixation is stationary, proximal convergence should remain unaltered. The gradient test is particularly suited to clinical uses where the prescription is to be altered for a specific object distance.

With the eyes dissociated by some means, the relative position of the visual axes in near vision is determined with the normal prescription in place. A further +1.00 DS lens is placed before each eye, reducing the stimulus to accommodation by 1.00 D. If the eyes diverge through 4Δ, the AC/A ratio is 4Δ/D. In the young patient, −1.00 DS lenses could also be used, the eyes now being expected to converge.

The gradient test may also be used in distant vision, but only negative lenses can be used since positive lenses would blur the fixation object. At either distance, the fixation object should be sufficiently detailed to stimulate accommodation. Typical results (Morgan, 1944) show a mean gradient of 4.0 ± 2.0.

Both these methods assume that the eyes accommodate exactly for the test object, but accommodation is usually under-active: the near bichromatic test shows that the green focus is more often closer to the retina than the red. Inattention will also probably produce a lower than normal accommodation level.

By measuring the accommodation level objectively, an AC/A response instead of an AC/A stimulus measurement is obtained. Using laser speckle refraction (*see* Chapter 19), Ramsdale and Charman (1988) confirmed the earlier results of Fincham and Walton (1957). The latter's results for a typical subject are shown in *Figure 9.7*. A Fincham Co-incidence Optometer was used, described in previous editions of this book.

The central line shows the subject's accommodation when the stimuli to convergence in dioptres and accommodation in metre angles were equal, as when viewing a real object. The accommodation is seen to lag slightly below the theoretical demand for objects closer than $-\frac{1}{3}$ m.

The left-hand curve shows the accommodative convergence, accommodation only being stimulated. As expected, the convergence produced is noticeably less than that occurring in normal vision, although it should also be noted that the measured accommodation rarely equalled the actual stimulus. Fincham and Walton point out that apparent fluctuations in the AC/A ratio measured using the stimulus value instead

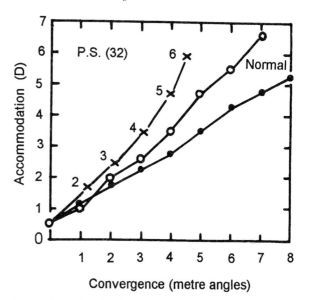

Figure 9.7.   Relationship between accommodation and convergence. The open circles show the accommodative response with equal stimuli to accommodation and convergence; the crosses the response of both accommodation and convergence, accommodation only being stimulated by the dioptric values indicated and the closed circles show convergence-induced accommodation. (Reproduced from Fincham and Walton, 1957, by kind permission of the publishers of *J. Physiol.*)

of the response value for accommodation may be due merely to inaccurate accommodation.

There is a voluminous literature on the subject of AC/A ratios. Among others, Alpern (1960) discusses many theoretical points, while Flom (1959) surveys many of the clinical aspects. A more recent review is given in the paper by Ramsdale and Charman (1988). It has been found that the type of refractive error may also influence the accommodative convergence. Rosenfield and Gilmartin (1987) investigated this possible link in emmetropes and two groups of myopes, those who became myopic before the age of 15 years and those who became myopic later. The early-onset myopes showed higher accommodative convergence than the later-onset myopes and the emmetropes.

Convergence-induced accommodation

Just as an alteration in the accommodative demand upon the eyes produces a change in their convergence, so a change in convergence may induce alterations in the level of accommodation. This alteration is known as convergence-induced accommodation, or sometimes convergence accommodation.

In order that the accommodation may take whatever value is induced by the convergence, the mechanisms which normally control the accommodation must be eliminated. Pinhole-sized artificial pupils of about 0.5 mm diameter are used, reducing the blur-circle diameter on the retina even when the image is several dioptres out of focus. As a result, the eye makes a negligible effort to bring the test object into focus. Two similar test objects are used, one for each eye, in an

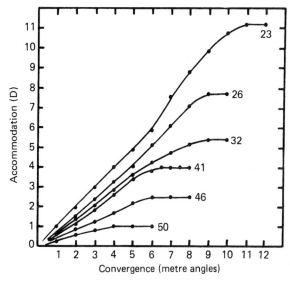

Figure 9.8. Convergence-induced accommodation: effect of age. (Reproduced from Fincham, 1958, by kind permission of the publishers of *Optician*.)

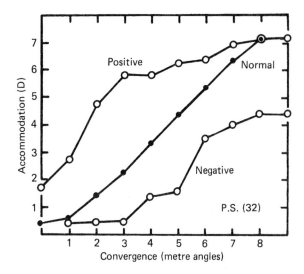

Figure 9.9. Positive and negative amplitudes of relative accommodation. (Reproduced in part from Fincham and Walton, 1957, by kind permission of the publishers of *J. Physiol.*)

instrument similar to a synoptophore (*see* page 203). Their relative positions control the convergence of the eyes. The dioptric state of the eye is measured, preferably with an objective optometer (*see* Chapter 18) or with a subjective optometer which can be viewed for only a fraction of a second at a time, again in order to prevent alterations in the level of accommodation.

Because of the difficulties in eliminating the dioptric clues to accommodation, convergence-induced accommodation cannot be studied accurately under clinical conditions. Dynamic retinoscopy (*see* Chapter 17), with a coarsely detailed fixation object such as a luminous pen torch bulb to reduce the need for exact focusing of the eyes, could perhaps be used.

Fincham and Walton (1957) measured the convergence-induced accommodation with an objective optometer. *Figure 9.7* shows their results for the same subject whose accommodative convergence was measured. The right-hand curve shows that less accommodation is produced when only convergence provides the stimulus than when dioptric clues are also available – the normal curve. A similar effect occurred when measuring accommodative convergence: the convergence produced was less than normal for the accommodation.

Figure 9.8 shows Fincham's (1958) results for several subjects of differing ages. The younger subjects have more accommodation induced by the same amount of convergence than the older subjects. This is to be expected, since the amplitude of accommodation declines with increased age.

Similar results have been found by Kent (1958) and Balsam and Fry (1959), among others.

Relative accommodation and convergence – accommodative facility

Approximately equal amounts of accommodation and convergence (in D and MA respectively) are used by the non-presbyopic emmetrope (or corrected ametrope) in viewing a near object. It is possible, however, to alter the stimulus to accommodation by placing additional positive or negative lenses before the eyes, the convergence remaining constant. The change in accommodation while maintaining clear single vision is called relative accommodation.

The results obtained by Fincham and Walton (1957) are shown in *Figure 9.9*. The central line labelled normal shows the objectively determined level of accommodation under normal conditions. The change in ordinate to reach the upper or lower curves at any particular convergence value gives the subjective relative amplitude or accommodation for the particular convergence value. It was found that accommodation continued to change slightly when the light vergence was altered beyond the subjective limit. This limit is reached when the subject reports that the test object begins to blur.

Figure 9.9 shows that the accommodation is most flexible between 3 and 5 MA of convergence. At high and low values of convergence, the relative amplitude is very much smaller. These amplitudes are useful when a patient's refractive correction is altered. An increasing myope will suddenly have to accommodate more than before when the spectacles are brought up to date, while the early presbyope will accommodate less. It is surprising, however, how little the oculomotor balance of low myopes (up to about 2.00 D) is altered by intermittent wear of the correction for close work. The AC/A ratio does not seem very significant with these patients.

Under clinical conditions, the relative amplitude of accommodation may be determined as follows. The patient observes a test object at the required distance, usually the N5 or J3 reading test types at his near working distance, with his distance correction in place. Plus spheres are then added binocularly until the patient reports that the test types have blurred. These extra lenses are

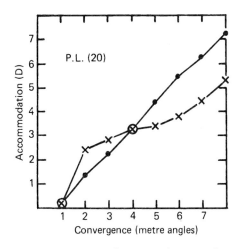

Figure 9.10. Accommodation as a function of convergence. The closed circles show convergence-induced accommodation through 0.5 mm artificial pupils, the crosses the inhibition of convergence-induced accommodation by a constant light vergence of −3.00 D through 3 mm artificial pupils. (Reproduced from Fincham and Walton, 1957, by kind permission of the publishers of *J. Physiol.*)

then removed and the process repeated with negative lenses, thus finding the maximum amount by which the accommodation may be relaxed and increased for fixed convergence and clarity of the test types. These results will, of course, include the depth of focus of the eye. In distance vision, only negative lenses may be added since positive lenses cause an immediate blur.

Although it is not a measure of relative accommodation, a clinical test that is also of use is to assess the flexibility of the linkage between accommodation and convergence. The patient observes N5 type and reports when it becomes clear when viewed binocularly through alternate positive and negative lenses of equal power, say 1.00 or 1.50 DS. Specially glazed 'flippers' are available for this. Some patients will take an appreciable time to refocus, whilst others will adjust very rapidly. This accommodation-rock technique, sometimes termed the accommodative facility, may be used as an orthoptic exercise to loosen the accommodation–convergence relationship.

The relative power of adjusting convergence of the eyes (in artificial situations) at a fixed level of accommodation is more properly discussed under the title of fusional reserves (*see* Chapter 10) and in texts on orthoptics. The subject views a finely detailed object through normal-sized pupils while the stimulus to convergence alone is altered. The limits of convergence and divergence of the eyes while the test object remains clear may then be found. The results of Fincham and Walton (1957), who measured objectively the actual accommodation in use, are shown in *Figure 9.10*. When the stimuli for convergence and accommodation were fairly similar, accommodation varied only slightly with changes in convergence. Convergence-induced accommodation changes were inhibited by the fixed light vergence, giving the nearly horizontal part of the curve. Once the difference between the actual accommodation and its dioptric stimulus was greater than about 1 D, the retinal blur was too great to allow the normal

control of accommodation to overcome the convergence-induced accommodation. The accommodative changes at both ends of the graph were accordingly much more rapid. This contrasts with the much more uniform slope of the convergence-induced accommodation graph where the accommodation is allowed to float freely with changes in the convergence stimulus.

Control of accommodation and convergence

On observing a near object, both accommodation and convergence are stimulated. The response of either can be considered as resulting from three factors. Thus, accommodation may be controlled jointly by a fast reflex reaction to the blur caused by the dioptric vergence stimulus, and secondly by a slower or tonic component possibly dependent on the amplitude of the reflex action and the stimulus from convergence. A similar hypothesis has been suggested for convergence. Various models of stimulus-response and cross-over networks between accommodation and convergence have been proposed by, among others, Schor and Cuiffreda (1983), Schor (1985), Rosenfield and Gilmartin (1987), Cuiffreda (1991), Hung (1992) and Schor *et al.* (1992). Arguments for and against a bioengineering approach to oculo-motor control, though not specifically dealing with convergence, have been discussed by Robinson (1986) and Steinman (1986).

A simplified and slightly modified version of Hung's (1992) and Hung *et al.*'s (1996) accommodation–convergence model is given in *Figure 9.11*. Taking the upper pathway for accommodation, the stimulus will be dependent on the difference between the dioptric vergence incident on the eye and the accommodation response. If this difference is less than the eye's depth of focus, the level of accommodation remains unaltered. Any greater difference (towards either an increase or a decrease) will cause the accommodation controller to change its response. The controller is assumed to have two systems, an immediate or transient response component and a sustained element. Thus, on receiving a demand for increased accommodation, the transient system stimulates the ciliary muscle. The output from the accommodation controller is fed back to the sustained element so that, providing the requirement remains constant, the output is increasingly produced by the sustained system and less by the transient.

Moreover, the longer the duration of the stimulus, the more the feedback increases the time constant of the sustained controller so that when the accommodative demand finally changes, the accommodation response continues for a short period of time which is somewhat proportional to the stimulus duration. Further inputs to the accommodation system are given by proximal factors (*see* Instrument myopia, page 135), tonic accommodation and the convergence-induced accommodation cross-linking from the convergence system.

A similar system operates for the vergence pathway. When measuring a heterophoria, the vergence pathway is effectively cut at the Panum's area box in the dia-

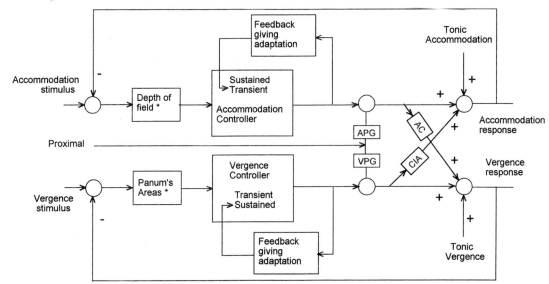

Figure 9.11. Bio-engineering model of the accommodation–convergence systems, simplified and modified from Hung *et al.* (1996). Key: * pathways open-looped here, i.e. cut, by a pinhole or occlusion respectively; AC, accommodative convergence; CIA, convergence-induced accommodation; APG and VPG, accommodation and vergence proximal controllers.

gram. Similarly, if accommodation is 'open-looped' by a small pinhole aperture, it is the depth of field box that acts as an opened switch.

Exercises

9.1 The eye of a patient with a PD of 65 mm adducts through 1Δ under cover in distance vision, while when fixating at $-\frac{1}{3}$ m, the eye adducts through 2Δ. Calculate the AC/A ratio.

9.2 (a) A patient shows 10Δ of divergence under cover (exophoria) in near vision. If the AC/A ratio is 4Δ/D, what change in lens strength would be expected to reduce the divergence to 4Δ? (b) Would the same change in lens help if the patient were also 10Δ exophoric in distance vision?

9.3 (a) A patient wearing his distance correction shows 6Δ of over-convergence under cover (esophoria) in near vision. If the AC/A ratio is 3Δ/D, what change in lens strength would be expected to reduce the convergence to 3Δ? (b) If the patient were also esophoric in distance vision, would the same change in lens strength help?

9.4 A 2 D uncorrected myope shows 6Δ of divergence under cover in near vision. What might the findings be when the correction is worn?

Note: the present writer (RBR) finds this approach too mechanistic. Because of proximal effects and the reliance on the dioptric values of accommodation stimuli not response (as used in Fincham and Walton's experiments), the AC/A ratio measure with the gradient test is frequently much less than the ratio found from calculations similar to those in question 1. Results around 2Δ/D may be more typical. Low myopes frequently show little change in eye co-ordination with or without the prescription in near vision. The technique of fixation disparity described in Chapter 10 may give more definite information for prescribing.

References

ALPERN, M. (1969) Part 1: Movements of the eyes. In *The Eye*, 2nd edn, Vol. 3 (Davson, H., ed.). New York and London: Academic Press

BALSAM, M.H. and FRY, C.A. (1959) Convergence accommodation. *Am. J. Optom.*, **36**, 567–575

CIUFFREDA, K.J. (1991) Accommodation and its anomalies. In *Visual Optics and Instrumentation*, Vol. 1 (Charman, W.N., ed.). In *Vision and Visual Dysfunction* (Cronly-Dillon, J.R., ed.). London: Macmillan

FINCHAM, E.F. (1958) The adjustment of the eyes for near vision. *Optician*, **136**, 471–480

FINCHAM, E.F. and WALTON, J. (1957) The reciprocal actions of accommodation and convergence. *J. Physiol., Lond.*, **137**, 488–508

FLOM, M.C. (1960) On the relationship between accommodation and accommodative convergence. *Am. J. Optom.*, **37**, 474–482, 517–523, 619–632

HOGAN, R.E. and GILMARTIN, B. (1985) The relationship between tonic vergence and oculomotor stress induced by alcohol. *Ophthal. Physiol. Opt.*, **5**, 43–52

HUNG, G.K. (1992) Adaptation model of accommodation and vergence. *Ophthal. Physiol. Opt.*, **12**, 319–326

HUNG, G.K., CIUFFREDA, K.J. and ROSENFIELD, M. (1996) Proximal contribution to a linear static model of accommodation and convergence. *Ophthal. Physiol. Opt.*, **16**, 31–41

KENT, P.R. (1958) Convergence accommodation. *Am. J. Optom.*, **35**, 393–406

MADDOX, E.E. (1886) Investigations on the relation between convergence and accommodation of the eyes. *J. Anat. Physiol., Lond.*, **20**, 565–584

MADDOX, E.E. (1907) *The Clinical Use of Prisms and the Decentring of Lenses*, 5th edn, pp. 158–177. Bristol: John Wright & Co.

MORGAN, N.W. JR. (1944) The clinical aspects of accommodation and convergence. *Am. J. Optom.*, **21**, 301–313

OWENS, D. and LEIBOWITZ, H. (1983) Perceptual and motor consequences of tonic convergence. In *Vergence Eye Movements: Basic and Clinical Aspects* (Schor, C.M. and Ciuffreda, K., eds), Ch. 3. London: Butterworths

PICKWELL, L.D. (1973) Eye movements during the cover test. *Br. J. Physiol. Optics*, **28**, 23–25

RAMSDALE, C. and CHARMAN, W.N. (1988) Accommodation and convergence: effects of lenses and prisms in 'closed-loop' conditions. *Ophthal. Physiol. Opt.*, **8**, 43–52

ROBINSON, D.A. (1986) The systems approach to the oculomotor system. *Vision Res.*, **26**, 91–99

ROSENFIELD, M. and GILMARTIN, B. (1987) Effect of a near-vision task on the response AC/A of a myopic population. *Ophthal. Physiol. Opt.*, **7**, 225–234

SCHOR, C.M., (1985) Models of mutual interactions between accommodation and convergence. *Am. J. Optom.*, **62**, 369–374

SCHOR, C.M., ALEXANDER, J., CORMACK, L. and STEVENSON, S. (1992) Negative feedback model of proximal convergence and accommodation. *Ophthal. Physiol. Opt.*, **12**, 307–318

SCHOR, C.M. and CIUFFREDA, K.J. (1983) *Vergence Eye Movements: Basic and Clinical Aspects*. London: Butterworths

STEINMAN, R.M. (1986) The need for an eclectic, rather than systems, approach to the study of the primate oculomotor system. *Vision Res.*, **26**, 101–112

10

Anomalies of binocular vision: heterophoria and heterotropia

Introduction

Binocular vision in its fullest sense can be achieved only with a well-developed and co-ordinated oculo-motor and neural system and with the optical functioning of each eye in reasonable adjustment. If one eye is markedly out of focus through uncorrected anisometropia, binocular vision must be impaired. Even when such an eye is corrected, difficulties may arise from unequal image sizes in the two eyes or different prismatic effects when viewing through peripheral parts of the correcting lenses (*see* Chapter 14). In this chapter we shall be looking at the various deviations from a perfectly co-ordinated oculo-motor system.

Heterophoria and heterotropia

As we saw in Chapter 8, single binocular vision requires the retinal images to fall on corresponding points in the two eyes. In general, the fine adjustments needed to maintain accurate bifoveal fixation are made by corrective reflex movements of the eyes, the stimulus being the avoidance of diplopia.

If, while fixating any stationary point, one of the patient's eyes is covered, the covered eye will probably turn so that its visual axis no longer passes through the fixation point (*Figure 10.1*) (in general, the effect of the cover is to dissociate the eyes, *see* pages 169–172). When the cover is removed, bifoveal fixation is rapidly regained. The anomaly thus revealed is known as heterophoria. If the visual axis of the covered eye remains exactly in line with the object viewed by the unoccluded eye, the condition is called orthophoria. Binocular vision is then maintained without the need for reflex fusional movements of the eyes. In clinical practice, the term orthophoria is extended to include all cases where the deviation under cover is insignificant, for example, less than 1Δ horizontally and 0.25Δ vertically. Nevertheless, a patient showing heterophoria of this amount will still need to use fusional movements to maintain binocular fixation. Moreover, though clinically orthophoric in distance vision, a patient may well be heterophoric in near vision.

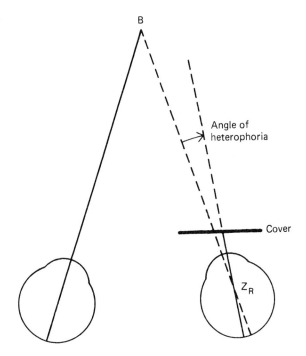

Figure 10.1. Exophoria showing divergence or abduction behind the cover.

Some patients do not achieve bifoveal fixation of any object, one eye showing a manifest deviation without being covered. Such patients are said to possess a squint,* strabismus or heterotropia. If the strabismic eye is covered while the patient looks at a fixed test object, neither the covered nor the uncovered eye will move. On the other hand, if the originally fixating eye is covered (*Figure 10.2*), the strabismic eye will turn through the angle of squint so that the image of the test object falls on the fovea (subject to various other factors to be discussed later in this chapter). At the same time the originally fixating eye, now under cover, makes a similar version movement.

---

* The term 'squint' is often incorrectly used by lay people to mean squeezing the eyelids together in order to reduce the retinal blurring in uncorrected ametropia.

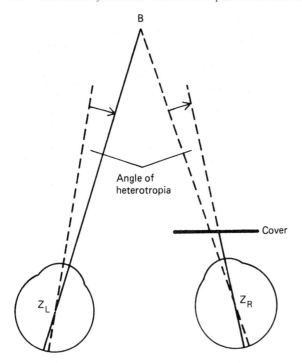

Figure 10.2. Left exotropia, showing adduction of the deviating left eye to take up fixation and corresponding abduction of the right eye behind the cover.

Table 10.1   Classification of heterophoria

Type	Movement of eye under cover	Common abbreviations
Esophoria	Adduction	SOP. Eso*
Exophoria	Abduction	XOP, Exo*
Hyperphoria	Elevation	See text
Hypophoria	Depression	See text

* The abbreviations Eso and Exo, together with Hyper, are understood to refer to phorias and not to tropias unless specifically stated.

Table 10.2   Classification of heterophoria

Type	Relative position of deviating eye	Common abbreviations
Esotropia	Adducted	SOT, EsoT
Exotropia	Abducted	XOT, ExoT
Hypertropia	Elevated	HyperT, see text
Hypotropia	Depressed	HypoT, see text

The above-described conditions can be briefly distinguished as follows:

(1) *Heterophoria.* When either eye of a heterophoric patient is dissociated, the eye deviates so that its visual axis no longer passes through the object of regard. Bifoveal fixation is restored on removal of the dissociative device. An orthophoric patient has a negligible deviation under cover or when dissociated.

(2) *Heterotropia.* The visual axes do not intersect at the object of regard, but the axis of the normally fixing eye does pass through the object of regard.

It is possible, indeed probable, that the angle of heterophoria varies with the distance of observation. The angle of heterotropia may also depend on the distance of fixation. Some patients may show a heterotropia for objects at one distance, yet only a phoria* at a different distance. The term 'latent strabismus' to describe a phoria is to be deprecated since it is relatively rare for a heterophoria to break down into a heterotropia after the age of about 6 years. The term oculo-motor (im)balance covers both heterophoria and heterotrophia.

Classification of heterophoria and heterotropia

The angle of heterophoria and heterotropia should be measured both in distance vision and at the patient's

habitual near working distance. This is not necessarily $\frac{1}{3}$ m, although unfortunately many of the instruments for measuring near heterophoria are designed for this distance.

Table 10.1 shows the classification of heterophoria with the terminology introduced by Stevens in 1886 (Stevens, 1906).

Consider a patient with hyperphoria of the right eye when covered. This means that the right eye tends to turn above the direction of regard of the left eye. If the left eye were covered instead, then the left eye would tend to turn below the right giving a left hypophoria. A right hyperphoria is the same as a left hypophoria.

Thus, when specifying a vertical phoria, one must also state which eye is regarded as deviating. To avoid confusion, clinical practice normally uses only the term hyperphoria. Thus a left hypophoria is recorded as right hyperphoria, abbreviated to R Hyper or $^R/_L$. The abbreviation Hyp should never be used, since it could easily be mistaken by another practitioner for hypophoria. The $^R/_L$ notation is to be preferred since it shows concisely and unambiguously the direction of the phoria. Left hyperphoria is written $^L/_R$. (Some other heterophorias will be discussed later.)

The heterotropias are classified in *Table 10.2*. The $^R/_L$ abbreviations may be adopted for tropias, a letter T denoting the deviating eye: for example, R hypertropia would be written as $^{RT}/_L$ and R hypotropia as $^L/_{RT}$.

With all the tropias both the angle and the eye that deviates must be recorded. It is also important to note whether the squint is unilateral or alternating and, if the latter, whether there is a preference for fixation by one eye. Some squinting patients can change fixation voluntarily from one eye to the other, while other patients change only if the originally fixating eye is covered. Other patients fixate with one eye in part of

---

* An accepted contraction, like tropia, in common clinical use.

the field of view and change to the other eye for the remainder.

Causes of an oculo-motor imbalance

Refractive

The uncorrected hypermetrope needs to accommodate in order to see clearly. Because of the close link between accommodation and convergence, the accommodative effort tends to induce adduction of the eyes – accommodative convergence. Thus, under-corrected hypermetropes tend to be esophoric. Conversely, under-corrected myopia makes a lower demand on accommodation than on convergence in near vision: exophoria in near vision is to be expected. This may be enough to give symptoms, even though each eye under monocular conditions would receive a perfectly focused image.

Anatomical

If one of the extra-ocular muscles is incorrectly attached to the globe, faulty muscle action is to be expected. If the medial rectus, for example, were attached too far from the limbus, its action might be reduced and an exo-deviation could be expected. The surgical treatment of strabismus is based on making anatomical corrections to the muscles, even when the strabismus is not primarily of muscular origin. Faulty positioning of check ligaments may also give rise to a motor anomaly.

Neurological

Some patients appear to have a natural excess of nervous energy – they are said to be highly strung. Similarly, some patients appear to have overactive convergence, and are therefore esophoric. Others may have a very poor (remote) near point of convergence, yet the motiliy test shows full power of adduction by the medial recti. The innervation for convergence is at fault, not the muscles themselves.

Pathological

This type includes both anatomical and neurological causes. In some patients, a particular muscle action or group of muscle actions may be affected by, for example, haemorrhage or nerve damage. The motility is usually incomitant, but in slight cases the resulting oculomotor imbalance may be only a phoria. In more severe cases a tropia will result. The sudden onset of a tropia in an adult produces diplopia, but in a young child double vision is readily prevented by suppression of one eye's image. The gradual breakdown of a heterophoria into a manifest deviation in an adult may also be unaccompanied by diplopia.

General debility and the side-effects of drugs such as tranquillizers can also cause or aggravate an oculomotor imbalance.

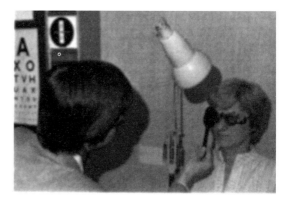

Figure 10.3.   The cover test.

The cover test

Objective cover test

This test, sometimes termed the cover–uncover test, is probably the most important of the tests for oculomotor imbalance. It may be carried out with fixation at any distance and with the patient wearing or not wearing his correction. If spectacles are habitually worn, it is pointless to do a cover test without them. The patient should observe a finely detailed test object, so that accommodation is sufficiently stimulated and accurate fixation is required. A good object for distance vision is a letter on the test chart from the line one size larger than the patient can just read with the poorer eye. The 'muscle spot light' (a bright illuminated spot 5–10 mm in diameter) should not, in general, be used as a fixation point, since it will not stimulate an under-corrected hypermetrope's accommodation. For near vision, a letter or small pattern on a card makes an ideal fixation stimulus. The card should be held at the patient's habitual reading or working position and the trial lenses must be carefully centred, both horizontally and vertically. Readjustment for near vision is usually necessary.

The examiner should first make sure that there is no strabismus present by placing the cover over the patient's right eye while observing the left eye (*Figure 10.3*). If the left eye moves to take up fixation, a left eye strabismus is demonstrated. The eye will move out or abduct in esotropia and move in or adduct in exotropia. The directions of movement in vertical tropias may similarly be deduced.

If a strabismus has been revealed, both eyes make a version movement when the cover is removed, the right eye fixating again. If no movement is seen on removing the cover, then the left eye remains fixating. Covering this eye will now produce a version movement, the right eye resuming fixation. This shows an alternating strabismus.

If, on covering the right eye initially, no movement of the left eye was seen, the left eye should be covered and the right eye watched. Movement of the right eye then demonstrates a tropia of that eye. The initial covering of the right eye had no effect, since the unimpeded left eye continued to fixate the test object.[*]

The examiner should then look for the presence of a heterophoria, although with practice it is possible to check for a tropia and a phoria with the same few movements of the cover. Thus, suppose that on covering the right eye no movement of the left eye is seen, but on removal of the cover the right eye makes a fusional movement to regain fixation of the test object, this shows that a heterophoria is present. If the return movement is inwards, then the eye had deviated outwards under cover, indicating exophoria. Similarly, if the eye moves down on removal of the cover, a right hyperphoria is revealed.

The left eye should now be covered. On removal of the cover this eye will adduct in exophoria, elevate in right hyperphoria.

To summarize:

(1) Cover RE while watching LE.
     Movement indicates an L tropia.
(2) Uncover RE
     (a) If movement seen in (1), watch for version movement of both eyes.
          Movement indicates an L tropia.
          No movement of either eye: alternating strabismus.
     (b) If no movement seen in (1), watch for movement of RE.
          Movement indicates heterophoria.
(3) Cover LE while watching RE.
     (a) If no movement seen in (1) but RE now moves, R tropia indicated.
     (b) If movement seen in (1) but RE now makes a return movement: alternating strabismus.
(4) Uncover LE.
     (a) If movement seen in (3), watch for version movement of both eyes. Movement indicates an R tropia.
     (b) If no movement seen in (3), watch for movement of LE.
          Movement indicates heterophoria.

If no movement is seen on any of these four steps, the patient is orthophoric (within the limits of observational accuracy).

The cover test needs practice and a good light on the patient's eyes but is much simpler to do than to describe. In order to demonstrate any heterophoria, the cover must be left in place for several seconds to allow the dissociated eye to deviate to its passive position. The cover is best removed in a swift vertical movement: a sideways removal of the cover may give the erroneous impression of an ocular movement in the opposite direction. It is imperative to watch the limbus and not the pupil margin

because the pupil size alters on removal of the cover. Because the lateral vertical borders of the limbus are easily seen between the patient's eyelids, it is much easier to detect horizontal than vertical movements of the eyes. For this reason it is essential to check instrumentally for vertical oculo-motor imbalances, or their resultant fixation disparity – *see* later in this chapter, especially as the eyes are much less tolerant of vertical errors.

Some writers suggest watching for movement of the eye behind the cover after occluding. This may be useful but has disadvantages:

(1) The movement of deviation in a heterophoria is much slower than the fusional refixation and thus more difficult to see.
(2) The speed of the recovery movement may be an indication of the control of the heterophoria: a quick movement suggests comfortable vision while a slow or jerky movement suggests discomfort.
(3) To allow observation, the cover must be held at an angle, so that the eye is less efficiently occluded. It is then possible that the retinal image of details seen peripherally by the occluded eye will be mentally fused with the image in the uncovered eye, holding the 'covered' eye in its normal position. In other words, the peripheral details form a 'binocular lock'.

With low phorias, it is sometimes easier to see the refixation movement of the eyes if the cover is repeatedly transferred from eye to eye, occluding each eye in turn for about a second. This tends to increase the angle of heterophoria in some patients, in which case the larger angle is probably the more significant. For the same reason, if a single rather than a repeated cover test is used with a heterophoric patient, it is better to hold the cover in place for several seconds to allow the heterophoria to build up than to record the 'instantaneous value'. Barnard and Thomson (1995) showed that the heterophoria in some subjects was still increasing after 10 s occlusion, so that a single period of 1–2 s occlusion is most unlikely to elicit the heterophoria. They point out that the cover test reveals the movement corresponding to the fast vergence controller (*see Figure 9.11*). Both repeated and prolonged cover testing may break a borderline heterophoria down into an apparent heterotropia. Thus in cases of strabismus, it may be advisable to do both a quick (2 s) and prolonged (10 s) cover to elicit the habitual and total angles of the heterotropia (*see* page 188).

With experience, it is possible to estimate the amount of movement of the corneal limbus and hence the angle of the heterophoria or heterotropia. If you get someone to look from one letter to another on the test chart you can work out the movement of the eye (in Δ). This is given by dividing the distance between the letters in centimetres by the observation distance in metres. A change in fixation from one end to the other of a 6 m line of letters viewed at 6 m is usually about 3Δ.

Small vertical phorias are more difficult to see, since vertical movements of the nasal and temporal limbi are much less obvious than a horizontal movement. For

---

[*] The occasional patient with a low-angle strabismus does not readily fixate with the deviating eye, which remains in the rotated position. If, with the normally fixating eye covered, the patient is asked to look at a different letter, the strabismus may become apparent because the eye turns through an unexpected angle: for example a diagonal movement when the letters are separated vertically.

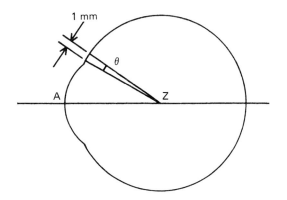

Figure 10.4. Conversion of linear limbus movement to angular measure.

this reason, the cover test should be supplemented with an instrumental measure of vertical heterophoria or fixation disparity.

Another method is illustrated in *Figure 10.4*. If the limbus is assumed to be 15 mm from the eye's centre of rotation Z, a movement of 1 mm of the limbus corresponds to a rotation θ of 1/15 rad. Hence

$$\theta \approx 4° \approx 7\Delta$$

since 1 rad is approximately 60°.

In fact, the distance from the limbus to Z would be nearer to 12.5 mm in most eyes, in which case a more accurate calculation of θ in the above example would give about 4.6° or 8.0Δ. Any spectacles worn by the patient may alter the apparent size of the movement, which will appear larger in high hypermetropia, smaller in myopia.

The deviation may also be measured by putting up a prism to neutralize the movement, so that with a tropia no movement of the normally deviating eye is seen when the dominant eye is covered, or, in a heterophoria, no movement on removing the cover. Consider, for example, the case of an esophore. The eye deviates in-

wards under cover and abducts when the cover is removed. *Figure 10.5* shows the right eye deviating behind the cover. A prism of the correct power placed base-out realigns the fixation axis, so that when the cover is removed, the image falls immediately on the fovea. No fusional movement is required. Thus, a more precise measurement of the deviation may be made than by estimation. A rotary prism or prism bar (explained in most texts on orthoptics) may be used to reduce the time taken.

Subjective cover test

This test was introduced in 1924 by Duane, who called it the parallax test.

The following remarks apply only to heterophoria. Sensory adaptations which would affect the results of this test occur in many heterotropias (*see* pages 185–189). *Figure 10.6* represents a case of esophoria, the right eye being covered. The cover is then transferred to the left eye. The image in the now-uncovered right eye will initially fall on the nasal retina and will be projected temporally to the right. The patient therefore sees the fixation object apparently jump to the right. The right eye will quickly rotate to return the image to the fovea, but this does not give rise to a sensation of movement, just as our surroundings are perceived as stationary when we move fixation.

Thus, in esophoria, the apparent movement is in the opposite direction to the movement of the cover, whereas in exophoria the apparent movement is in the same direction. You can confirm for yourself that the fixation object appears to jump downwards in R hyperphoria and upwards in L hyperphoria when the cover is

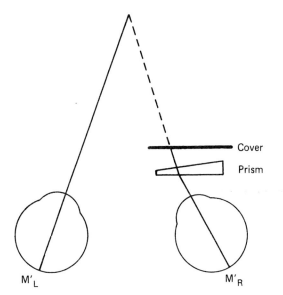

Figure 10.5. Measurement of an esophoric deviation by means of a prism behind the cover.

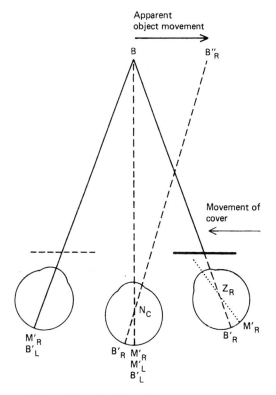

Figure 10.6. Principle of the subjective cover test.

passed from right to left. In all cases the direction of movement is opposite to the right eye's deviation under cover, which can be measured by adding prisms with their base in the direction of the recovery movement until the object appears stationary. It should be noted that the subjective direction of movement is the same as that of the refixation.

This subjective movement is sometimes erroneously termed the φ-phenomenon. This term should be reserved for the apparent motion when different retinal elements in one or both eyes are stimulated consecutively by similar images formed from different objects. Certain advertisements make use of this process: a series of electric lamps light up one after the other to give the impression of a single moving light. The subjective cover test is similar, but relies solely on cerebral perception and integration between the different layers representing the two eyes. The φ-phenomenon could involve retinal processing and certainly need not involve changing representation from one layer to another in the striate cortex, but only from one part to another within the same layer.

Instrumentation for measuring heterophoria

Dissociation techniques

The only method of dissociating the eyes mentioned so far has been to cover one eye, thus virtually eliminating any area of overlap of the visual fields and hence reducing the stimulus to fusion. The covered eye is then free to deviate from its active to its passive position, in response to refractive, anatomical and innervational factors. In general, instruments for investigating the oculo-motor imbalance rely instead on dissociating the two visual images. The methods used include:

(1) *Selective screening.* Some parts of the visual field are seen by one eye, adjacent parts by the other eye (for example, the Maddox wing and similar tests).

(2) *Distortion.* The image in one eye is distorted to such an extent that fusion is virtually eliminated, as by the Maddox rod.

(3) *Prismatic dissociation.* For example, von Graefe's method in which a vertical imbalance of about 4–6Δ is induced by a prism. This is too large for the eyes to overcome, so diplopia is produced. A horizontal phoria may then become manifest. A similar device is the Maddox biprism, consisting of two prisms of about 5Δ placed base to base so as to divide the pupil of one eye. Monocular diplopia is produced and again the eye may deviate. These techniques have become obsolete.

(4) *Tests with independent objects.* In effect, different objects are presented to each eye by means of red/green dissociation (*see* page 148), crossed Polaroid techniques as used in fixation disparity devices (*see* page 174) or instruments of the synoptophore type (*see* page 203).

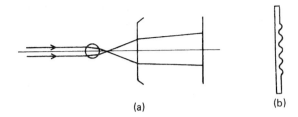

Figure 10.7. (a) The Maddox rod, giving a vertical streak on the retina, (b) the Maddox multiple rod or groove.

It is more logical to describe these tests when classified according to the distance of fixation.

Tests in distance vision

The test most commonly used is the Maddox rod, sometimes called the Maddox multiple rod or groove. This gives dissociation by distortion. It originally consisted of a glass rod of diameter about 3 mm forming an extremely powerful cylindrical lens. If placed horizontally, as shown in cross-section in *Figure 10.7(a)*, rays in a vertical plane from a distant illuminated aperture (the spot or muscle light) are brought to a focus just behind the rear surface of the rod and then diverge. Since the rod is held close to the patient's eye, the rays remain divergent on entering the eye and form a vertical streak on the retina. Because the single rod had to be placed very carefully in front of the patient's pupil, it has been replaced by the multiple rod or groove (*Figure 10.7b*) which has a similar optical effect but is easier to position and gives a brighter streak. (This modern form is still generally called a Maddox rod.) The Maddox rod is usually made of either red or green material: this both enhances dissociation and aids recognition of the streak by the patient. The red rod is usually preferred for distance fixation, the green for near, to correspond with the eye's usual lead or lag of accommodation at the two distances.

The patient views the distant muscle light with one eye while the rod is in front of the other. It is useful to follow the routine of always placing the rod before one particular eye, say the right. The vertical streak seen by the patient when the rod is horizontal enables the horizontal deviation of the eye to be measured.

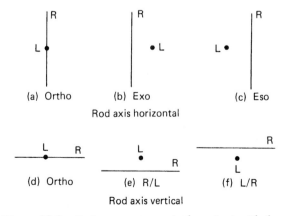

Figure 10.8. Various appearances to the patient, with the Maddox rod before the right eye.

Figure 10.8 illustrates the various appearances with the Maddox rod placed horizontal before the right eye. In orthophoria (*Figure 10.8a*), the streak appears to pass through the spot seen by the left eye. In exophoria (*Figure 10.8b*), the right eye abducts, so that the image of the streak falls on the temporal side of the fovea. By projection it is thus seen to the left of the spot. The opposite occurs in esophoria (*Figure 10.8c*). To measure the deviation, prisms are now placed in front of the same eye as the Maddox rod with their base in the same direction as the displaced streak until the streak passes through the spot. In general, the results are often 'bracketed' by finding the powers which just under- and over-correct the deviation. To measure vertical deviations, the rod is then turned through a right angle to give a horizontal streak. This will be seen passing through the spot in orthophoria (*Figure 10.8d*), below the spot in R hyperphoria (*Figure 10.8e*) and above it in L hyperphoria (*Figure 10.8f*).

Because a spotlight does not demand the most critical focusing by the eye, the test does not necessarily give a true indication of the horizontal heterophoria present. Another possibility, despite the completely different shape and colour of spot and streak, is that a small element of fusion may exist. The eyes may then not be completely dissociated. As a check, a cover is additionally placed in front of one of the patient's eyes and he is asked to say whether the streak is to the left or right of (or above or below) the spot immediately the cover is removed. The Maddox rod is then providing a marker rather than acting as a dissociating device.

There are several devices which can help to determine the correct prism power rapidly. A prism bar, Risley variable prism or even a single 10Δ rotating prism may be used. The latter is placed with its base-apex line at right-angles to the rod, in which setting the streak is apparently displaced along itself. The prism may then be rotated until the streak is seen to pass through the spot. The resolved component of prism power at right-angles

to the streak gives the angle of heterophoria. Calibrated holders for prism and rod are made.

Another method is to use a tangent scale, a technique simplified by Freeman in the 1950s. A green Maddox rod is held before the patient's right eye while the left eye views a scale of red transilluminated numbers (*Figure 10.9*). The white light at the centre of the scale produces the streak, while the red numbers and green-coloured rod eliminate the additional streaks that would otherwise have been caused had white numbers been used. The scale, calibrated in prism dioptres for the assumed testing distance, is placed obliquely, and hence may be used to measure both horizontal and vertical deviations. Odd numbers are used on one side of the spot and even numbers on the other, allowing the practitioner to tell immediately in which direction the eye has deviated. The patient is asked to say through what number, or between what numbers, the spot appears to pass. Otherwise, for example, he may reply '3' instead of 'between 2 and 4', thus misleading the examiner. It is essential that the Maddox rod be accurately placed horizontally or vertically to prevent inaccuracies in measurement.

The symbol ⊖ is often used to denote orthophoria in the vertical direction, ⬮ in the horizontal direction, and ⊕ for both. They indicate the positions of spotlight and streak.

Tests in near vision

Correct centration of the trial lenses is essential before a near heterophoria is measured. A general-purpose correction may be left centred at the distance PD, but a true near correction should be centred to correspond to the near PD. For the presbyopic patient, the reading addition must be in place. If a trial frame is used, it should be adjusted vertically and the bottom rim angled in towards the face so that the patient can look downwards through the centre of the lenses without obliquity. Equivalent adjustments, where possible, should be made if a refractor head is used. Measurement of the state of the eyes in near vision taken in a horizontal visual plane through a refractor head may not be realistic.

The Maddox rod may again be used. The Freeman–Archer oblique tangent scale for distance vision, described above, has also been scaled down for use at 330 mm, but the red figures used perhaps over-stimulate the accommodation, resulting in a falsely esophoric (or low exophoric) reading. On the other hand, the use of the Maddox rod with a small spot of light such as a torch bulb under-stimulates the accommodation, giving an over-estimate of exophoria.

A popular test based on selective screening of a test card is the Maddox wing test (*Figure 10.10*), introduced in 1912. A vertical arrow is presented to one eye and a horizontal tangent scale to the other to give the measurement of the horizontal phoria. A horizontal arrow and vertical scale are used to measure the vertical imbalance. The scales are mounted at the fixed viewing distance of $\frac{1}{3}$ m, much closer than most patients read, so the results obtained are not necessarily significant.

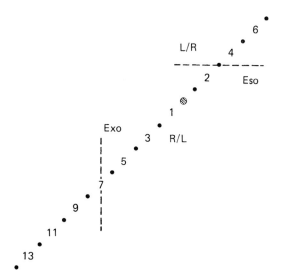

Figure 10.9. The Freeman–Archer oblique tangent scale (Birmingham Optical Group Ltd): illustration refers to near unit.

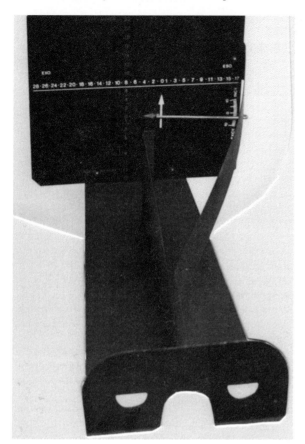

Figure 10.10.   One model of the Maddox wing test. The lower-right scale is for cyclophoria.

Early models used relatively large numbers on the tangent scale, giving an exophoric bias to the measurements because accommodation and hence accommodative convergence were under-stimulated. Recent models have much smaller figures.

Fixation disparity

The cover test and instrumental tests already described for the investigation of the oculo-motor balance give a measure of the total imbalance when the eyes are completely dissociated. The phenomenon of fixation disparity needs negligible dissociation of the eyes to be demonstrable, yet helps the practitioner to decide the significance of the total imbalance.

Though binocular fixation is based on corresponding points, it was shown on pages 154–156 that there is an element of flexibility in the system. As indicated in *Figure 10.11*, binocular single vision is possible, provided that the retinal image Q'_L in the left eye falls within Panum's fusional area surrounding the retinal receptor corresponding to Q'_R in the right eye. This is as true for images in the fovea as in the parafovea or peripheral retina. It is therefore possible for one eye to maintain fixation while the second eye deviates through only a fraction of a degree, up to 15 minutes of arc. This deviation in binocular vision is called a fixation disparity. It should not be regarded as a heterotropic devia-

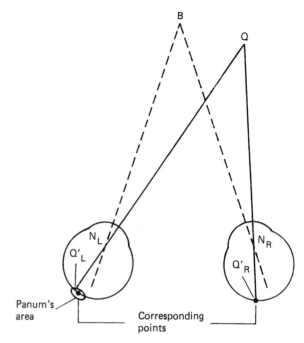

Figure 10.11.   Panum's areas. The eyes are fixating B. A neighbouring element Q will be seen singly, provided that its image in the left eye falls in the area around the point corresponding to Q'_R.

tion since it is a departure within physiological limits from normal bifoveal fixation.

In a case of true heterophoria, advantage may habitually be taken of fixation disparity to give partial relief by allowing one eye to deviate slightly from the position of accurate fixation. The fixation disparity units developed by Mallett (1964, 1983) for distance and near vision provide a simple method of investigation, the principle of which is illustrated in *Figure 10.12*. The letter **X** is seen by both eyes, but the markers above and below it are polarized at right-angles. Viewing through the analysing visor, the patient sees the upper marker only with his left eye and the lower marker with his right eye.

Since the right eye of our hypothetical subject is exactly fixating the **X**, the right eye's marker will be seen precisely below the **X**, as illustrated by the projection from the cyclopean eye. On the other hand, the marker for the left eye is imaged, like the **X**, fractionally to the temporal side of the visual axis. Unlike the **X**, which is projected as though from the fovea because of fusion within Panum's area, the left marker is projected to the right and appears out of line with the **X** and lower marker.

The fixation disparity of the object **X** is demonstrated by the misalignment of the two markers. The image of the **X** may be said to have slipped across the retina of the left eye – hence the older and less-apt term for fixation disparity: 'retinal slip' (Ames and Gliddon, 1928).

The value of the relieving or aligning prism that realigns the workers, thus eliminating the fixation disparity is sometimes termed the 'associated heterophoria'. This

---

* Institute of Optometry Marketing Ltd.

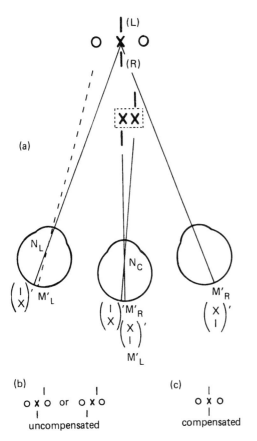

(a)

(b)

o x o   or   o x o

uncompensated

(c)

o x o

compensated

Figure 10.12. (a) Diagrammatic representation of fixation disparity in exophoria. The fixation letter **X**, foveal lock circles **OO** and markers are situated in a vertical plane perpendicular to the plane of the diagram. **OXO** is seen binocularly, the upper marker by the left eye and the lower by the right eye. The binoculus projects to the distance of the object plane but is shortened here for clarity. (b) The appearance in uncompensated exophoria and (c) when compensated.

term (deprecated by Mallett, pers. comm. 1993) is contradictory, since heterophoria implies dissociation.

It must be emphasized that the angle of disparity, if any, is small since it is governed by the angular size of Panum's fusional areas at the fovea. The Mallett fixation disparity units* contain central detail which may be fused binocularly, whereas the apparatus used by Ogle (1950) presented, in the main, peripheral details only. Thus Ogle's apparatus is likely to demonstrate fixation disparity more frequently and of larger angle than the Mallett units. This is also true for some other clinical tests for fixation disparity (*see* Pickwell *et al.*, 1988).

Mallett's apparatus was developed to help the practitioner decide when relief from heterophoria should be prescribed. The magnitude of a heterophoria as demonstrated by dissociation tests is not necessarily an indication of the need for help. One patient may be able to overcome a large angle of heterophoria quite comfortably, while another patient will be given symptoms by a small heterophoria. A heterophoric patient who is symptom-free is said to have a compensated heterophoria and is unlikely to show a fixation disparity. Conversely, a patient with symptoms caused by binocular vision problems has an uncompensated heterophoria and will probably show a fixation disparity. The only ob-

jective assessment is the speed of the fusional recovery movement in the cover test: a rapid movement suggests good control, a slow movement poor control of the heterophoria.

Aligning prisms for heterophoria should be placed before the eye showing the disparity with their base in the direction of the marker's movement, thus allowing the eye to deviate while keeping the image on the fovea. In the example above, the left eye showed an exophoric fixation disparity. Base-in prism should hence be added before this eye until the two marks are aligned. This minimum prism may then be prescribed. It is probably better to divide equally a prism of more than 2Δ, thereby avoiding the more noticeable aberrations of a single stronger prism.

With horizontal heterophorias, partial compensation is sometimes possible by altering the spherical part of the correction. In near vision, an esophoric disparity may be reduced by a positive spherical addition, either in a separate near correction or conventional bifocals. An esophoric disparity in distance vision cannot be relieved in the same manner because the extra spherical power will fog acuity; refraction under cyclopegia should be considered in case there is significant latent hypermetropia. An esophoria which is significantly greater in near than in distance vision is termed a convergence excess. The opposite condition of divergence excess is characterized by greater exophoria (or exotropia) in distance vision than in near vision. An exophoric disparity in either or both distance and near vision may be helped by adding equal minus spheres before each eye. The extra accommodation so stimulated will produce accommodative convergence and help reduce the exophoria. The reserves of accommodation must be more than adequate, so this method must not be regarded as universal; each patient must be considered in the light of the findings. Such a negative addition should be regarded as a middle term arrangement to allow 'passive' development of the fusional abilities, both neurological and muscular. The negative addition is progressively reduced with time. 'Active' treatment of both esophoria and exophoria by orthoptic exercises may also be undertaken, but such treatment falls outside the scope of this book.

Since the Polaroid visor is effectively a neutral density filter of luminous transmittance about 25%, similar to a typical sunglass, it is essential that extra illumination be provided on the fixation disparity panel and its surrounds. The latter are seen binocularly and contribute to the binocular lock. In poor illumination, a falsely high proportion of patients will appear to need prismatic help.

The original design of apparatus for distance vision could be rotated through 90° in order to check for the presence of an uncompensated vertical heterophoria. Care should be taken to ensure that the trial frame (if used) is level: a frame containing right and left +5.00 DS and tilted so that one lens is 2 mm higher than the other will induce a 1Δ vertical error. Such a tilt is quite easily obtained should one of the frame sides be caught up in the patient's hair. With a refractor unit, the patient's head must be level. The distance

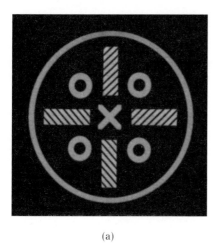

(a)

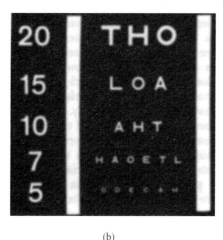

(b)

Figure 10.13. (a) The Mallett dual fixation disparity unit. (b) The Mallett near-vision suppression test. The numbers, which are normally blue, indicate the angle subtended at the eye when the chart is held at 35 cm. The central letters and the two bars are seen binocularly. (Illustration by courtesy of Mr R.F.J. Mallett.)

unit is available for near-vision examination providing separate displays for horizontal and vertical disparities, while somewhat similar devices are produced by other companies.

Some patients with heterophorias only just maintain fusion, but are symptom-free because fine details in the image falling near the fovea of one eye are suppressed, that is, the brain disregards the information. This is demonstrated if the marker for one eye constantly disappears. However, this does not always indicate suppression but in some cases may be due to only retinal rivalry. If the patient is asked to blink several times, the line may reappear. Especially in near vision, the practitioner should check by covering the eye seeing the opposite marker that the disappearing marker is not simply occluded by a badly fitting trial frame.

Sometimes a suppression area is only on one side of the fovea, so that if the marker's image falls in this zone, it will not be seen. Thus in esophoria, the image of one of the horizontal markers for examining vertical disparity may be imaged on the nasal retina. Reversing the analysing visor will now interchange the markers so that the image falls on the temporal side of the fovea, in which case it may be seen. The same tactic may be used if the two markers form a fused strip through the central **X**.

If diplopia occurs, the practitioner should use a dissociation test to assess the heterotropia (or 'broken-down' heterophoria) and incorporate relieving prisms in the correction to obtain single binocular vision of the unit before adding the visor. The prism may then be verified (either increased or decreased) in the normal manner.

If the patient's record shows that a prismatic correction was incorporated in their last spectacles, it is sensible to check the fixation disparity through their present lenses before occluding one eye, whether to check the visual acuity or to perform the cover test. This avoids the risk of breaking down an unstable binocularity – the actual prismatic correction in the present spectacles can then be measured on the focimeter if the lenses are positioned on the instrument at the patient's PD.

Some patients may need prism for distance vision but not near vision, or vice versa. The required prism can be checked at the other distance to see whether or not adverse fixation disparity is induced. With anisometropic bifocal wearers, the need for specialized dispensing (*see* pages 263–265) may be verified by checking for vertical fixation disparity using lowered gaze through their present spectacles. A more typical angle of depression will be obtained with these whether or not they are bifocals (or single vision distance or near spectacles) than with trial lenses.

With the demand for larger frames in dispensing, the unit may also be used to gauge any possible intolerance to poor centration. Equally, the prescriber should consider whether accurate centration of lenses to the patient's PD is necessary for the exophoric myope or the esophoric hypermetrope, but must also bear in mind the possible problems of prism distortion (*see* pages 238–246) and peripheral distortion through large lenses (*see* page 256).

An alternative test for suppression is a series of letters

unit, introduced in 1994 and illustrated in *Figure 10.13(a)*, demonstrates both horizontal and vertical disparity simultaneously (Mallet and Radnam-Skibin, 1994).

An alternative test for a vertical imbalance in distance vision is the Turville infinity balance technique described on pages 106–107. With the pair of concentric circles as test object, the strip is placed so that one set is seen by each eye. Any vertical imbalance tends to result in an apparent vertical displacement of the circles. Prism is then added to level their appearance. This test tends to be more sensitive than the fixation disparity units since there is no foveal lock, only a parafoveal lock formed by the surrounding details on the test chart. Horizontal imbalance cannot be examined by this technique. In esophoria, the ring spacing appears to increase, while in exophoria the rings may be fused into one. Base-in prism may then be added to separate the rings, but this is little guide to its need in everyday life.

A scaled-down version of the Mallett fixation disparity

or words of graded sizes transilluminated by polarized light. Some letters of each size are visible to both eyes, others to one eye only (*Figure 10.13b*). All the letters on the top line may be visible, but on the remaining smaller lines, the letters for one eye may not be seen. It is often better not to prescribe prismatic help for such patients, even though the fixation disparity markers may not be suppressed and indicate a need for prism.

One useful advantage of the fixation disparity units is that binocular vision is maintained, the two visual axes being correctly aligned or very nearly so. This eliminates a possible error of tests using complete dissociation: when a large, slightly paretic heterophoria is present, the eye may make a secondary movement of elevation in abducting or adducting. In the fixation disparity test, the lateral movement is minimal because of the binocular lock, so there may now be no tendency for a vertical deviation. The vertical error shown by full dissociation is of very much less significance from the standpoint of prescribing prisms.

A fixation disparity is best recorded in terms of the prism power and base setting required for alignment, not as the type of causative heterophoria. Thus, 2Δ base-down L should be recorded, rather than 2Δ L hyperphoric disparity. This reduces the possibility of error when incorporating into the final prescription. Since the test does not provide complete dissociation, the findings should not be called a heterophoria, nor should the usual orthophoric symbol of a line through a circle be used to denote no fixation disparity. This condition may be recorded, instead, by a line through an **X**: for example, compensation in the horizontal direction would be denoted by a vertical line through an **X**, or simply recorded as comp H or CH.

Fusional reserves*

Just as there are reserves of accommodation, so the binocular system has reserves of fusional movements. Consider the two eyes fixating a test stimulus, such as a letter on the chart, at 6 m. If a 2Δ prism is placed base-out before each eye, the image seen by the right eye is displaced to the left and that by the left eye to the right. The eyes will probably make the fusional movement of relative convergence needed to maintain single vision, accommodation remaining approximately steady. If the base-out prism is gradually increased, for example, by means of refractor-head prisms or a variable prism stereoscope, the eyes will continue to converge. This convergence will induce accommodation, the patient eventually reporting that the test object has blurred. The prismatic power in place at this moment is recorded as the 'blur point'. The prism power may be increased still further until fusion is no longer possible and binocular fixation breaks down. The patient reports that the test object has gone double – the 'break point'. If the prism power is now reduced, a state will be reached

Table 10.3 Typical values of fusional reserves

Direction	Fixation distance	Fusional reserve (in Δ)		
		Blur point	Break point	Recovery point
Positive (convergence)	Distance	4	20	12
	Near	8	30	20
Negative (divergence)	Distance		8	4
	Near		15	8
Vertical	Both		4	2

when binocular single vision is regained – the 'recovery point'. These results are known as the positive fusional reserves for distance vision.

In the unusual event of a heterophoria in which single vision is not possible without prismatic assistance, the prismatic power at the fusion point is also recorded.

The negative fusional reserves of abduction or divergence are obtained with base-in prism before each eye. In distance vision there is now no blur point since there is no 'negative' accommodation, provided that the patient is fully corrected or hypermetropic.

The vertical reserves may be measured by adding separate prisms or a Risley variable prism before one eye. Some variable-prism stereoscopes have special test-card holders to adjust the relative vertical position of the test cards. A synoptophore may also be used.

The entire process can be repeated in near vision, though the vertical reserves are normally the same for both. A typical set of values is given in *Table 10.3*.

Although the fusional reserves are of great importance in the orthoptic treatment of heterophoria and heterotropia, their investigation has several disadvantages in routine examination.

(1) It often gives the patient a headache;
(2) the results may not be repeatable, improving with practice;
(3) the measurements may be affected by the rate of change in the prism powers;
(4) measurement of the negative fusional reserves made immediately after the positive will be inaccurate because extreme exertion in one direction will leave a neural or muscular tonus, reducing the effort in the opposite direction.

Despite these disadvantages, techniques for prescribing relieving prisms in heterophoria based on fusional reserves are widely used in some countries (Borish, 1970).

Incidence of heterophoria

The great majority of the population in the UK enjoy bifoveal fixation, only some 2–4% having strabismus. The findings of Tait (1951) on the incidence of horizontal phorias are shown in *Figure 10.14*. In distance vision, about 70% are clinically orthophoric, though esophoria and exophoria up to 8Δ are both fairly

---

*These have occasionally been called ductions, but this term should be reserved for movements of one eye.

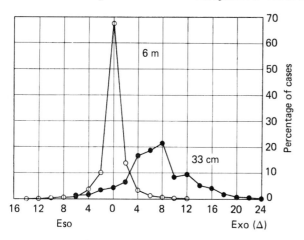

Figure 10.14. The distribution of horizontal heterophoria in ocularly comfortable subjects, redrawn from Tait (1951). (By kind permission of the publishers of *Am. J. Ophthal.* ©1951 by the Ophthalmological Publishing Co.)

common. Larger angles may well be encountered and are not necessarily pathological. In near vision, exophoria is seen to be the typical condition.

Vertical heterophorias are much smaller, seldom more than 1Δ and rarely more than 2Δ. A small vertical heterophoria is, however, much more likely to give symptoms than the same deviation laterally, because the vertical fusional reserves are very much smaller than the horizontal.

As already noted, convergence is usually the dominant function in near vision. It must be highly accurate to avoid diplopia, whereas the eye's depth of focus allows some latitude in the accommodation. In the course of a near muscle balance test, the dominant convergence function is no longer fully stimulated. The accommodation is stimulated partly by the proximal factor and partly by monocular clues such as the eye's chromatic aberration.

The ease and accuracy of the accommodation influence the amount of accommodative convergence. This, taken in conjunction with the proximal convergence and any distance heterophoria, determines the oculomotor imbalance in near vision.

Vertical heterophoria is much less likely to alter between distance and near vision. Slight incomitancy and relative vertical prism effects in anisometropia (*see* Chapter 14) may, however, cause differences in the angle of a vertical heterophoria as the gaze depresses for close work.

Many patients are exophoric both in distance and near vision or esophoric in both. The angle of deviation, however, may not be the same at the two distances. A patient under 40 years of age, with adequate refractive correction, often appears to show little difference between the distance and near phoria when estimated by the cover test. The Maddox wing test often shows the pointer wandering relative to the scale as accommodation and hence accommodative-convergence fluctuate, but the mean reading in near vision is often about 6Δ relatively more exophoric than the distance heterophoria measured with the Maddox rod. This normal difference is known as physiological exophoria. It corre-

sponds to the lag shown by the accommodative convergence line, the graph to the left of the normal curve in *Figure 9.7*.

Freier and Pickwell (1983) found that physiological exophoria (measured with the Maddox rod for distance, and Maddox wing test or rod and tangent scale for near vision) increased with age from approximately none at ages up to 15 to about 6Δ at 65 or thereabouts. They did not find that presbyopic near additions made a significant contribution to this.

A person in the 40–50 age group may be esophoric in near vision because of the declining power of accommodation: excessive innervational effort is needed to obtain a satisfactory focus if the correction worn, if any, is out of date. An increase in near addition may well cause the patient to become exophoric, even apparently uncompensated on the fixation disparity units. A near exophoric disparity when the addition has been increased should be regarded with caution.

The older patient may have declining reserves of convergence. If, because of failing acuity he also needs to read closer with a higher than normal near addition, he may then show a high near exophoria needing prismatic help. A useful guide is the incorporation of one prism dioptre base in each eye for every dioptre of near addition, as in prismatic binocular loupes (*see* page 250).

Convergence insufficiency denotes a very high relative exophoria in near vision with a 'normal' imbalance in distance vision. In general, but not always, such patients have a poor near point of convergence. Divergence excess denotes a high exophoria or even exotropia in distance vision, but a normal imbalance in near vision.

Symptoms of heterophoria

The symptoms produced by heterophoria are not necessarily related to the size of the angle when the eyes are dissociated. One patient may be troubled by a small heterophoria, while another may have good fusional reserves and be able to cope with a much larger amount.

Typical symptoms are headaches, a feeling of tired or 'pulling' eyes, intermittent blurred vision, and jumbling of the letters of words. Those relatively rare patients whose heterophoria breaks down into an intermittent heterotropia may experience diplopia. Bright light appears to aggravate heterophoric asthenopia.

The continual nervous effort required to control a heterophoria may give rise to headaches. The lateral heterophorias tend to give frontal headaches.

In exophoria they occur during periods when critical vision is in use, for example, during work. Esophoria tends to cause apparently unrelated headaches, even the day after concentrated use of the eyes. The hyperphorias tend to give occipital headaches. There are many possible causes of headaches and it may be that an ocular component is one of several, each capable of triggering a tension headache.

The reason for the tired or pulling feeling around the eyes is probably fatigue. Blurred vision may result from inhibition or spasm of convergence-induced accommodation in esophoria and exophoria respectively. Blurred vision can also be caused by very small angles of diplopia, but this is often reported as a jumbling of the letters. In a word such as 'falling', it is possible for the left eye to fixate the first letter 'l', while the right eye fixates the second. Fusion of these two letters could result, but the remainder of the word would appear confused since the images in the two eyes are incorrectly superimposed. As a result, binocular acuity may be somewhat lower than the monocular acuity, whereas in the normal patient binocular acuity is usually the better. This was demonstrated experimentally with induced fixation disparity by Jenkins *et al.* (1992), the expected 11% increase in binocular acuity over the mean monocular acuity being reduced to the monocular level with 6Δ base-out each eye, a 6% reduction with 4Δ base-in.

Every time a different object is fixated, the eyes have to make a fusional movement at the instant of refixation. Symptoms are likely to be worse when the visual task requires constant changes of fixation. Dynamic tasks such as reading, when fixation passes from one line to the next, or looking out of a train or car window to watch the ever-changing scene, are more likely to cause trouble from this source than watching television, which involves much smaller angular movements of the eyes. For this reason, the incorporation of a small horizontal prism in the prescription for a dyslexic patient may reduce the jumbling of letters (*see* Exercise 10.10).

Similarly, the patient's vision may be disturbed following changes in the distance of fixation. This is perhaps most likely where the oculo-motor balance differs significantly between distance and near vision.

Since dizziness or vertigo may occur with an incomitant heterophoria, the ocular motility should be tested in patients with this symptom. In the normal eye, a change in the pattern of innervation to the extraocular muscles is associated with a particular movement of the image across the retina. If this relationship is disturbed, for example, by a paresis of the right lateral rectus muscle, the right eye will no longer abduct as far on command as it did before. The resulting imbalance between innervation and retinal image movement makes the patient's surroundings appear to move. If the paresis is not too great, the patient may still have single binocular vision with an incomitant heterophoria rather than a heterotropia and diplopia.

Other causes of vertigo are variations in the blood supply to the brain and middle-ear defects, while some patients are worried initially by the magnification changes resulting from alterations to their spectacle prescription, especially to the astigmatic component.

A head tilt may also be produced in a heterophoric patient. Motility testing frequently shows that in depressed gaze the visual axes tend to converge, while in elevation divergence occurs. In pronounced cases, this type of motility is termed a V-pattern, while the opposite type of deviation is an A-pattern. An esophoric patient may then tend to tip his face downwards in order to obtain an elevated plane of regard with respect to the face, thus reducing the tendency for convergence. Conversely, the exophoric may tip his chin up. Head tilts may also occur in version heterophorias (*see* page 183), ocular muscle paresis or for psychological reasons.

With many patients, it is difficult to decide whether their symptoms are refractive or oculo-motor in origin. These two are not exclusive and simultaneous treatment of both may be required. Blurring of vision may also be caused by pathology anywhere in the visual system, while headaches, even those immediately around the eyes, may have a non-ocular cause. It is part of the ophthalmic practitioner's duty to consider these many other causes and refer for medical investigation when the ophthalmic findings do not appear an adequate cause.

Treatment of heterophoria

It is possible to give only a few general guidelines on when and how to help a heterophoric patient, since the decision has to be based on the experience of the practitioner. Having discovered the patient's symptoms, the first step is an accurate refraction and then the measurement of the oculo-motor balance. If an esophoric finding is obtained in the young patient, it is often advisable to recheck the refraction under cycloplegia to verify that there was no large error of latent hypermetropia or pseudo-myopia present.

In general, there should be no need to treat the oculo-motor imbalance either by refractive, prismatic or orthoptic means in the absence of symptoms. Fixation-disparity tests may be used to help decide whether or not a heterophoria is significant, but no hard and fast rule can be given. The authors' experience with the Turville infinity balance and the fixation disparity units is that a number of apparently symptom-free patients show an uncompensated heterophoria, while some patients have an apparently compensated heterophoria, and yet are happier with prismatic help. Pickwell *et al.* (1991) investigated the fixation disparity in 383 patients. The group was subdivided by age and whether they were symptomatic or asymptomatic for distance and near vision. In distance vision, horizontal fixation disparity measured with the present spectacles or unaided, as appropriate, showed a similar distribution in both symptomatic and asymptomatic people for all age groups, suggesting that fixation disparity was a poor indicator of symptoms. In near vision, they concluded that an exophoric fixation disparity requiring 2Δ or more was indicative of symptoms for the under-40 age group, 3Δ for the 40–59 age group, but that for the 60 and over group, many asymptomatic patients showed a need for 4Δ or more base-in aligning prism. Obviously, some of the symptomatic patient's symptoms may have been caused by refractive changes or non-ocular reasons.

This confirms the present writer's (RBR) approach, in which indications for vertical aligning prism and base-out prism (or near additions) are nearly always prescribed, while small exophoric deviations, especially in near vision, are ignored unless confirmed empirically by increased comfort or clarity viewing the chart or

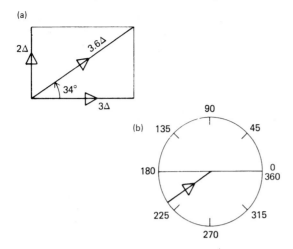

Figure 10.15. (a) Compounding vertical and horizontal prisms into a single oblique prism. (b) Use of the 360° protractor for specifying prism base setting.

near test types, or better recovery in the cover test. If only a small prism is indicated, it may be worth reversing it so as to increase the heterophoria. If comfort is unimpaired, prismatic help is probably unnecessary.

Patients showing deep suppression of one eye are almost certainly best left without prismatic aid.

Orthoptic treatment is best reserved for those patients who are under about 30 years of age. It is particularly useful for those patients who may thereby avoid the need for spectacles (for more details, refer to Evans, 1997; Edwards and Llewellyn, 1988, or other texts).

Inaccurate optical centration, whether horizontal or vertical, is an important possible source of discomfort with spectacles. For example, a pair of plus lenses with their optical centres several millimetres too wide could give enough base-out prism effect to decompensate an exophoria or to create discomfort because of the extra convergence needed. This is more likely to happen in near vision because of the greater possibility of centration errors (*see* Exercise 10.4 on page 189) and higher positive lens powers.

In Great Britain and some other countries, the term centration distance CD is used to denote the intended distance between the right and left optical centres, or between the two points at which prescribed prism is to be measured. It is important when ordering spectacles always to state the required centration distance (and also the vertex distance if the lens powers are numerically over about ±5.00 D).

When a prismatic component is added to a prescription, it is written after the lens power, for example:

R + 4.00/−2.50 × 140 4Δ base-in CD 64

The base setting of the prism is specified as up, down, in (towards the nose) or out, as the case may be. If prism power is needed in both the horizontal and vertical directions, it is customary to give the vertical component first, as in the example:

L + 2.00/−1.00 × 20 2Δ base-down and 3Δ base-in CD 61

Oblique prisms can be specified in two different ways. One is to state the orientation in standard axis notation,

followed by the word up or down to resolve the ambiguity as to the position of the base. For example, the prism combination specified in the last example could be compounded into the single prism 3.60Δ base 34 down (*Figure 10.15a*). Alternatively, if the 0–360° protractor is used, the same prism would be completely specified by 3.60Δ base 214 (*Figure 10.15b*).

The dominant eye

Although the majority of patients have binocular vision, this must not be interpreted as meaning that the two eyes are equally important. Similarly, there are few ambidextrous people. In most cases, ocular and hand dominance are both right or both left, which is to be expected since the dominant side of the body tends to be related to the functionally more important, but opposite, cerebral hemisphere. Hughes (1953) found that some 15% of his sample population were left dominant, although about half of these had become right-handed through education. Genuine crossed dominance of hand and eye does occur.

The dominant eye is the one which contributes most to the visual percept: it is easier in general to suppress the non-dominant eye. Thus, when lining up two objects, for example, one relies on the dominant eye even if the non-dominant eye is kept open. Again, it is usually the dominant eye which is used with monocular instruments, such as a camera or focimeter.

Clinically, it is useful to know which is the dominant eye. Some patients are uncomfortable if their dominant eye is fractionally blurred, for example over-plussed by 0.25 DS relative to the other eye. Later on in life, senile lens or macular changes cause more worry if the dominant eye shows the greater deterioration in acuity. On the other hand, a small uncorrected or residual refractive error in the non-dominant eye only may possibly not give any discomfort.

There are many different methods aimed at identifying the dominant eye. On pages 156–157, about the cyclopean eye, it was shown that our two separate uniocular views are fused unconsciously into a single mental percept, which could be regarded as the projection or view from the cyclopean eye. This imaginary eye is, in general, not situated midway between the two eyes but is positioned nearer to the dominant eye. Alignment tests for dominance are based on this displacement. The patient clasps both hands together with the forefingers outstretched together. The patient is then asked to swing the hands up to point at a distant object, or perhaps at the practitioner's eye, the practitioner standing on the opposite side of the room. Because both hands are held together, hand dominance is eliminated while the fingers are instinctively lined up with the object and the cyclopean eye. The hands will therefore tend to be placed nearer in line with the dominant eye and often the patient will then move them over to give an exact line with the dominant eye. Similar tests, which are also held in both hands, are Parson's cone or manoptoscope and the Dolman card. They use a screening aperture which allows the patient to see the fixation object with only one eye. The aperture is lined up instead of the hand.

Carter (1960) and Mallett (1964) have independently found that the eye which shows a fixation disparity is nearly always the non-dominant eye. Some patients show a disparity in both eyes. If no disparity is seen, it may be induced for this purpose by adding equal prism before each eye until a displacement is shown. The results of these workers suggests that marked ocular dominance is less common than alignment tests would predict.

A further and objective method of determining ocular dominancy is to investigate either the convergence–divergence movements of the eyes, or the near point of convergence. Two pencils of different colours are held up in the median plane before the patient's eyes, say at 150 and 500 mm, and the patient is asked to look at first one and then the other. The faster moving eye is the dominant eye. In determining the near point of convergence, at some point the non-dominant eye often ceases to adduct and suddenly abducts. In practice, these two tests may be indeterminate because the speed of movement in the two eyes may be so similar as to render judgement impossible.

Some patients, especially anisometropes, may have acquired a different ocular dominance in near and distance vision. Consider an uncorrected unilateral low myope: the emmetropic eye is likely to be used for distance vision, the myopic eye for near vision.

When the dominant eye has been identified, the Turville infinity balance test can be used to ensure that the dominant eye has, if possible, the better acuity. The non-dominant eye should not, however, be deliberately fogged.

Some patients, as a result of occupational conditions or hand dominance, may place close work significantly to one side: this may be worth considering when ordering the insetting of bifocal segments (*see* Hughes, 1953 for further references on this subject).

Tonic convergence and heterophoria

Referring to *Figure 9.2*, tonic convergence is that produced by the natural tonus in the extra-ocular motor system, bringing the eyes from the position of anatomical rest to the fusion-free or dissociated position. Because the position of anatomical rest is unknown, tonic convergence is measured both clinically and experimentally from the parallel position for distance fixation. In the dark, a position of convergence to about 110 cm occurs (*see* page 159).

This tonus can be reduced by prolonged occlusion, as opposed to the few seconds of the normal dissociation test. Dowley (1987) found a much wider spread of horizontal heterophoria in his subjects after 5.5 h of occlusion, than initially. He postulated, therefore, that there was an adaptive mechanism bringing the oculo-motor system towards orthophoria.

Conversely, the effect of working at an exceptionally close distance (20 cm) was found by Wolf *et al.* (1987) and Ehrlich (1987) to give a short-lived esophoric shift.

Ehrlich's results showed that this shift was greater in subjects who were exophoric rather than esophoric before commencing the near vision task, and in those who had to accommodate more from their natural accommodative resting state, thus inducing more accommodative convergence.

Yekta *et al.* (1987) and Pickwell *et al.* (1987) found an increase in exophoria and exophoric fixation disparity (both in angular amount and aligning prism) after a day's study or half an hour's close reading at 20 cm. This again was interpreted to indicate fatigue of the visual system.

Adaptation to prisms and lenses has been studied by North and Henson (1981, 1982, 1985) and North *et al.* (1986), among others. In general they found that if, for example, base-in prism is placed before the eyes, an immediate shift to esophoria occurs when measured through the prism. This rapidly declines over a minute, the heterophoria returning towards its initial level despite the presence of the prism. The longer the period of adaptation to the prism, the longer the decay back to the original phoria on removal of the prism. This confirms the idea of a fast and slow controller of tonic vergence (*see* end of Chapter 9).

Clinically, this might suggest that the patients having an uncompensated heterophoria would obtain no relief from a prescribed prism. They point out, however, that patients with oculo-motor symptoms may be poorer at adapting to prisms, though these findings were not supported by Pickwell and Kurtz (1986). In another approach, Tunnacliffe and Williams (1985, 1986) measured the contrast sensitivity (*see* pages 51–55) under binocular conditions. They found a significant drop in the binocular contrast sensitivity function compared with the monocular in the presence of an unwanted 0.5 or 1Δ vertical prism, or a horizontal prism of 2Δ or more outside the region between the active to passive position, for example, 6Δ base-in when there is only 4Δ of exophoria. They concluded that despite an adaptation to heterophoria as established by dissociation tests, the visual system was under-performing. This in turn may be of significance when sizeable prismatic effect is induced in a spectacle correction because of poor centration. An excellent review article on prism adaptation is given by Sethie (1986).

Cyclophoria

Types of cyclophoria

The heterophorias so far described have been either lateral, vertical or, when these two coexist, oblique. It is also possible for the eyes to show a torsional heterophoria. Such deviations around the line of sight when the eyes are dissociated are called cyclophorias. By analogy with the classification of ocular torsion, the best of several methods of classifying cyclophoria is as follows:

(1) *Incyclophoria.* The upper vertical meridian of either eye rotates inwards towards the median plane when dissociated (*Figure 10.16a*).

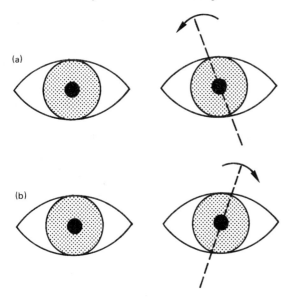

Figure 10.16. Examiner's view of (a) incyclophoria and (b) excyclophoria.

(2) *Excyclophoria.* The upper meridian of either eye rotates outwards away from the median plane when dissociated (*Figure 10.16b*).

Subjectively, the visual scene will appear to tilt in the opposite direction to the phoria. In theory, this could be demonstrated by the subjective cover test. Cyclophoria may frequently coexist with vertical deviations due to the torsional actions of the vertically acting extra-ocular muscles. The possible causes of cyclophoria are similar to those of the other heterophorias, namely: re-fractive, anatomical, neurological and pathological. To these we may add proximal, while refractive cyclophoria also needs explanation. The importance of refractive cy-clophoria has been exaggerated by many authors. Their argument is as follows. In general, a spectacle lens produces a magnification of the retinal image, equal in all directions if the lens is spherical. A cylindri-cal component of a lens, however, magnifies only in the direction perpendicular to the cylinder axis.

In general, a line viewed through an astigmatic spec-tacle lens incorporating a minus cylinder appears tilted towards the cylinder axis. *Figure 10.17* illustrates an ex-ample in which only the left lens is astigmatic. A vertical line is therefore imaged vertically on the right retina, whereas the retinal image in the left eye is tilted towards

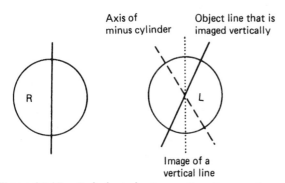

Axis of minus cylinder

Object line that is imaged vertically

R

L

Image of a vertical line

Figure 10.17. Cyclophoria due to an astigmatic correction at an oblique axis.

the cylinder axis, in this case, with the top inwards. In order for a line to be imaged on the vertical meridian of the retina of a newly corrected patient, it would have to be tilted top outwards, suggesting excyclophoria.

Since real surroundings, as opposed to test objects for cyclophoria, cannot be tilted so that the retinal images fall on corresponding meridians, the eyes make a com-pensatory torsional movement. After a period of time, this becomes habitual, resulting in a cyclophoria. In the example shown in *Figure 10.17*, the compensatory movement would be an inward rotation of the upper vertical meridian, resulting in an incyclophoria .

The major fallacy of this argument is that it ignores the scissors nature of astigmatic distortion in the cor-rected eye. As shown in *Figure 13.8* on page 235, a hor-izontal line also appears tilted towards the minus cylinder axis, that is, in the opposite direction to the tilt of the vertical line. Thus if the patient were tested for cy-clophoria with horizontal instead of vertical lines, the opposite results would now be found. The preponder-ance of vertical lines in our surroundings, for example, buildings, trees, the upright limbs of letters, perhaps gives some slight plausibility to the theory.

The tilt shown in the diagrams is greatly exaggerated for ease of illustration. For example, if the astigmatic lens were:

$$\text{plano}/-4.00\,\text{DC}\times135$$

fitted at 16 mm from the eye's entrance pupil, it can be shown (equation 13.20 on page 235) that the apparent tilt of distant horizontal and vertical lines would be just less than $2°$ in each case. Other factors being equal, the tilt is approximately proportional to the cylinder power. Assuming that the ocular astigmatism is due to the cornea, the tilt in the uncorrected eye is negligible since the cornea is so close to the entrance pupil. A full discussion of astigmatic line rotation will be found on pages 234–236.

To summarize on refractive cyclophoria, the condition is induced on correction and depends on the orientation of the test lines for cyclophoria relative to the axes of as-tigmatism. The uncorrected astigmat should not be troubled, but on first correction with spectacle lenses and on subsequent changes, difficulties may occur. These may not be due to cyclophoria but far more likely to changes in spatial perception arising from distortion of the image (*see*, for example, Ogle and Madigan, 1945).

Proximal cyclophoria is the term introduced by Rab-betts (1972) to describe that cyclophoria produced in near vision as a secondary effect of convergence and de-pression of the eyes. Because the eyes are no longer in the primary position, some false torsion (*see* pages 149–152) is expected, equal and opposite in direction in the two eyes. Cyclophoria is therefore predicted, but, in gen-eral, a lesser amount is found experimentally. Hermans (1944) gives results of a detailed survey of 104 subjects with no detected visual defect. He determined the cyclo-phoria at angles of elevation and depression up to $40°$ and monocular convergence up to $10°$. In the primary position there was almost zero cyclophoria. At the pos-ition normally used in near vision, a depression of about $20°$ and convergence of about $4°$ by each eye,

Figure 10.18. Synoptophore slides for cyclophoria.

less than 0.5° of cyclophoria was found, compared with 0.7° predicted by the standard false torsion equations. In positions of greater convergence or depression, and especially convergence in elevated gaze, higher amounts of cyclophoria were found.

Measurement of cyclophoria

There is no standard clinical test for cyclophoria. This is partly because very few patients have significant amounts of cyclophoria, while fewer still have symptoms. In any case there is very little that can be done to help such patients by direct treatment of the condition, although the symptoms can perhaps be relieved as described below. Ames invented a spectacle device for the correction of cyclophoria (Lancaster, 1928) but it was necessarily complicated and has fallen into disuse.

In theory, Maddox rods may be placed before both eyes with their axes accurately vertical, thus giving a horizontal line. A vertical prism of about 5Δ will then produce vertical separation of the lines, since it is greater than the comfortable fusional reserve of most patients. If one line appears tilted with respect to the other, one of the rods may be rotated to give parallelism. The angle and direction of the required rotation gives the cyclophoria. In practice, it is not possible to place the rods in the trial frame with sufficient accuracy, while those mounted in a refractor head are incapable of rotation.

Test slides (*Figure 10.18*) are available for mounting in a synoptophore, and a similar design could be used with a hand stereoscope. A horizontal line is seen by one eye, while a pair of lines, one above and one below, are seen by the other eye. In order to reduce the effects of secondary muscle actions, horizontal and vertical heterophorias are kept under control by the fixation dots seen binocularly. As a result, the parallel lines seen by one eye can be positioned close to the central line seen by the other eye, increasing the accuracy of the test. If the test line(s) for one eye can be rotated about the fixation point, the cyclophoria can be measured, preferably by the bracketing method. Starting from a tilted position, the setting is recorded at which the patient reports that parallelism has been restored and the process is then repeated from the opposite direction.

The Maddox wing test incorporates a rotatable marker seen by the right eye which can be set parallel with the horizontal line viewed by the left eye (*Figure 10.10*).

The fixation disparity units can be used to detect the presence of cyclophoria, which is inferred if one of the monocular markers appears tilted. (Some patients erroneously call a displacement of one of the markers in a horizontal or vertical disparity a tilt.) If there is high astigmatism at an oblique axis, the test should be repeated with the markers at right angles to their original direction. An opposite tilt confirms that the effect is due to astigmatic distortion, while a tilt in the same direction confirms that it is due to cyclophoria.

In the presence of a pronounced cyclophoria, a monocular refraction can give incorrect values for the astigmatic axes. Binocular refraction is therefore preferable, especially when the astigmatism is marked. Moreover, the eyes will orientate themselves as they prefer with regard to the astigmatic scissors distortion: parallelism of vertical contours in the field of view may be more important than parallelism of horizontal contours. Because of the close relationship between hyperphoria and cyclophoria, a patient suspected of having cyclophoria should be very carefully checked for hyperphoria, relieving prism being prescribed as necessary. This alone may be enough to relieve symptoms, especially if the astigmatic axes are verified under binocular conditions with the prismatic power in place.

A complicating factor in the measurement of cyclophoria may be that the meridians of the retina which perceptually relate to horizontal and vertical may not be truly horizontal and vertical. If so, the corresponding vertical meridians of the retinae will not be parallel, while the horizontal meridians through the foveae may not be in a straight line. The zero position for a cyclophorometer would have to allow for this deviation. One method of ascertaining the relationship of the corresponding vertical meridians of the two retinae is to compare the true (plumb-line) vertical and the retinal images that give a perceptual stereoscopic vertical. Rabbetts (1972) found that the objective and stereoscopic verticals coincided with no tilt of the retinal images, showing that the perceptually vertical meridians of the retinae were truly vertical.

Other oculo-motor defects

Dissociated vertical deviation

In right hyperphoria, the right eye deviates upwards under cover and the left eye downwards. In dissociated vertical divergence, the covered eye always moves upwards, whichever eye is covered, although the angles of deviation behind the cover may be different. On removal of the cover, the eye returns to its normal position, the uncovered eye not having moved unless the condition is associated with a horizontal heterotropia. The cause is probably defective supra-nuclear innervation of the oculo-motor nuclei. This condition has also been termed 'alternating hyperphoria' or 'alternating sursumduction'.

Version heterophorias

The heterophorias described earlier in this chapter were all vergence phorias. If, however, there is defective innervation to or by the supra-nuclear centres controlling version movements, there will be a bilateral limitation of movement in the affected direction of gaze, hence the term 'gaze palsy'. These are not shown by the dissociative tests described earlier in this chapter, but will be evident in the motility test. Thus, a patient may be unable to elevate the eyes as far as normal above the horizontal plane, giving a resultant tendency for the eyes to have a passive position in a plane distinctly depressed below the horizon: kataphoria. The patient will probably develop a head tilt, chin up (compare with pages 148 and 179), so that the eyes are depressed with respect to the head when the plane of fixation is straight ahead. Even in the normal subject, the range of elevation of the eyes is less than that of depression (*Figure 8.17*) and it is possible that the range of elevation reduces further with increasing age. Conversely, in anaphoria the eyes will tend to be elevated, depression being limited.

These unfamiliar terms can be avoided by describing the condition as a gaze palsy, with deficiency of gaze up or down. Lateral gaze palsies may also occur.

Nystagmus

Most patients can fixate an object steadily for a long time if the physiological movements of the eye which are too small for direct observation are disregarded. A few patients are unable to maintain fixation, their eyes showing perpetual involuntary movements to and fro. The movement is usually similar in direction and amount in the two eyes, but the speed of movement in one direction is frequently slower than the return movement. These oscillations may be lateral, vertical, oblique or torsional and are denoted by the term 'nystagmus'. The physiological optokinetic nystagmus induced by watching a moving object has already been introduced on page 38.

In some patients, nystagmus is produced by an obvious defect: for example, congenital opacities in the media prevent a good retinal image. As a result, the fovea and visual acuity may not develop fully, thus causing a poor fixational reflex. A similar result occurs in an albinotic eye because of light scatter in the eye and neural misrouting to the brain. Defective visual pathways to the cerebral cortex may again cause nystagmus if the lesion occurred in infancy or young childhood.

Other patients with nystagmus show no obvious cause. Their nystagmus will increase in frequency or amplitude on occluding either eye. Vision and refraction are therefore best determined by employing a binocular method such as the Humphriss fogging method, but with a +1.50 or +2.00 DS lens chosen in relation to the acuity.

End-position nystagmus may occur in extreme positions of gaze, as in motility testing. Small nystagmoid movements may often be seen, especially in the presence of paresis of an extra-ocular muscle. Acquired nystagmus may also occur in patients with defective co-ordination of the innervation, while miners' nystagmus was partly caused by spending long periods of time in low illumination. (For a further discussion of this defect of motility, *see* for example Lyle and Bridgeman, 1959; Walsh and Hoyt, 1969.)

Heterotropia (strabismus)

The essential difference between heterophoria and heterotropia is that in heterophoria, bifoveal fixation of the object of regard is maintained, whereas in heterotropia one eye deviates and the image in that eye does not fall on the fovea.

The nomenclature of heterotropia according to the direction of deviation of the eye follows that of heterophoria and has already been discussed. The deviation may be:

(1) *Unilateral.* The deviating eye takes up fixation only when the normally fixating eye is covered and deviates again immediately the cover is removed.
(2) *Alternating.* Either eye may fixate. Alternating strabismus is much less common than unilateral.

Some patients with alternating strabismus may change fixation readily from eye to eye: sometimes this can be achieved voluntarily and sometimes the direction of gaze determines which eye fixates. A few patients with a unilateral strabismus retain fixation with the normally deviating eye when the cover is removed during the cover test. Immediately the point of fixation is moved or the patient blinks, however, the dominant eye regains fixation. These tropias should not be classed as alternating.

All heterotropic patients may additionally be classified according to whether the deviation is intermittent or continuous. In a similar fashion to the development of visual acuity, the very young infant probably does not have binocular vision but develops this during the first few months of life. During this period, intermittent deviations of the eyes from binocular fixation can often be seen. After this first 6 months or so, co-ordinated movements of the two eyes should be well developed, with approximate bifoveal fixation. Some children appear never to have reached a stage where both visual axes become parallel in distance vision, but always manifest a deviation. It is probable, however, that most patients with heterotropia have at some time attained bifoveal fixation, only to lose it later.

In the early stages of the development of a squint, the deviation may often be intermittent. Bifoveal vision may be present most of the time, but when the patient is tired, ill, or, in the accommodative type of strabismus, paying critical attention to the object of regard, the deviation may then appear.

Strabismus may be subdivided yet again according to whether the angle of deviation is constant (comitant or concomitant) or variable. Particularly if the strabismus is of muscular origin or if secondary muscular changes (*see* page 189) are pronounced, the angle of squint may vary with the direction of gaze; for example, if there is a paralysed right lateral rectus muscle, there may be a marked right esotropia on looking to the right, yet the eyes may be almost straight when looking to the left. Such a strabismus is incomitant, described on page 148. Different primary and secondary deviations may also be shown, depending on which eye is fixating.

Causes of heterotropia

In many respects, the causes of a heterotropia are similar to those of heterophoria, but the deficiency or deficiencies may be more pronounced or the ability to overcome the difficulties may be less well developed.

Refractive

A hypermetropic error may cause esophoria, but should the patient become ill, much more nervous energy may be needed to provide sufficient accommodation to correct the error. There will simultaneously be a greatly increased esophoria which the debilitated person may not be able to control. The deviation becomes manifest as an esotropia. Thus, the parents of a strabismic child often say that an illness such as measles caused the squint at an age between $2\frac{1}{2}$ and 4 years. The illness was merely the trigger and not the basic cause. If such a child is promptly refracted under cycloplegia and a full refractive correction worn, the strabismus is rapidly cured. An accommodative squint of this kind is often called a Donders' squint.

Unfortunately, if several months or even years elapse before the child is brought for examination, the refractive correction may only reduce the angle of strabismus. Secondary sensory and motor sequelae to the deviation (described below) prevent an immediate elimination of the strabismus.

Anatomical

Any anatomical defect within the orbit can predispose to a strabismus. A small obstacle following trauma in an adult, for example, may cause only a heterophoria, but in the infant may prevent binocular vision ever being attained.

Neurological

In addition to any defects at or below the oculo-motor nuclei, the influence of the higher neural paths must be remembered. Defects in the reflex paths such as those of fixation, or those originating in the middle ear or a failure of co-ordination between various centres, may all contribute or predispose to a strabismus. Central co-ordination may temporarily be affected during the childhood infectious diseases, giving yet another difficulty to the uncorrected hypermetropic child.

Pathological

Anatomical damage to the lateral walls of the orbit, the lateral recti or the sixth cranial nerve may be caused by the use of forceps during birth. Transient pathology such as a haemorrhage in an extra-ocular muscle in childhood may induce a strabismus, even though no trace of pathology may be detected later.

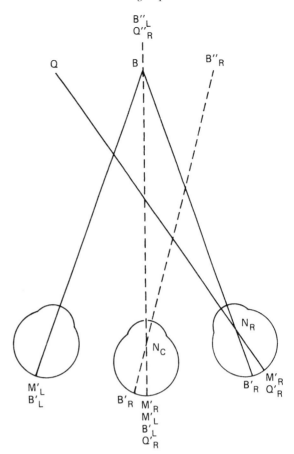

Figure 10.19. The projection through the cyclopean eye of the retinal images in right esotropia: normal retinal correspondence.

Sensory sequelae to strabismus

Suppression and amblyopia

Figure 10.19 represents the eyes of a patient with right esotropia viewing a fixation object B. The image of B in the deviating eye falls on the nasal retina and should therefore be projected temporally. As a result the patient should see B in diplopia; indeed, this is what happens in a strabismus of sudden onset in an adult. It is the image of object Q which falls on the fovea of the deviating eye and would therefore be seen superimposed on B, giving rise to confusion.

Moreover, if normal retinal correspondence (the relationship between corresponding points described on pages 154–157) is maintained, every object in the field of view of the left eye that forms an image on the retina of the right eye will be seen in diplopia. This may be inferred from *Figure 10.20*.

In consequence, in the patient young enough for changes to occur, the brain will tend to disregard the image of the deviating eye – a process known as suppression. Because the central region of the retina has the highest acuity and largest representation in the occipital cortex, it is in this area that the most pronounced or deepest suppression will occur. Suppose two different objects, such as the letters F and L suggested by Javal, are presented one to each eye of a heterotropic patient

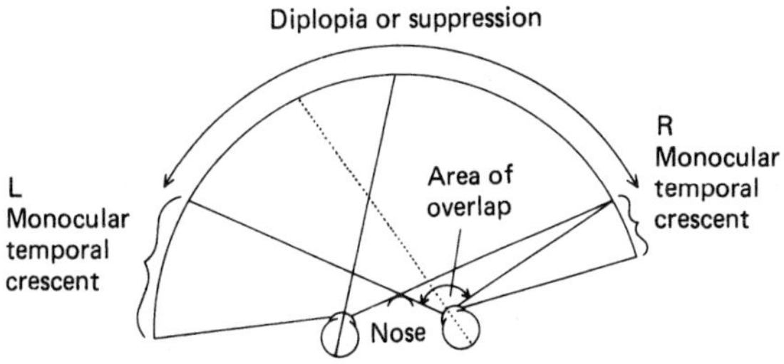

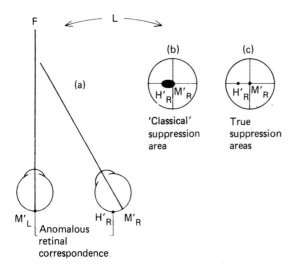

Figure 10.20. Field of diplopia in R esotropia (prior to secondary changes).

by means of a synoptophore (an instrument discussed on page 203). The normally fixating eye will see the letter F (*Figure 10.21a*) but the right eye will not seen the letter L. If the position of the letter L is moved relative to the eye, it may be possible to plot an area of suppression. This area will be affected by the nature and angular subtense of the test objects, but will include a large region around the macula M'_R and the point H'_R on the retina of the deviating eye that would receive the image of the fixation object in normal viewing conditions (*Figure 10.21b*).

This test is utterly unrealistic in that a patient does not in normal life have different objects presented to the two eyes. The results of such tests, commonly described in older texts on orthoptics, cannot be used to predict the state of the patient's binocular vision in normal surroundings. If suppression is investigated under conditions which cause little disturbance to normal vision, the large area found with the cruder techniques will shrink to a minute area at the fovea of the deviating eye and possibly another at H'_R (*Figure 10.21c*). One method that could be used is to project a spot of polarized light on to a metallic screen with the patient wearing an analysing visor so arranged that the fixating eye cannot see the spot. An unpolarized picture is simultaneously projected on to the screen to provide detail seen binocularly. Alternatively, the Stanworth synoptophore may be used (Mallett, 1970a,b).

The area of suppression tends to vary with the type of strabismus and depends on the nature of the correspondence between the elements of the two retinae. In virtually all patients, the fovea of the deviating eye is suppressed. As a result of this active inhibition, the acuity in this eye does not develop. It either remains retarded at the acuity level reached by the age of onset of the strabismus or may even deteriorate. This reduced acuity is known as strabismic amblyopia and has already been discussed on pages 42–43. It must be emphasized that amblyopia is a monocular condition, while suppression occurs when both retinae are stimulated. Even under the most artificial conditions, the deviating eye ceases to be suppressed when the normally fixating eye is occluded (the only exception to this may be the fovea). Some authorities regard amblyopia not as an undeveloped fovea, but as a fovea so greatly inhibited that the central portion no longer operates even in monocular vision. The reduced acuity then results from using a parafoveal area (*see* pages 36–37). Only if the strabismus is intermittent, alternating or of late onset will there be no amblyopia. Active treatment by refractive correction and occlusion of the better eye are necessary to reduce the amblyopia in cases of constant unilateral strabismus.

Anomalous retinal correspondence

In the young patient of less than 3–5 years of age, the onset of strabismus is followed temporarily by suppression. Provided that the angle of deviation remains approximately constant, the retinal correspondence is shifted, so that the fovea of the deviating eye no longer

Figure 10.21. Suppression in strabismus. (a) Presentation of Javal FL to a patient with right esotropia. (b) 'Classical' suppression area on the retina. (c) True suppression areas when measured under conditions of normal vision.

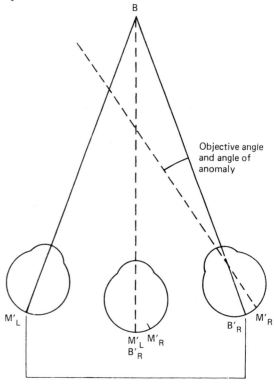

Figure 10.22. Harmonious anomalous retinal correspondence: objective angle equal to angle of anomaly.

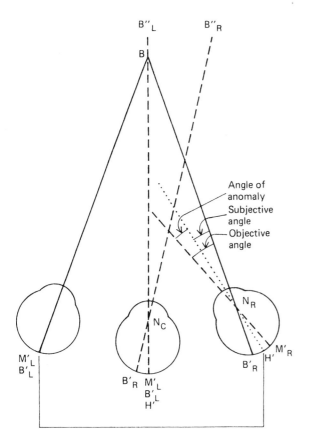

Figure 10.23. Unharmonious retinal correspondence: objective angle equals subjective angle plus angle of anomaly.

corresponds to that of the fixating eye. In *Figure 10.22*, point B'_R now corresponds to M'_L and so on for the remainder of the retina. A new retinal correspondence has been produced so that images in the two eyes again fall on corresponding points. This is called an anomalous (or abnormal) retinal correspondence (ARC). In this particular case, the ARC is said to be harmonious because the images fall on the 'adjusted' corresponding points. In such patients, diplopia will not exist in normal conditions so that suppression will be minimal. The harmonious ARC acts as a positive factor allowing a partial return to binocular vision.

Patients with a consolidated harmonious ARC may have reasonable stereoscopic acuity if, say, the three-needle test is used (*see* Chapter 11). Since stereoscopic vision is regarded as the highest grade of binocular vision, it is not strictly correct to describe the strabismic patient possessing this faculty as not having binocular vision. For this reason, the authors have preferred to use the term 'bifoveal fixation' to describe the attribute of the normal, but quite frequently, heterophoric, patient.

The angle through which the retinal correspondence has been shifted from the normal is called the angle of anomaly.

Because the retinal images fall on corresponding points, the deviating eye projects them in the same direction as the fixating eye. When this eye is covered, no apparent movement of the surroundings will be seen. Thus, in harmonious ARC, the subjective angle of the

heterotropia is zero, while the objective angle equals the angle of anomaly.

Some patients show an unharmonious ARC, in which the angle of anomaly does not equal the angle of deviation. In *Figure 10.23* the left fovea M'_L corresponds with point H' on the right retina. Object B is imaged nasally to H' at B'_R and hence is projected temporally to B''_R. The subjective angle of the strabismus is $B'_R \hat{N}_R H'$, or the angle through which the eye must turn before B is imaged on H'. The objective angle is the angle between the visual axis and BB'_R. The angle of anomaly could be determined in theory by using a synoptophore and asking the patient to superimpose two similar slides. The cover test will then reveal the angle of anomaly. In practice, the patient will probably show suppression to avoid diplopia.

Unharmonious ARC in real life may be due to a change in angle of deviation of a mature patient's strabismus after a deeply ingrained harmonious ARC had been developed. *Figure 10.23* represented a patient whose angle had increased. It is instructive to draw a similar diagram for a patient whose angle has decreased, perhaps by surgical intervention, to show that the direction of diplopia is apparently paradoxical, that is, crossed in an esotropia. The conditions of examination may produce an apparently unharmonious ARC in a patient with harmonious ARC. This is discussed below.

Tests for strabismus and retinal correspondence

The only satisfactory test for strabismus is the objective cover test, already described on pages 169–171. The prism recovery test described under the screening of young children (*see* page 371) and, to some extent, the presence or absence of stereopsis (*see* Chapter 11) may also be employed to evaluate a patient's binocular status. A few patients are unable to straighten their deviating eye; they may have extremely poor fixation or be too unco-operative to examine with the cover test. The angle of strabismus may be estimated in these cases by asking the patient to fixate a small bright light, an instinctive act if this is the only light in a dark room. The relative positions of the corneal reflexes in the two eyes may then be observed: the Hirschberg test. According to Lyle and Bridgeman (1959), the deviation is 10–15° (17–27Δ) when the reflex appears on the margin of the pupil (assumed to be 4 mm in diameter); about 25° (47Δ) when halfway between pupil margin and limbus and 45° when on the limbus. Alternatively, a displacement of 1 mm in the position of the reflex relative to the centre of the pupil may be equated to a deviation of about 22Δ in an adult (Brodie, 1987; Eskridge *et al.*, 1988), and because of the steeper cornea, to around 27Δ in an infant (Eskridge *et al.*, 1990). This test, like the cosmetic appearance of a strabismus, is influenced by the angle λ between the visual and pupillary axes (*see* page 221).

Another casual method is to compare the relative amounts of sclera seen on either side of the cornea in each eye. If there is much less nasal sclera than usual

Table 10.4 Example of calculation of angles of anomaly

Angle	Habitual angle in play (Δ)	Total angle in play (Δ)
Objective angle	15	22
Subjective angle	0	7
Angle of anomaly	15	15

in one eye, an esotropia is suggested. Some children have a very shallow bridge to the nose, giving an abnormally wide fold of skin on either side of it. This is termed 'epicanthus' and can give a misleading impression of esotropia, although such patients may indeed have esotropia as well as the epicanthus.

Whereas the subjective cover test may be used in heterophoria to measure the angle of deviation, the presence of ARC in a heterotropic patient gives a subjective angle different from the objective angle. Only if normal retinal correspondence and normal projection are maintained by the squinting eye will the fixation object appear to jump through the objective angle when the fixating eye is covered. In harmonious ARC there will be no apparent movement of the object on covering the good eye. Nevertheless, if the cover test were repeated several times, it is possible that the objective angle of the strabismus would change. This gives the important concepts of:

(1) *Habitual angle of strabismus.* The objective angle normally maintained by the patient under undisturbed conditions.
(2) *Total angle of strabismus.* The objective angle following prolonged or repeated dissociation of the eyes.

(The difference between the habitual and total angles implies that the ARC may induce some motor fusion to hold the eyes at the habitual angle.)

In the presence of a consolidated harmonious ARC, the change from the habitual to the total angle of strabismus does not normally affect the angle of anomaly. For example, if a patient with 15Δ of habitual esotropia was found to have a total angle of 22Δ, the fixation object in this latter state would appear to jump through 7Δ, but this is not an indication of unharmonious ARC. As shown in *Table 10.4*, the angle of anomaly remains 15Δ.

Another cause of a false indication of an unharmonious ARC is the proximal convergence induced by measuring strabismus with instruments such as the synoptophore. The test objects are viewed at optical infinity, but the proximal convergence induced by looking into an instrument which is obviously close to the eyes may increase the habitual angle of an esotrope in a manner similar to the above example.

Perhaps the simplest and least unnatural test for ARC is the Bagolini striated glass (Bagolini and Capobianco, 1965). These lenses produce a faint streak of light at right-angles to the striations when a small bright source of light is viewed through them. Unlike the Maddox rod, they enable the surroundings to be seen quite clearly, only a slight reduction in visual acuity

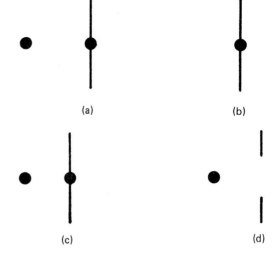

Figure 10.24. Appearance of the streak when the Bagolini striated glass is placed before the right eye in R esotropia: (a) normal retinal correspondence, (b) harmonious ARC, (c) unharmonious ARC, (d) unharmonious ARC and partial suppression. Note the narrower separation in (c) compared with (a).

being caused. Normal vision is thus virtually undisturbed.

The patient views a spot of light such as a naked torch bulb in an illuminated room. When the strabismus is unilateral, only one Bagolini glass is needed. This is placed before the deviating eye to produce a vertical streak. It is useful to demonstrate the streak to the patient by first holding the glass for a few moments before the fixating eye.

If the patient has normal retinal correspondence, the streak and the spot of light seen by the deviating eye will probably be suppressed to avoid diplopia. If there is no suppression, the spotlight will be seen in diplopia with the streak passing through the diplopic image (*Figure 10.24a*).

In harmonious ARC, only one spot will be seen with the streak passing through or very close to the spot (*Figure 10.24b*). The streak often passes within 0.5Δ of the spot rather than exactly through it. This should be regarded as a type of fixation disparity and not an unharmonious ARC. The Bagolini glasses show that a very high proportion of strabismic patients have harmonious ARC.

When unharmonious ARC is present, the spot will in theory be seen in diplopia (*Figure 10.24c*), but the angle of diplopia will not correspond with the objective angle. The streak will again pass through the diplopic image of the spot.

In some patients, suppression of the retinal area in the squinting eye that receives the image of the fixation object is so marked that the streak will not be seen at all, or sometimes shows a gap (*Figure 10.24d*). Thus, the diplopia of a true unharmonious ARC may be masked.

Some patients may change fixation to the normally deviating eye in order to see the streak, which will then pass through the light. For this reason the Bagolini glass should be used with a cover test to verify that the eye behind the glass is still deviating. To check for ARC in the vertical direction, the glass is rotated to give a horizontal streak.

In alternating strabismus, two glasses must be used, placed obliquely so that the streaks form an 'X' (St. Andrew's cross). In harmonious ARC, these will intersect at the spot of light whichever eye is fixating.

Uncertainty about the size of the subjective and objective angles in the strabismic patient makes a full study of ARC somewhat time consuming. Moreover, the false conditions of examination with an instrument such as a synoptophore with its reduced field of view may cause the patient to change from, say, harmonious ARC back to normal retinal correspondence. Hence, the various tests for ARC allow the depth of a patient's ARC to be graded. Patients with deep ARC may need to be given treatment for this before dealing with the angle of deviation, whereas ARC may be ignored if only slightly developed.

Motor sequelae to strabismus

Some strabismus is directly due to anatomical or neurological abnormalities. Even if the extra-ocular muscles were anatomically and physiologically normal before the onset of strabismus, months or years of deviation may eventually produce secondary changes in the muscles. In a high esotropia, for example, the lateral rectus may be permanently elongated while the medial rectus remains in contracture. Eventually, the ability of the eye to abduct may become restricted. A motility test might initially show relatively little disproportion between the left and right eyes, although the fields are laterally displaced. Later on, the fields may take an appearance similar to that produced by an extra-ocular muscle palsy. In the presence of a well-established ARC that does not break down on investigation of the motility, the subjective angle recorded will differ from the objective angle. As a result of both motor and sensory changes, deviation that might have been readily cured by refractive and/or orthoptic means soon after onset may become very difficult to cure after only a few years.

Examination and treatment of the strabismic patient

The examination must include a thorough history of the patient: type of birth, whether premature or if forceps were needed; age at the onset of the strabismus; childhood illnesses; any previous treatment including spectacles, occlusion, orthoptics, surgery; whether parents or relations have strabismus or have to wear spectacles (or contact lenses).

A thorough refractive examination of the patient is essential. With a young child, it is necessary to use objective methods such as retinoscopy to determine the distance refractive error and dynamic retinoscopy to check that full reserves of accommodation are present. The child should then be refracted again under cycloplegia; 1% cyclopentolate should be adequate, with 2 drops in each eye probably being indicated if the irides are exceptionally dark in colour.

Those hypermetropes whose esotropia is refractive in origin will show a reduced angle or may become heterophoric with correction of the error. Even when the angle is not totally eliminated, constant wear of the correction must be ordered, since the residual angle may decrease still further with time. If left uncorrected, the child may develop motor changes, making later treatment less likely to succeed.

If amblyopia is present, occlusion should be prescribed together with a refractive correction. If the error is at all large, occlusion alone without spectacles is a waste of time.

Patients with convergence excess, that is, those who show (greater) esotropia in near vision, may be further helped by bifocals, while exotropic patients may be able to control their deviation better if given a negative spherical addition to their lenses (somewhat as suggested on page 175).

The study of heterotropia covers many facets, not all of which have been mentioned in this chapter. For example, false projection and classical eccentric fixation of several prism dioptres of eccentricity* have purposely been ignored as being outside the scope of the present text.

Exercises

10.1 A $+3.00\,$DS bilateral hypermetrope is orthophoric with spectacles and has an AC/A ratio of $3\Delta/$D. What is the predicted heterophoria in distance and near vision at 40 cm without spectacles?

10.2 (a) A $-4.00\,$DS bilateral myope is 6Δ exophoric in distance and near vision. Discuss whether his spectacles need to be accurately centred to PD, and if not, what latitude in optical centration would be admissible in dispensing? (b) Repeat the above, but for an exophoric hypermetrope.

10.3 (a) A $+5.00\,$D bilateral hypermetrope has a fixation disparity of 1Δ base-up right eye. What decentration of each lens is required to correct the disparity? (b) Repeat the above, but for a $-2.00\,$D myope.

10.4 A patient's prescription is R and L $+4.00\,$DS, add $+2.00\,$DS. Separate pairs are dispensed, both with incorrect centration distances of 70 mm instead of the correct 64 and 61 mm. What is the induced prismatic effect in each case?

10.5 The Freeman–Archer tangent scale shown in *Figure 10.9* is viewed by a patient with 10Δ of esophoria. The rod before the right eye is tilted through $5°$ anticlockwise. What is the false hyperphoria reading?

10.6 A patient views a fixation disparity unit at 6 m. One of the markers appears displaced through 20 mm. What is the angular fixation disparity and the displacement on the retina of a $+60\,$D reduced eye?

10.7 Draw the appearance of bilateral fixation disparity for both horizontal and vertical markers in incyclophoria.

10.8 The spectacle correction BE $+4.50\,$DS add $+1.50\,$D is made up as: (a) Executive-type bifocals; (b) plastics bifocals with each segment geometrically inset 2 mm. Given a separation of 64 mm between distance optical centres, what is the distance between the near optical centres of each pair and what

---

* Most amblyopes may be regarded as having a very small angle eccentric fixation, indicated by the reduction in visual acuity shown in *Figure 3.16*.

is the horizontal prismatic effect at the segment centre of each lens?

10.9 Repeat Exercise 10.8 for the prescription BE +12.00 DS add +3.00 D in plastics bifocals only.

10.10 A (dyslexic) patient suffers from slight diplopia and confusion when reading. If the print of these exercises is read from a distance of 300 mm, calculate the horizontal prism needed to displace the image in one eye by the equivalent of the width of four letters.

References

AMES, A.J.R. and GLIDDON, G.H. (1928) Ocular measurements. *Trans. Sect. Ophthal. Am. Med. As. 1928*, 102–175

BAGOLINI, B. and CAPOBIANCO, N.M. (1965) Subjective space in comitant squint. *Am. J. Ophthal.*, **59**, 430–442

BARNARD, N.A.S. and THOMSON, W.D. (1995) A quantitative analysis of eye movements during the cover test – a preliminary report. *Ophthal. Physiol. Opt.*, **15**, 413–419

BORISH, I.M. (1970) *Clinical Refraction*, 3rd edn. Chicago: Professional Press

BRODIE, S.E. (1987) Photographic calibration of the Hirschberg test. *Invest. Ophthalmol. Vis. Sci.*, **28**, 736–742

CARTER, D.B. (1960) Studies in fixation disparity. III: The apparent uniocular components of fixation disparity. *Am. J. Optom.*, **37**, 408–419

DOWLEY, D. (1987) The orthophorization of heterophoria. *Ophthal. Physiol. Opt.*, **7**, 169–174

EDWARDS, K.H. and LLEWLLYN, R.D. (1988) *Optometry*. London: Butterworths

EHRLICH, D.L. (1987) Near vision stress: vergence adaptation and accommodative fatigue. *Ophthal. Physiol. Opt.*, **7**, 353–357

ESKRIDGE, J.B., PERRIGIN, D.M. and LEACH, N.E. (1990) The Hirschberg test: correlation with corneal radius and axial length. *Optom. Vis. Sci.*, **67**, 243–247

ESKRIDGE, J.B., WICK, B. and PERRIGIN, D. (1988) The Hirschberg test: a double-masked clinical evaluation. *Am. J. Optom. Phys. Opt.*, **65**, 745–750

EVANS, B.J.W. (1997) *Pickwell's Binocular Vision Anomalies*, 3rd edn. Oxford: Butterworth-Heinemann

FREEMAN, H. (c.1950) The Freeman Near Vision Unit. London: R. Archer & Sons Ltd

FREIER, B.E. and PICKWELL, L.D. (1983) Physiological exophoria. *Ophthal. Physiol. Opt.*, **3**, 267–272

HERMANS, T.G. (1944) Torsion in persons with no known eye defect. *Am. J. Ophthal.*, **27**, 153–158

HUGHES, H. (1953) An investigation into ocular dominancy. *Br. J. Physiol. Optics*, **10**, 119–143

JENKINS, T.C.A., PICKWELL, L.D. and ABD-MANAN, F. (1992) Effect of induced fixation disparity on binocular visual acuity. *Ophthal. Physiol. Opt.*, **12**, 299–301

LANCASTER, W.D. (1928) The Ames spectacle device for the treatment of cyclophoria, with a report of a successful case. *Archs Ophthal., N.Y.*, **57**, 332–338

LYLE, T.K. and BRIDGEMAN, G.J.O. (1959) *Worth and Chavasse's Squint*, 9th edn. London: Baillière, Tindall & Cox

MALLETT, R.F.J. (1964) The investigation of heterophoria at near and a new fixation disparity technique. *Optician*, **148**, 547–551, 574–581

MALLETT, R.F.J. (1969) Binocular vision in strabismus. *Ophthal. Optn*, **9**, 812–824

MALLETT, R.F.J. (1970a) The Stanworth synoptoscope in the investigation and treatment of strabismus. *Ophthal. Optn*, **10**, 556–558, 571–573

MALLETT, R.F.J. (1970b) Anomalous retinal correspondence – the new outlook. *Ophthal. Optn*, **10**, 606–608, 621–624

MALLETT, R.F.J. (1983) A new fixation disparity test and its applications. *Optician*, **186**(4815), 11–15

MALLETT, R.F.J. and RADNAN-SKIBIN, R. (1994) The new dual fixation disparity test. *Optom. Today*, **34**(5), 32–34

NORTH, R.V. and HENSON, D.B. (1981) Adaptation to prism induced heterophoria in subjects with abnormal binocular vision or asthenopia. *Am. J. Optom.*, **58**, 746–752

NORTH, R.V. and HENSON, D.B. (1982) Effects of orthoptics upon the ability of patients to adapt to prism induced heterophoria. *Am. J. Optom.*, **59**, 983–986

NORTH, R.V. and HENSON, D.B. (1985) Adaptation to lens-induced heterophorias. *Am. J. Optom.*, **62**, 774–780

NORTH, R.V., SETHI, B. (née DHARAMSHI) and HENSON, D.B. (1986) Effects of prolonged forced vergence upon the adaptation system. *Ophthal. Physiol. Opt.*, **6**, 391–396

OGLE, K.N. (1950) *Researches in Binocular Vision*. Philadelphia: W. B. Saunders Co

OGLE, K.N. (1962) The optical space sense. In *The Eye*, Vol. 4 (Davson, H., ed.). New York and London: Academic Press

OGLE, K.N. and MADIGAN, L.F. (1945) Astigmatism at oblique axes and binocular stereoscopic spatial localisation. *Archs Ophthal., N.Y.*, **33**, 116–127

PICKWELL, L.D., GILCHRIST, J.M. and HESLER, J. (1988) Comparison of associated heterophoria measurements using the Mallett test for near vision and the Sheedy Disparometer. *Ophthal. Physiol. Opt.*, **8**, 19–25

PICKWELL, D., JENKINS, T. and YEKTA, A.A. (1987) The effect on fixation disparity and associated heterophoria of reading at an abnormally close distance. *Ophthal. Physiol. Opt.*, **7**, 345–347

PICKWELL, L.D. and KURTZ, B.H. (1986) Lateral short-term prism adaptation in clinical evaluation. *Ophthal. Physiol. Opt.*, **6**, 67–73

PICKWELL, L.D., KAYE, N.A. and JENKINS, T.C.A. (1991) Distance and new readings of associated heterotrophoria taken on 500 patients. *Ophthal. Physiol. Opt.*, **11**, 291–296

RABBETTS, R.B. (1972) A comparison of astigmatism and cyclophoria in distance and near vision. *Br. J. Physiol. Optics*, **27**, 161–190

SETHI, B. (1986) Vergence adaptation; a review. *Doc. Ophthalmol.*, **63**, 247–263

STEVENS, G.T. (1906) *The Motor Apparatus of the Eyes*. Philadelphia: F. A. Davis Co.

TAIT, E.F. (1951) Accommodative convergence. *Am. J. Ophthal.*, **34**, 1093–1107

TUNNACLIFFE, A.H. and WILLIAMS, A.T. (1985) The effect of vertical differential prism on the binocular contrast sensivity function. *Ophthal. Physiol. Opt.*, **5**, 417–424

TUNNACLIFFE, A.H. and WILLIAMS, A.T. (1986) The effect of horizontal differential prism on the binocular contrast sensitivity function. *Ophthal. Physiol. Opt.*, **6**, 207–212

WALSH, F.B. and HOYT, W.F. (1969) *Clinical Neuro-Ophthalmology*, 3rd edn, Vol. 1, pp. 130–349. Baltimore: Williams and Wilkins Co.

WOLF, K.S., CIUFFREDA, K.J. and JACOBS, S.E. (1987) Time course and decay of effects of near work on tonic accommodation and tonic vergence. *Ophthal. Physiol. Opt.*, **7**, 131–135

YEKTA, A.A., JENKINS, T. and PICKWELL, D.I. (1987) The clinical assessment of binocular vision before and after a working day. *Ophthal. Physiol. Opt.*, **7**, 349–352

Stereopsis and the stereoscope

Perception of depth and stereopsis

Monocular clues to depth perception

Though retinal local sign enables us to determine the direction of objects relative to the fixation axis, on its own it gives no indication of the distances of objects from the observer. A person with only one eye is able to judge the relative distances of objects in space by using various monocular clues to depth perception. Good coordination of the two eyes results in binocular vision in its highest form: stereoscopic vision or stereopsis. This enables us to judge the relative distances of objects with great precision, even in the absence of monocular clues.

Monocular clues are discussed in many textbooks on vision (for example, Davson, 1980) and will merely be summarized here.

(1) *Size*. The size of the retinal image varies directly with the angular subtense of the object and is also inversely proportional to the object distance. In normal circumstances, an image decreasing in size is not interpreted as a shrinking object but as an object of constant size moving away (a phenomenon known as size constancy). The distance of an object, provided it is familiar, can thus be judged by accumulated experience. The geometrical perspective of buildings provides a similar clue.

(2) *Overlap*. Nearer objects obstruct the view of more distant objects.

(3) *Aerial perspective*. Scattering of light in the atmosphere makes distant objects appear less clearly defined and often tones them with blue.

(4) *Shading*. The direction of illumination gives rise to shadows, thus giving texture to the surface.

(5) *Parallax*. As the observer moves, nearer objects appear to move in the opposite direction, further objects in the same direction as the observer. Moving objects show their own passage through the surroundings even in the absence of observer motion. Parallax and apparent size are probably the most important elements in driving.

(6) *Accommodation and convergence*. Although accommodation is adjusted to focus upon a near object, it is of little help in judging distance. Convergence, although a binocular function, is also of little aid.

The possibility of another mechanism serving specifically as an aid to depth perception of approaching or retreating objects has recently been postulated. Researches by Regan and Beverley (1978) have suggested the existence of 'looming detectors' in the visual system. These are neurons or groups of neurons, some sensitive to an increase and others to a decrease in the retinal image size of moving objects.

Stereoscopic vision

Stereoscopic vision is the ability to judge the relative distances of objects from the observer by means of binocular vision only. This ability depends on very small disparities between the retinal images in the two eyes.

In *Figure 11.1*, the object Q on the horopter through B, to which point both eyes are directed, is imaged on the corresponding points Q'_L and Q'_R. Point H, at the limit of Panum's fusional space, is imaged at H'_R coincident with Q'_R and at H'_L at the edge of Panum's area centred on Q'_L. It is this small disparity, $Q'_L H'_L$ which gives rise to stereopsis.[*]

For the purpose of analysis, *Figure 11.2* illustrates the more general case in which the two given object points Q and H are not in alignment with either eye. The line joining the right and left nodal points plays an important role as the common base of the two relevant triangles. Its length $2a$ clearly varies with the state of convergence, but can be taken without serious error as equal to the inter-pupillary distance under the same conditions. According to our sign convention, the distance ℓ from the inter-nodal base line to the object Q is negative and the distance $\Delta\ell$ is positive.

The small angle ϕ_Q subtended by the base line at Q is the binocular parallax of Q, while the angle ϕ_H is the binocular parallax of H. They are expressed in radians by the approximations

$$\phi_Q = -2a/\ell$$

---

[*] This is not meant to imply that stereopsis is possible only if the retinal images of a given point fall within Panum's areas. Ogle (1962) has shown that stereopsis is possible, even with images significantly outside these areas.

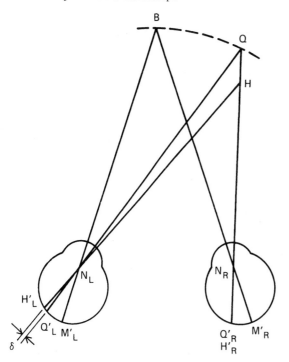

Figure 11.1. The retinal disparity δ associated with the depth QH in object space.

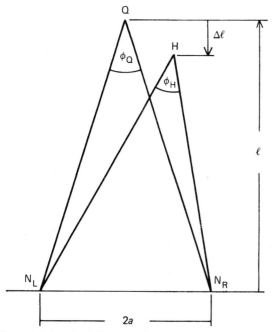

Figure 11.2. The difference in binocular parallax, θ_Q and θ_H respectively, of object Q and H at different distances.

and

$$\phi_H = -2a/(\ell + \Delta\ell)$$

with a and ℓ in the same units. The difference $(\theta_H - \theta_Q)$ is known as the relative binocular parallax and is given by

$$\phi_H - \phi_Q = \frac{-2a\Delta\ell}{\ell(\ell + \Delta\ell)} \tag{11.1}$$

$$\approx -2a\Delta\ell/\ell^2 \tag{11.1a}$$

if the quantity $\ell\Delta\ell$ is ignored as small in comparison with ℓ^2.

It can be seen from *Figure 11.1* that the relative binocular parallax in this case is the angle $H'_L N_L Q'_L$ and that this angle determines the total linear disparity δ between the positions of the retinal images of the two given points. In this case the disparity occurs in the left eye only, but if both object points were situated in the median plane the disparity δ would be equally divided between the two eyes.

Stereoscopic acuity is expressed in seconds of arc as the smallest angle η of relative binocular parallax that can be perceived. It can be determined from equation (11.1) by finding the smallest distance $\Delta\ell$ that can be seen as a difference in depth at a given object distance ℓ.

One method of measurement is the three-needle test. The subject views three vertical wires, the two outer ones being fixed in a fronto-parallel plane while the middle one is movable back and forth along the median plane. To obviate the important clue of parallax, the subject's head must be held still by some means. The three wires must be seen against a uniform background with their tops and bottoms screened so that the vertical angular subtense of all three remains constant. Fractional changes in the apparent width of the middle wire as it is moved may still provide a clue. To counteract this effect the wires may be replaced by the straight inner edges of two surfaces whose outer edges are screened from view. One edge is kept fixed while the other may be moved. A forced-choice statistical approach is normally used.

The forced-choice approach was introduced for a two-needle test by Howard (1919). In the Dolman modification often used in the USA, the subject moves the second rod by remote control into the same apparent plane as the first rod. The mean error in positioning in a series of trials is taken as a guide to stereo-acuity. Larson (1985) shows that the Howard–Dolman approach is much less satisfactory than the forced-choice approach.

The stereoscopic acuity of a trained observer is about 5 seconds of arc and can even be as fine as 2 seconds under favourable conditions. It improves with time allowed for observation up to about 1 second. Stereoscopic acuity is of the same order as vernier acuity, and both are much keener than line-width acuity. If η is taken as 5 seconds and the nodal point 16.7 mm from the retina, the disparity shown in *Figure 11.1* is as little as 0.0004 mm, much less than the diameter of a single retinal cone.

In equation (11.1a) the relative binocular parallax $(\theta_H - \theta_Q)$ is in radians. If it is replaced by its minimum perceptible value η in seconds of arc and the appropriate conversion factors are applied, the equation can be rearranged to give

$$\Delta\ell = \pm\frac{\eta\ell^2}{206 \times PD} \tag{11.2}$$

in which the denominator $2a$ has been replaced by the PD in millimetres. For example, given $\eta = 5$ seconds, $\ell = -1$ metre and PD = 65 mm, $\Delta\ell$ is found to be $\pm3.7 \times 10^{-4}$ m or ±0.37 mm. For other values of η, the value of $\Delta\ell$ would vary in proportion.

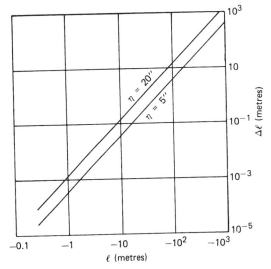

Figure 11.3. The minimum perceptible depth difference $\Delta\ell$ as a function of object distance ℓ for two values of the stereoscopic acuity. Both co-ordinates are scaled logarithmically.

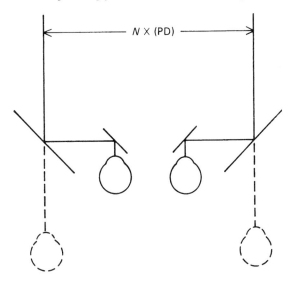

Figure 11.4. Optical arrangement of the telestereoscope.

It can also be seen from equation (11.2) that the minimum detectable depth $\Delta\ell$ is directly proportional to the square of the observation distance and inversely proportional to the base line or PD. *Figure 11.3* shows on logarithmic scales $\Delta\ell$ plotted against ℓ for two different stereoscopic acuities, 5 and 20 seconds of arc, the PD being taken as 65 mm. Since $\Delta\ell$ is proportional to ℓ^2, the scale factor for ℓ is twice that for $\Delta\ell$.

It may be further deduced that beyond a certain distance (sometimes known as the stereoscopic range), differences in depth, however great, cannot be perceived. This is the distance at which the base line subtends the same angle η as the subject's stereoscopic acuity. Beyond this distance, the binocular parallax of any object must be less than the angle η. Consequently, the relative binocular parallax must also be less than η, which by definition is the smallest perceptible value. For a PD of 65 mm, the limiting distance is about 2700 m when $\eta = 5$ seconds of arc but reduces to about 670 m when η has the poorer value of 20 seconds of arc.

Stereoscopic acuity declines:

(1) with increasing lateral separation of the test objects,
(2) at increasing angular distances from fixation.

In this latter respect it is similar to visual acuity, except that the maximum may occur at about 21 minutes of arc or slightly less from the central fovea. Measurements at various angles from fixation were made by Ogle (1962). At 6° from fixation he found stereoscopic acuity to diminish by a factor in the neighbourhood of 10–15.

Telestereoscopes, rangefinders and binocular telescopes

Equations (11.1) and (11.1a) show that depth perception can be improved by increasing the base line.

Another method is to magnify the retinal images, thus increasing the disparities on which stereoscopic vision depends (*Figure 11.1*).

The telestereoscope devised by Helmholtz consists essentially of two pairs of mirrors (*Figure 11.4*) so arranged that the inter-nodal base line is increased by the factor N. At the same time, the relative binocular parallax and the greatest distance distinguishable from infinity are also increased by the factor N. At the same time, the least perceptible difference in depth is decreased by the factor N.

These effects are enhanced if, in addition, a telescopic system magnifying M times is incorporated in each side of the instrument. The factor MN should now be included in the numerator of equations (11.1) and (11.1a) and in the denominator of equation (11.2). In theory, the least perceptible separation $\Delta\ell$ for a given distance ℓ should now be $1/MN$ times the corresponding value for the naked eyes. In practice, however, the magnification factor M is not as effective as predicted.

Optical rangefinders, which combine the two expedients just described, are of two different types: the coincidence and the stereoscopic. The former type combines half the field of view from each of the two separate viewing points and measures the adjustment needed to bring them into coincidence. The stereoscopic type depends upon the fact that if two marks, one placed before each eye, are seen stereoscopically, the apparent distance of the single percept depends on the lateral separation of the marks. These are adjusted to place the fused percept in the apparent plane of the object viewed. For further technical and descriptive detail, *see* Jacobs (1943), Patrick (1969) or Horne (1980).

Ordinary prism binoculars also give some enhancement of stereopsis. In those models using the conventional Porro prism erecting system, the separation of the objectives is usually at least 1.5 times the PD. With an 8× magnification, the product MN would have the value 12. It was shown earlier that the stereoscopic range of a person with stereoscopic acuity of 20 seconds of arc and PD 65 mm was about 670 m. With the binoculars just described, the range would be increased to 8040 m or approximately 8 km.

A coefficient of stereoscopic relief R may be defined as

$$R = N/M = \frac{\text{base-line magnification}}{\text{image magnification}}$$

A normal three-dimensional appearance of objects will be seen in binocular instruments if R is approximately equal to unity, as in unaided binocular vision.

Alteration of perspective

In general, perspective is altered when objects are viewed through magnifying devices, whether monocular or binocular. *Figure 11.5* illustrates schematically two objects of equal height at J and K viewed by an unaided observer stationed at A. The ratio of their angular subtenses at A is equal to KA/JA (1.5 in the drawing). If the observer now moves to the nearer point B, the ratio becomes KB/JB, which is clearly greater (2.0) than before. If the scene were viewed from A, through a telescope magnifying M times, the apparent angular subtense of each object would be multiplied by M, but the ratio would remain KA/JA. Nevertheless, the perspective is changed because the subjective effect of the magnification is to place the observer nearer to the scene, say, at B where the ratio ought to have the value KB/JB. The telescope has apparently diminished the relative height of the nearer object. With binocular telescopes, another effect of the angular magnification is to increase the convergence normally required when viewing near objects.

Changes in perspective are often more noticeable in photography. A comparison of photographs of the same scene taken through a wide-angle lens and a telephoto lens will show completely different perspective if the object distance is adjusted so that the image of the principal feature has the same size on each negative. Provided that the camera lens does not introduce distortion, pictures of a scene photographed from the same point through lenses of different focal lengths will all have the same perspective (*see*, for example, the illustrations in Langford, 1971, or other books on photography). For a correct impression of perspective, a photograph should be viewed from a distance given by the product of camera lens focal length and enlargement (ratio of print size to negative). The print then subtends the same angle at the eye as the original did at the camera lens. On the same principle, a projected image

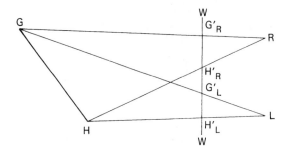

Figure 11.6. A basic method for producing a stereogram of the tilted line object GH.

should ideally be viewed from a distance v given by

$$v = (f'_c/f'_p)d \tag{11.3}$$

where f'_c is the focal length of the camera lens, f'_p the focal length of the projector lens and d the distance of the screen from the projector.

The stereoscope

To simulate the slightly different images obtained by the two eyes, a real three-dimensional scene or object can be photographed or drawn from two different viewing points. The resulting pair of two-dimensional pictures, called a stereogram or stereopair,* can then be viewed in a stereoscope, a special instrument enabling the observer to obtain a single three-dimensional percept of the original scene.

Figure 11.6 illustrates the two eyes (R and L) viewing an obliquely placed wall GH through a window WW. Because GH is tilted, its projection $G'_L H'_L$ on the window from the left viewpoint is smaller than the right projection $G'_R H'_R$. It is this difference, however small, in a pair of stereocards which gives rise to the retinal image disparities and hence to stereopsis. The points GH need not be the extremities of a single object but could also represent two separate objects at different distances.

If these two projections are now substituted for GH, a subject with normal stereoscopic vision could obtain a three-dimensional impression. There would, however, be certain difficulties. The eyes may be unable to accommodate for such a small viewing distance, especially since the convergence of the visual axes must remain the same as when viewing the actual distant object. Furthermore, it may be disconcerting for the subject to be strongly accommodating while apparently viewing a distant scene. Also, the size of the stereoscopic pair ($G'_R H'_R \ G'_L H'_L$) is limited because the two projections must not overlap. It was to overcome these drawbacks that the stereoscope was invented.

Figure 11.7 illustrates the principle of the reflecting stereoscope invented by Wheatstone in 1838. The two mirrors VV allow the separate halves of the stereogram to be placed at a convenient distance from the eyes while keeping them of relatively large size. The points

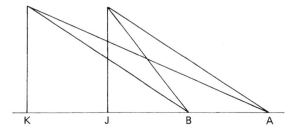

Figure 11.5. Perspective: angular subtense as a function of object distance; KA/JA<KB/JB.

---

* The term 'stereopair' is better used to denote a specific pair of R and L *points* presented stereoscopically.

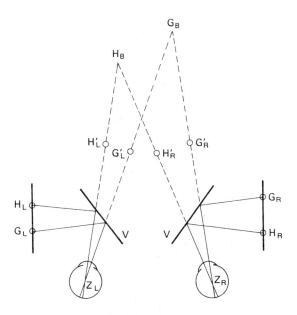

Figure 11.7. Principle of the Wheatstone stereoscope (1838).

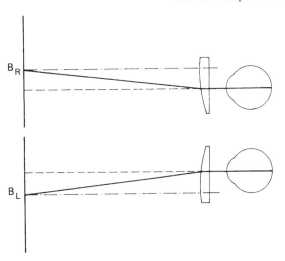

Figure 11.9. The increased card size of the Brewster–Holmes stereoscope (1861) (cf. *Figure 11.8*).

G_L, G_R represent a stereopair, as do H_L, H_R. They are imaged at G'_L, G'_R and H'_L, H'_R respectively. In the stereogram, the distance separating G_L and H_L is smaller than that between G_R and H_R. To see G_L and G_R singly, the two visual axes must lie along $Z_L G'_L$ and $Z_R G'_R$, intersecting at G_B. This is the hypothetical point which, viewed directly, would require the two eyes to converge exactly as in the diagram with the stereoscope in use. For this reason it was termed by Bennett (1977/78) the equivalent binocular object (point). It represents the position which the perceived image seen with the stereoscope might be expected to occupy. The same reasoning applies to the equivalent binocular object point H_B which is at a shorter distance from the eyes, thus giving a three-dimensional impression.

Several other designs, one using a single plano prism, were later introduced by Brewster, whose classic work on the subject appeared in 1856. The best-known model, which he called the lenticular stereoscope and first described in 1849, achieved an enormous success as a form of home entertainment. It is illustrated schematically in *Figure 11.8*. In essence, it consists of a box, one side housing two centred collimating lenses laterally adjustable to suit the viewer's PD. The other side held the stereogram, which could be a transparency.

The lenses allowed the pictures to be seen at optical infinity and without convergence. It can be seen from *Figure 11.8* that with this arrangement the distance $B_R B_L$ between the centres of the right and left pictures, which limits the picture width, is the same as the distance between the optical centres of the lenses.

As recalled by Fincham (1948), this model was modified and improved in 1861 by Oliver Wendell Holmes, more widely known as writer than as ophthalmologist. The lenses were decentred outwards, becoming spheroprisms, and the stereogram holder was mounted on a central bar along which it could slide, thus adjusting the distance of the image to suit the user's vision. The instrument could also be hand held comfortably.

As shown by *Figures 11.8* and *11.9*, the incorporation of the base-out prisms increases the maximum picture size merely by increasing the distance between the optical centres of the lenses. Owing to these various improvements, the Brewster–Holmes stereoscope has been the design most widely found in clinical use. Usually the lenses are of power +5.25 D with their optical centres 85 mm apart.

Even though enjoying good stereoscopic acuity, some patients find that it takes a little time for the three-dimensional effect to emerge. Familiarity with the stereoscope pictures or the objects portrayed may help to speed the process.

Strong evidence that retinal image disparity is a sufficient as well as a necessary condition for stereopsis is provided by 'random dot' stereograms. According to Shipley (1971) the first stereogram of this type was devised in 1954 by Aschenbrenner, using a simple but ingenious method of construction.[*] The right and left halves are apparently the same but, in fact, contain corresponding portions laterally displaced with respect to the background. As a result, these areas appear to stand out or recede from the background despite the

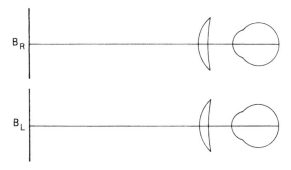

Figure 11.8. Principle of the Brewster stereoscope (1849).

---

[*] In fact, random dot stereograms constructed from small black circles of different sizes, somewhat similar to Ishihara colour plates, had been marketed by Carl Zeiss (Jena) before 1930.

absence of any extraneous clues as to their size, shape or position.

The stereogram reproduced in *Figure 11.10* was constructed from identical portions cut from two photocopies of a piece of Harris tweed – a material with a pronounced weave. When viewed stereoscopically, a face will be seen. The nose appears in front of the cheeks, tilting towards the viewer. This effect was achieved by superimposing identical strips of the photocopy on the right and left halves of the stereogram, both strips being equally decentred inwards with an additional slight inward tilt at the bottom. The eyes also stand forward, while the strips for the mouth, being decentred outwards, should (but may not) be seen as a cavity behind the plane of the face. Letratone material LT 134 and 136 can be used in the same way.

Computer-generated stereograms on the random dot principle have recently become familiar through the work of Julesz (1960).

More recently, computer programs for generating random dot stereograms have been devised by Fowler (1985), Graham (1985) and Burek (1985).

Some of the more recent theories of stereopsis, derived partly from the need to explain random dot stereopsis, are summarized by Gilchrist (1988).

Optics of the Brewster–Holmes stereoscope

Basic principle

The basic principle of the instrument is illustrated in *Figure 11.11*. In the state of adjustment shown, the stereogram has been moved forwards from the anterior focal plane of the stereoscope lenses so that the conjugate image plane lies at a desired finite distance. The points (G_R, G_L) and (H_R, H_L) are two stereopairs; G_R and H_R are imaged by the right lens at G'_R and H'_R while G_L and H_L are imaged by the left lens at G'_L and H'_L. Their positions can be determined graphically by straight lines drawn from the optical centres O_R and O_L of the stereoscope lenses through the given object points.

When the right visual axis is directed towards G_R and the left towards G'_L they intersect at G_B as though the naked eyes were fixating a single object point in this position. By a similar construction, the point H_B can be located.

If the picture viewed is a reproduction of a real object or scene as distinct from an abstract geometrical drawing, the perspective should, if possible, approximate to that which would be seen under natural conditions. To maintain the correct angular relationships if photography is used, the lateral separation of the two camera positions should be the same as the viewer's PD and the magnification (enlargement) m of the prints should satisfy the relationship

$$m = \frac{\text{Focal length of stereoscope lenses}}{\text{Focal length of camera lens}} \quad (11.4)$$

If a greatly enhanced sensation of depth is required when the stereogram is viewed, the distance between the two camera positions should be increased like the base line of the telestereoscope. This occurs in aerial photography when the two positions may be separated by several kilometres. For the accurate measurements required in cartography, both the camera and stereoscope lenses should be very free from distortion (Horne, 1980).

A detailed mathematical analysis of perspective in binocular projection can be found in Helmholtz's classic treatise (1924).

Use in clinical practice

In clinical practice, the stereoscope is mainly used as a device for presenting different test objects or stimuli to each eye. These may be designed to test or exercise the muscular fusional reserves or to examine the quality of the perceptual fusional process, for example, with the Javal FL card. To describe any such tests as 'stereoscopic' would be misleading: the term 'stereoscope test' would be preferable.

When the stereoscope is used in this way, any disturbance of the normal relationship between accommodation and convergence should be avoided. To meet this

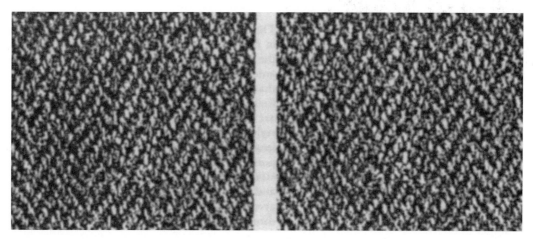

Figure 11.10. A 'Harris Tweedogram' or a random dot stereogram constructed from identical pieces cut from photocopies of Harris Tweed.

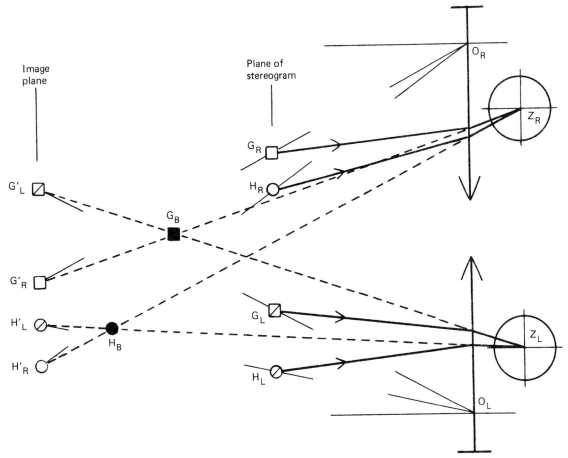

Figure 11.11.   Arrangement and optical principles of the Brewster–Holmes stereoscope.

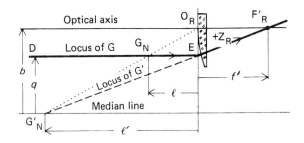

Figure 11.12.   Diagrammatic construction to find the position of the test card required to place the image of the point G_N on the median line.

requirement, both right and left test objects must be imaged on the median line or at equal distances to the same side of it.

If the separation between corresponding details on the test card is smaller than that of the optical centres of the stereoscope lenses, the correct adjustment of the instrument can be found graphically, as shown in *Figure 11.12*. This shows that part of the instrument used by the right eye. The lens of power F and optical centre O_R distant b from the median line is assumed to be thin. For ray construction it is replaced by a straight line. As the test card is moved towards the observer, the centre G of the right test object, at a distance q from the median line, moves along the line DE parallel to the optical axis of the stereoscope lens. If DE is imagined as an

incident ray, the refracted ray passes through the second principal focus F'_R of the lens. Wherever G is situated, its image G' must therefore lie on the line EF'_R produced either way. The required position G_N of the test object is such that G'_N lies on the median line at its intersection with $F'_R E$ produced backwards. A line drawn from G'_N to O_R intersects DE at the desired point G_N.

From the similar triangles in the diagram it can be seen that

$$\frac{b-q}{f'} = \frac{q}{-\ell'}$$

or

$$(b-q)F = -qL'$$

This gives

$$L' = \{1 - (b/q)\}F \tag{11.5}$$

and

$$L = L' - F = -(b/q)F \tag{11.6}$$

These relationships are independent of the position of the observer's eyes.

Assuming that, as is usual, $F = +5.25\,\text{D}$ and $2b = 85\,\text{mm}$, with $q = 30\,\text{mm}$, we should have

$$L' = \{1 - (42.5/30)\}5.25 = -2.19\,\text{D}$$

and

$$L = -7.44\,\text{D}$$

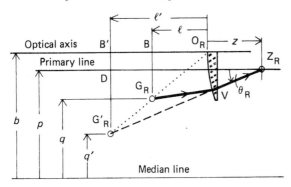

Figure 11.13. Diagram for analysis of convergence and accommodation through the Brewster–Holmes stereoscope.

Measured from the lens plane, the accommodation required would be $-L'$ or approximately 2.25 D

The above construction could be reversed to find the necessary value of q to place the image on the median line at a desired distance from the lens.

Convergence and accommodation

The general analysis in this section is abridged from Bennett (1970). *Figure 11.13* shows the optical arrangement for the right eye, with the following distances all measured from the median line:

b to the optical axis of the stereoscope lens,
p to the primary line of sight,
q to a given point GR on the stereogram,
q' to G'_R the image of G_R formed by the stereoscope lens.

The first three of these distances are invariably regarded as positive. In general, G'_R does not lie on the median line and the distance q' is regarded as negative if it lies on the opposite sign of the median line.

To receive a sharp image of G_R the eye must exert the necessary amount of accommodation and converge so that the visual axis is directed towards the image point G'_R. The ray path through the eye's centre of rotation is then $G_R V Z_R$.

Convergence

Let the convergence of the eye in prism dioptres be denoted by C. It can then be seen from the diagram that

$$C = \theta_R = \frac{G'_R D}{DZ_R} = \frac{p - q'}{-\ell' + z}$$

Putting $L' = 1/\ell' = (L + F)$ and $Z = 1/z$, gives

$$C = \frac{(p - q')(L + F)Z}{L + F - Z} \qquad (11.7)$$

A more useful expression is obtained if q' is replaced by other known quantities. From the similar triangles in *Figure 11.13* having a common vertex at O_R the optical centre of the lens, we get

$$BG_R/BO_R = B'G'_R/B'O_R$$

or

$$\frac{b - q}{-\ell} = \frac{b - q'}{-\ell'}$$

from which

$$(b - q)L = (b - q')(L + F)$$

and

$$q' = \frac{qL + bF}{L + F} \qquad (11.8)$$

When this expression is substituted for q' in equation (11.7), we get

$$C = \frac{\{(p - q)L + (p - b)F\}Z}{L + F - Z} \qquad (11.9)$$

This gives the uniocular convergence in prism dioptres when p, q and b are in centimetres.

Accommodation

To sufficient accuracy, the accommodation required is the reciprocal of the distance in metres from the image plane to the eye's centre of rotation. Hence

$$A = \frac{1}{-\ell' + z} = \frac{L'Z}{L' - Z}$$
$$= \frac{(L + F)Z}{L + F - Z} \qquad (11.10)$$

Convergence/accommodation ratio (C/A)

On dividing equation (11.9) by (11.10) we obtain the general relationship

$$C/A = \frac{(p - q)L + (p - b)F}{L + F} \qquad (11.11)$$

A simpler and more enlightening expression can be derived from equations (11.7) and (11.10), giving

$$C/A = p - q' \qquad (11.12)$$

The normal relationship between convergence and accommodation requires G'_R to lie on the median line. In this event, $q' = 0$ and $C/A = p$ (compare this equation with (9.6) in which $\hat{C}$ denotes the total convergence by both eyes). If expression (11.8) for q' is equated to zero, we obtain the condition that

$$L = -(b/q)F$$

This is the same as equation (11.6) derived earlier from a graphical construction.

This value of L gives the position of the stereogram along the axis of the instrument so that a given stereo-pair defined by the distance $2q$, is seen under the normal C/A ratio. Maddox called this position the 'neutral point'. If the stereogram is placed further from the eyes, the image point G'_R then lies on the remote side of the median line. The distance q' thus assumes a negative value, so that $(p - q')$, the measure of C/A, becomes greater than p. Conversely, when the stereogram is moved nearer than the neutral point, G'_R shifts to the near side of the median line, making q' positive in sign and $(p - q')$ less than p. Negative fusional reserves of convergence are brought into play. Alternatively, the card holder is left in a position to simulate a distant or near object, and cards having detail at steadily decreasing or increasing values of *q* are used in order to stimulate relative convergence or divergence respectively. Typical cards are the Wells, Bradford (Pickwell) and London Refraction Hospital stereograms (Mallett, 1988).

Control over the *C/A* ratio can be achieved by separating the two halves of the stereogram and mounting each one on its own adjustably angled rail. Their separation then varies to a predetermined degree as the viewing distance, which can be kept the same for each eye, is altered. By this means, the *C/A* ratio can be maintained at any desired value for all viewing distances. This is the principle of the Asher–Law stereoscope. For details of this and of the Barrett relative accommodation stereoscope, *see* Bennett (1970).

Fixation with crossed or uncrossed axes: the autostereoscopic effect

Single vision as opposed to double vision occurs when the two retinal images are positioned similarly with respect to the two foveae. This is normally achieved by correct alignment of the two eyes, but when viewing any pattern with detail repeated at regular horizontal intervals, for example, wallpaper with vertical lines, it is possible for the eyes to over-converge so that the right eye fixates detail to the left of similar detail fixated by the left eye. This is the principle underlying the 'three cats' orthoptic exercise for developing positive relative convergence – *see* Evans (1997). The effective binocular object is then situated in the plane containing the intersection of the visual axes. Micropsia then results – the angular subtense of detail of size *s* is then s/d, where *d* is the distance to the wall, whereas the brain would expect it to subtend s/ℓ, where ℓ is the smaller distance to the effective binocular object. Since s/d is less than s/ℓ, the brain interprets this as a reduction in size. A similar effect when accommodation is weak is noted on page 119).

The term 'autostereogram' has been given to diagrams producing this effect, for example, computerized random dot constructions as described by Tyler (1983) and popularized in books such as Horibuchi (1994). *Figure 11.14* shows the method for designing an autostereogram for crossed visual axes. When viewed in crossed convergence, the repeated letter C forms the background, while the wider spacing of the letter Ds means that they are perceived to be closer. A similar process can be used for diagrams for uncrossed visual axes, again with a narrower spacing for the part to be perceived closer. Orthoptic exercises for developing convergence based on autostereograms are being developed by B.J.W. Evans (pers. comm., 1996).

Additional methods of producing stereoscopic relief

Unaided vision

Since it is not always convenient to use a stereoscope, other methods of obtaining stereoscopic reproduction

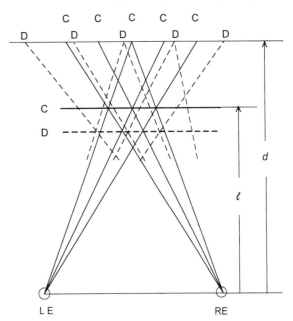

Figure 11.14. Principles of the autostereogram.

are of interest. If the stereogram is small, the separation being no bigger than the inter-pupillary distance, some people can fuse a stereogram unaided. This requires them to relax their convergence while maintaining accommodation.[*] With the visual axes approximately parallel, the right eye fixates the right half and the left eye the left half of the stereogram. The entire card is, in fact, viewed in crossed physiological diplopia so that four pictures may be seen initially. If the convergence is adjusted, the two centre pictures can be superimposed to give a stereoscopic percept. This appears to be distant, yet nevertheless larger than one of the single pictures viewed at the same distance from the eyes. The angular subtense is the same in both cases, but when the perceived image seems further away its size is accordingly judged to be greater.

Alternatively, the visual axes may be crossed so as to view the stereogram in uncrossed diplopia, the right and left pictures having been interchanged. In this case, the single percept will appear to be relatively small though closer to the eyes because of the greater convergence required. Without practice it may be difficult to make these relative adjustments of accommodation and convergence.

Anaglyphs

An anaglyph is a stereogram produced by the method described by Rollman (1853). The right and left views are printed superimposed on a white ground, but one in red and the other in green ink. One eye looks through a green filter, so that the green ink cannot be seen against the apparently white ground, whereas the red printing appears black. The other eye looks through a

---

[*] With a reading correction in use, some presbyopes find it possible to diverge sufficiently to fuse a stereogram of larger size.

red filter and therefore sees as black the picture printed in green. A vivid though substantially monotone stereoscopic impression can be created in this way. Extensive use of anaglyphs is made in the work by Gregory (1970).

One disadvantage of this method is that the red and green colours induce an 0.50 D difference in refraction between the two eyes. This may have a significant effect in studies involving monocular blur. A further drawback is that some people have difficulty in integrating the right and left retinal images if they are in complementary colours. For these reasons, monocular suppression could possibly result. It might be possible to use narrow spectral band filters of relatively similar colour, but whose transmission curves hardly overlap, for example, a bluish-green and yellow–green.

Use of polarized light

Somewhat like an anaglyph, a stereogram can be constructed from two superimposed views, each printed or reproduced in such a way that the light entering the eye is substantially plane polarized. The right and left planes of polarization are mutually perpendicular and the composite picture, a vectograph, has to be viewed through an analysing visor. This technique allows only black and white tones to be used. However, if two transparencies are made and separately projected with polarized light on to a metallic diffusing screen, the original colours can be retained. An analysing visor is still required.

Other methods

Various methods whereby single coloured pictures, up to quite large sizes, can be made to give a three-dimensional impression when viewed normally without a visor have been described by Dudley (1951). In one technique, for example, the picture is composed of narrow vertical strips presenting alternative right and left viewpoints. A prismatic Fresnel-type grid permanently superimposed on the picture ensures that each strip is seen only by the eye intended.

Pseudoscopy

Pseudoscopy is an induced impression of relief in reverse, nearer objects appearing further away than more distant ones. The simplest way of producing this effect is to interchange the two halves of a stereogram. In *Figure 11.15(a)* the stereogram would be seen three-dimensionally as a pyramid viewed from above with its apex towards the observer. When presented as in *Figure 11.15(b)*, the pyramid would appear to be hollow towards the viewer. Another possibility is illustrated in *Figure 11.15(c)*, in which each half of the original stereogram has been reversed right to left. The three-dimensional appearance is again that of a hollow pyramid, but laterally reversed.

An optical arrangement for producing reversal of relief when a real object or scene is viewed is called a pseudoscope. The first was devised in 1838 by

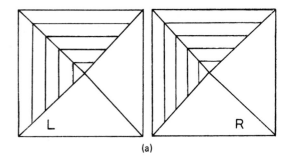

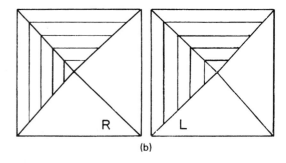

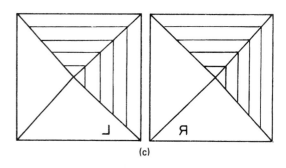

Figure 11.15. Simulation of reversed relief or pseudoscopy with stereocards: (a) normal view of a pyramid, apex towards observer; (b) pseudoscopic view obtained by interchanging cards; (c) pseudoscopic view obtained by laterally reversing the individual cards.

Wheatstone, who used a pair of Dove reflecting prisms, one before each eye with the two reflecting (hypotenuse) faces turned inwards. In effect, this is equivalent to the arrangement in *Figure 11.15(c)*. To generalize, pseudoscopy is possible when there is a contradiction between relative binocular parallax and the right and left viewpoints, either of these entities being reversed from the normal situation.

The mirror pseudoscope invented by Stratton in 1898 is shown diagrammatically in *Figure 11.16*. It avoids the lateral inversion of the Wheatstone model. By an arrangement of two plane mirrors, the right and left viewpoints are reversed; the effect of the double reflection is to image the viewer's left eye in the position shown. In near vision, the result of the increased path length to this eye is a smaller visual angle and hence a smaller retinal image than in the fellow eye. This drawback can be obviated by various symmetrical arrangements of four mirrors, two before each eye (von Rohr, 1920).

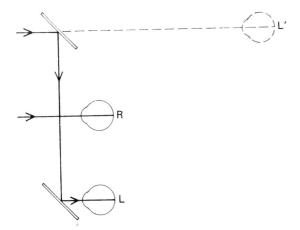

Figure 11.16. Arrangement of the Stratton pseudoscope (1898).

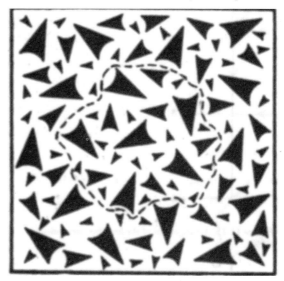

Figure 11.17. One pattern from the Frisby stereotest (1978). The portion enclosed by the broken line is on the opposite side of the plate. (With acknowledgements to Professor Frisby and Clement Clarke International Ltd.)

In general, pseudoscopic vision is most easily obtained with geometrical constructions or objects which can themselves be seen in either form; for example, a bucket which may have its open end either facing or turned away or an embossed surface which could have either raised or hollow relief. An everyday scene or an object such as a house is unlikely to give a pseudoscopic impression because it could not be accepted psychologically, being contrary to all past experience.

Clinical tests for stereopsis

While tests for stereopsis are relevant to certain occupational requirements, they may also be used as a test for the quality of binocular vision. If this is poor, good stereopsis cannot occur. Hence the presence of reasonable stereopsis may be used as a screening test to confirm that binocular vision is present and that there will probably be little amblyopia. The three-needle test described on page 192 is excellent for laboratory use, but the care required to obtain accurate results makes it unsuitable for general clinical use.

Stereotests for distance vision

Some test chart projectors have a vectographic slide enabling the presence of stereopsis in distance vision to be verified, though possibly at only a single angular disparity. Rutstein *et al.* (1994) describe the Mentor binocular vision testing system: the patient wears spectacles with computer controlled liquid crystal lenses allowing alternating vision between the eyes at 60 cycles/s while the computer simultaneously alternates the VDU display. As this frequency is above the critical fusion frequency, a steady display is perceived.

The Frisby test

The Frisby stereotest introduced in 1978 consists of a square transparent plate on which four similar patterns are apparently printed on one side (*Figure 11.17*). In fact, the central part of one of the patterns, enclosed within the dotted ring superimposed on the diagram, is printed on the other side of the plate. There are three plates of thickness 6, 3 and 1 (or 1.5) mm. The patient views the thickest plate first against a uniform white background and has to say which of the four patterns has the centre in relief, either forwards or backwards. For young patients, this can be expressed as 'find the ball' or 'find the hole'. The plate may be turned over or rotated so as to alter the position of the pattern with relief. If the patient is successful with the 6 mm plate, the thinner plates are shown in turn or the observation distance increased. At a 40 cm observation distance, the three plates show a relative binocular parallax of approximately 340, 170 and 55 (or 88) seconds of arc respectively. These figures can be checked using equation (11.2), after allowing for the 'reduced thickness' (t/n) of the plates and assuming the PD to be 65 mm. Intermediate values of stereoscopic acuity can be tested by varying the working distance (*see* Exercise 11.10).

Because of its dot-like structure, the Frisby test is sometimes mistakenly termed a random dot test. It relies, however, on real three-dimensional clues, not disparities within a stereopair.

To avoid the assistance given by parallax in tests using real three-dimensional objects, the patient's head and the plates should be kept still, though it is surprisingly difficult to identify the pattern with the relief by movement. This possible source of error does not arise with tests using anaglyphs or vectographs. On the other hand, anaglyphs have the disadvantages mentioned on pages 199–200.

The Titmus Wirt test

The Titmus Wirt Test introduced in 1971 makes use of vectographs. The right and left eye pictures are polarized at $45°$ and $135°$ respectively and viewed through a correspondingly oriented spectacle analyser. As a gross test for stereopsis, a greatly enlarged picture of a housefly has been used. Very young children may respond to this but not to less interesting though more scientific presentations. These include a graded set of nine pictures each comprising four circles arranged in diamond formation. One of the circles in each group is designed to stand forward in relief when seen binocularly through the visor. At a viewing distance of 40 cm, the stereo-acuity needed to identify the forward circle ranges from 800 to 40 seconds of arc.*

Young children might manage another test in which three rows of animal pictures are presented. In each row, one of the animals appears to stand forward, representing stereo-acuities of 400, 200 and 100 seconds of arc.

A polarized test incorporating a column of geometric shapes is incorporated in the Mallett near fixation disparity unit.

The TNO test

Anaglyphic separation is used in the Dutch TNO† test, introduced in 1972. Demonstration plates showing butterflies and geometric shapes in relief serve to explain the test. Monocularly, they appear to be a random display of dots, printed in red and green, the picture emerging only in binocular vision through the visor provided which has a red filter for the right eye, green for the left. To measure the stereo-acuity from 480 down to 15 seconds of arc,† test plates intended for use at 40 cm are used. They show circles with one sector remaining in the plane of the background; the patient has to identify its position.

The Randot test

The Randot stereo test utilizes vectographic dissociation. Rather like the Titmus Wirt test, it includes a series of 10 groups of three circles, one in each pattern designed to appear standing forward. At a distance of 40 cm, the range covered‡ is from 400 to 20 seconds of arc. It also has a similar set of animal pictures, while a third set of plates use random dot stereograms, with various hidden geometric shapes having disparities of 500 or 250 seconds of arc.

With both the Wirt and the TNO tests, reversing the visor (or turning the TNO book upside down) reverses the relief, the test figure receding from the background. Some patients, especially those with fixation disparity, may find their ability to obtain the three-dimensional impression affected by the direction in which the relief is presented. Displacement towards the eyes is usually seen more readily than away from them. This may be caused by separate neural channels for perceiving these

two types of relief: Birch *et al.* (1982) showed that appreciation of forwards relief developed in infants earlier than perception of depth, while Richards (1971) found mature subjects who could see only forwards relief or depth. Alternatively, as with fixation disparity testing, suppression areas on only one side of the fovea will affect relief more in one direction than the other. Larson (1990) sensibly suggests that stereo-acuity for both advancing and receding reliefs should be measured and recorded, with the best result taken as the stereo-acuity.

If finer levels of acuity are required from the vectographic or anaglyphic tests, they may be held at a greater distance, or as suggested by Reading and Tanlami (1982), the anaglyphic test rotated in its own plane to reduce the horizontal component of its disparity. The plates must not be turned too far, as Charman and Jennings (1995) found that if the TNO test is rotated through a right-angle so that the disparities are vertical instead of horizontal, the presence of the test figure could often still be identified, though obviously without stereoscopic relief, possibly because of binocular rivalry. They questioned whether some of the coarse stereopsis results reported for subjects with poor binocular vision were perceived by the same mechanism. If a patient does not pass one test, the cause may be a lack of comprehension rather than poor stereopsis, and another test should be tried.

The Lang Stereotests

The Lang Stereotest,§ introduced in 1982, utilizes a series of tiny vertical cylindrical strips to present random dot stereograms. The first edition shows a cat (1200 seconds of arc), star (600 seconds) and cat (550 seconds), while the second shows an elephant (600 seconds), car (400 seconds) and moon (200 seconds), together with a control picture of a star which may be seen with monocular vision. Both editions are available. Because the optical arrangement is directional, the test has to be held fairly precisely in a fronto-parallel plane at about 40 cm. As no polarizing or anaglyphic visor is required, the test is suitable for infants down to about 6–8 months. At this age, stereoscopic vision may be recognized from the child's fixational eye movements or attempts to grasp the objects.

Dynamic random dot stereograms

Anaglyphic dissociation of computer-generated random dot stereograms displayed on computer screens has been combined with a preferential looking test (*see* page 38) to investigate the development of stereo-acuity in infants.

---

* The complete range is 800, 400, 200, 140, 100, 80, 60, 50 and 40 seconds of arc.

† Institute for Perception TNO, 3769 ZG Soesterberg, The Netherlands. The complete range is 480, 240, 120, 60, 30 and 15 seconds of arc.

‡ The complete range is 400, 200, 140, 70, 50, 40, 30, 25 and 20 seconds of arc.

---

§ In the UK, the Lang, Frisby, Titmus and Randot tests are obtainable through Clement Clarke International Ltd, Edinburgh Way, Harlow, Essex CM20 2TT.

Comparison of tests

Simons (1981), Hall (1982) and Heron *et al.* (1985) have made comparisons of the various clinical stereotests. The different tests gave different values for the mean stereo-acuity. In both studies, some subjects were found to achieve finer stereo-acuities with the Frisby test than with the other clinical tests. Heron and colleagues found the Frisby test to be understood by young children, and to have the least variability in its scores. Simons found the Frisby test to give lower acuities than the other stereotests. He pointed out that the separation between the figure and background is larger in this test than the other clinical tests, resulting in the lower score. Hall, however, reported that some patients with poor binocular vision could achieve a coarse stereoscopic acuity with this test but none at all with the vectographic or anaglyphic tests – this may result from parallax or from the reflection of the printing ink off the surface of the plate if the light source is badly positioned showing the Frisby pattern, while conversely, suppression with the other tests may result in their poorer performance. Heron and colleagues found that the TNO and Randot tests were unable to measure acuities finer than about 20 seconds of arc because the necessary increase in the testing distance meant that the dot structure became too fine to resolve.

An obvious conclusion to be drawn from the various studies is that the statistical, forced-choice approach of the two- or three-needle test results in finer acuities than the clinical tests. Moreover, the results found for the latter vary significantly. It would appear necessary for the clinician to establish his/her own norms.

Development of stereopsis

Held *et al.* (1980), cited by Heron *et al.* (1985), used preferential looking techniques (*see* page 38) to demonstrate stereo-acuities of 60 seconds of arc or better in children aged 5–6 months. Using the Frisby test, Heron and colleagues found that the median stereo-acuity was 27.5 seconds at 3 years of age, improving to 16.5 seconds at 7 years. The adults they examined showed acuities of 8 seconds. Because the other tests used could not record acuities much finer than about 20 seconds of arc, both adults and older children obtained the same scores. This could be misinterpreted to mean that the children had attained adult values for stereo-acuity.

Williams *et al.* (1988), using the TNO test, found that acuities of 60 seconds of arc or better were attained by 52.7% of their 7-year-old children and 83.5% of their 9 year olds. The numbers for 30 seconds of arc or better were 4.0% and 24.7% respectively, while at age 11, 3.4% achieved 15 seconds of arc.

Stereopsis and age

Like visual acuity, stereo-acuity also appears to decline slightly with age. Yap *et al.* (1994) using a two-needle test found mean stereo-acuities of 8.37 seconds of arc for a 20–29-year-old group, 9.18 seconds for a 30–49 age group and 11.21 seconds for a 50–67 year olds. Re-duced retinal illuminance because of pupillary miosis and loss of transparency of the eye were eliminated as the cause.

Stereopsis and refraction

As binocular vision is necessary for stereopsis, tests for this may be used to identify patients with strabismus – not always easy if the angle of deviation is small. Williams *et al.* (1988) found that their strabismic patients either showed no stereopsis on the TNO test, or managed only the demonstration plates or the 480 seconds of arc test plate. Hall (1982) similarly found very poor stereoscopic ability for his non-binocular subjects on the TNO, Titmus, Frisby and two-needle tests.

Many studies have been made of the fall in stereoscopic acuity with monocular or binocular blur. This may be relevant when screening for monocular or binocular errors, or to the deficit produced in a presbyopic contact lens wearer who is corrected for near vision in one eye, distance in the other (Larson and Lachance, 1983; McGill and Erickson, 1988; Collins and Bruce, 1994).

Levy and Glick (1974) found the stereoscopic acuity to drop from 40 seconds of arc to 60 seconds with monocular blur to 20/40, and to 120 seconds with further blurring to 20/120. Also with monocular blurring, Lovasik and Szymkiw (1985) found a drop in stereoacuity from about 25 to 40 seconds, with only 0.5 D of blur on the Titmus circles, and with 1.0 D of blur on the Randot test. With these two tests, aniseikonia of 2% and 6% respectively gave the same drop in stereopsis. A moderate degree of depth judgement could be maintained in the presence of 2.0 D of blur. For small degrees of blur they found the acuity measured by the Titmus test to deteriorate about 1.8 times as fast as with the Randot test.

Goodwin and Romano (1985), Simons (1984), Wood (1983) and Schmidt (1994) all demonstrated a greater drop in stereo-acuity with monocular than binocular blur. Goodwin and Romano found only a small drop in acuity with blur to 20/25 (6/7.5), but at 20/30 (6/9) the acuity was 78 seconds with binocular blur compared with 358 seconds monocularly. When blurred to 20/40 (6/12), the results were 136 and 378 seconds respectively. For blurs of 20/50 or worse, the binocular and monocular values were similar. Using diffusive rather than out-of-focus blur, Simons found the monocular acuity to be about three times as bad as that with binocular blur to 20/100 (6/30). The difference between subjects is demonstrated by Wood; one subject showed only a slight drop in stereo-acuity on a two-needle test at up 2.0 D of blur, while his other two subjects showed increasing deterioration at more than 0.5 or 1.0 D of blur.

The synoptophore

Various trade names have been used to denote the type of orthoptic instrument commonly known as a synopto-

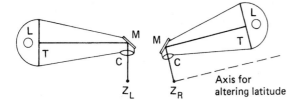

Figure 11.18. Optical arrangement of the synoptophore.

phore. A history of this instrument and associated terminology has been given by Revell (1972).

As indicated by *Figure 11.18*, the synoptophore is a much modified Wheatstone stereoscope. The test transparencies TT are illuminated by small lamp bulbs LL and imaged at infinity by the collimating lenses CC. They are seen by the subject after reflection at the silvered mirrors MM. Each tube is pivoted about a vertical axis through Z, the assumed position of the eye's centre of rotation. This makes it possible to alter the stimulus to convergence and to measure the horizontal angle of strabismus. The pivot separation is adjustable to suit the subject's PD. Each tube may also be tilted upwards or downwards about a horizontal axis passing through Z and parallel to the axis of the tube. By this means a vertical oculo-motor imbalance can be measured. In addition, both tubes can simultaneously be tilted up or down in order to exercise the eyes or measure deviations in elevated or depressed planes of gaze. The transparency holders can also be raised or lowered to measure vertical imbalances, while torsional movements are obtained by rotating the transparency holders about their centres.

Although the transparencies are imaged at infinity, proximal convergence and accommodation are induced by the known physical nearness of the test objects. A reduction in proximal effects was one of the advantages claimed for the modified design due to Stanworth (1958). The mirrors MM are replaced by transparent glass plates PP (*Figure 11.19*) which allow the subject to fixate on a wall or screen at 3–6 m from the instrument. It is against this background that the transparencies are seen. To prevent blurring, the collimating lenses are moved to the position shown and their power

modified accordingly. In order that corresponding detail on the right and left transparencies should appear superimposed, the tubes must be converged to the plane of the fixation wall or screen: 1Δ each if the distance is 3 m.

The variable prism stereoscope

The rotary or Risley prism (known in France as the Crétès and in Germany as the Herschel prism) is a device for producing continuously variable prism power. It consists of two plano prisms of equal power, mounted almost in contact in a carrier disc which can be placed in a standard trial frame or fitted to a refractor head.

The principle is illustrated in *Figure 11.20* in which the two prisms are shown side by side instead of superimposed. In the zero setting (*Figure 11.20a*), the prisms have their bases opposed. To obtain a desired prism power, the prisms are mechanically rotated in opposite directions through an equal angle θ. In the position shown in Figure 11.20b, one prism has its base up and to the left, while the base of the other is down and to the left. The vertical components cancel out but the horizontal ones are additive, giving a resultant with its base to the left. If the power of each of the single prisms is denoted by P, it can be seen from the diagram that the total power of the resultant prism is simply $2P \sin\theta$. Had the initial rotations been reversed in direction, the resultant would have been the same but with its base to the right.

The diagram also shows that the resultant prism effect

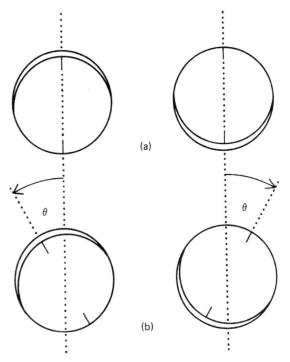

Figure 11.20. The rotary or Risley prism. The two component prisms are drawn side by side for clarity. (a) Zero setting: bases opposed; (b) setting after each prism has been rotated through θ in opposite directions from the zero position: base of resultant prism to the left.

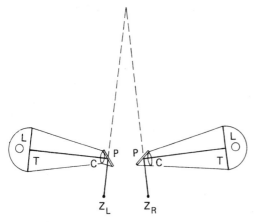

Figure 11.19. Principle of the Stanworth synoptophore (1958), using partially reflecting mirrors.

is invariably perpendicular to the zero setting. The device must therefore be appropriately orientated in the trial frame or refractor head. In the simpler models, the carrier disc is graduated to indicate the power of the resultant prism, the maximum value frequently being 30Δ.

The variable prism stereoscope (VPS) incorporates two Risley prisms, so geared that equal amounts of base-in or base-out prism can be placed before each eye. A total of 60Δ is thus available.

When the VPS is used to measure fusional reserves, the prism power is initially set at zero while the patient observes a single vertical line of letters at 6 m, or, in near vision, a card placed in the holder provided.

To use the instrument as a stereoscope, a septum should be positioned so as to prevent either eye from seeing the opposite half of the stereogram. Also, to maintain the normal relationship between accommodation and convergence, base-out prism should be placed before each eye. Otherwise, instead of converging to a point in the plane of the card, each eye might even have to diverge in order to fixate a pair of corresponding points. If, for example, the separation of these points is 7 cm and the viewing distance is $\frac{1}{3}$ m, the total base-out prism required is 21Δ.

The stereocomparator

If the right and left halves of a stereogram are identical, no impression of relief can arise. The converse is also true and this is the principle of the stereocomparator. If two flat objects are viewed in a stereoscope, for example, a genuine bank note and a forgery, any detail which is not in exact register between the two will appear in stereoscopic relief, either forward or backwards.

Holography

The stereoscope enables a three-dimensional percept to be obtained by binocular viewing of a two-dimensional stereocard. Holography, a technique of recording on a photographic plate the fringes formed when light reflected off the object interferes with a reference beam, produces a genuinely three-dimensional image. Clinical applications may follow.

Virtual reality

Computer-generated graphics coupled with miniature visual display units, one for each eye mounted with collimating lenses in a helmet, enable almost realistic three-dimensional scenes to be presented to the wearer. Feedback from sensors attached to the helmet and wearer enable the scene to alter in response to the individual's actions. This is a field in rapid development at present, with potential for education, design and simulation of flight or surgery for example.

Exercises

11.1 Taking η as 10 seconds of arc and the PD as 65 mm, ta-

bulate from equation (11.2) the values of $\Delta\ell$ for ℓ = 0.2, 0.5, 1.0, 5, 10, 20, 30, 50 and 100 m (minus signs omitted).

11.2 A depth difference of 0.5 mm is just noticeable at a distance of 1 m. What is the corresponding stereoscopic acuity for an observer with a PD of: (a) 60 mm, (b) 70 mm?

11.3 A slit lamp's binocular microscope has a working distance of 100 mm and an objective separation (between centres) of 25 mm. At magnifications of 10× and 20×, what is the least perceptible difference in depth corresponding to an observer's stereoscopic acuity of 20 seconds of arc?

11.4 A slit lamp's binocular microscope is formed by a nominally achromatic objective to collimate the light from the object, followed by a binocular prismatic telescope to magnify the image (*see Figure 16.4* on page 304). Explain why a yellow object might appear further away than a blue object in the same plane.

11.5 An observer with PD of 65 mm views an object at −5 m. Find the convergence required when viewing: (a) with the unaided eyes and (b) through a prismatic binocular with magnification 10× and objective separation 80 mm. What effect has the latter on ocular co-ordination?

11.6 Using the conventional Brewster–Holmes stereoscope, what is the required separation of corresponding details on the stereo-cards to avoid disturbing the accommodation/convergence relationship, the stimulus to accommodation in the lens plane being: (a) −1.00 D, (b) −4.00 D?

11.7 A stereoscope test is made with detail separation of 54 mm for use with the normal Brewster–Holmes stereoscope in the −3.00 D position. From first principles, find the binocular (total) convergence/accommodation ratio when the card is placed in: (a) the −1.00 D and (b) the −5.00 D positions. Assume a PD of 65 mm, ocular centres of rotation 35 mm behind the lenses and accommodation referred to the stereoscope lens plane.

11.8 The Brewster–Holmes stereoscope is used in the −3.00 D position to exercise fusional reserves. What is (a) the binocular convergence and (b) the binocular convergence/accommodation ratio for detail separations of (i) 49 mm, (ii) 64 mm? (assumptions as in Exercise 11.7).

11.9 Explain, with diagrams and typical numerical values, why the stereoscopic acuity corresponding to one particular thickness plate of the Frisby test varies with the PD of the observer, while the Titmus vectographic test gives an invariant angular acuity. What does vary between observers with different PDs when viewing a particular Titmus test? Assume a constant observation distance.

11.10 A Frisby plate (a) and a Titmus vectographic plate (b) both correspond to a stereoscopic acuity of η at a distance ℓ. If this distance is now doubled, what is the new corresponding value of stereoscopic acuity for each plate?

11.11 A Brewster–Holmes stereoscope has lenses (to be assumed thin) of power +5.50 D, their optical centres being 84 mm apart. Two corresponding points on a stereogram placed 125 mm from the lens plane are 49 mm apart, equally spaced from the median line. Determine (a) the convergence (expressed in prism dioptres) which an emmetropic subject would need to exert in order to fuse the two image points, (b) the distance from the lens plane at which the two visual axes would then intersect. Assume the subject to have an interocular distance of 58 mm, the eyes' centres of rotation being 30 mm behind the lens plane. Either calculation or a scale diagram may be employed.

11.12 An autostereogram is constructed with detail separations of C = 15 mm and D = 17 mm, as in *Figure 11.14*. If viewed with (a) crossed convergence and (b) uncrossed convergence with the paper at 350 mm from the eyes' centre of rotation, calculate the apparent distances to the binocular percepts of C and D. Assume a PD of 65 mm.

References

BENNETT, A.G. (1970) The optics of the prism stereoscope as a clinical instrument. *Ophthal. Optn*, **10**, 391–394, 399–402

BENNETT, A.G. (1977/78) Binocular vision through lenses and prisms. *Optician*, **174**(4511), 7–11; (4512), 7–12; **176** (4560), 8

BIRCH, E.E., GWIAZDA, J. and HELD, R. (1982) Stereoacuity development for crossed and uncrossed disparities in human infants. *Vision Res.*, **22**, 507–513

BREWSTER, D. (1856) *The Stereoscope: Its History, Theory, and Construction*. London: John Murray

BUREK, H. (1985) Improved random dot stereograms. *Optician*, **190**(5010), 18–19; (5011), 39, 41

CHARMAN, W.N. and JENNINGS, J.A.M. (1995) Recognition of TNO stereotest figures in the absence of true stereopsis. *Optom. Vis. Sci.*, **72**, 535–536

COLLINS, M.J. and BRUCE, A.S. (1994) Factors influencing performance with monovision. *J. Brit. Contact Lens Assoc.*, **17**, 83–89

DAVSON, H. (1980) *The Physiology of the Eye*, 4th edn. London: Churchill Livingstone

DUDLEY, L.P. (1951) *Stereoptics: An Introduction*. London: Macdonald & Co.

EVANS, B.J.W. (1997), *Pickwell's Binocular Vision Anomalies*, 3rd edn. Oxford: Butterworth-Heinemann.

FINCHAM, W.H.A. (1948) A note on the stereoscope. *Optician*, **116**, 569

FOWLER, C. (1985) Producing random dot stereograms on a microcomputer. *Optician*, **189**(4979), 22–23

GILCHRIST, J. (1988) The psychology of vision. In *Optometry*, pp. 36–37 (Edwards, K. and Llewellyn, R. eds). London: Butterworths

GOODWIN, R.T. and ROMANO, P.E. (1985) Stereoacuity degradation by experimental and real monocular and binocular amblyopia. *Invest. Ophthalmol. Vis. Sci.*, **26**, 917–923

GRAHAM, I. (1985) An alternative program for stereo image patterns. *Optician*, **189**(4999), 27–28, 33

GREGORY, R.L. (1970) *The Intelligent Eye*. London: Weidenfeld & Nicolson

HALL, C. (1982) The relationship between clinical stereotests. *Ophthal. Physiol. Opt.*, **2**, 135–143

HELMHOLTZ, H. VON (1924) *Physiological Optics*, Vol. 3, pp. 281–400. English translation: J.P.C. Southall (ed.). New York: Optical Society of America. Reprinted: New York: Dover Publications, 1962

HERON, G., DHOLAKIA, S., COLLINS, D.E. and McGLAUGHLAN, H. (1985) Stereoscopic threshold in children and adults. *Am. J. Optom.*, **62**, 505–515

HORIBUCHI, S. (ed.) (1994) *Stereogram*. Boxtree, London; Cadence Books, USA

HORNE, D.F. (1980) *Optical Instruments and their Applications*. Bristol: Adam Hilger

HOWARD, H.J. (1919) A test for the judgement of distance. *Am. J. Ophthal.*, **2**, 656–675. Cited in Larson, *op. cit.*

JACOBS, D.H. (1943) *Fundamentals of Optical Engineering*, pp. 249–281. New York and London: McGraw-Hill

JULESZ, B. (1960) Binocular depth perception of computer-generated patterns. *Bell Syst. Tech. J.*, **39**, 1125–1162

LANGFORD, M.J. (1971) *Basic Photography*. London and New York: Focal Press

LARSON, W.L. (1985) Does the Howard–Dolman really measure stereoacuity? *Am. J. Optom.*, **62**, 763–767

LARSON, W.L. (1990) An investigation of the difference in stereoacuity between crossed and uncrossed disparities using Frisby and TNO tests. *Optom. Vis. Sci.*, **67**, 157–161

LARSON, W.L. and LACHANCE, A. (1983) Stereoscopic acuity with induced refractive errors. *Am. J. Optom.*, **60**, 509–513

LEVY, N.S. and GLICK, E.B. (1974) Stereoscopic perception and Snellen visual acuity. *Am. J. Ophthal.*, **78**, 722–724

LOVASIK, J.V. and SZYMKIW, M. (1985) Effects of aniseikonia, accommodation, retinal illuminance, and pupil size on stereopsis. *Invest. Ophthalmol. Vis. Sci.*, **26**, 741–750

McGILL, E. and ERICKSON, P. (1988) Stereopsis in presbyopes wearing monovision and simultaneous vision bifocal contact lenses. *Am. J. Optom.*, **65**, 619–626

MADDOX, E.E. (1927) The bearing of stereoscopes on the relation between convergence and accommodation. *Br. J. Ophthal.*, **11**, 331–337

MALLETT, R. (1988) The management of binocular anomalies. In *Optometry*, pp. 270–286 (Edwards, K. and Llewellyn, R., eds). London: Butterworths

OGLE, K.N. (1962) The optical space sense. In *The Eye*, Vol. 4 (Davson, H., ed.). New York and London: Academic Press

PATRICK, F.B. (1969) Military optical instruments. In *Applied Optics and Optical Engineering*, Vol. 5, pp. 221–230 (Kingslake, R., ed). New York and London: Academic Press

READING, R.W. and TANLAMI, T. (1982) Finely graded binocular disparities from random-dot stereograms. *Ophthal. Physiol. Opt.*, **2**, 47–56

REGAN, D. and BEVERLEY, K.I. (1978) Looming detectors in the human visual pathway. *Vision Res.*, **18**, 415–421

REVELL, M.J. (1972) A history of the synoptophores. *International Optical Congress 1970*, pp. 13–26. London: British Optical Association

RICHARDS, W. (1971) Anomalous stereoscopic depth perception. *J. Opt. Soc. Am.*, **61**, 410–414

ROHR, M., VON (1920) *Die Binokularen Instrumente*, 2nd edn. Berlin: Julius Springer.

ROLLMANN, W. (1853) Zwei neue stereoskopische Methoden. *Pogg. Annln.*, **89**, 350–351

RUTSTEIN, R.P., FUHR, P. and SCHAAFSMA, D. (1994) Distance stereopsis in orthophores, heterophores, and intermittent strabismics. *Optom. Vis. Sci.*, **71**, 415–421

SCHMIDT, P.P. (1994) Sensitivity of random dot stereoacuity and Snellen acuity to optical blur. *Optom. Vis. Sci.*, **71**, 446–471

SHIPLEY, T. (1971) The first random-dot texture stereogram. *Vision Res.*, **11**, 1491–1492

SIMONS, K. (1981) Stereoacuity norms in young children. *Arch. Ophthalmol.*, **99**, 439–455

SIMONS, K. (1984) Effects on stereopsis of monocular versus binocular degradation of image contrast. *Invest. Ophthalmol. Vis. Sci.*, **25**, 987–989

STANWORTH, A. (1958) Modified major amblyoscope. *Br. J. Ophthal.*, **42**, 270–287

STRATTON, G.M. (1898) A mirror-pseudoscope and the limit of visible depth. *Psychol. Rev.*, **5**, 632–638

TYLER, C.W. (1983) Sensory processing of binocular disparity. In *Vergence Eye Movements: Basic and Clinical Aspects*. (Schor, C.M. and Ciuffreda, K.J., eds). Boston: Butterworths

WHEATSTONE, C. (1838) Contributions to the physiology of vision. *Phil. Trans. R. Soc.*, **128**, 371–394

WILLIAMS, S., SIMPSON, A. and SILVA, P.A. (1988) Stereoacuity levels and vision problems in children from 7 to 11 years. *Ophthal. Physiol. Opt.*, **8**, 386–389

WOOD, I.J.C. (1983) Stereopsis with spatially-degraded images. *Ophthal. Physiol. Opt.*, **3**, 337–340

YAP, M., BROWN, B. and CLARKE, J. (1994) Reduction in stereoacuity with age and reduced retinal illuminance. *Ophthal. Physiol. Opt.*, **14**, 298–301

The schematic eye

Schematic eyes in general

The object of a schematic eye is to provide a basis for theoretical studies of the eye as an optical instrument. In designing such an eye, complexities not of fundamental importance must be ignored, but the degree to which the refracting system can be simplified varies in different fields of investigation. For example, replacing the cornea with a single refracting system would not affect the size of the retinal image but would make the design unsuitable for the study of Purkinje images.

An excellent account of earlier schematic eyes, together with a detailed table of comparative dimensions, has been given by Swaine (1921). The specification introduced by Listing (1851) became a basis for subsequent modifications by Helmholtz and Wüllner. All these versions gave the eye as a whole an equivalent power in excess of +64.5 D, the refractive index of the homogeneous crystalline lens having been assigned too high a value.

A different approach was adopted by Matthiessen, whose three versions of the schematic eye all retained a stratified structure and refractive index variation typical of the actual crystalline lens. Even so, he arrived at a total equivalent power greater than +67 D.

In his *Optique Physiologique*, published in 1898, Tscherning detailed two different models of a relaxed schematic eye, one a three-surface and the other a four-surface system. Tscherning was, in fact, not only the first to include the back surface of the cornea but also the first to measure its radius of curvature *in vivo*. He assigned a lower refractive index to the crystalline than his predecessors, and in consequence the equivalent power of his four-surface system was +58.38 D, which is much nearer to an average value.

In a sense, the two schematic eyes of Gullstrand (1909) represent opposite extremes. The No.1 version has six refracting surfaces, whereas the No.2 consists of a single-surface cornea and a 'thin' crystalline lens. Like Helmholtz and Matthiessen, Gullstrand also provided a separate version (of each of his models) representing the eye when strongly accommodated. The equivalent power of the No.1 eye was +58.64 D in the relaxed and +70.57 D in the accommodated state. For the No.2 simplified eye the corresponding values were +59.74 D and +70.54 D. Both eyes were given the same axial length of 24 mm, the No.1 version having

+1.00 D of hypermetropia while the No.2 version was emmetropic.

For general purposes, the three-surface eye put forward by Listing is undoubtedly the best and the version devised by Emsley (1936) on the basis of Gullstrand's data has been widely accepted. This eye was used in the two previous editions of this book, but has now been replaced by a new version. Like Emsley's eye, this is emmetropic in its relaxed state.

Three other schematic eyes of recent origin are worthy of mention. Le Grand (1945) has modified the constants of Tscherning's four-surface system in the light of subsequent researches, the equivalent power becoming +59.94 D. He has also modified the constants of Gullstrand's No.2 eye to provide a simplified version having the same power (+59.94 D). Ivanoff (1953) has produced an updated version of Listing's three-surface model.

For practical purposes, slight differences between different schematic eyes of the same basic construction are of little consequence. Furthermore, as Ivanoff has so justly remarked, the degree of accuracy to which theoretical calculations on the subject are usually carried is not matched by our knowledge, the justification for it being the avoidance of an accumulation of errors.

A comprehensive review of many schematic eyes is also given by Smith (1995).

The cornea

Gullstrand's No.1 schematic eye represents both surfaces of the cornea (*Figure 2.8*), their radii of curvature being +7.7 and +6.8 mm respectively and the axial thickness t being 0.5 mm. The refractive index n_2 of the corneal substance is given as 1.376 and that of the aqueous humour n_3 as 1.336. This gives

Front surface power

$$F_1 = 376/ + 7.7 = +48.83 \,\text{D}$$

Back surface power

$$F_2 = \frac{1336 - 1376}{+6.8} = -5.88 \,\text{D}$$

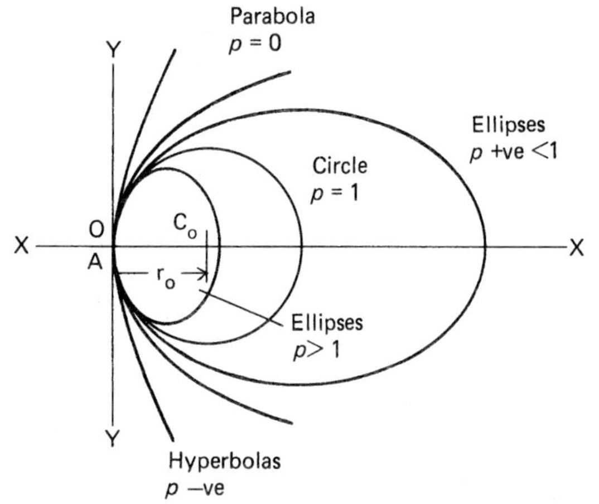

Figure 12.1. Conic sections all having the same radius of curvature r_o at the pole. A schematic aspherical cornea showing peripheral flattening or steepening of curvature is formed by revolution of the curve about the *x*-axis.

Equivalent power

$$F = +48.83 - 5.88$$

$$- [(0.0005/1.376) \times 48.83 \times (-5.88)]$$

$$= +43.05 \, \text{D}$$

The distance e of the first principal point from the vertex of the front surface is found from

$$e = \frac{t}{n_2} \times \frac{F_2}{F} = -0.050 \, \text{mm}$$

while the distance e' of the second principal point from the vertex of the second surface is found from

$$e' = \frac{-tn_3}{n_2} \times \frac{F_1}{F} = -0.551 \, \text{mm}$$

Consequently, both principal points are situated in front of the cornea, the first 0.050 and the second 0.051 mm from the front vertex. This means that they very nearly coincide with each other as well as with the first surface of the cornea. The single-surface cornea used in some schematic eyes is an optically legitimate simplification.

Because of its peripheral flattening, an ellipsoid has been suggested as a better schematic representation of the front surface of the cornea than the conventional spherical figure. *Figure 12.1* shows an ellipse with its major axis coincident with the *x*-axis of Cartesian coordinates and its vertex A at the origin O. The point C_o is the centre of a sphere of radius r_o having the same curvature as the ellipsoid at its vertex A. Following Baker (1943), the equation of *any* conic section symmetrically placed with its vertex at O may be written as

$$y^2 = 2r_o x - px^2 \tag{12.1}$$

in which p is a parameter defining any one of the entire family of conics having the same vertex radius r_o. For a circle, $p = 1$, while for a parabola $p = 0$. Intermediate values of p define ellipses of different dimensions and shape and negative values of p define a family of hyperbolas. For the purposes of certain calculations on the schematic eye, a single-surface cornea represented in

profile by equation (12.1) is a useful concept. A *p*-value in the neighbourhood of 0.6–0.8 is probably the best approximation to a typical cornea. (Corneal topography is discussed in greater detail on pages 391–397.)

Since XX in *Figure 12.1* is a unique axis of symmetry of the convex ellipsoid, the cornea as a whole could not be a centred system unless the paraxial centre of curvature of the back surface were also situated on XX. This may not occur, in which case the cornea itself will not possess a true optical axis.

The crystalline lens

Schematic representations

For the purpose of a schematic eye, the crystalline lens with its complicated refractive index variations must be replaced by something very much simpler. In his No.1 schematic eye, Gullstrand represented it by the mathematically based approximation shown in the upper part of *Figure 12.2*. It consisted of a homogeneous nucleus of refractive index 1.406, surrounded by a cortex of refractive index 1.386. Both the aqueous and vitreous humours were considered to have a refractive index of 1.336. The radii of curvature of the four refracting surfaces were, in order, +10, +7.911, −5.76 and −6 mm, while the axial thicknesses were 0.546, 2.419 and 0.635 mm, giving a total thickness of 3.6 mm. Calculation shows the equivalent power of the system to be +19.11 D, the first and second principal points being respectively 2.080 and 2.205 mm from the anterior pole of the lens, which is 3.6 mm from the anterior corneal vertex.

If the crystalline lens were conceived instead as a homogeneous biconvex element with the same radii of curvature and axial thickness as before, it may be shown that the refractive index would need to be very nearly 1.409 in order to have the same equivalent

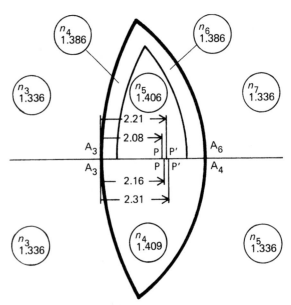

Figure 12.2. A schematic crystalline lens. The upper figure shows the Gullstrand No. 1 lens, the lower figure a homogeneous lens of the same equivalent power, outer radii and thickness.

power of +19.11 D. As shown in the lower part of *Figure 12.2*, the principal points would shift only slightly, now being 2.159 and 2.305 mm from the anterior pole.

The more complex structure undoubtedly shows the main effect of the refractive index variation of the actual crystalline lens but for most other purposes a simpler representation is adequate. In fact, in his No.2 (simplified) schematic eye, Gullstrand reduced the lens to a hypothetical one of equivalent power +20.53 D and of zero thickness, situated 5.85 mm from the corneal vertex. This is approximately the mean position of the principal points of the lens of his No.1 eye.

In the schematic eye adopted in this text, the radii of curvature of the homogeneous lens have been increased to 11.0 and −6.476 mm, while the axial thickness has increased to 3.7 mm. A refractive index of 1.422 gives an equivalent power of +20.83 D, slightly more than in the Gullstrand four-surface lens.

Effect of a tilted crystalline

Comparisons between measured corneal astigmatism and the cylinder correction found by refraction suggest that the crystalline lens tends to make a contribution of 'against the rule' astigmatism.

If the crystalline is tilted with respect to the visual axis, the resulting obliquity of incidence gives rise to oblique astigmatism, even though the surfaces are perfectly spherical. For a narrow pencil passing obliquely through the centre of a thin lens of power F, the astigmatic effect A can be determined from the well-known approximation

$$A = \theta^2 F \qquad (12.2)$$

where θ is the angle (in radians) between the incident pencil and the optical axis of the lens.

Applied to the tilted crystalline lens, this expression over-estimates the astigmatism for reasons explained elsewhere (Bennett, 1984). Calculation by a more accurate method, in which a pencil is traced from the fovea through the tilted lens to the cornea, gives the results shown graphically in *Figure 12.3*. It will be noted that a tilt of around 14° is needed to produce lenticular astigmatism of 0.50 D. To give rise to astigmatism against the rule, the lens must be tilted about a *vertical* axis. The results plotted in *Figure 12.3* relate to the relaxed Bennett–Rabbetts version of the crystalline lens.

According to Tscherning (1890), the crystalline lens is usually tilted from 3° to 7° about a vertical axis, the temporal side moving towards the cornea. There is often a tilt about a horizontal axis as well, the upper part of the lens moving forward by up to 3°.

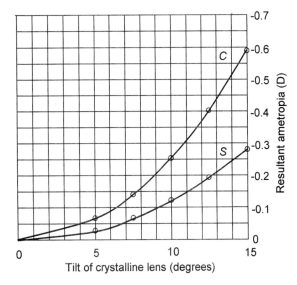

Figure 12.3. The effect on ametropia of a tilt of the Bennett–Rabbetts schematic crystalline lens.

tions of this work. The dimensions of this eye in its relaxed state are given in Appendix B.

Now, more than 50 years later, we believe that changes are needed. The most compelling reason is the value of 4/3 chosen by Emsley for the refractive indices of the humours, possibly to simplify mental arithmetic in the pre-calculator age. Unfortunately, it is not a realistic value. The figure of 1.336 adopted by Gullstrand is much more defensible and is routinely used in calculations on intra-ocular implants. We have therefore reinstated it.

Another cogent argument is that some of the present dimensions have remained unchanged for generations and were originally based on a very small number of experimental determinations. In particular, the values of 10 and −6 mm for the radii of curvature of the outer surfaces of the crystalline lens go back to Listing's model of 1851. During the past few decades, several large-scale investigations using new techniques of greater reliability have provided a mass of data on ocular dimensions. This is the solid basis on which our schematic eye is founded. Only a brief summary of these conclusions is given below. More detailed explanations have been provided in a separate publication (Bennett and Rabbetts, 1989).

Equivalent power of eye

Since the spread of results closely straddles +60 D, which is the power allotted to the reduced eye, this value in round figures should also be adopted for the schematic eye.

The Bennett–Rabbetts schematic eye

In his *Visual Optics*, first published in 1936, Emsley rendered a valuable service by introducing his version of the three-surface schematic eye. As it combined dimensions from the two Gullstrand models, we termed it the Gullstrand–Emsley eye when using it in the first two edi-

Corneal radius

Although no change has been made from the Gullstrand–Emsley value of 7.8 mm, the new index of 1.336 for the aqueous humour increases the surface power from 42.73 D to 43.08 D.

Table 12.1   The Bennett–Rabbetts schematic eye, relaxed, accommodated and elderly

Quantity		Relaxed	2.5 D	5.0 D	7.5 D	10.0 D	Elderly
			Accommodation				
Radii of curvature							
cornea	r_1	+7.80	+7.80	+7.80	+7.80	+7.80	+7.80
crystalline: first surface	r_2	+11.00	+8.60	+7.00	+6.00	+5.20	+9.25
crystalline: second surface*	r_3	−6.47515	−5.909	−5.504	−5.063	−4.750	−6.130
Axial separations							
depth of anterior chamber	d_1	3.60	3.475	3.37	3.28	3.21	2.95
thickness of crystalline	d_2	3.70	3.825	3.93	4.02	4.09	4.45
depth of vitreous body	d_3	16.79	16.79	16.79	16.79	16.79	16.69
overall axial length †		24.09	24.09	24.09	24.09	24.09	24.09
Mean refractive indices							
air	n_1	1	1	1	1	1	1
aqueous humour	n_2	1.336	1.336	1.336	1.336	1.336	1.336
crystalline	n_3	1.422	1.422	1.422	1.422	1.422	1.406
vitreous humour	n_4	1.336	1.336	1.336	1.336	1.336	1.336
Surface powers							
cornea	F_1	+43.08	+43.08	+43.08	+43.08	+43.08	+43.08
crystalline: first surface	F_2	+7.82	+10.00	+12.29	+14.33	+16.54	+7.57
crystalline: second surface	F_3	+13.28	+14.55	+15.63	+16.98	+18.10	+11.42
Equivalent powers							
crystalline	F_L	+20.83	+24.16	+27.38	+30.63	+33.78	+18.71
eye	F_o	+60.00	+62.85	+62.62	+68.40	+71.12	+58.45
Equivalent focal lengths of eye							
first (PF)	f_o	−16.67	−15.91	−15.24	−14.62	−14.06	−17.10
second (P'F')	f'_o	+22.27	+21.26	+20.36	+19.53	+18.79	+22.85
Distances from corneal vertex							
first principal point	A_1P	+1.51	+1.62	+1.71	+1.80	+1.87	+1.33
second principal point‡	A_1P'	+1.82	+1.95	+2.05	+2.15	+2.23	+1.61
first nodal point	A_1N	+7.11	+6.97	+6.83	+6.71	+6.60	+7.07
second nodal point	A_1N'	+7.42	+7.29	+7.17	+7.06	+6.95	+7.36
entrance pupil	A_1E	+3.05	+2.93	+2.83	+2.75	+2.68	+2.44
exit pupil	A_1E'	+3.70	+3.56	+3.44	+3.33	+3.25	+3.01
first principal focus	A_1F	−15.16	−14.29	−13.53	−12.82	−12.19	−15.78
second principal focus	A_1F'	+24.09	+23.21	+22.41	+21.68	+21.01	+24.47
Refractive state (principal point)	K	0	−2.50	−5.00	−7.50	−10.00	+1.00
Distance of near point from corneal vertex			−398.5	−198.3	−131.6	−98.1	

All linear distances are in millimetres and powers in dioptres.

* This radius is specified to three or more places of decimals solely to 'fine-tune' the resulting refractive state, and does not imply that an eye has to be constructed to this degree of precision.

† The accurate value of 24.0859 was used in the reversed ray traces for the accommodating and elderly eyes.

‡ Rounding errors explain the apparent differences between PP' and NN' for the various eyes.

Crystalline lens

Available data strongly suggest that the present radii of 10.0 and −6.0 mm are too short. More realistic values for a young adult would be in the neighbourhood of 11.0 and −6.5 mm. We have fine-tuned the latter to −6.47515 mm and fixed the refractive index at 1.422 in order to arrive at the exact power of 60.00 D for the eye as a whole. The equivalent power of the lens itself is 20.83 D, which is well below Emsley's figure of 21.76 D but justified by available data, as is the proposed increase in centre thickness from 3.6 to 3.7 mm.

Axial length of eye

The axial length for emmetropia resulting from the combination of the other dimensions is 24.09 mm. This, too, is consistent with published data which point to a mean value of 24.0 mm or slightly in excess of it.

The complete set of dimensions is given in *Table 12.1*,

while the positions of its cardinal points in the relaxed state are illustrated in *Figure 2.17*.

The reduced eye

To produce a power of 60.00 D with a refractive index of 1.336, the radius of curvature of the reduced eye surface is 5.6 mm. Its second principal focal length, which is also the axial length for emmetropia, is 22.27 mm (both rounded off to two decimal places). The pupil is assumed to be coincident with the refracting surface.

Calculation of optical constants: conventional method

For the schematic eye in general, the conventional approach is first to determine the equivalent power F_C of the cornea and the position of its principal points (P_1, P'_1) from standard expressions. Next, the equivalent power F_L of the crystalline and its principal points (P_2,

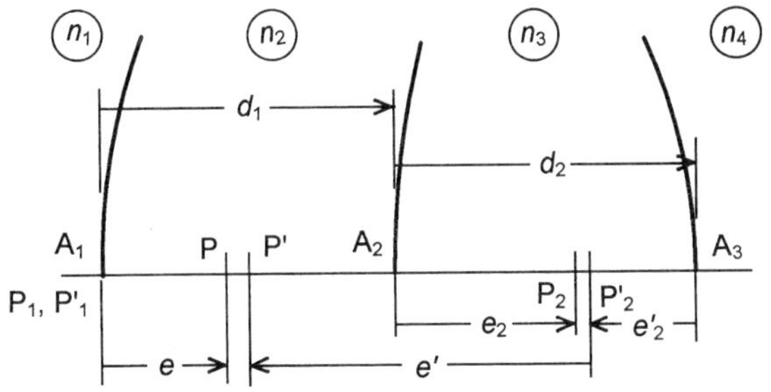

Figure 12.4. Position of the principal points P, P′ of the Bennett–Rabbetts schematic eye and of its components: P_1, P_1' coincident with A_1 (cornea); P_2, P_2' (lens).

P$_2'$) are similarly determined. The two systems are then combined, making use of the familiar relationship

$$F = F_1 + F_2 - \frac{d}{n} F_1 F_2 \tag{12.3}$$

in which F is the equivalent power of a combination of two systems of equivalent power F_1 and F_2 *optically* separated by a reduced distance d/n in metres. In this case, d is measured from the second principal point of the cornea to the first principal point of the lens.

When the cornea is represented by a single surface, the calculation becomes simplified because the equivalent power of the cornea is that of the single surface and the two principal points coincide with its vertex. *Figure 12.4* illustrates the above procedure applied to the Bennett–Rabbetts relaxed eye, the result being as follows:

Surface powers

$$F_1 = \frac{1000(n_2 - n_1)}{r_1} = \frac{336}{+7.8} = +43.077\,D$$

$$F_2 = \frac{1000(n_3 - n_2)}{r_2} = \frac{86}{11} = +7.818\,D$$

$$F_3 = \frac{1000(n_4 - n_3)}{r_3} = \frac{-86}{-6.475} = +13.282\,D$$

Equivalent power of crystalline (F_L)

$$F_L = F_2 + F_3 - \frac{d_2 F_2 F_3}{1000 n_3}$$

$$= +21.100 - 0.270 = +20.830\,D$$

Principal points of crystalline (P_2, P_2')

$$e_2 = A_2 P_2 = \frac{n_2 d_2 F_3}{n_3 F_L} = +2.217\,mm$$

$$e_2' = A_3 P_2' = \frac{-n_4 d_2 F_2}{n_3 F_L} = -1.305\,mm$$

Equivalent power of eye (F_o)

$$P_1' P_2 = P_1' A_2 + A_2 P_2 = d_1 + e_2$$

$$= 3.600 + 2.217 = 5.817\,mm$$

and

$$F_o = F_1 + F_L - \frac{(d_1 + e_2) F_1 F_L}{1000 n_2}$$

$$= +43.077 + 20.830 - 3.907 = +60.000\,D$$

Position of eye's principal points (P, P')

$$e = P_1' P = A_1 P = \frac{n_1(d_1 + e_2) F_L}{n_2 F_o} = +1.511\,mm$$

$$e' = P_2' P' = \frac{-n_4(d_1 + e_2) F_1}{n_2 F_o} = -4.176\,mm$$

$$A_1 P' = A_1 A_2 + A_2 A_3 + A_3 P_2' + P_2' P'$$

$$= 3.600 + 3.700 - 1.305 - 4.176$$

$$= +1.819\,mm$$

Equivalent focal lengths of eye (f_o, f_o')

$$f_o = PF = -1000\,n_1/F_o = -16.667\,mm$$

$$f_o' = P'F' = 1000\,n_4/F_o = +22.267\,mm$$

Position of nodal points (N, N')

As explained in Chapter 2, the nodal points of any refracting system are symmetrically positioned such that N′F′ = FP and NN′ = PP′. This gives

$$A_1 N = +7.111\,mm$$

and

$$A_1 N' = +7.419\,mm$$

Overall length of emmetropic eye ($A_1 F'$)

$$A_1 F' = A_1 P' + P'F'$$

$$= +1.819 + 22.267 = 24.086\,mm$$

Alternative method of calculation

A simpler method of calculation is based on the theorem that the equivalent power F of any refracting system can be found from the expression

$$F = \frac{L_1' L_2' L_3' \cdots}{L_2 L_3 \cdots} \quad \text{when } L_1 = 0 \tag{12.4}$$

Thus, a parallel incident pencil is traced through the system by 'step-along' methods. Applied to the Bennett–Rabbetts schematic eye, this procedure gives the results shown in *Table 12.2*.

Table 12.2 'Step-along' method of calculating equivalent power of eye

Routine		Relaxed eye	Accommodated eye (10.00 D)
L_1'	$= F_1$	$+43.077$	$+43.077$
L_2	$= \dfrac{L_1'}{1 - (d_1/n_2)L_1'}$	$+48.734$	$+48.050$
L_2'	$= L_2 + F_2$	$+56.552$	$+64.589$
L_3	$= \dfrac{L_2'}{1 - (d_2/n_3)L_2'}$	$+66.309$	$+79.325$
L_3'	$= L_3 + F_3$	$+79.591$	$+97.431$
ℓ_3' (mm)	$= 1000\, n_4/L_3'$	$+16.786$	$+13.712$
F_o (from equation 12.4)		$+60.000$	$+71.120$

In the above sequence of equations, d_1 and d_2 are in metres.

The distance A_1P' of the second principal point from the corneal vertex can be found at once because

$$A_1P' = A_1F' + F'P' = (d_1 + d_2 + \ell_3') - f_o'$$

To locate the first principal point, however, it is necessary to trace a parallel incident pencil through the system in the reverse direction, which gives the position of the first principal focus F as an intermediate step.

The accommodated schematic eye

As the eye accommodates, both surfaces of the crystalline lens, but especially the anterior, become more steeply curved. At the same time, the axial thickness increases and the lens moves slightly forward into the anterior chamber. In the Bennett–Rabbetts schematic eye, as in Gullstrand's original, the back vertex of the lens is assumed to remain stationary. In the 10 D accommodated state the axial thickness increases by 0.39 mm from 3.7 to 4.09 mm and the depth of the anterior chamber accordingly decreases by 0.39 mm to 3.21 mm. Many versions of schematic eyes also adopt an increase in the refractive index for the crystalline lens with accommodation. From the experimental data of Garner *et al.* (1997b), Garner *et al.* (1997a) concluded that there was no significant difference between the lens index at different levels of accommodation. The figures for the accommodated eye in *Table 12.1*, which perhaps should be regarded as provisional, have been based both upon this assumption and on the proportional changes to the lens found by Garner *et al.* (1997b).

The effect of accommodation on the position of the eye's principal points is relatively small. Both move towards the retina by approximately 0.4 mm in the 10 D accommodated state. The value of K', measured dioptrically from the new position of the eye's second principal point, is then increased by about 1.1 D. At the same time, both nodal points move approximately 0.5 mm towards the cornea. *Figure 12.5*, drawn to scale, shows these relative movements.

It can be seen from *Table 12.1* that whereas the equivalent power of the crystalline lens in the 10 D accommodated state has increased by 12.95 D from

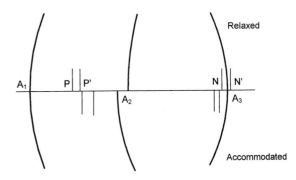

Figure 12.5. Comparison of the positions of the principal points P, P′ and nodal points N, N′ of the Bennett–Rabbetts schematic eye in its relaxed (upper) and fully accommodated (lower) states.

$+20.83$ to $+33.78$ D, the equivalent power of the eye has increased by only 11.12 D. This results from the separation between the two main components of the eye's refracting system. To a first approximation we can take the power of the cornea as $+43$ D and its mean distance from the first principal point of the lens as 5.8 mm, ignoring the variation in this distance with accommodation. The equivalent power F_e of the eye would then be expressed by

$$F_e \approx +43 + F_L - \frac{0.0058 \times 43 \times F_L}{1.336} \approx 43 + 0.81\, F_L$$

Consequently, a change of ΔF_L in the power of the crystalline would produce a change of about $0.8\Delta F_L$ in the equivalent power of the eye.

Since the standard schematic eye is emmetropic in its relaxed state, its refractive condition K in an accommodated state can be taken to indicate the amount of ocular accommodation that has been brought into play when measured at the eye's first principal point.

The schematic 'elderly' eye

As will be discussed in Chapter 21, the crystalline lens grows in thickness throughout life. Experimentally, the positions of both the anterior and posterior surfaces of the lens relative to the cornea are measured by ultrasound (*see* Chapter 20). The results show some variation in the ageing changes of the ocular dimensions. Koretz *et al.* (1989) found no significant shift in the position of the posterior lens surface, though the lens increased in thickness by 0.13 mm per decade. Over a 50-year span, Lowe (1970) found that the anterior chamber depth reduced by 0.65 mm while the lens thickness increased by about 0.73 mm. If, for simplicity, this is rounded up to 0.75 mm, the rear surface moves back by 0.10 mm, which was within the range of his experimental findings. The resulting lens thickness of 4.45 mm fits in with Weale's (1982) review. Similar results were found by Hemenger *et al.* (1995) in their groups of 48 young eyes (mean age 22 years) and 48 older eyes (mean age 54 years). Over this smaller time interval, the anterior chamber depth reduced by 0.4 mm (3.8 to 3.4 mm), while the lens increased in thickness by 0.75 mm (3.6 to 4.35 mm). The posterior surface of their sample thus moved 0.4 mm towards the retina.

Since the equatorial diameter of the lens stays approximately constant in adult life, the increased thickness is accompanied by a steepening of the radii of curvature, as shown by Brown's (1974) photographic evidence. Using ophthalmophakometry (*see* pages 398–401) and allowing for the effects of the natural lens' refractive index gradients, Hemenger and colleagues calculated the young lens to have radii of 11.2 and −6.45 mm while the older lens to be 9.3 and −6.15 mm, somewhat steeper than Brown's results.

Despite the change in lens shape towards an accommodated form with age, the typical eye's refractive error alters either little or slightly towards hypermetropia (excluding eyes with nuclear sclerosis cataract). This contradiction was studied by Pierscionek (1990), who showed that the nucleus of the crystalline lens had a uniform refractive index, only the cortex having an index gradient. Changes in this gradient are the probable explanation for the lack of a myopic shift. With a homogeneous lens in the schematic eye shown in the extreme right column of *Table 12.1*, the notional refractive index of the lens has therefore been reduced compared with the young eye, and again the radius of the posterior surface has been fine-tuned to achieve the required hypermetropia of +1.00 D.

The eye in infancy

There is insufficient information at present to develop schematic eyes for the infant and child. Wood *et al.* (1996) both review previous data and used video keratophakometry to calculate the crystalline lens parameters of 27 infants. The median results were a refractive error of +1.50 D, corneal power of +43.5 D and lens radii of 8.7 and −5.6 mm. A notional index of 1.49 was required to give the necessary lens power of 46.7 D. Since these radii are only slightly steeper than those of the adult eye having a power of around +21 D, they suggest that it is predominantly a change in this notional index (or, in real life, the index gradient of the lens) that falls to maintain near emmetropia as the axial length grows from about 17 mm at birth to its adult size.

Other vertebrates' eyes

On the basis of published data supplemented by much original work, Coile and O'Keefe (1988) have constructed schematic eyes for six domesticated animals. Both corneal surfaces were included and the lens assumed to be homogeneous. The equivalent powers of the cat, dog, and pig eyes are all very close to a mean value of 78.5 D. At the other end of the range are the horse (39.5 D) and the cow (47.7 D). Nearest to the human eye is the sheep's (61.3 D). The last row in the tabulated specifications gives the equivalent focal length of the eye in air, not the retinal image size as stated.

The cat appears to be emmetropic. The dog and the cow are slightly myopic and the pig rather more so, about −1.50 D. The horse has about +0.50 D of hypermetropia and the sheep about +1.50 D. Calculation of all the optical constants of these eyes was carried out by computer, using a program devised by the same team (O'Keefe and Coile, 1988). References to schematic eyes for other mammals are given in Oswaldo-Cruz *et al.* (1979) and Hughes (1979), while Hodos and Erichsen (1990) describe an adaptation to the focusing of bird's eyes to enable them to keep both the ground and the horizon in focus.

Schematic eyes for research

A number of schematic eyes have been designed for use in research, the general aim being to provide a model exhibiting typical values of one or more of the aberrations of real eyes. Aspherizing the refracting surfaces and departing when necessary from accepted values of refractive indices are the expedients mainly used.

In the design by Lotmar (1971), based on Le Grand's schematic eye, the front surface of the cornea was given a contour based on a study by Bonnet and the back surface of the lens was made paraboloidal. Ray tracing showed the model to have spherical aberration and peripheral astigmatism of the order required.

The eye constructed by Pomerantzeff *et al.* (1984) was designed to have the same spherical aberration as the mean value obtained from experimental measurement of 50 emmetropic subjects. The cornea was aspherized to produce a partial correction of its own spherical aberration, but the main focus of interest was on the crystalline lens. This was treated as a homogeneous nucleus surrounded by 200 or more extremely thin layers varying in refractive index and asphericity. Smith *et al.* (1991) developed two schematic lenses, with both aspheric surfaces and a gradient refractive index. These were developed further to investigate the refractive index gradient in older eyes (Smith *et al.*, 1992). A similar lens was used by Patel *et al.* (1993) to provide a model eye for predicting the optical performance after laser ablation refractive surgery (*see* pages 417–419). By careful choice of lens parameters, they obtained an eye corrected for spherical aberration. In 1995, the same team investigated the refractive index of the corneal stroma, to find a slight decrease from the anterior (1.380) to the posterior surface (1.373), with the epithelium having the higher index of about 1.401.

A model having the same spherical and longitudinal chromatic aberration as the typical real eye was designed by Navarro *et al.* (1985). One necessary step was to compile a table of notional refractive indices for the various ocular media at four different wavelengths from 365 to 1014 nm. The front corneal surface was made ellipsoidal ($p = 0.75$), the back surface remaining spherical. Following the indications of Howcroft and Parker (1977), the front surface of the lens was made hyperboloidal and the back surface paraboloidal. Of particular interest is the method adopted to determine the change in the radii of curvature, thickness and notional refractive index of the lens when the eye accommodates. Each of these quantities was defined by a formula containing the amount of accommodation (A) in use. For

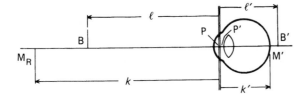

Figure 12.6. Measurement of conjugate distances from the eye's principal points.

example, the anterior radius (r_3) of the lens, taken as 10.2 in the relaxed eye, assumes the new value $r_3(A)$ given by

$$r_3(A) = 10.2 - 1.75 \log_e (A + 1)$$

When $A = 4\,\text{D}, r_3(A)$ thus becomes 7.38 mm.

A very different aim was pursued by Kooijman (1983), whose model was designed for the study of light distribution on the retina. Liou and Brennan (1996) demonstrated that most schematic eyes showed significantly more spherical aberration than the average real eye. The reduction of spherical aberration in the Bennett–Rabbetts schematic eye from aspherizing the cornea is shown in *Figure 15.6*.

Paraxial relationships

The fundamental equations

$$L' = L + F_e$$
$$K' = K + F_e$$

and

$$L' = h(L/L') \quad \text{or} \quad h(K/K')$$

apply to the schematic eye provided that the distances ℓ and ℓ', or k and k', whichever applies, are measured from the first and second principal points respectively, as in *Figure 12.6*. It is important to remember that in the schematic eye the distance k' does not represent the overall axial length, as it does in the reduced eye.

Example (1)

A schematic eye with the relaxed Bennett–Rabbetts optical system has an axial length of 26 mm. What is its refractive state?

$$k' = P'M' = P'A_1 = A_1M' = -1.82 + 26 = 24.18\,\text{mm}$$

$$K' = 1000 n_4/k' = 1336/24.18 = +55.25\,\text{D}$$

$$K = K' - F_o = 55.25 - 60.00 = -4.75\,\text{D}$$

$$k = PM_R = 1000/K = -210.63\,\text{mm}$$

The distance A_1M_R from the corneal vertex to the far point is found from

$$A_1M_R = A_1P + PM_R = 1.51 - 210.63 = -209.12\,\text{mm}$$

Example (2)

An object 30 mm high is situated at a distance of 500 mm from the corneal vertex of the Bennett–Rabbetts unaccommodated schematic eye. Determine the position and size of the optical image.

Measured from the first principal point P

$$\ell = -(500 + 1.51) = -501.51\,\text{mm}$$

so that

$$L = 1000/\ell = -1.99\,\text{D}$$

$$L' = L + F_o = -1.99 + 60.00 = +58.01\,\text{D}$$

$$\ell' = 1336/L' = +23.03\,\text{mm}$$

This distance is measured from the second principal point P', which is +1.82 mm from the corneal vertex A_1. The image distance from A_1 is therefore

$$23.03 + 1.82 = 24.85\,\text{mm}$$

and

$$h' = hL/L' = -1.029\,\text{mm}$$

Blurred imagery

Entrance and exit pupils

As indicated in Chapter 2, the entrance and exit pupils of the eye play an important role in the study of blurred imagery. The entrance pupil is the image of the real pupil formed by the cornea. Hence, taking the centre E_o of the pupil as an object for the cornea of the Bennett–Rabbetts eye we should have

$$L = 1336/-3.60 = -371.11\,\text{D}$$

$$L' = L + F_1 = -371.11 + 43.08 = -328.03\,\text{D}$$

$$\ell' = 1000/L' = -3.048\,\text{mm}$$

$$m = L/L' = 1.131$$

The entrance pupil is therefore some 3.05 mm behind the corneal vertex, while the magnification is 1.13.

Since the edge of the iris forming the pupil boundary is in approximately the same plane as the front vertex of the crystalline, it is self-conjugate by refraction at this surface. Accordingly, the exit pupil can be located by considering refraction at the posterior surface only. Hence

$$L = 1442/-3.70 = -384.32\,\text{D}$$

$$L' = L + F_3 = -384.32 + 13.28 = -371.04\,\text{D}$$

$$\ell' = 1336/L' = -3.601\,\text{mm}$$

$$m = L/L' = 1.036$$

The exit pupil is thus situated just within the crystalline lens, at a distance of $(3.70 - 3.60)$ or 0.10 mm from its anterior pole. Its size is the fraction $1.036/1.131$ or 0.916 of that of the entrance pupil.

With respect to the optical system of the eye as a whole, the entrance and exit pupils are conjugate points. An incident ray directed towards the centre E of

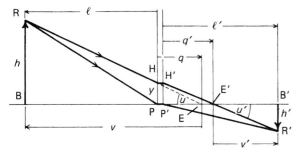

Figure 12.7. Measurement of conjugate distances v, v' from the entrance and exit pupils E, E'.

the entrance pupil would be refracted by the cornea so as to pass through the centre E_o of the real pupil; then, after refraction by the crystalline, it would emerge as though from the centre E' of the exit pupil (*see Figure 2.11*).

Paraxial relationships referred to pupils

If any one pair of conjugate foci is known, they can be used as reference points for the determination of any other pair. Thus, instead of the eye's principal points, the entrance and exit pupil centres may be used as origins of measurement. The familiar paraxial formulas then require surprisingly little modification.

In Figure 12.7, P and P' denote the principal points and E and E' the centres of the entrance and exit pupils of an eye.

The distance of E from P is denoted by q and the distance of E' from P' by q'. If n is the refractive index of the first medium (assumed to be air) and n' that of the last medium (the vitreous body), we can replace q and q' by their dioptric equivalents Q and Q', obtained from

$$Q = n/q \quad \text{and} \quad Q' = n'/q'$$

An incident ray directed towards E, from the extremity of an object BR, meets the first principal plane at H. According to a well-known principle of ray construction, the refracted ray must leave the second principal plane at a point H' at the same height y from the axis as H. This ray must also pass through E' since this is conjugate with E. Let B'R' be the image of BR formed by the eye. Then the incident ray RP must give rise to the refracted ray P'R'.

The next step is to find the relationship between the object distance v, measured from the entrance pupil, and the image distance v' measured from the exit pupil. Expressing these distances dioptrically we should have

$$V = n/v \quad \text{and} \quad V' = n'/v'$$

From similar triangles in *Figure 12.7*

$$h/y = BE/PE = -v/q = -Q/V$$

and

$$h'/y = B'E'/P'E' = -v'/q' = -Q'/V'$$

which gives

$$\frac{h'}{h} = \frac{VQ'}{V'Q}$$

If ℓ and ℓ' are the object and image distances measured (as is normal) from P and P' respectively, then

$$\frac{h'}{h} = \frac{n\ell'}{n'\ell} = \frac{n(q'+v')}{n'(q+v)} = \frac{n\{(n'/Q') + (n'/V')\}}{n'\{(n/Q) + (n/V)\}}$$

$$= \frac{(V' + Q')VQ}{(V + Q)V'Q'}$$

Equating the two expressions for h'/h gives

$$VV'^2Q^2 = V^2V'Q'^2 + VV'QQ'^2 - VV'Q^2Q'$$

which, when divided by $VV'QQ'$ becomes

$$\frac{V'Q}{Q'} = \frac{VQ'}{Q} + Q' - Q \tag{12.5}$$

Let the magnification of the system for the two given conjugates be denoted by m_E, so that

$$m_E = Q/Q' = q'/n'q \tag{12.6}$$

From the laws of conjugate foci we also have

$$Q' - Q = F_o$$

When these substitutions are made in (12.5) we get

$$m_E V' = V/m_E + F_o \tag{12.7}$$

It is evident from the derivation of this expression that E and E' can refer to any pair of conjugate points. If these were the principal points, for which the magnification is unity, the expression would simplify to its familiar form, V and V' becoming L and L'.

In the case of the Bennett–Rabbetts unaccommodated schematic eye it has already been established that

$$A_1P = +1.511 \, mm$$

and

$$A_1E = +3.048 \, mm$$

so that

$$q = PE = A_1E - A_1P = +1.537 \, mm$$

$$Q = 1000/+1.537 = +650.62 \, D$$

$$Q' = Q + F_o = +650.62 + 60.00 = +710.62 \, D$$

$$m_E = Q/Q' = 0.9156$$

For this value of m_E, equation (12.7) becomes

$$0.916V' = 1.092V + 60.00 \tag{12.8}$$

or

$$V' = 1.192V + 65.50 \tag{12.9}$$

The next step is to establish a relationship between the angle u subtended by the object at the centre E of the entrance pupil and the angle u' subtended by the image at the centre E' of the exit pupil. In *Figure 12.7*

$$u = PH/PE = y/q$$

and

$$u' = P'H'/P'E' = y/q'$$

from which

$$u'/u = q/q' = nQ'/n'Q = n/n'm_E$$

and

$$u' = \left(\frac{n}{n'm_E}\right)u \tag{12.10}$$

Finally, from *Figure 12.7* we can also obtain an expression for the transverse magnification h'/h. In this diagram, the angles u and u' are both positive in accordance with the sign convention set out in Chapter 2. Hence

$$u = -h/v = -hV/n$$

and

$$u' = -h'/v' = -h'V'/n'$$

which gives, using equation (12.10)

$$\frac{h'}{h} = \frac{n'u'V}{nuV'} = \frac{V}{m_E V'} \tag{12.11}$$

For the Bennett–Rabbetts unaccommodated schematic eye we have $n = 1$, $n' = 1.336$, and $m_E = 0.9156$. With these substitutions expression (12.10) becomes

$$u' = 0.817\,u \tag{12.12}$$

and expression (12.11) becomes

$$h'/h = 1.092\,V/V' \tag{12.13}$$

It must be emphasized that these last two expressions, together with (12.8) and (12.9), refer to the Bennett–Rabbetts schematic eye in its unaccommodated state. Calculations using the assumed values of d_1, d_2, r_2 and r_3 for the states of accommodation given in *Table 12.1* show that the coefficients of u in equation (12.12) progressively decrease (2.50 D: 0.809, 5.00 D: 0.802, 7.50 D: 0.796 and 10.00 D: 0.790) as the eye accommodates. As a result, the *basic* size of the retinal image of an object at any distance becomes very slightly smaller as accommodation is brought into play.

Blurred retinal images

Blurred retinal images in the reduced eye have already been discussed in Chapter 4. The same basic principles will now be applied to the schematic eye. In *Figure 12.8*, an object BQ (not shown), situated on the optical axis of a myopic schematic eye, gives rise to the sharp optical image B′Q′ formed in front of the retina. The diagram indicates the pencils of rays, limited by the exit pupil H′J′, which focus at B′ and Q′ and proceed to form blur circles on the retina. The centres of these circles are determined by the rays E′B′ and E′Q′ from the

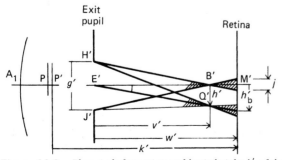

Figure 12.8. Blur-circle formation and basic height h'_b of the retinal image in a myopic schematic eye.

centre E′ of the exit pupil. As explained in Chapter 4, the basic height of the retinal image is the distance between the centres of the limiting blur circles. If g is the diameter of the entrance pupil (not shown); g' the diameter of exit pupil; $v' = E'B'$ the distance of the optical image from E′; $w' = E'M'$ the distance of the retina from E′; $h' = B'Q'$ the optical image height; h'_b the basic height of the retinal image and j the diameter of the retinal blur circles; then, from *Figure 12.8*, the quantities h'_b and j can be found from

$$h'_b = (w'/v')h' \tag{12.14}$$

and

$$j = g'\left(\frac{v' - w'}{v'}\right) \tag{12.15}$$

Example (3)

A 60 m Snellen test letter is viewed from a distance of 3 m by a myope of ocular refraction -4.00 D. Find the dimensions of the blurred retinal image, taking the optics of the Bennett–Rabbetts unaccommodated eye with a 4 mm entrance pupil.

The magnification of the exit pupil, given by equation (12.6), was found to be 0.916 for this eye. Consequently, its diameter g' is 4×0.916 or 3.664 mm.

The image distance P′B′, measured from the eye's second principal point P′, is found from

$$L' = L + F_e = -0.33 + 60.00 = +59.67\,\text{D}$$

and thus

$$P'B' = 1336/59.67 = 22.39\,\text{mm}$$

From *Table 12.1*, the distance P′E′, equal to $A_1E' - A_1P'$), is seen to be 1.88 mm. Hence

$$v' = 22.39 - 1.88 = 20.51\,\text{mm}$$

The value of k' is obtained from

$$K' = K + F_e = -4.00 + 60.00 = +56.00\,\text{D}$$

so that

$$k' = P'M' = 1336/56.00 = 23.86\,\text{mm}$$

and

$$w' = k' - P'E' = 23.86 - 1.88 = 21.98\,\text{mm}$$

The height of a 60 m Snellen letter, which subtends an angle of 50 minutes of arc (or 0.8333°) at 6 m, is

$$6000 \times \tan 0.8333° = 87.27\,\text{mm}$$

and the sharp image height h' is therefore

$$h' = hL/L' = 87.27 \times (-\tfrac{1}{3})/59.67 = -0.488\,\text{mm}$$

Then, from equation (12.14)

$$h'_b = -(21.98/20.51) \times 0.488 = -0.523\,\text{mm}$$

and, from equation (12.15),

$$j = 3.664\left(\frac{20.51 - 21.98}{20.51}\right) = -0.263\,\text{mm}$$

The minus sign indicates that in this case the optical image lies in front of the retina, the blur circles being formed by rays which have crossed over in the optical image plane.

Since the blur ratio j/h_b' is approximately 0.5, the probability is that the letter would be read.

It is interesting to compare these results with those obtained from the standard reduced eye of power $+60$ D. In this example, $K = -4.00$ D and $L = -0.33$ D, so that $K' = +56$ D and $L' = +59.67$ D. Expression (4.19) (for the reduced eye) then gives

$$h_b = hL/K' = 87.27 \times (-\tfrac{1}{3})/56 = -0.519 \text{ mm}$$

while equation (4.16) gives

$$j = 4\left(\frac{56 - 59.67}{56}\right) = -0.262 \text{ mm}$$

Projected blurs

If θ' denotes the angular subtense of a blurred retinal image at the centre of the exit pupil, the corresponding angle θ in object space (with its vertex at the centre of the entrance pupil), can be found by substituting θ and θ' for u and u' in expression (12.10). This results in

$$\theta = \left(\frac{n' m_E}{n}\right)\theta' \tag{12.16}$$

$$= 1.223\,\theta' \tag{12.17}$$

for the Bennett–Rabbetts unaccommodated schematic eye.

For the reduced eye having a refractive error K, it was shown that the angular subtense θ of the projected blurred image of a distant object point is gK prism dioptres where g is the pupil diameter in centimetres. The corresponding expression for the schematic eye is

$$\theta \approx gK(1 + K/Q') \tag{12.18}$$

where g is the diameter of the entrance pupil.[*] In many cases the term K/Q' would be entirely negligible.

The Purkinje images

Theoretical considerations

The Purkinje images, named after the celebrated Czech physiologist, are reflections from the various refracting surfaces of the eye.

When light is incident on a refracting surface, a small proportion undergoes reflection, the reflected light being plane polarized to a degree determined by the angle of incidence. It was Fresnel who deduced the equations for what is now called the 'reflectance' (ρ) or fraction of the incident light that is reflected. For angles of incidence up to about $15°$, the degree of polarization is negligible and the reflectance can be found from the simplified expression

$$\rho = \left(\frac{n_2 - n_1}{n_2 + n_1}\right)^2 \tag{12.19}$$

where n_1 and n_2 are the refractive indices of the first and second media respectively. Equation (12.19) shows that the reflectance increases as the difference between the two refractive indices increases. In the eye, by far the biggest index change is at the front surface, so that the first reflection, from the anterior surface of the cornea, is about 100 times as bright as any of the others.

Light entering the eye undergoes further partial reflections at the back surface of the cornea and at the outer surfaces of the crystalline lens. It is customary to designate the images so produced as Purkinje I, II, III and IV, the Roman numerals denoting the refracting surfaces in the order in which they occur.

For studying Purkinje I (also called the 'corneal reflex'), we can regard the anterior surface of the cornea as a convex mirror. Any convex mirror gives rise to a virtual, erect and diminished image of any real object, the image moving towards the mirror and growing larger as the object approaches the mirror. Ultimately, object and image coincide at the vertex of the mirror. If the anterior radius of the cornea is taken as $+7.8$ mm, the focal plane is situated at half this distance, that is, 3.9 mm, behind the vertex, giving the surface a catoptric power of some -256 D. This is so high that Purkinje I remains substantially in the focal plane until the object distance is quite short. For example, if an object were as close as 100 mm its Purkinje I image would have moved only 0.15 mm from the focal plane.

To form the remaining Purkinje images, the incident light is first refracted by all the surfaces in front of the one acting as a mirror and then, after reflection, is refracted again by these same surfaces in reverse order before emerging from the eye. Calculating the position and size of these images is made simpler by using the equivalent mirror theorem. This states that a system comprising one or more refracting surfaces followed by a plane or spherical mirror can be simplified for calculation to an 'equivalent' spherical mirror. The vertex and centre of curvature of the equivalent mirror coincide, respectively, with the images of the vertex and centre of curvature of the actual mirror formed by the refracting elements.

In its simplest form, a system of the type under discussion can be represented, as in *Figure 12.9*, by a thin plus lens in front of a convex mirror with its vertex at A and its centre of curvature at C. The off-axis point Q is an object for the system and Q_1' is its image formed by the lens alone. If A and C are taken as object points for the lens, the rays AQ_1 and CQ_1 directed towards Q_1 must, of necessity, pass through Q after refraction, since Q and Q_1' are conjugates. Moreover, if the refracted rays are produced backwards from Q, the points A' and C' at which they meet the axis must be respectively the images of A and C formed by the lens.

We now revert to Q as an object point for the system, its first image (formed by the lens) being Q_1'. To find the second image Q_2' formed by reflection, we take $Q_1'A$ and $Q_1'C$ as incident rays, the first being reflected along the symmetrical path AG and the other, which meets the

---

[*] This expression is left as an exercise for the student to derive by projection into object space via the centres of the exit and entrance pupils.

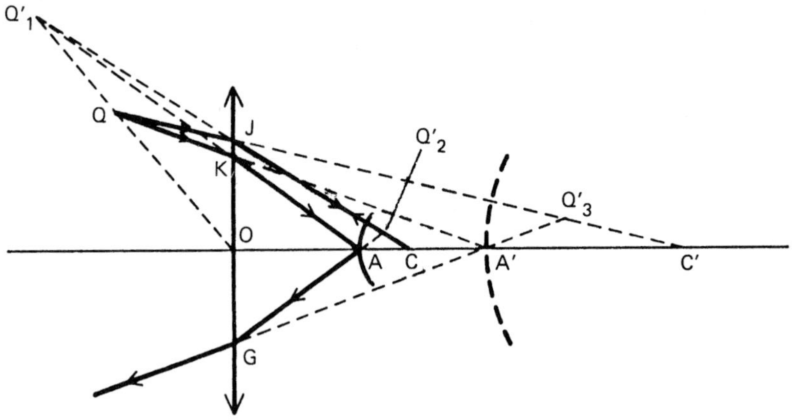

Figure 12.9. The equivalent mirror, shows as a broken curve, that replaces the system formed by the thin lens at O and mirror at A.

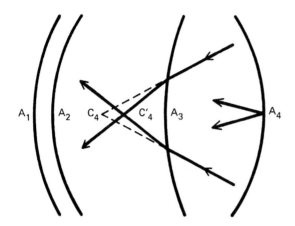

Figure 12.10. Equivalent mirror theorem applied to reflection at the posterior surface of the crystalline lens.

surface normally, being returned along its own path. Hence, Q'_2 is located at the (virtual) intersection of AG and CQ'_1. Finally, these reflected rays are refracted by the lens, from which they emerge in the directions $A'G$ and $C'Q$. The final image Q'_3 lies at the virtual intersection of these two ray paths. These ray paths determine the final image of Q and are precisely those which would result from replacing the system by a single spherical mirror with its vertex at A' and its centre of curvature at C'.

When applying this procedure to Purkinje IV (*Figure 12.10*), it will be found that A_4 and C_4 lie on opposite sides of the front surface of the crystalline, which is the refracting surface next in line. In this case, C_4 must be regarded as a *virtual* object towards which a pencil of rays is travelling *in the crystalline lens* before being intercepted. As shown in the diagram, the front surface of the crystalline then forms a real image C'_4. However, this is only an intermediate image of C_4 because further refractions at the two surfaces of the cornea are to follow.

Given a relatively distant object, the size of the image formed by reflection is proportional to the focal length of the mirror, which is one-half of the radius of curvature. If the object subtends an angle u (in radians), the height h' of the image is given by

$$h' = uf' = u(r/2) \tag{12.20}$$

Since the radius of curvature r_1 of the cornea can be measured directly with a keratometer, it can be used as a basis of calculation. Thus, if h'_k denotes the height of the kth Purkinje image and r'_k is the radius of curvature of the corresponding equivalent mirror,

$$h'_k = u(r'_k/2)$$

and since, for the same object

$$h'_1 = u(r_1/2)$$

it follows that

$$r'_k = r_1 h'_k/h'_1 \tag{12.21}$$

This is the basis of the comparison method of phakometry described on page 398.

Typical dimensions and properties

Le Grand's schematic eye is a suitable one for calculations on the Purkinje images because it incorporates the four surfaces responsible. Le Grand himself (1945) has calculated the positions and relative sizes of the images, given an object distance of 500 mm. His results are included in *Table 12.3*, together with similar calculations (by the authors) for an object at infinity. These latter computations covered the fully accommodated as well as the relaxed eye. For convenient reference the dimensions of Le Grand's schematic eye are summarized below.

Relaxed eye

Radii of curvature +7.8, +6.5, +10.2, −6.0 mm
Axial separations 0.55, 3.05, 4.0 mm
Refractive indices 1, 1.3771, 1.3374, 1.42, 1.336

Eye accommodated 6.96 D

Radii of curvature +7.8, +6.5, +6, −5.5 mm
Axial separations 0.55, 2.65, 4.5 mm
Refractive indices 1, 1.3771, 1.3374, 1.427, 1.336

Using Fresnel's formula, Le Grand also calculated the relative brightness of the Purkinje images, taking account of the pre-corneal tears film (which he assumed to be homogeneous) and of the lens capsule, which has a slightly lower refractive index than the adjacent

Table 12.3 The Purkinje images (calculated from Le Grand's schematic eye)

Image No.	Relative brightness	Unaccommodated eye				Eye accommodated 6.96 D (distant object)	
		Distant object		Object at 500 mm			
		Image position (mm)	Relative size	Image position (mm)	Relative size	Image position (mm)	Relative size
I	1	+3.900	1	+3.870	1	+3.900	1
II	0.010	+3.605	0.820	+3.585	0.821	+3.605	0.820
III	0.008	+10.726	1.971	+10.610	1.945	+6.200	1.102
IV	0.008	+4.625	−0.763	+4.325	−0.762	+5.237	−0.773

Image positions expressed as their distances from the anterior corneal vertex.

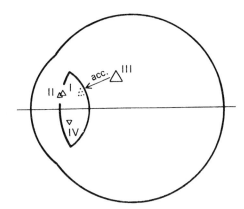

Figure 12.11. Relative positions and sizes of the Purkinje images of a distant object positioned 20° above the optic axis.

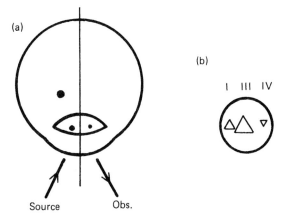

Figure 12.12. (a) Relative positions of the Purkinje images – images of a distant object positioned 20° above the optic axis. (b) The appearance within the pupil.

layers of the crystalline itself. His results are shown in the second column of *Table 12.3*, taking the corneal reflectance of 2.1% as a basis of comparison.

Clark and Carney (1971) found experimentally a corneal reflectance of up to 8% and postulated the actual multi-layer structure of the tears film as the explanation. The epithelial index of 1.401 mentioned above would give a reflectance of 2.8%.

Figure 12.11 shows the positions and relative sizes of the Purkinje images of a distant object inclined at 20° from the optical axis. Purkinje II, being slightly smaller than I and just in front of it, is normally indistinguishable from I, though Tscherning has described a simple technique of observation. With the eye in its relaxed state, Purkinje III is nearly twice the size of I, but as accommodation is brought into play it becomes smaller and moves forward into the crystalline. Accommodation affects Purkinje IV, which is inverted, to a much lesser extent. Its size remains about three-quarters of that of Purkinje I and it moves a short distance towards the retina.

Purkinje III is of notoriously poor quality. This is attributed to the 'orange peel' nature of the surface structure of the lens. The defects of this image are no doubt accentuated by its greater size.

Figure 12.12 illustrates the Purkinje images I, III and IV, the object being an illuminated triangle lying to one side of the eye's optical axis. If the observation is made from the other side as indicated in the diagram, the Purkinje images will be seen in approximately the relative positions shown on the right.

Several important uses have been found for the Purkinje images, principally in measuring or calculating the various optical dimensions of the eye. There are also some useful clinical applications in establishing the direction of the patient's gaze or of the examiner's own position relative to the patient's visual axis.

If two small light sources are placed in the same vertical line, one above and one below the eye's fixation axis, the three pairs of visible Purkinje images (I, III, and IV) will usually appear to be out of vertical alignment. Tscherning attributed this to a tilt of the crystalline lens. The angle alpha can be measured by this means (*see* page 397). An extensive study of the effects of both a tilt and an off-axis displacement of the cornea and crystalline lens on the observed positions of the Purkinje images has been made by Clement *et al.* (1987). Each surface was assumed to be of a specified conicoidal form. One of the points which emerged was that Tscherning's assumption was right. The method used in this study was a skew ray tracing system specially developed for this purpose but having further possible applications in the field of ocular dioptrics.

Secondary ghost images

The reflected pencils responsible for the Purkinje images undergo further reflections at the various surfaces they meet on their outward path. However, it is only at the front surface of the cornea that the reflectance is high enough for visible effects to be possible when the twice-reflected light reaches the retina. Account must therefore be taken of a secondary set of ghost images arising from reflection at the front surface of the cornea, acting as a concave mirror. If formed sufficiently close to the retina, the images so arising could (under suitable conditions) be perceived as such by the subject.

For purposes of reference we shall designate the ghost image formed by a first reflection at the back surface of the cornea as Purkinje V, which is associated with Purkinje II. Similarly, Purkinje VI and VII are associated with III and IV respectively.

Calculation shows that Purkinje V is situated well beyond the retina, while VI lies within the crystalline lens. Neither could be perceived recognizably. On the other hand, VII could be formed quite close to the retina and even in sharp focus. The deciding factor is the front corneal radius which determines the catoptric power Z_1 of this surface when acting as a concave mirror, given by Bennett (1968a) in the form

$$Z_1 = 2000 \, n_2/r_1 \qquad (12.22)$$

when r_1 is in millimetres. In the case of Le Grand's schematic eye, for which $n_2 = 1.3771$, this expression would become

$$Z_1 = 2754.2/r_1 \qquad (12.23)$$

Thus, a relatively small difference in r_1 would make an appreciable difference in the value of Z_1.

In the emmetropic schematic eye, Purkinje VII would lie approximately 7 mm in front of the retina, too far out of focus to be discernible. To place the image on the retina, the convergence of the pencil reflected from the cornea must be reduced, which will occur if the cornea were flatter.

A corneal radius in the neighbourhood of 8.4 mm is required to place Purkinje VII on the retina of an eye of otherwise average dimensions. Such an eye would have several dioptres of hypermetropia. It is worth noting that Tscherning, one of the pioneers in the investigation of this topic, made the observation that myopes find it difficult to see Purkinje VII (*see* Tscherning, 1924, for further details of his experiments).

Purkinje VII is erect on the retina and would therefore appear inverted to the subject. Its perceived size when in focus would be about three-quarters of that of the object seen by direct refraction.

The eye's optical centration

In Le Grand's memorable phrase, the subject of the eye's optical centration is 'confus et délicat'. The plethora of terms and conflicting definitions in this field was comprehensively reviewed by Martin (1942). Martin reduced the number of terms to an essential minimum, at the same time defining them with the necessary (or possible) degree of precision, a course we shall adopt here.

Optical axis

Since the eye is not a centred optical system, it does not possess a true optical axis. Using his ophthalmophakometer, Tscherning nevertheless found it possible to establish an axis of observation, relative to the subject's visual axis, such that all the Purkinje images of a test object appear in approximate alignment. This axis of observation can be taken as the closest approximation possible to a true optical axis. At least it has the merit of being experimentally ascertainable.

Visual axis

Names have been given to two different ray paths to the fovea. The ray path via the nodal points N and N′ has traditionally been called the visual axis, while the ray path via the centres E and E′ of the entrance and exit pupils is generally called the principal line of sight or simply the line of sight. Both paths are shown in *Figures 12.13* and *12.14*. Applied to the ray path via the nodal points, the term 'visual axis' is clearly a misnomer and should be transferred to the ray path via the pupils. In the first place, the ray from the fixation point to the centre of the entrance pupil is the true axis of the pencil of rays which actually enters the eye and stimulates the retina. Secondly, the statement that the rays from the fixation point to E and N are, in any case, parallel in distance vision applies only to the emmetropic eye (*Figure 12.13*). The situation that arises in the myopic eye is illustrated in *Figure 12.14*. If rays are traced backwards from the fovea M′ to E′ and N′, the refracted rays will emerge from the eye as though from E and N respectively, but in this case they cannot be parallel. They are bound to intersect at the eye's far point M_R since, by definition, this is the point conjugate with the fovea. Any fixation point such as B must clearly lie on the line passing through E and M_R because this is the incident path of the ray which finally impinges on the fovea. Thus, in general, the so-called visual axis

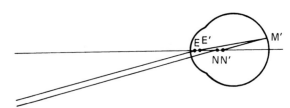

Figure 12.13. The visual axis through the entrance and exit pupils E, E′ and the nodal axis through the nodal points N, N′ of the emmetropic eye (not to scale). In emmetropia, the two axes are parallel in object space.

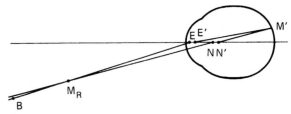

Figure 12.14. The myopic eye. Reverse trace from the fovea through the exit and entrance pupils and through the nodal points, showing their intersection at M_R (not to scale).

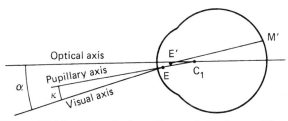

Figure 12.15. The optical, pupillary and visual axes of the eye (not to scale).

would not even pass through the fixation point. Thirdly, the visual axis as traditionally defined, besides being a concept of limited utility, cannot be located in practice.

It is therefore suggested that the ray path to the fovea via the nodal points should be renamed the nodal axis, and that the term visual axis should apply to the ray path to the fovea via the pupil centres. As already indicated on page 13, it will be used in this sense throughout the present work.

Angle alpha

This angle, which can be measured with Tscherning's ophthalmophakometer, is the angle between the eye's optical axis and its visual axis. It is taken as positive when the visual axis in object space lies on the nasal side of the optical axis (*see* page 397).

Pupillary axis

This can be defined as the line from the centre of the entrance pupil which meets the (single surface) cornea normally. It thus passes through C_1, the centre of curvature of this surface (*Figure 12.15*).

Typically, the pupil is thought to be decentred nasally from the optical axis by about 0.25 mm, in which case both the entrance and exit pupils would lie on the nasal side of the optical axis. Even a displacement as small as 0.25 mm would create an angle of some 3° between the pupillary and optical axes.

There is also evidence to suggest that when the pupil contracts, it does not do so symmetrically. Its geometrical centre moves slightly nasalwards – a fact of some significance in the study of chromatic stereopsis (*see* Chapter 15).

Angle kappa (or lambda)

As introduced by Landolt, this term denoted the angle between the pupillary axis and the visual axis as then understood (i.e. the nodal axis). More recently, the angle kappa has been used (by Le Grand, for example) to denote the angle between the pupillary axis and the principal line of sight or visual axis as redefined above. The same angle has also been called 'angle lambda' by some American writers.

A simple means of measuring the angle kappa (in its modern sense) or angle lambda has been described by Loper (1959). A circular fluorescent lamp is mounted so as to surround the object glass of a sighting telescope. A fixation object movable laterally along a scale in nearly the same plane as the lamp is used to direct the subject's gaze until the first Purkinje image of the lamp appears centrally within the subject's pupil. The displacement of the fixation object from the axis of observation divided by the distance of the scale from the subject's eye gives the tangent of the angle kappa (or lambda).

Iris-perpendicular axis

Subjective judgement of the direction of gaze is undoubtedly aided by mentally constructing an axis through the pupil centre, perpendicular to the iris. This is a particularly useful clue when the corneal reflex is not visible because of diffuse illumination or obliquity of observation. Another clue, mentioned on page 187, is the extent of sclera visible on each side of the cornea.

Corneal reflection PD gauge

For distance PD measurement, these devices use a simple telecentric system. A small observation aperture is situated at the anterior focal point of a converging lens of about 80 mm width. The subject views the image formed at infinity of a small illuminated ring surrounding the observation aperture. Since only rays substantially parallel to the optical axis can pass through this aperture after refraction by the lens, measuring errors due to parallax are obviated. For each eye independently, the observer moves a vertical fiducial wire so as to bisect the corneal reflection of the annular source. As can be seen from *Figure 12.15*, the centre of this reflected image must lie in the ray parallel to the visual axis and passing through C_1, the centre of curvature of the cornea. Because of the angle alpha (assumed to be positive), the PD thus measured will be slightly smaller than the distance between the centres of the eyes' entrance pupils, unless the pupils are decentred nasally. Because of this, it may be preferable to move the fiduciary wire to bisect the pupil. For measuring the near PD, the lens is moved closer to the aperture and set to a scale, so that the source image is formed at the given near distance.

An ordered range of variants

In general, the optical dimensions of the various schematic eyes represented mean values as suggested by available data. When studying ametropia and optical imagery in the ametropic eye – and even in emmetropia, for that matter – the known variations in these dimensions must be taken into account. The values listed in *Table 12.4* were compiled mainly on the basis of Stenström's classic study (1946) of 1000 eyes *in vivo*.

Table 12.4 Standard values and ranges of main ocular dimensions

Dimension	Symbol	Standard value	Range
Corneal radius (mm)	r_1	7.80	7.0 to 8.8
Corneal power*(D)	F_1	+43.08	+38 to +48
Depth of anterior chamber (mm) (including corneal thickness)	d_1	3.60	2.9 to 4.5
Equivalent power of lens (D)	F_L	+20.83	+16 to +29
Equivalent power of eye (D)	F_e	+60.00	+51 to +71

* Evaluated from the radius, assuming a single surface cornea and a refractive index of 1.336.

Table 12.5 Variants of the Bennett–Rabbetts schematic crystalline lens

Dimension	Lens A (low power)	Lens B (standard)	Lens C (high power)
Radii of curvature			
r_2	+14.25	+11.00	+7.82
r_3	−8.50	−6.475	−4.60
Axial thickness (d_2)	2.90	3.70	4.50
Surface powers			
F_2	+ 6.04	+ 7.82	+11.00
F_3	+10.12	+13.28	+18.70
Equivalent power (F_L)	+16.03	+20.83	+29.04
Position of principal points from anterior pole			
first	+1.72	+2.22	+2.72
second	+1.87	+2.40	+2.90
Assumed depth of anterior chamber (d_1)	4.10	3.60	3.00

All linear dimensions are in millimetres and powers in dioptres.

If the 'standard' cornea and crystalline lens are each supplemented by two others, one from each end of the tabulated range, the permutation of these two sets of variables will produce nine different feasible optical systems. Stenström did not measure the radii of curvature of the lens surfaces, but for our present purpose it will be legitimate to assume that they maintain the same ratio (11:6.475) as in the 'standard' eye. On this basis, a set of hypothetical crystalline lenses has been constructed, the dimensions of the middle one being those of the Bennett–Rabbetts schematic eye. Their dimensions are given in *Table 12.5*. This table also gives an ar-bitrary value of d_1 (depth of anterior chamber) which the eye is assumed to have in each case.

The set of variant schematic eyes derived from this approach is detailed in *Table 12.6*. In addition to the dimensions, the table also gives the positions of the principal points and of the entrance and exit pupils, together with the axial length required for emmetropia. This is seen to vary from 20.83 to 27.67 mm. It is interesting to note that Sorsby *et al.* (1957) found the axial length of 90 emmetropic eyes to vary from 21 to 26 mm.

Given a set of hypothetical eyes as tabulated, it is a simple matter to calculate the axial length required in each case to produce various degrees of spherical ametropia. *Table 12.7* gives the results of such a study, the ametropia being expressed as the spectacle correction needed at 14 mm from the eye's first principal point.

These results were used to construct the graph in *Figure 12.16*. It was found possible to draw a series of curved lines passing very close to all the points plotted for a particular refractive error. To a reasonable approximation, the graph shows the range of possible combinations of equivalent power and axial length producing various degrees of ametropia. It can also be used in reverse. For example, an equivalent power of +69 D and an axial length of 27 mm would result in a spectacle refraction of approximately −20 D.

Determination of the equivalent power of the eye

A method for the determination of the equivalent power of the crystalline lens and of the eye, based on the shape of the schematic eye's lens, is given in Chapter 20.

Table 12.6 Variants of the Bennett–Rabbetts schematic eye

Corneal power Lens	+38.01 A (low power)	B (standard)	C (high power)	+43.08 A (low power)	B* (standard)	C (high power)	+48.00 A (low power)	B (standard)	C (high power)
r_1	+8.84	+8.84	+8.84	+7.80	+7.80	+7.80	+7.00	+7.00	+7.00
r_2	+14.25	+11.00	+7.82	+14.25	+11.00	+7.82	+14.25	+11.00	+7.82
r_3	−8.50	−6.475	−4.60	−8.50	−6.475	−4.60	−8.50	−6.475	−4.60
d_1	4.10	3.60	3.00	4.10	3.60	3.00	4.10	3.60	3.00
d_2	2.90	3.70	4.50	2.90	3.70	4.50	2.90	3.70	4.50
F_1	+38.01	+38.01	+38.01	+43.08	+43.08	+43.08	+48.00	+48.00	+48.00
F_2	+6.04	+7.82	+11.00	+6.04	+7.82	+11.00	+6.04	+7.82	+11.00
F_3	+10.12	+13.28	+18.70	+10.12	+13.28	+18.70	+10.12	+13.28	+18.70
Equivalent power of eye (F_e)	+51.38	+55.39	+62.32	+56.10	+60.00	+66.76	+60.68	+64.48	+71.07
Focal lengths									
f_e	−19.46	−18.05	−16.04	−17.83	−16.67	−14.98	−16.48	−15.51	−14.07
f'_e	+26.00	+24.12	+21.44	+23.82	+22.27	+20.01	+22.01	+20.72	+18.80
Principal points									
A_1P	+1.36	+1.64	+2.00	+1.24	+1.51	+1.86	+1.15	+1.41	+1.75
A_1P'	+1.67	+2.00	+2.41	+1.51	+1.82	+2.21	+1.37	+1.67	+2.03
Pupils									
A_1E	+3.47	+3.00	+2.46	+3.54	+3.05	+2.49	+3.60	+3.09	+2.52
A_1E'	+4.22	+3.70	+3.01	+4.22	+3.70	+3.01	+4.22	+3.70	+3.01
Axial length for emmetropia	+27.67	+26.12	+23.85	+25.32	+24.09	+22.22	+23.39	+22.39	+20.83

* This column corresponds to the 'standard' eye.
All linear dimensions are in millimetres and powers in dioptres.

Table 12.7 Axial lengths (in mm) of the variant schematic eyes detailed in *Table 12.6* when exhibiting various amounts of spherical ametropia

Spectacle refraction	Power of cornea (F_1)								
	+38.01			+43.08			+48.00		
	Lens A (low power)	Lens B (standard)	Lens C (high power)	Lens A (low power)	Lens B (standard)	Lens C (high power)	Lens A (low power)	Lens B (standard)	Lens C (high power)
+10.00	22.87	21.94	20.48	21.23	20.47	19.25	19.85	19.22	18.19
+5.00	25.21	23.99	22.14	23.24	22.25	20.73	21.60	20.79	19.51
0	27.67	26.12	23.85	25.32	24.09	22.22	23.39	22.39	20.83
−5.00	30.27	28.35	25.58	27.48	25.97	23.72	25.23	24.00	22.16
−10.00	33.02	30.66	27.36	29.74	27.90	25.25	27.11	25.65	23.48
−15.00	35.94	33.08	29.17	32.08	29.88	26.78	29.04	27.32	24.80
−20.00	39.03	35.60	31.02	34.52	31.93	28.33	31.02	29.01	26.13
−25.00	42.32	38.24	32.91	37.06	34.03	29.90	33.06	30.73	27.46

The spectacle refraction is the distance correction that would be needed at 14 mm from the eye's first principal point or approximately 12.5 mm from the corneal vertex.

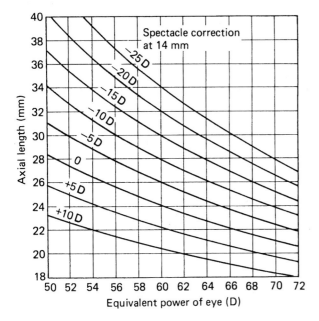

Figure 12.16. Graph showing possible combinations of axial length and equivalent power required to produce various spectacle refractions at 14 mm from the eye's first principal point (compiled from the data of *Tables 12.6* and *12.7*).

The aphakic eye

The distance correction

Etymologically, the term 'aphakia' denotes the absence of the (crystalline) lens. Its surgical removal because of cataract is by far the most common cause of this condition, but the term is also applied to cases in which the lens has become displaced from the pupillary area (subluxation) and plays no part in the eye's refracting system.

The equivalent power of the aphakic eye is that of the cornea alone. As we have already noted, the principal points of the typical cornea very nearly coincide with each other and with the vertex of its front surface. We may thus regard the aphakic schematic eye as having only one refracting surface, the power of which is given to a fair degree of accuracy by the keratometer.

Removal of the crystalline lens entails a drastic reduction in the power of the eye's optical system and, in most cases, the need for a strong plus correction. In the Bennett–Rabbetts schematic eye the axial length is 24.09 mm and the power of the single corneal surface is +43.08 D. Thus

$$K' = 1336/24.09 = +55.46 \text{ D}$$

$$K = K' - F_e = +55.46 - 43.08 = +12.38 \text{ D}$$

To correct this eye for distance, a spectacle lens with its back vertex 12 mm from the cornea would need to have a back vertex power of approximately +10.75 D, since

$$k = 1000/+12.38 = +80.78 \text{ mm}$$

and

$$f'_{sp} = k + d = +92.78 \text{ mm}$$

Thus

$$F_{sp} = 1000/+92.78 = +10.78 \text{ D}$$

Older operation techniques for cataract extraction with long incisions and their necessary sutures often left some deformation of the cornea, resulting in significant astigmatism, though this often decreased postoperatively.

The post-cataract correction needed in a particular case is clearly related to the previous refractive state of the eye, but this is not the only determining factor. The optical dimensions of the given eye also play an important role. As a result, the relationship between the post-cataract spectacle correction F_a and the previous spectacle refraction F_{sp} shows a spread of some 3–5 D on each side of the mean. This can be seen from *Figure 12.17*, which was constructed by calculating the post-cataract corrections needed by a range of variant schematic eyes having the refractive errors and axial lengths similar to those shown in *Table 12.7*.

In *Figure 12.17*, the central unbroken line refers to eyes having the optical system of the Bennett–Rabbetts

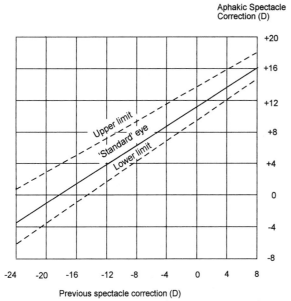

Aphakic Spectacle
Correction (D)

Upper limit

'Standard' eye

Lower limit

Previous spectacle correction (D)

Figure 12.17. Approximate power of the aphakic spectacle correction needed at 12 mm vertex distance as a function of the correction before operation.

eye. A reasonable approximation to this curve is given by the linear equation.

$$F_a = 0.6\,F_{sp} + 10.75 \tag{12.24}$$

It can be seen from the graph that eyes in this category having some 18–20 D of myopia would become nearly emmetropic (apart from any astigmatism) after extraction of the crystalline. This procedure was, in fact, proposed by Fukala (1890) in cases of high myopia, but was not well received.

The near correction

Because removal of the crystalline lens deprives the eye of its mechanism of accommodation, a near addition is invariably required; factors relevant to the prescribing of such additions have already been discussed on pages 119–121.

Visual problems in aphakia

Though surgery has restored their sight, aphakics have a number of visual problems. The loss of accommodation is not usually a serious blow because the majority of aphakics are elderly and already have a greatly depleted amplitude. A more serious disturbance is the considerable increase in the size of the retinal image when a spectacle correction is worn. As shown by Bennett (1968b) when all the relevant factors (including variations in ocular dimensions) are taken into account, the spectacle-corrected aphakic may have a retinal image from about 17 to 53% larger than in his previous refractive state. An average figure would be in the neighbourhood of 30–35%. In unilateral aphakia, this enormous disparity between the two eyes would make single binocular vision impossible. With a contact lens correction, the increase in the retinal image sizes ranges from zero in the eye previously strongly hypermetropic to about

10% in near emmetropia and 35% in extreme cases of antecedent myopia. All these results, shown graphically in *Figure 14.3*, are further discussed on pages 262–263 with particular reference to unilateral aphakia.

A number of other problems, described by an aphakic ophthalmologist (Woods, 1952), arise from the unintended but unavoidable effects of high-powered spectacle lenses. These subsidiary effects of lenses are discussed in detail in Chapter 13.

Intra-ocular lenses

Replacing the natural crystalline with an artificial lens of similar power in a similar position would leave the eye in a much more normal optical state. The term pseudophakia to denote this ocular condition has found general acceptance.

After Harold Ridley's pioneer work in fitting posterior chamber implants, development turned to the anterior chamber as a more convenient site. Thanks to the work of Strampelli and many others, the surgical and optical problems posed by this procedure have been greatly reduced. Nevertheless, posterior chamber implants (of new designs placed in the original lens capsule) have now returned to favour in order to avoid the possibility of damage to the corneal endothelium and anterior chamber angle.

When in position, the front vertex of an anterior chamber implant is about 2.0–2.5 mm from the back surface of the cornea. For a posterior implant, the corresponding distance is about 3.0–4.0 mm. No differences of principle are involved and the following discussion embraces both types.

In general, only spherical surfaces are used, but the form of the lens varies in different designs. In addition to the corneal power, the overall axial length of the eye should be determined, the latter usually by ultrasonography. While the intention is frequently to aim at emmetropia or low myopia, a residual error similar to that in the patient's other eye to avoid anisometropia may be a wiser option, especially if cataract surgery is not likely to be needed in this eye for some time. Auxiliary spectacles may be needed to correct pre-existing corneal astigmatism, residual errors of refraction and the lack of accommodation. Moreover, the controlled use of an auxiliary lens gives a useful means of varying the size of the retinal image (*see* pages 262–263 on unilateral aphakia).

If the thickness of the implant is ignored, the required power F (*in situ*, not in air) can be found to a reasonably close approximation by the step-along vergence method illustrated in *Figure 12.18*. The intended auxiliary lens (if any), placed at a vertex distance d from the single surface cornea, is of power F'_{sp} and its effective power at the cornea is

$$E = \frac{F'_{sp}}{1 - dF'_{sp}} \tag{12.25}$$

The implant is at a distance d_1 from the cornea and the refractive index n' of the ocular medium is taken as 1.336. The measured power of the cornea is F_c and the

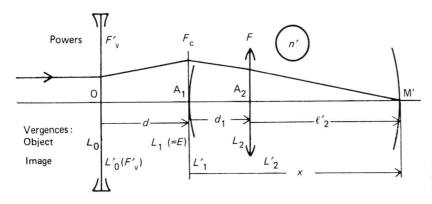

Figure 12.18. Step-along method of calculation to determine the power F of a thin intra-ocular implant.

overall axial length of the eye is x. All axial distances are in metres.

Given a distant object, the vergence at the eye is E. Thus

$$L'_1 = E + F_c$$

and

$$L_2 = \frac{E + F_c}{1 - (d_1/n')(E + F_c)} \tag{12.26}$$

After refraction by the implant, the pencil has the vergence L'_2, equal to n'/ℓ'_2, and will focus on the retina provided that

$$\ell'_2 = x - d_1$$

so that

$$L'_2 = \frac{n'}{x - d_1} = \frac{1}{(x/n') - (d_1/n')} \tag{12.27}$$

Let $X = n'/x$. Then, by substitution in equation (12.27),

$$L'_2 = \frac{X}{1 - (d_1/n')X} \tag{12.28}$$

The required power F of the implant can now be found from equations (12.26) and (12.27), since

$$F = L'_2 - L_2$$

$$= \frac{X}{1 - (d_1/n')X} - \frac{E + F_c}{1 - (d_1/n')(E + F_c)}$$

$$= \frac{X - E - F_c}{\{1 - (d_1/n')X\}\{1 - (d_1/n')(E + F_c)\}} \tag{12.29}$$

By expanding the denominator and ignoring terms in $(d_1/n')^2$, this expression can be simplified with little loss of accuracy to

$$F = \frac{X - E - F_c}{1 - (d_1/n')(X + E + F_c)} \tag{12.30}$$

Although the implant is usually inserted as part of the cataract operation, an anterior chamber lens could be inserted into an aphakic eye later as a second operation. In this case, the overall length of the eye expressed as X dioptres can be determined fairly accurately without recourse to ultrasonography. In addition to the corneal power F_c, it is necessary to determine the spectacle refraction and convert it into the ocular refraction K. The value of X can then be found from

$$X = K + F_c \tag{12.31}$$

Practical approximate formulae

A better formula than equation (12.30) can be derived for calculating the required power of an implant if its thickness is ignored and if it is intended to make the eye emmetropic. Let F_c denote the corneal power, d the distance from the corneal vertex to the implant but this time in millimetres, and x the axial length, also in millimetres. Then, assuming parallel incident light, the vergence L_2 at the implant is

$$L_2 = \frac{F_c}{1 - d(F_c/1336)}$$

After refraction by the implant, the vergence L'_2 needed to place the focus on the retina is

$$L'_2 = \frac{1336}{x - d}$$

Consequently, the required power F of the implant is

$$F = L'_2 - L_2 = \frac{1336}{x - d} - \frac{F_c}{1 - d(F_c/1336)} \tag{12.33}$$

For example, if $F_c = 43.08$ D, $d = 5.6$ mm, and $x = 24.09$ mm, so that $(x - d) = 18.59$ mm,

$$L'_2 = 1336/18.49 = 72.25 \text{ D}$$

$$L_2 = \frac{43.08}{1 - 5.6(43.08/1336)} = 52.57 \text{ D}$$

$$F = 72.25 - 52.57 = +19.68 \text{ D}$$

If a planoconvex lens is fitted with its plane surface to the cornea, its reduced thickness should be added to d when using simplified equations such as equation (12.33).

Errors in determining or estimating the values of x and d would have the following effects on the calculated power of the implant for the typical eye:

Error in d (only)	*Approximate error in power*
Each 0.1 mm too deep	0.14 D too strong
Each 0.1 mm too shallow	0.14 D too weak

Error in x only	
Each 0.1 mm too long	0.30 D too weak
Each 0.1 mm too short	0.30 D too strong

Equation (12.33) can be adjusted in various ways to compensate for systematic inaccuracies arising in practice. A comparison of several such formulae has been made by Sanders and Kraff (1984), Olsen *et al.* (1990) and Douthwaite (1993).

The SRK formula

This simple formula, devised by Retzlaff et al. (1981), was the outcome of an entirely different approach. Expressed in the symbols used in this chapter, it becomes

$$F = A - 2.5 - 0.9 F_c \quad (x \text{ in mm}) \qquad (12.34)$$

in which A is a numerical term differing for each lens type and manufacturer. For anterior chamber implants, the mean value of A approximates to 115, while for posterior chamber implants it is about 116.8. A table of values is given by Sanders and Kraff (1984).

It is noteworthy that a specified value for the anterior chamber depth is not required, being reflected in the variation of the numerical term A. Thus, in the numerical example above, if a lens with an A constant of 119.0 is implanted in the schematic eye, the power F of the implant for emmetropia is +20.00 D.

The SRK formula was based on a statistical analysis of several thousand cases from various practitioners, covering many different implant designs. It is a regression formula, with the coefficients of corneal power and axial length calculated to give the best fit for the entire available sample. Its main advantage is that, being derived from case records, it takes account of systematic measuring errors and uncertainties such as postoperative corneal curvature changes and anterior chamber depth.

While coping well with eyes of average axial length, the SRK formula was less accurate in predicting the implant power required for longer and shorter eyes. Sanders et al. (1988) suggested correction factors for modifying the constant A for eyes with axial length outside the range 22.0–24.5 mm.

Although the SRK formulae have worked well, they have not been based on the vergences within the eye, as described above. They therefore (Retzlaff et al., 1990) developed a theoretically based formula, SRK/T, though even this had various multiplying factors derived from a regression analysis of pre- and postoperative results. It includes correction factors for axial length in long eyes, an estimated value for the postoperative anterior chamber depth calculated from the (corrected) axial length and keratometry findings, and retinal thickness.

Lens form and image size

Intra-ocular lenses are less than 1 mm thick and their principal planes will be about 0.12 mm apart and will lie towards the front, centre or rear surface depending on the implant lens form, that is, on whether it has most of its power on the front surface, is equiconvex, or has a near plano front surface power.

In view of the uncertainties involved in implantation and the fact that their principal points are only about 0.12 mm apart, they may almost be regarded as 'thin' lenses.

The draft Standard ISO 11979: Intra-ocular lenses – Part 1 – Terminology classifies their strength on the basis of their equivalent power. The A constant in the SRK formulae for any particular design will take account of the lens form and the average anterior chamber depth after implantation.

The principal points of the lens in the Bennett–Rabbetts 'elderly' schematic eye shown in Table 12.1 lie approximately 2.58 and 2.74 mm behind the anterior lens pole. A posterior chamber implant designed to lie approximately 5.5 mm behind the front surface of the cornea will therefore have its principal plane situated close to those of the crystalline lens it replaces, and so will have little effect on the equivalent power of the eye as a whole. There will then be little effect on the retinal image size, provided that there is little change in the patient's refractive error. For example, if the Bennett–Rabbetts schematic eye is provided with a thin implant at 5.6 mm depth, the required power as shown above is +19.68 D. This gives an equivalent power to the eye as a whole of 59.20 D, giving a relative image size 1.3% larger than the previously emmetropic young schematic eye. Anterior chamber implants, however, give a significantly greater image size.

Where a patient's fellow eye is nearly emmetropic, or where both eyes will need implant operations within a short space of time, the surgeon will probably aim to choose an implant lens that subsequently renders the patient emmetropic or mildly myopic. Where a patient's fellow eye retains good vision and has a significant refractive error, the surgeon should aim to duplicate that error or perhaps slightly reduce it, otherwise anisometropia (Chapter 14) will result. In the neighbourhood of emmetropia, the implant power should be decreased by about 1.5 D for every dioptre of residual hypermetropia that is desired, and conversely, increased for myopia. For larger residual errors, decreases of 1.65 D or increases of 1.35 D per dioptre will be more accurate.

Exercises

12.1　A schematic eye suggested by W. Swaine consists of two thin lenses in air, separated by 4 mm. The first, representing the cornea, has a power of +43.00 D and the second representing the crystalline lens, has a power of +20.50 D. Find: (a) the equivalent power of this eye, (b) the positions of its principal points, (c) the axial length needed for emmetropia.

12.2　Assume that the schematic eye detailed in Question 12.1 has the correct axial length for emmetropia (17.81 mm) and that the power of the second lens is increased by 5.00 D to represent the maximum effort of accommodation. Find: (a) the position of the near point, (b) the increase in the equivalent power of the eye. How do you reconcile these results?

12.3　If the Bennett–Rabbetts unaccommodated schematic eye had an axial length of 26.00 mm, all other details being unchanged, what would be the precise values of K and K'? At what distance from the corneal vertex would the eye's far point be situated?

12.4　Assuming the optical system of the Bennett–Rabbetts unaccommodated schematic eye, determine the axial length corresponding to a principal point refraction of −2.50 D.

12.5　A possible mechanism for accommodation was thought to be a forward axial shift of the crystalline lens. Calculate the refractive state (measured at the corneal vertex) of the relaxed Bennett–Rabbetts schematic eye following a 1.0 mm advancement of the lens.

12.6　Recalculate the data of Table 12.1 for a relaxed, emmetropic eye with a changed refractive index of 1.333 for the aqueous and vitreous humours, all other dimensions except depth of vitreous body remaining the same.

12.7　An uncorrected myopic eye with a 3 mm entrance pupil and the optics of the Bennett–Rabbetts schematic eye views a car at 100 m. If the rear lights are 1.5 m apart and the retinal blur circles just touch, what is the ametropia?

12.8 In a given eye, the radii of curvature of the first and second surfaces of the cornea are 7.8 and 6.9 mm respectively. The cornea is 0.6 mm thick and has a refractive index of 1.376. Find the size and position of the eye's entrance pupil, assuming the real pupil to have a diameter of 4.5 mm, the depth of the anterior chamber to be 3.2 mm and the refractive index of the aqueous humour to be 1.336.

12.9 A myopic eye has its crystalline lens removed and is then found to be emmetropic. What was the previous spectacle refraction, assuming the optical system of the Bennett–Rabbetts schematic eye with the spectacle plane 12 mm from the cornea?

12.10 An aphakic eye is corrected for distance by a thin lens of power + 12.50 DS placed $13\frac{1}{3}$ mm from the cornea. How far and in what direction would this lens have to be shifted to allow the eye to see distinctly at $\frac{1}{3}$ m from the cornea?

12.11 A Bennett–Rabbetts schematic eye is rendered aphakic and is subsequently corrected by a plano-convex spectacle lens 8.0 mm thick (with its convex surface forward) at a vertex distance of 12 mm. Calculate, and draw a scale diagram showing, the positions of the cardinal points of the system. Assume a refractive index of 1.523 for the spectacle lens.

12.12 The image size in a corrected aphakic eye is proportional to the equivalent focal length (in air) of the system. At what distance should a patient with a corrected aphakic eye (as in the previous example) view a 1 m Bjerrum screen, so that the blind spot will be plotted at the correct distance from the centre of the screen?

12.13 Ultrasonography gives the length of an eye as 20.00 mm, while the corneal radius is measured as 7.60 mm. Assuming an index of 1.336 for the ocular humours and a single surface cornea, find: (a) the aphakic ocular refraction, (b) the power of the 'thin' implant needed at 3.5 mm from the cornea to give emmetropia.

12.14 (a) An aphakic eye is represented schematically by a single surface cornea of radius of curvature 7.6 mm, the axial length being 24.50 mm and the refractive index 1.336. What distance correcting lens would be needed at 13 mm from the cornea? (b) Compare the size of the retinal images in this corrected aphakic eye with those formed in the schematic emmetropic eye of power +60 D.

12.15 Draw a diagram to 5× scale showing the iris perpendicular axis and the pupillary axis for the right eye, given a corneal radius of 8.0 mm, anterior chamber depth of 3.5 mm and pupillary decentration of 1 mm temporally.

12.16 Draw a diagram similar to *Figure 12.15* to show the ray path of a corneal reflection PD gauge for an emmetropic eye. Assume the PD gauge to be set for distance vision, an exaggerated angle alpha of +15° and the pupil to be centred on the optical axis of the eye.

References

BAKER, T.Y. (1943) Ray tracing through non-spherical surfaces. *Proc. Phys. Soc.*, **55**, 361–364

BENNETT, A.G. (1968a) *Emsley and Swaine's Ophthalmic Lenses.* London: Hatton Press

BENNETT, A.G. (1968b) The corrected aphakic eye: a study of retinal image sizes. *Optician*, **155**, 106–111, 132–135

BENNETT, A.G. (1984) Astigmatic effect of a tilted crystalline lens. *Ophthal. Optn*, **24**, 793–794

BENNETT, A.G. (1988) A method of determining the equivalent powers of the eye and its crystalline lens without resort to phakometry. *Ophthal. Physiol. Opt.*, **8**, 53–59

BENNETT, A.G. and RABBETTS, R.B. (1988) Schematic eyes – time for a change? *Optician*, **196**(5169), 14–15

BENNETT, A.G. and RABBETTS, R.B. (1989) Letter to the Editor (on proposals for new reduced and schematic eyes). *Ophthal. Physiol. Opt.*, **9**, 228–230

BROWN, N. (1974) The change in lens curvature with age. *Exp. Eye Res.*, **19**, 175–183

CLARKE, B.A.J. and CARNEY, I.G. (1971) Refractive index and reflectance of the anterior surface of the cornea. *Am. J. Optom.*, **48**, 333–343

CLEMENT, R.A., DUNNE, N.C.M. and BARNES, D.A. (1987) A method for ray tracing through schematic eyes with off-axis components. *Ophthal. Physiol. Opt.*, **7**, 149–152

COILE, D.C. and O'KEEFE, L.P. (1988) Schematic eyes for domestic animals. *Ophthal. Physiol. Opt.*, **8**, 215–220

DOUTHWAITE, W.A. (1993) The intraocular lens. In *Cataract, Detection, Measurement and Management in Optometric Practice* (Douthwaite, W. A. and Hurst, M. A., eds), pp. 114–127. Oxford: Butterworth-Heinemann

EMSLEY, H.H. (1936) *Visual Optics*. London: Hatton Press

FUKALA, V. (1890) Operative Behandlung der höchstgradigen Myopie durch Aphakie. *Albrecht v. Graefes Arch. Ophthal.*, **36**(2), 230–244

GARNER, L.F. and SMITH, G. (1997a) Changes in equivalent and gradient refractive index of the crystalline lens with accommodation. *Optom. Vision Sci.*, **74**, 114–119.

GARNER, L.F. and YAP, M.K.H. (1997b) Changes in ocular dimensions and refraction with accommodation. *Ophthal. Physiol. Opt.*, **17**, 12–17

GULLSTRAND, A. (1909) Appendix 11.3. The optical system of the eye. In Helmholtz, H. von, *Physiological Optics*, Vol. 1, pp. 350–358. English translation: J.P.C. Southall (ed.). New York: Optical Society of America. Reprinted 1962: Dover Publications, New York

HEMENGER, R.P., GARNER, L.F. and OOI, C.S. (1995) Change with age of the refractive index gradient of the human ocular lens. *Invest. Ophthalmol. Vis. Sci.*, **36**, 703–707

HODOS, W. and ERICHSEN, J.T. (1990) Lower-field myopia in birds: an adaptation that keeps the ground in focus. *Vision Res.*, **30**, 653–657

HOWCROFT, M.J. and PARKER, J.A. (1977) Aspheric curvatures for the human lens. *Vision Res.*, **17**, 1217–1223

HUGHES, A. (1979) A useful table of reduced schematic eyes for vertebrates which includes computed longitudinal chromatic aberration. *Vision Res.*, **19**, 1273–1275

IVANOFF, A. (1953) *Les Aberrations de l'Oeil*. Paris: Editions de la Revue d'Optique

KOOIJMAN, A.C. (1983) Light distribution on the retina of a wide-angle theoretical eye. *J. Opt. Soc. Am.*, **73**, 1544–1550

KORETZ, J.F., KAUFMAN, P.L., NEIDER, M.W. and GOECKNER, P.A. (1989) Accommodation and presbyopia in the human eye – aging of the anterior segment. *Vision Res.*, **29**, 1685–1692

LE GRAND, Y. (1945) *Optique Physiologique*, Vol. I. Paris: Editions de la Revue d'Optique. English translation: S.G. El Hage (1980) Springer, Berlin, Heidelberg and New York

LIOU, H.L. and BRENNAN, N.A. (1996) The prediction of spherical aberration with schematic eyes. *Ophthal. Physiol. Opt.*, **16**, 348–354

LISTING, J.B. (1851) Dioptrik des Auges. In *Handwörterbuch der Physiologie*, Vol. 4. (Wagner, R., ed.). Brunswick: Vieweg

LOPER, L.R. (1959) The relationship between angle lambda and the residual astigmatism of the eye. *Am. J. Optom.*, **36**, 365–377

LOTMAR, W. (1971) Theoretical eye model with aspherics. *J. Opt. Soc. Am.*, **61**, 1522–1529

LOWE, R.F. (1970) Anterior lens displacement with age. *Br. J. Ophthalmol.*, **54**, 117–121

MARTIN, F.E. (1942) The importance and measurement of angle alpha. *Br. J. Physiol. Optics*, **3**, 27–45

NAVARRO, R., SANTAMARÍA, J. and BESCÓS, J. (1985) Accommodation-dependent model of the human eye with aspherics. *J. Opt. Soc. Am. A*, **2**(8), 1273–1281

O'KEEFE, L.P. and COILE, D.C. (1988) A BASIC computer program for schematic and reduced eye construction. *Ophthal. Physiol. Opt.*, **8**, 97–100

OLSEN, T., THIM, K. and CORYDON, L. (1990) Theoretical versus SRK I and SRK II calculation of intraocular lens power. *J. Cataract Refract. Surg.*, **16**, 217–224

OSWALSO-CRUZ, E., HOKOÇ, J.N. and SOUSA, A.P.B. (1979) A schematic eye for the opossum. *Vision Res.*, **19**, 263–278

PATEL, S., MARSHALL, J. and FITZKE III, F.W. (1993) Model for predicting the optical performance of the eye in refractive surgery. *Refract. Corneal Surg.*, **9**, 366–375

PATEL, S., MARSHALL, J. and FITZKE III, F.W. (1995) Refractive index of the human corneal epithelium and stroma. *J. Refract Surg.*, **11**, 100–105

PIERSCIONEK, B.K. (1990) Presbyopia – effect of refractive index. *Clin. Exp. Optom.*, **73**, 23–30

POMERANTZEFF, O., PANKRATOV, M., WANG, G.J. and DUFAULT, P. (1984) Wideangle optical model of the eye. *Am. J. Optom.*, **61**, 166–176

RETZLAFF, J., SANDERS, D.R. and KRAFF, M.D. (1981) *A Manual of Implant Power Calculation: SRK Formula*, Medford, Oregon: published by the authors

RETZLAFF, J., SANDERS, D.R. and KRAFF, M.D. (1990) Development of the SRK/T intraocular lens implant power calculation formula. *J. Cataract Refract. Surg.*, **16**, 333–340

SANDERS, D.R. and KRAFF, I.C. (1984) Determination of proper intraocular power for implant patients: intraocular lens power calculation formulas, A-scan instruments, and techniques for use. In *Cataract and Intraocular Lens Surgery*, Vol. 1 (Ginsberg, S.P., ed.), pp. 44–59. Amsterdam: Kugler Publications

SANDERS, D.R. RETZLAFF, K.A. and KRAFF, M.D. (1988) Comparison of the SRK II $^{(TM)}$ formula and other second generation formulas. *J. Cataract Refract. Surg.*, **14**, 136-141

SMITH, G. (1995) Schematic eyes: history, description and applications. *Clin. Exp. Optom.*, **78**(5), 176–189

SMITH, G., ATCHISON, D.A. and PIERSCIONEK, B.K. (1992) Modeling the power of the aging human eye. *J. Opt. Soc. Am. A*, **9**, 2111–2117

SMITH, G., PIERSCIONEK, B.K. and ATCHISON, D.A. (1991) The optical modelling of the human lens. *Ophthal. Physiol. Opt.*, **11**, 359–369

SORSBY, A., BENJAMIN, B., DAVEY, J.B., SHERIDAN, M. and TANNER, J.M. (1957) Emmetropia and its aberrations. *Spec. Rep. Ser. Med. Res. Coun.*, No. 293

STENSTÖM, S. (1946) Untersuchungen über die Variation und Kovariation der optischen Elemente des menschlichen Auges. *Acta Ophthal.*, suppl. 26. English translation: D. Woolf. *Am. J. Optom.*, **25**, 218–232, 1948

SWAINE, W. (1921) Geometrical optics – VII: paraxial schematic and reduced eyes. *Optn Scient. Instrum. Mkr*, **62**, 133–136

TSCHERNING, M. (1890) Etude sur la position du cristallin de l'oeil humain. In (Javal, L.E., ed). *Mémoires d'Ophtalmométrie*. Paris: Masson

TSCHERNING, M. (1924) *Physiologic Optics*, 4th edn (trans. C. Weiland). Philadelphia: Keystone Publishing Co.

WEALE, R.A. (1982) *A Biography of the Eye*. London: H. Lewis

WOOD, I.J.C., MUTTIO, D.O. and ZAONIA, K. (1996) Crystalline lens parameters in infancy. *Ophthal. Physiol. Opt.*, **16**, 310–317

WOODS, A.C. (1952) The adjustment to aphakia. *Am. J. Ophthal.*, **35**, 118–122

Further reading

BARNES, D.A., DUNNE, M.C.M. and CLEMENT, R.A. (1987) A schematic eye model for the effects of translation and rotation of ocular components on peripheral astigmatism. *Ophthal. Physiol. Opt.*, **7**, 153–158

DUNNE, M.C.M. (1993) Model for co-ordination of corneal and crystalline lens power in emmetropic human eyes. *Ophthal. Physiol. Opt.*, **13**, 397–399

DUNNE, M.C.M., BARNES, D.A. and CLEMENT, R.A. (1987) A model for retinal shape changes in ametropia. *Ophthal. Physiol. Opt.*, **7**, 159–160

13

Subsidiary effects of correcting lenses; magnifying devices

Principal subsidiary effects

In natural vision, object space is the same for each eye, apart from the slight difference in viewpoints. Wearing spectacles creates an entirely different visual situation. A common object space is now replaced by two separate image fields formed by the right and left lenses. As a result, spectacle lenses give rise to a number of subsidiary effects. In particular, they may alter

(1) Monocularly
   (a) The size and possibly the shape of the retinal image.
   (b) The amount of accommodation needed in near vision.
(2) Binocularly
   (a) The ocular rotations needed to place the retinal image of a given point in space on the fovea of each eye.
   (b) The relationship between accommodation and convergence (see Chapter 9).

In general, these side-effects are caused by the lens–eye separation and the fact that the lens does not move with the eye. Consequently, they are either absent or are much less pronounced when contact lenses are worn.

In this chapter we shall also be looking at the various effects of plano prisms, fields of view through spectacle lenses and the optics and clinical use of lenses, and optical systems designed to magnify the retinal image in normal visual tasks. The aberrations or image defects of ophthalmic lenses will also briefly be discussed.

Spectacle magnification

Definitions

Spectacle magnification relates to the change in the retinal image size in any given eye as a result of wearing either a spectacle or a contact lens.

The retinal image in the uncorrected ametropic eye is not necessarily blurred, because in hypermetropia it could be brought into focus given sufficient accommodation. To cover both possibilities, we take the size of the retinal image in the uncorrected eye to be its basic height, which is independent of the degree of blurring (see Chapter 4, page 69). Spectacle magnification SM may therefore be defined as the ratio

$$SM = \frac{\text{Retinal image size in corrected eye}}{\text{Basic height of retinal image in uncorrected eye}}$$

(13.1)

In this context; the word 'corrected' simply implies that a lens is being worn, irrespective of the degree to which it 'corrects' the ametropia.

The basic height of a retinal image is determined by the limiting ray through the centre of the eye's exit pupil. As we saw in Chapter 12, the angle u' which this ray makes with the optical axis bears a constant ratio (for any given eye) to the angle u made with the optical axis by the conjugate incident ray directed towards the centre of the entrance pupil. Thus the basic height of the retinal image is directly proportional to the angular subtense of the object at this point.

This enables spectacle magnification to be defined in more general terms as the ratio of the angular subtense at the eye's entrance pupil of the image formed by the lens to that of the object viewed directly without change of position.

Distance vision: single lens

Figure 13.1 shows a plus lens of meniscus form, A_2 being its back vertex, F' its second principal focus, and P and P' its first and second principal points respectively. Let F_1 and F_2 denote the front and back surface powers, t the centre thickness in metres and n the refractive index of the material.

Then its equivalent power F is given by the expression

$$F = 1/f' = F_1 + F_2 - (t/n)F_1F_2$$

(13.2)

and its back vertex power, denoted by F'_v rather than F'_{sp} since the theory is applicable to both spectacle and contact lenses, by

$$F'_v = 1/f'_v = \frac{F_1}{1 - (t/n)F_1} + F_2 = FS$$

(13.3)

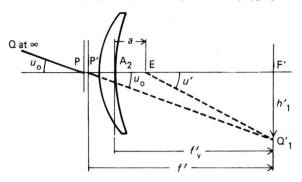

Figure 13.1. Spectacle magnification in distance vision: the ratio of the angular subtense u' of the image height h'_1, at the centre E of the eye's entrance pupil to that u_o of the distant object.

where

$$S = \frac{1}{1 - (t/n)F_1} \tag{13.4}$$

The quantity S is known as the 'shape factor' because the centre thickness and front surface power determine the profile of a cross-section of the lens.

In *Figure 13.1*, E is the centre of the eye's entrance pupil and a its distance A_2E from the back vertex of the lens. Suppose Q to be the extremity of a distant object situated on the optical axis. Its image Q'_1 formed by the lens is the intersection with the second focal plane (through F') of the ray from P' parallel to the incident ray QP. The entire image, of height h'_1, subtends an angle u' at E such that

$$u' = \frac{-h'_1}{EF'} = \frac{-h'_1}{f'_v - a} = \frac{-h'_1 F'_v}{1 - aF'_v}$$

Using equation (13.3) we can rewrite this last expression as

$$u = \frac{-h'_1 FS}{1 - aF'_v} = -h'_1 FSP$$

where

$$P = \frac{1}{1 - aF'_v} \tag{13.5}$$

The quantity P is called the power factor. The object itself would subtend at E an angle u_o given by

$$u_o = -h'_1 P'F' = -h'_1/f' = -h'_1 F$$

The spectacle magnification, being the ratio of u' to u_o, is given by

$$SM = \frac{u'}{u_o} = \frac{-h'_1 FSP}{-h'_1 F}$$

$$= PS = \frac{1}{\{1 - aF'_v\}\{1 - (t/n)F_1\}} \tag{13.6}$$

By using equation (13.3), an alternative expression for the shape factor S can be obtained in the form

$$S = 1 + \frac{t}{n}(F'_v - F_2) \tag{13.7}$$

This is sometimes more convenient.

Table 13.1 Spectacle magnification: typical values (distance vision, $a = 0.016$ m)

Details of lens			Shape factor (S)	Power factor (P)	Spectacle magnification (PS)
F'_v	t (mm)	F_1			
−20.00	0.7	0	1.000	0.758	0.758
−15.00	0.7	0	1.000	0.806	0.806
−10.00	0.8	+3.00	1.002	0.862	0.864
−5.00	0.8	+4.49	1.002	0.926	0.928
0	1.8	+5.96	1.007	1.000	1.007
+5.00	4.5	+10.19	1.031	1.087	1.121
+10.00	7.0	+12.27	1.060	1.190	1.261
+15.00	8.5	+13.84	1.084	1.316	1.426

Numerical values

Table 13.1 has been compiled to give an idea of the range of typical values of spectacle magnification and its components.

In computing the power factor, the distance a from the back vertex of the lens to the eye's entrance pupil was taken as 0.016 m. Average values were assigned to the front surface power F_1 and centre thickness t, on which the shape factor principally depends, and the refractive index of the material was taken as 1.523. Possible differences in this value would have a relatively slight effect on the value S.

Spectacle magnification can conveniently be expressed in percentage terms. For example, values of 1.12 and 0.96 could be expressed as +12 and −4% respectively.

In the case of contact lenses, the value of a can be taken as 0.003 m and so the power factor P would vary from about 0.94 on a −20 D lens to 1.03 on a +10 D lens. Over the same range of powers, the shape factor would vary from about 1.01 to no more than 1.02.

The fact that the spectacle magnification of contact lenses remains much closer to unity over the whole range of powers is one of the principal ways in which they differ optically from spectacle lenses.

A generalized approach

A more general method of calculating spectacle magnification is needed in those rare cases when the correction is a combination of two or more lenses. It could, of course, be applied to a single lens as well.

In a system of k surfaces, the last two in order are $(k - 1)$ and k, shown in *Figure 13.2*. The emergent ray is directed towards B'_k (in this case the centre of the eye's entrance pupil) and makes a small angle u'_k with the optical axis. Prior to this last refraction, the ray made an angle u_k with the optical axis and was directed towards the axial point B_k, conjugate with B'_k. The point of incidence G_k is at a height y_k from the axis.

If we denote the dioptric distances of B'_k and B_k from the last vertex by L'_k and L_k respectively, then

$$u'_k = y_k/\ell'_k = \frac{y_k L'_k}{n_{k+1}}$$

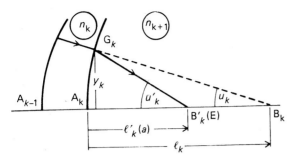

Figure 13.2. Refraction by a series of coaxial surfaces, A_{k-1} and A_k being the poles of the penultimate and last surfaces.

and

$$u_k = y_k/\ell_k = \frac{y_k L_k}{n_k}$$

Since B'_k is used here to represent the centre E of the eye's entrance pupil, the distance $A_k B'_k$ is not only the last image distance ℓ'_k but is also the distance previously denoted by a. Hence $L'_k = 1/a$.

The angular magnification m_k at this last refraction is the ratio u'_k/u_k, i.e. the ratio of the apparent angles made by the object after and before refraction. Thus

$$m_k = \frac{u'_k}{u_k} = \frac{n_k}{n_{k+1}} \times \frac{L'_k}{L_k}$$

Similarly, at the previous surface

$$m_{k-1} = \frac{n_{k-1}}{n_k} \times \frac{L'_{k-1}}{L_{k-1}}$$

and so on until, at the first surface

$$m_1 = \frac{n_1}{n_2} \times \frac{L'_1}{L_1}$$

The spectacle magnification is the product of all the separate values of m. All the refractive indices except the first and last cancel out, so that

$$SM = \frac{n_1}{n_{k+1}} \times \frac{L'_k L'_{k-1} \dots L'_1}{L_k L_{k-1} \dots L_1} \qquad (13.8)$$

If the first and last media are the same, as is usually the case, this expression simplifies to

$$SM = \frac{L'_k L'_{k-1} \dots L'_1}{L_k L_{k-1} \dots L_1} \qquad (13.9)$$

where $L'_k = 1/a$, as also in equation (13.8).

The required values of L and L' at each surface can be found from a backward paraxial trace through the system, beginning with the known value of L'_k. The following example using a single lens illustrates the above method.

Example (1)

Find the spectacle magnification, given that $F'_v = +8.00\,D$, $F_2 = -3.00\,D$, $n = 1.523$ and $t = 6.0\,mm$. The eye's entrance pupil is to be taken as 16 mm from the back vertex of the lens.

We can find F_1 from the expression

$$F_1 = \frac{F'_v - F_2}{1 + (t/n)(F'_v - F_2)}. \qquad (13.10)$$

derived from equation (13.3). This gives $F_1 = +10.54\,D$. Starting from $a = 16\,mm = 0.016\,m$, we have

$$L'_2 = 1/a = 1/0.016 = +62.50\,D$$

$$L_2 = L'_2 - F_2 = +65.50\,D$$

$$L'_1 = \frac{L_2}{1 + (t/n)L_2} = +52.06\,D \qquad \text{(from equation 2.11)}$$

and

$$L = L'_1 - F_1 = +41.52\,D$$

which gives

$$SM = 1.1964 \qquad \text{(from equation 13.9)}$$

Using the analysis explained on pages 229–230, we should arrive at

$$S = 1.0433 \qquad \text{(from equation 13.4 or 13.7)}$$

$$P = 1.1468 \qquad \text{(from equation 13.5)}$$

from which

$$SM = PS = 1.1964$$

Pupil magnification

The pupil seen on looking at a naked eye is the entrance pupil, the image of the real pupil formed by the cornea. A correcting lens, in turn, forms a second image which becomes the entrance pupil of the lens–eye system. To distinguish between them we will call these first and second images of the real pupil the ocular entrance pupil and the effective entrance pupil respectively. Their respective diameters will be denoted by g and g_e.

The linear magnification of the ocular entrance pupil by the correcting lens is the ratio g_e/g. We shall now show that this ratio, the pupil magnification, is numerically equal to the spectacle magnification.

In *Figure 13.3*, HJ represents the ocular entrance pupil and H′J′ the effective entrance pupil, the image of HJ formed by a lens having k surfaces. If we reverse the direction of the light, at the same time interchanging

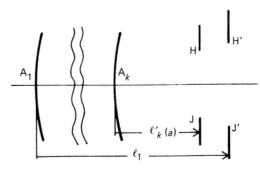

Figure 13.3. Imagery of the pupil by a lens system. HJ is the ocular entrance pupil. Its image H′J′ formed by the lens system becomes the effective entrance pupil.

object and image, H'J' becomes a virtual object for the lens and HJ its real image. The distance a of HJ from the back vertex of the lens then becomes the last image distance ℓ'_k, so that $L'_k = 1/a$. The paraxial formula (2.10) for linear magnification then gives

$$m = \frac{h'}{h} = \frac{HJ}{H'J'} = \frac{g}{g_e} = \frac{L_1 L_2 \dots L_k}{L'_1 L'_2 \dots L'_k}$$

and thus

$$\frac{\text{pupil}}{\text{magnification}} = \frac{g_e}{g} = \frac{L'_1 L'_2 \dots L'_k}{L_1 L_2 \dots L_k} \qquad (13.11)$$

where $L'_k = 1/a$.

This is mathematically identical with the general expression (13.9) for spectacle magnification. The principle of equation (13.9) has been used by García *et al.* (1995) to develop a matrix formulation, together with numerical examples, for both spectacle and relative spectacle (*see* page 236) magnification.

The importance of pupil magnification is its effect on the amount of light admitted to the eye. This is proportional to the area of the relevant entrance pupil, and thus to the square of its diameter. For example, if a myope wears a spectacle correction with a spectacle magnification of 0.9, then

$$g_e = 0.9\,g \quad \text{and} \quad g_e^2 = 0.81\,g^2$$

The amount of light admitted to the eye is thus reduced by nearly 20%. A contact lens correcting the same subject would have a spectacle magnification of the order of 0.97, giving $g_e^2 = 0.94\,g^2$ – a reduction of only 6%. Thus, for the same real pupil diameter (to which g remains proportional in any given eye), more light would be admitted. The reverse applies to hypermetropia.

Spectacle magnification in near vision

The spectacle magnification of a lens used in near vision is a product of three factors: the power and shape factors already defined, and a third which might be called the 'proximity factor'.

Figure 13.4 depicts an object BR and its virtual image B'R' formed by a lens. The centre of the eye's entrance pupil is at E, and E'_L is its image formed by the lens.

Since E and E'_L are conjugate points, the incident ray RS directed towards E'_L gives rise to the refracted ray TE.

The object subtends an angle u at E, while the image subtends an angle u'. Consequently, the spectacle magnification is the ratio u'/u. If Q were a *distant* object point on the same ray path RS, all the rays from Q reaching the lens would make the same angle u_o with the optical axis, while the image of Q would be seen in the direction ET, making an angle u' with the optical axis. Hence, for distance vision, the spectacle magnification – shown previously to be the product of the power and shape factors – would be the ratio u'/u_o. Thus we obtain

$$\text{SM (near vision)} = u'/u$$

$$= \frac{u'}{u_o} \times \frac{u_o}{u} = PS \times \frac{u_o}{u}$$

$$= PSN \qquad (13.12)$$

where N is the proximity factor u_o/u.

An accurate expression for N in terms of the known object distance and the quantities defining the lens has been given by Ogle (1936). It is, however, too cumbersome for practical use. Calculation from first principles by finding the position and size of the image formed by the lens would be both easier and quicker.

Since the value of N is in any case very close to unity, an approximate expression is adequate for all practical purposes. To obtain this we imagine the lens, of power F'_v, to be of negligible thickness and situated at the back vertex A_2 of the real lens, from which the object distance ℓ is measured. We also consider E'_L, at a positive distance a' from A_2, to be a virtual object point for light passing through the lens from left to right in *Figure 13.4*. The point E, at a distance a from A_2, is then the real image of E'_L formed by the lens. The paraxial law of conjugate foci then gives

$$1/a' - 1/a = F'_v$$

which gives

$$a' = \frac{a}{1 - aF'_v} = a + a^2 F'_v + \dots \qquad (13.13)$$

when the binomial expansion is taken as far as terms in a^2.

From the diagram it can be seen that

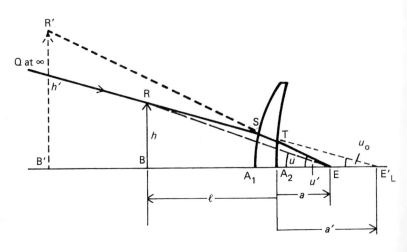

Figure 13.4. Derivation of expression for spectacle magnification in near vision.

$$u_o = \frac{h}{\mathrm{BE}'_L} = \frac{h}{-\ell + a'}$$

and

$$u = \frac{h}{\mathrm{BE}} = \frac{h}{-\ell + a}$$

so that

$$N = \frac{u_o}{u} = \frac{-\ell + a}{-\ell + a'} = \frac{1 - aL}{1 - a'L}$$

The binomial expansion of this expression up to the second power of a and a' gives

$$N \approx (1 - aL)(1 + a'L + a'^2 L^2 + \ldots)$$
$$= 1 + (a' - a)L + a'(a' - a)L^2$$

Finally, on substituting the value of a' from equation (13.13) in this last expression and neglecting terms in a^3 and higher powers, we get

$$N = 1 + a_2 F'_v L \qquad (13.14)$$

If L is taken as $-3.00\,\mathrm{D}$ and an average value of 16 mm or 0.016 m is assigned to a, equation (13.14) becomes

$$N = 1 - 0.000\,8\,F'_v$$

N is thus a negligible factor, except for high-power lenses.

The astigmatic eye

When the effects of blurring are excluded, the retinal image in the uncorrected astigmatic eye is slightly distorted because of the different magnification in the two principal meridians. If the astigmatism is attributed to the cornea alone, the exit pupil remains the same for both principal meridians. The following simple analysis can then be made.

Figure 13.5 represents part of a schematic eye with an astigmatic cornea. As before, the subscript α has been used to denote the principal meridian of steeper and β the meridian of flatter corneal curvature. Ray paths in these meridians have been superimposed on the same diagram, bold lines referring to the steeper meridian and thinner lines to the flatter. In *Figure 13.5*, E_o, E_α

and E_β denote the centres of the real pupil, the entrance pupil for the steeper meridian and the entrance pupil for the flatter meridian respectively. Surprisingly at first sight, E_β is nearer than E_α to the corneal vertex A_1.

A distant object, for example a circle with its centre on the optical axis of the eye, subtends an angle $2u$. The rays from each extremity then make an angle u with the axis. In the steeper meridian, a ray QR directed towards E_α, passes, after refraction, through E_o and emerges from the crystalline lens as though from E'. In the flatter meridian, a ray JK directed towards E_β is also refracted through E_o and emerges from the lens as though from E'. It can be seen from the diagram that the retinal image is larger in the meridian of steeper corneal curvature.

The entrance pupil being the image of the real pupil formed by the cornea, it seems logical to denote the distances $\mathrm{A}_1\mathrm{E}_\alpha$ and $\mathrm{A}_1\mathrm{E}_\beta$ by d'_α and d'_β respectively.

Because the rays RE_o and $\mathrm{E}_o\mathrm{V}$ are conjugate, as are the rays KE_o and $\mathrm{E}_o\mathrm{W}$, it follows from the paraxial law of refraction that

$$\mathrm{VA}_3/\mathrm{WA}_3 = \mathrm{RA}_1/\mathrm{KA}_1$$

The following relationship can also be deduced from *Figure 13.5*

$$\mathrm{VA}_3/\mathrm{WA}_3 = u'_\alpha/u'_\beta$$

and

$$\mathrm{RA}_1/\mathrm{KA}_1 = d'_\alpha/d'_\beta$$

which gives

$$u'_\alpha/u'_\beta = d'_\alpha/d'_\beta \qquad (13.15)$$

Example (2)

Find the distortion of the basic retinal image in an uncorrected eye with 1.00 D of corneal astigmatism with the rule. Assume the constants of the Bennett–Rabbetts schematic eye for the horizontal meridian.

Horizontal meridian
$F_1 = +43.08\,\mathrm{D}$
$d_1 = 3.6\,\mathrm{mm}$

Vertical meridian
$F_1 = +44.08\,\mathrm{D}$
$d_1 = 3.6\,\mathrm{mm}$

from which

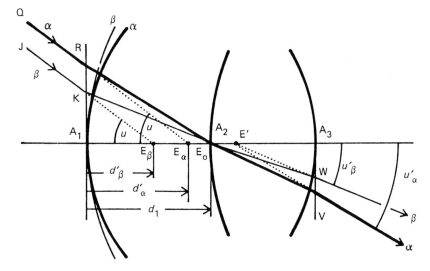

Figure 13.5. A schematic eye with astigmatic cornea: subscripts α and β refer to its stronger and weaker principal meridians respectively. Ray paths from a distant object through the centre of the pupil are shown for both meridians.

$d'_\beta = +3.048$ mm $d'_\alpha = +3.058$ mm

and

$u'_\alpha/u'_\beta = 3.058/3.048 = 1.003$

giving percentage distortion = 0.3%.

A general expression for the percentage distortion may be deduced as follows. The law of conjugate foci gives

$$d' = \frac{1}{1.336/d_1 - F_1}$$

Differentiating

$$\frac{\Delta d'}{\Delta F_1} = \frac{1}{(1.336/d_1 - F_1)^2} = d'^2$$

In this context, d' represents the lesser quantity d'_β, the increment $\Delta d'$ the difference $(d'_\alpha - d'_\beta)$ and ΔF_1 the corneal astigmatism. Hence

$$d'_\alpha - d'_\beta = d'^2_\beta \times \text{Ast}$$

and

$$\text{percentage distortion} = 100\frac{d'_\alpha - d'_\beta}{d'_\beta}$$

$$= 100\, d'_\beta \times \text{Ast} \qquad (13.16)$$

If d'_β is taken as 0.003 m this last expression shows the distortion to be about 0.3% per dioptre of astigmatism.

It should be borne in mind that ray paths through the pupil centres determine only the basic height of the retinal image, that is the distance between the centres of the limiting blur formations. In the astigmatic eye, the blurred image of a point is generally elongated. As a result, the distortion of the basic retinal image could well be masked, accentuated or even reversed by the effects of blurring.

In the corrected astigmatic eye, distortion of the sharp retinal image arises from the unequal spectacle magnification in the two principal meridians. Equation (13.5) for the power factor leads to the binomial approximation

$$P \approx 1 + aF'_v$$

If we ignore the slight difference in the value of a for the two principal meridians, the meridional difference ΔP can be expressed as

$$\Delta P = aC \qquad (13.17)$$

since C, the cylinder power of the lens, is the meridional difference in F'_v.

For a spectacle lens we can taken 0.016 m as an average value for a, in which case

$$\Delta P = 0.016C$$

This represents a distortion of 1.6% for every dioptre of cylinder power. For contact lenses, this figure reduces to about 0.3% per dioptre.

A similar method of approximation can be applied to equation (13.4) for the shape factor, giving

$$S \approx 1 + (t/n)F_1$$

and

$$\Delta S \approx (t/n)C_1$$

where C_1 is the cylinder power incorporated in the front surface of the lens. Thus, the meridional difference ΔP is accentuated by a small difference ΔS in the shape factor if the front surface of the lens is cylindrical or toroidal. If, however, the lens is a 'minus base' toric with a spherical front surface, the shape factor is the same for both principal meridians. This is one of the arguments used in favour of minus base torics.

Astigmats of moderate and high degree may complain of distortion, for example, circles appearing to be elliptical, when changing from spectacle to contact lenses. Paradoxically, their troubles arise because they have become habituated to the distortion of spectacle lenses and have initial difficulty in adapting to the relatively undistorted retinal images obtained with contact lenses.

Calculation of spectacle magnification becomes more complicated when the principal meridians of the correcting lens and those of the cornea (and possibly of the other refracting surfaces) are all at variance. Rigorous solutions have been formulated from two different approaches, one employing matrix methods (Keating, 1982) and the other paraxial ray tracing procedures (Bennett, 1986).

Astigmatic line rotation

In general, a straight line viewed through an astigmatic lens appears to have rotated through an angle which changes as the lens itself is rotated. This well-known effect is the result of the different spectacle magnifications in the two principal meridians of the lens. To a sufficient degree of accuracy, an analysis can be made without taking the thickness of the lens into account. This enables an expression for spectacle magnification to be obtained in a much simpler form.

In *Figure 13.6*, the near object BQ subtends an angle u at the eye's entrance pupil E, while its image B'Q' formed by a thin lens of power F subtends an angle u'. Thus

$$\text{SM} = u'/u = \frac{h'}{-\ell' + a} \times \frac{-\ell + a}{h}$$

and, since $h'/h = L/L'$ and $L' = L + F$

$$\text{SM} = \frac{L(-\ell + a)}{L'(-\ell' + a)} = \frac{1 - aL}{1 - aL'}$$

$$= \frac{A - L}{A - L - F} \qquad (13.18)$$

when the distance a from the back vertex of the lens to the entrance pupil is replaced by its dioptric equivalent A, equal to $1/a$.

For an astigmatic lens, if F_m denotes the power along the 'minus axis' or principal meridian of higher plus or lower minus power, F_p the power along the 'plus axis' (having the lower plus or higher minus power), M_m and M_p the spectacle magnifications in these meridians

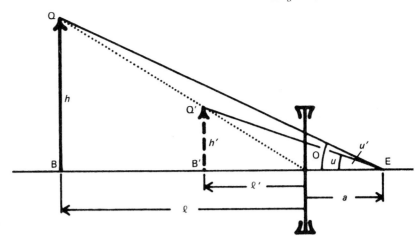

Figure 13.6. Spectacle magnification of a thin lens in near vision.

and μ the ratio M_m/M_p, then

$$\mu = \frac{M_m}{M_p} = \frac{A-L}{A-L-F_m} \times \frac{A-L-F_p}{A-L}$$

$$= \frac{A-L-F_p}{A-L-F_m} \qquad (13.19)$$

It is possible to derive a simple relationship between the actual and apparent directions of a straight line viewed through an astigmatic lens. Because M_p and M_m have different values, the proportions of a rectangle with its sides parallel to the principal meridians of the lens will apparently be altered. Thus, OSQT in *Figure 13.7* will appear as OS'Q'T' such that

$$y'/y = M_m \quad \text{and} \quad x'/x = M_p$$

As a result the diagonal OQ making an acute angle φ with the plus axis OP will appear in the different direction OQ' making an angle φ' with OP. From the

diagram,

$$\tan \phi = y/x$$

and

$$\tan \phi' = y'/x' = \frac{yM_m}{xM_p} = \mu \tan \phi \qquad (13.20)$$

The values of the quantities in equation (13.19) may be such that μ has negative as well as positive values. When the lens is held relatively close to the eye, A has a positive value generally high enough to make both the numerator and the denominator of equation (13.19) positive in sign. Since $F_m > F_p$, the value of μ is greater than unity in this case. When this occurs, the apparent movement of the limbs of a crossline chart when the lens is rotated is of the familiar 'scissors' type. This is illustrated in *Figure 13.8* which shows the appearance after the plus axis of the lens has been rotated through a small clockwise angle from the horizontal.

The horizontal limb of the chart now makes a positive acute angle ϕ_H measured from the plus axis. Since $\mu > 1, \phi'_H > \phi_H$ and so this line appears to have made an 'against' movement, that is a rotation in the opposite

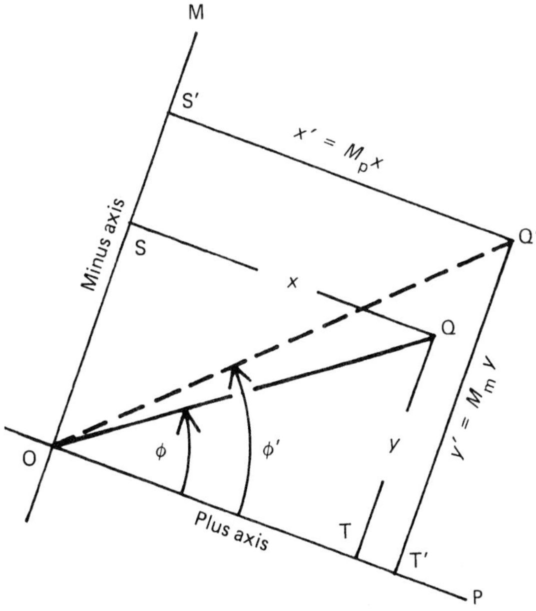

Figure 13.7. Spectacle magnification of an astigmatic lens derived from the distortion of a rectangle with its sides along the principal meridians.

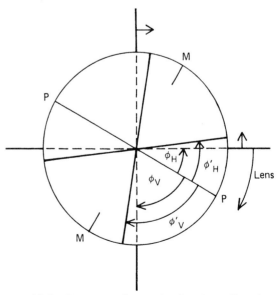

Figure 13.8. Derivation of expression for scissors distortion of a crossline chart viewed through an astigmatic lens.

direction to that of the lens. With the lens in the same position, the acute angle ϕ_V from the plus axis to the vertical meridian is negative in sign, equal to $90° - \phi_H$ but ϕ_V' is a larger angle since $\mu > 1$. Consequently, the vertical line of the chart appears to have made a 'with' movement. The rotation test, as it is called, is a very simple and reliable means of distinguishing an astigmatic from a spherical lens and of locating its principal meridians. An against movement identifies the plus axis and a with movement the minus axis.

It can be deduced from equation (13.20) that as ϕ increases a 'turning point' is reached beyond which ϕ' increases at a slower rate than ϕ. In consequence, the direction in which the given line appears to rotate is reversed, the line seen through the lens returning to its true direction when $\phi = 90°$.

Other forms of apparent movement can be produced when A and L are given suitable values. For example, when the value of $(A - L)$ is intermediate between F_m and F_p, μ assumes a negative value. As a result, ϕ and ϕ' become opposite in sign and there are no turning points. Both limbs of the crossline continue to rotate in the same direction as the lens is turned, at the same time making a scissors movement.

Pure rotation without scissors effect occurs when $\mu = -1$, resulting in ϕ and ϕ' remaining numerically equal though opposite in sign. The necessary condition is that

$$A - L - F_p = -(A - L - F_m)$$

or

$$A = L + \frac{F_m + F_p}{2} \tag{13.21}$$

This is the value of A when the eye is placed at the distance from the lens at which the circles of least confusion are formed. Both limbs of the crossline then appear to rotate at twice the speed of the lens, always remaining mutually perpendicular.

If $A = L + F_m$ the value of μ becomes infinity, so that ϕ' is $90°$ irrespective of the value of ϕ. This means that *any* line viewed through the lens will then appear parallel to the minus axis and remain parallel to it as the lens is rotated.

In a similar way, if $A = L + F_p$, the value of μ (and hence of ϕ') becomes zero. As a result, the apparent direction of any line must always be parallel to the plus axis.

Relative spectacle magnification

Relative spectacle magnification is the ratio of the retinal image size in the corrected ametropic eye to that in a specified emmetropic schematic eye. It thus compares the given corrected eye with a hypothetical standard.

Given the same distant object, the images formed by two different lenses or optical systems are inversely proportional in size to the respective equivalent powers. Hence, if the equivalent power of the reference eye is denoted by F_o and that of the given lens–eye system by

F^*, the relative spectacle magnification RSM is the ratio

$$\text{RSM} = F_o/F^* \tag{13.22}$$

Suppose that the given eye, of equivalent power F_e is corrected by a *thin* lens of back vertex power F_v, placed with its vertex at a distance d from the eye's first principal point. Then, in accordance with a well-known formula for equivalent power

$$F^* = F_v' + F_e - dF_v'F_e \tag{13.23}$$

As with spectacle magnification, the form and thickness of the lens can be allowed for by introducing the shape factor S. On this basis, the expression for relative spectacle magnification becomes

$$\text{RSM} = F_oS/F^* = \frac{F_oS}{F_v' + F_e - dF_v'F_e} \tag{13.24}$$

This is a general relationship and particular cases can be examined by assigning the appropriate value to F_e. Unfortunately, a reliable determination of the eye's equivalent power is outside the scope of normal clinical practice.

If the back vertex of the spectacle lens coincides with the eye's anterior focal point, the distance d becomes equal to $1/F_e$, in which case the value of F^* (equation 13.23) is seen to reduce to F_e. Then, on the assumptions that $F_e = F_o$ as in 'axial' ametropia, and that the shape factor is negligible, the relative spectacle magnification becomes unity. This result is known as Knapp's law.

Equation (13.24) can be put in a more significant form by making use of the expressions

$$F_e = K' - K \qquad \text{(from equation 4.2)}$$

and

$$F_v' = \frac{K}{1 + dK} \qquad \text{(from equation 4.10)}$$

When these substitutions are made in equation (13.24) it becomes

$$\text{RSM} = \frac{(1 + dK)F_oS}{K'} \tag{13.25}$$

The equivalent power F_o of an emmetropic eye is equal to the quantity K_o'. Thus

$$F_o/K' = K_o'/K' = k'/k_o'$$

where k' and k_o' are the distances from the second principal point to the retina in the ametropic and reference eyes respectively. This relationship enables equation (13.25) to be written in the form

$$\text{RSM} = AES \tag{13.26}$$

where

$$A = \text{ametropia factor} = 1 + dK \tag{13.27}$$

$$E = \text{elongation factor} = k'/k_o \tag{13.28}$$

and

$$S = \text{shape factor defined by equation (13.4)}$$

On the basis of normally available clinical data, the value of E can only be conjectured, but could be estimated from ultrasonography (*see* pages 378–380).

Plano prisms

Definitions and sign conventions

Prism power

The power of an ophthalmic plano prism is the deviation in prism dioptres of a ray at normal incidence on either surface, the wavelength being that for the d-line of the helium spectrum (587.6 nm). The deviation for this specified ray path is slightly greater than the minimum, which occurs when the ray path through the prism is symmetrical.

The main effect of an ophthalmic prism is to alter the ocular rotation that would otherwise be required to place the retinal image of a given point of regard on the fovea. The amount by which the rotation is altered may be called the effective prism power.

Sign convention for prism base settings

A sign convention for prism base settings is needed in order to arrive at universally valid expressions. The accepted convention is:

(1) *Horizontal prisms.* Base-out is positive; base-in is negative.
(2) *Vertical prisms.* Base-down is positive; base-up is negative.

When required for mathematical treatment, the sign of the deviation undergone by a ray on passing through a prism must be taken as that of the prism base setting. Thus, the deviation produced by a base-up prism (negative) is itself of negative sign.

Sign convention for image displacements and ocular rotations

The deviation of a ray on passing through a plano prism could be expressed in terms of a transverse displacement δ in a plane at a distance q from the prism. The following sign convention applies not only to these displacements but also to ocular rotations:

(1) *Horizontal image displacements or ocular rotations.* Inwards is positive; outwards is negative.
(2) *Vertical image displacements or ocular rotations.* Upwards is positive; downwards is negative.

If the displacement is measured from a point on the incident ray, the distance q is regarded as negative, being measured against the direction of the incident light. If the displacement is measured on the refracted ray, q is regarded as positive. In *Figure 13.9*, for example, the point J on the incident ray is imaged at J$'$ on the refracted ray produced backwards. In this case, δ is positive because the deviation is upwards, whereas q is negative. On the other hand, the point K$'$ on the refracted ray path can be taken as the image of K on the original ray path produced. The displacement δ is now negative because downwards, but q is positive.

For small angles of incidence, the deviation produced by a prism can be regarded as equal to the power of the

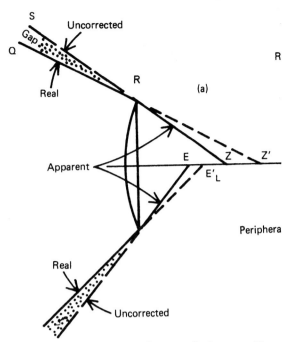

Figure 13.9. Sign convention for image displacement δ by a plano prism of power P (in prism dioptres): (a) incident ray from left, (b) incident ray from right.

prism P in prism dioptres. From the definition of the prism dioptre it follows that

$$P = -100\delta/q \qquad (13.29)$$

if δ and q are in the same units, or

$$P = -\delta/q \qquad (13.30)$$

if δ is in centimetres and q is in metres.

The minus sign is needed to conform to the various sign conventions. This can be seen from *Figure 13.9* in which the prism can be viewed as base-down for either eye or base-out for the left eye, P thus being positive in either case. We also have

$$\delta = -qP \qquad (13.31)$$

where δ is in centimetres and q is in metres.

Despite first appearances, the sign convention for ocular rotations is in harmony with that for prism base setting. For example, a prism base-down (P positive) induces an upward ocular rotation (also positive), and so on.

Effective prism power

It has long been recognized that the effective power of a plano prism in near vision is less than its nominal power. The same is also true of a prism incorporated in a correcting lens of minus power, whether by decentration or otherwise. In *Figure 13.10*, a prismatic spherical lens is represented by its optical equivalent in the form of a thin centred lens of power F in contact with a separate plano prism of power P. Given an axial object point B at any distance, the lens will form an axial image point B$'_1$ according to

$$L' = L + F$$

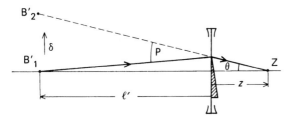

Figure 13.10. Effective power in near vision of a prism when incorporated in a minus spectacle lens.

The image B'_1 becomes an object for the prism which forms a second image B'_2 displaced through a distance δ in the direction of the apex. The ocular rotation θ needed to fixate B'_2 represents the effective prism power.

It can be seen from the diagram that

$$\theta = \frac{\delta}{-\ell' + z}$$

whereas

$$P = \delta / - \ell'$$

Thus

$$\theta = \left(\frac{-\ell'}{-\ell' + z} \right) P = \left(\frac{Z}{Z - L'} \right) P$$

$$= \left(\frac{Z}{Z - L - F} \right) P \qquad (13.32)$$

For all negative values of F, the effective power of the prism is less than its nominal value. The difference is of little significance in prescribing, because the same effect would arise with combinations of trial lenses and prisms used in subjective testing.

When the lens is of positive power and the near object distance such that L' is negative, the effective prism power is again less than its nominal value. On the other hand, if L' is positive, the images B'_1 and B'_2 are formed behind the lens and the effective prism power becomes greater than its nominal value. This result agrees with equation (13.32), which is valid generally. It is left to the student to construct a diagram on the lines of *Figure 13.10* to illustrate the case where L' is positive.

In the case of a plano prism, the image point B' in *Figure 13.10* would be replaced by the object point B itself at a dioptric distance L from the lens. On putting $F = 0$ in equation (13.32), we then have

$$\theta = \left(\frac{Z}{Z - L} \right) P \qquad (13.32a)$$

For all normal values of Z and L, the effective power of a plano prism in near vision is in the neighbourhood of 5–10% less than its nominal power.

Prism distortion and magnification

If a square grid is viewed through a flat plano prism with its back surface approximately normal to the primary line of the eye, a typical distortion pattern may be observed. The effect is enhanced by tilting the prism so as to bring its base closer to the eye than the apex. The

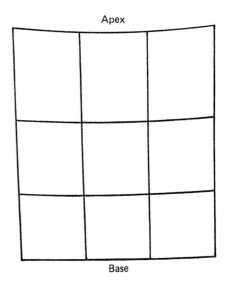

Figure 13.11. Prism magnification and distortion. Appearance of a square grid viewed through a base-down flat plano prism with its base tilted towards the eye.

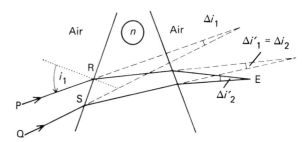

Figure 13.12. Ray trace through a flat plano prism of a narrow bundle of rays initially enclosing the small angle Δi_1.

image of the grid seen through a tilted base-down prism would then appear somewhat as shown in *Figure 13.11*. Three different features of the image distortion can be distinguished. The first is the elongation in the direction of the base–apex line. Reversing the tilt so as to bring the apex nearer to the eye produces the opposite effect. This elongation or compression of the image is known as 'prism magnification'. Since it varies with the angle of incidence, the magnification is not uniform. Another element of the distortion is the varying curvature of straight lines perpendicular to the base–apex direction. This effect is known as 'prism metamorphopsia'. Perhaps the least noticeable aspect of prism distortion is the fanning out of lines parallel to the base–apex direction, the divergence being away from the base of the prism. It is interesting to note that tilting the apex of the prism nearer to the eye does *not* reverse the direction of the curvature and fanning effects.

A simple expression for prism magnification can be obtained from *Figure 13.12*, showing a flat plano prism of refractive index n surrounded by air. An incident ray PR makes an angle of incidence i_1, with the first surface, while a neighbouring ray QS makes the slightly larger angle of incidence $(i_1 + \Delta i_1)$. After the first refraction, the angle between the rays is $\Delta i'_1$, equal to Δi_2, since the refracted rays from the first surface become the inci-

Table 13.2 Deviation and prism magnification (plano prisms 4Δ in flat and meniscus forms; $z = 27$ mm, $n = 1.523$)

Ocular rotation		*Type of prism*			
		Flat		*Meniscus ($F_2 = -6.00$ D)*	
		Deviation	*Prism magnification*	*Deviation*	*Prism magnification*
+30° } towards apex		4.78	1.039	4.82	1.024
+15°		4.13	1.014	4.35	1.008
0°		4.00	0.996	4.00	0.996
−15° } towards base		4.35	0.977	3.73	0.986
−30°		5.38	0.945	3.45	0.977

The back surface of the prism is normal to the primary of the eye.

dent rays at the second. After refraction at this surface, the angle between the rays becomes $\Delta i_2'$ and they meet at E where an observer's eye is placed.

It can be seen from the diagram that an object subtending an angle Δi_1, would appear to subtend an angle $\Delta i_2'$ when viewed through the prism. Thus, for any given ray path, the ratio $\Delta i_2'/\Delta i_1$ is the prism magnification.

Differentiating the basic expression for refraction, we obtain

$$n' \cos i' \Delta i' = n \cos i \, \Delta i$$

Applied to each surface of the prism in turn, this yields

$$\frac{\Delta i_1'}{\Delta i_1} = \frac{\cos i_1}{n \cos i_1'}$$

and

$$\frac{\Delta i_2'}{\Delta i_2} = \frac{\Delta i_2'}{\Delta i_1'} = \frac{n \cos i_2}{\cos i_2'}$$

which gives

$$\frac{\Delta i_2'}{\Delta i_1} = \frac{\cos i_1 \cos i_2}{\cos i_1' \cos i_2'} \tag{13.33}$$

This reduces to unity for the symmetrical ray path giving minimum deviation.

Prism magnification and distortion are not very noticeable with most plano prisms as normally mounted for ophthalmic use or in testing. Some idea of the magnitudes involved can be seen from *Table 13.2* which is based on accurate ray-trace data. It lists the deviation and prism magnification at various ocular rotations of a 4Δ prism, both in flat and meniscus form (back surface power −6.00 D). The latter form is superior because it makes the various ray paths more symmetrical and the angles of incidence more uniform.

A further modest improvement would result from tilting the prism through some 5–10° so that its apex moves nearer to the eye.

A mathematical analysis of prism distortion was published by Ogle (1951, 1952), the treatment being restricted to untilted prisms (i.e. with the back surface normal to the primary line of the eye). Using the same approach as Ogle, Adams *et al.* (1971) compared the various computed distortions of conventional ophthalmic prisms with those of the Fresnel type. Neither variety showed overall superiority.

If a pair of flat plano prisms is arranged as in *Figure 13.13*, each contributes an element of meridional

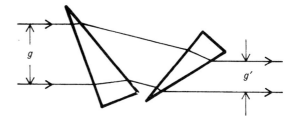

Figure 13.13. Optical arrangement of Brewster's teinoscope using prism magnification.

magnification, but the deviation and chromatic aberration produced by the first prism are neutralized by the second. At the same time the asymmetry of the magnification is largely eliminated. An arrangement of this kind 'for extending or altering the lineal proportions of objects' was devised by Brewster (1813) who called it a teinoscope. The principle found a recent application in the motion-picture industry in order to 'squeeze' a horizontally wide-angle view into a frame of standard size and proportions, the process being reversed when the film was projected.

It was shown by Bennett (1951) that the meridional magnification of a teinoscope is equal to the ratio g/g' of the widths of a parallel incident pencil of rays and of the conjugate emergent pencil. This property was already well known in reference to telescopes consisting of lenses.

Prismatic effects of lenses

General expressions for prismatic effects

A ray passing through any point of a lens other than its optical centre undergoes a deviation known as the 'prismatic effect of the lens' at that point. For clinical purposes, the magnitude P of the prismatic effect, measured in prism dioptres, can be found with sufficient accuracy from Prentice's rule

$$P = cF \tag{13.34}$$

where c is the distance in centimetres of the given point from the optical centre and F the power of the lens. Prentice's rule is an approximation based on paraxial theory applied to a thin lens. It also assumes that the prismatic effect is independent of the direction of the incident ray.

In the case of a spherical lens, the base–apex direction of the prismatic effect lies in the meridian containing the given point and the optical centre of the lens. The base is towards the optical centre of a plus lens and away from the optical centre of a minus lens.

The above applies to a spherical lens or to the spherical component of an astigmatic lens. Prentice's rule is applicable also to cylindrical surfaces, where the distance c is now the length of the perpendicular from the given point to the cylinder axis and F is the cylinder power. The base–apex line of the prismatic effect is in the meridian perpendicular to the cylinder axis, the base being towards the axis of a plus cylinder and away from the axis of a minus cylinder.

For the solution of specific problems on astigmatic lenses, various useful graphical constructions have been devised. They are explained in most textbooks on ophthalmic lenses. For the purpose of analysis or for routine practical use, such as computer programming, mathematical formulae are needed. Two different systems may be used.

Rectangular co-ordinates

The point at which the prismatic effect is to be calculated is defined by its co-ordinates (x, y) with respect to horizontal and vertical meridians through the optical centre of the lens. Regard must be paid to the following sign convention, which is the same for right and left lenses:

> x positive inwards, negative outwards
> y positive upwards, negative downwards

These distances are both to be expressed in centimetres.

The prismatic effect at the point (x, y) is obtained in terms of its horizontal component H and vertical component V, both in prism dioptres. The following sign convention applies:

> H positive base-out, negative base-in
> V positive base-down, negative base-up

Let S be the spherical power of the lens, C the cylindrical power of the lens, ϕ for the right lens be $180° -$ cylinder axis in standard notation and for the left lens, the cylinder axis in standard notation.

Then

$$H = Ax + By \tag{13.35}$$

and

$$V = Bx + Dy \tag{13.36}$$

where

$$A = S + C \sin^2 \phi \tag{13.37}$$

$$B = C \sin \phi \cos \phi \tag{13.38}$$

and

$$D = S + C \cos^2 \phi \tag{13.39}$$

Example (3)

Find the prismatic effect at a point 8 mm below and 2 mm inwards from the optical centre of the lens

> R − 3.00 DS/−2.00 DC axis 60

From the given data, $x = +0.2$, $y = -0.8$ and $\phi = (180 - 60) = 120°$ which gives

$$A = -3.00 - 2.00 (\sin^2 120°) = -4.50$$

$$B = -2.00 (\sin 120° \cos 120°) = +0.866$$

and

$$D = -3.00 - 2.00 (\cos^2 120°) = -3.50$$

giving

$$H = (-4.50 \times 0.2) + (0.866 \times -0.8) = -1.59\Delta \text{(base in)}$$

and

$$V = (0.866 \times 0.2) + (-3.50 \times -0.8) = +2.97\Delta \text{(base down)}$$

Polar co-ordinates

In this system, the given point is defined by its distance c (in centimetres) from the optical centre of the lens and the acute angle ϵ from the cylinder axis to the meridian containing the given point. The normal mathematical sign convention applies, the anticlockwise direction being positive. Similarly, the prismatic effect is obtained in terms of its magnitude P and the angle ψ from the cylinder axis to the base–apex meridian of the prismatic effect. There are two separate calculations to be made in the following order:

$$\tan \psi = \left(\frac{S + C}{S} \right) \tan \epsilon \tag{13.40}$$

and

$$P = |cS(\cos \epsilon / \cos \psi)| \tag{13.41}$$

One further item of information is needed. It is not enough to know, for example, that the base–apex meridian is $130°$; the prism base setting (i.e. whether base up or base down) along this meridian must also be known. A way of resolving this ambiguity when the answer is not obvious is described in this solution of Example (3).

Let the optical centre be denoted by O and the given point by Q. A preliminary calculation shows that the meridian OQ is at $104°$ in standard notation, so that

$$\epsilon = 104 - 60 = 44°$$

while

$$c = OQ = \sqrt{0.8^2 + 0.2^2} = 0.825 \text{ cm}$$

Then, from equation (13.40)

$$\psi = \arctan (-5.00/ - 3.00) \tan 44° = +58°$$

so that the base–apex meridian is $(60+58)$ or $118°$, while from equation (13.41)

$$P = |(0.825 \times -3.00)(\cos 44° / \cos 58°)|$$

$$= 3.36\Delta$$

In the absence of the cylinder, the prismatic effect at Q would be base down along $104°$, that is, base *away from* the optical centre because the spherical power is of minus sign. The rule is that the same condition must apply to the modified base setting of the prism. In this case, the base must still be away from the optical centre, along the 118° meridian. Thus

$$P = 3.36\Delta \text{ base 118 down}$$

This will be found to resolve into the horizontal and vertical components already obtained in Example (3). For mixed lenses (principal powers opposite in sign), this method is unsuitable.

Ocular rotation factor

The prismatic effects of spectacle lenses alter the ocular rotations required for fixation. If θ_o denotes the ocular rotation from the primary line needed to fixate a given point viewed directly and θ the rotation needed when the point is viewed through a spectacle lens, then the ratio θ/θ_o is the ocular rotation factor, ORF. In the case of a thin centred spherical lens, it takes a comparatively simple form.

In *Figure 13.14*, in which Q is the point of fixation, the relationship between the angles θ_o and θ is of exactly the same form as between u and u' in *Figure 13.6*, the difference being that z and Z now take the place of a and E. So we can simply rewrite equation (13.18) as

$$\text{ORF} = \frac{\theta}{\theta_o} = \frac{Z - L}{Z - L - F} \tag{13.42}$$

Thus the ocular rotation factor is akin to, but numerically different from, spectacle magnification. In most cases the two values would not differ by more than 10%, usually less than this.

Visual points

The visual point is the intersection of the visual axis with the back surface of the lens, or the lens itself if assumed thin, in a specified direction of the gaze. In cases of anisometropia the right and left ocular rotation factors are different. Difficulties may then arise, especially if large vertical rotations are needed for binocular fixation. A common method of assessing the situation is to assume arbitrary positions for the right and left visual points and to compare the prismatic effects at those points. For example, in considering the optical suitability of various types of bifocals, it is customary to assume a mean position of the near visual points as being 8 or 10 mm below and 2 mm inwards from the optical centre of the distance portion, the same for both lenses.

Suppose that in a given case the vertical prismatic effects at the near visual points are found to be R 4.4Δ base down and L 6.9Δ base down. The relative prismatic effect or imbalance is therefore 2.5Δ base down L, and it is assumed that the eyes would need to make vertical rotations differing by this amount. There are, in fact, two sources of inaccuracy in this procedure. A numerical example illustrating this will be given later, but in the meantime, the following relationships can readily be deduced from *Figure 13.14*. Rotations and prismatic effects are in prism dioptres throughout. Any units, provided they are the same for all, may be used in expressions containing only distances, but distances must be in centimetres whenever they appear in expressions also containing dioptric powers or vergences.

Ocular rotation θ_o for the unaided eye

$$\theta_o = \frac{100h}{-\ell + z} = \frac{-hLZ}{Z - L} \tag{13.43}$$

Ocular rotation θ for the corrected eye

$$\theta = \frac{100h'}{-\ell' + z} = \frac{-h'L'Z}{Z - L'}$$

$$= \frac{-hLZ}{Z - L - F} \tag{13.44}$$

Distance OV (c)

$$c = \frac{h'z}{-\ell' + z} = \frac{-hL}{Z - L - F} \tag{13.45}$$

Prismatic effect P at visual point

$$P = cF = \frac{-hLF}{Z - L - F} \tag{13.46}$$

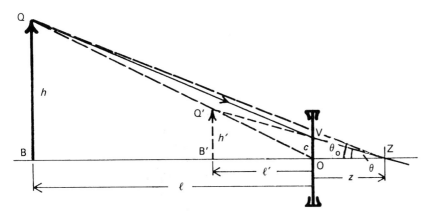

Figure 13.14. Ocular rotation factor. The ratio of the angle θ subtended by the image point Q' at the eye's centre of rotation Z to the angle θ_o subtended by the object point Q.

Effective change in ocular rotation $(\theta - \theta_0)$

$$\theta - \theta_0 = -hLZ\left(\frac{1}{Z - L - F} - \frac{1}{Z - L}\right)$$

$$= \frac{-hLFZ}{(Z - L - F)(Z - L)}$$

which, with the aid of equation (13.46), can be simplified to

$$\theta - \theta_0 = cF\left(\frac{Z}{Z - L}\right) \qquad (13.47)$$

This last result is similar to the relationship expressed by equation (13.32a) for the effective power of a plano prism. In both cases the deviation at the lens or prism has to be multiplied by the factor $Z/(Z - L)$ to obtain the ocular rotation.

Students may find it instructive to make a drawing and work from first principles. The appropriate expression can then be used to check the result.

Example (4)

A subject wearing centred lenses R -5.00 DS L -9.00 DS fixates an object point 120 mm below the level of the primary line of sight in a plane at one-third of a metre from the lenses. The centre of rotation of the eye is 25 mm from the lens. Determine the downward ocular rotations required for fixation.

The calculations are as described above, and the basic data and results are tabulated below.

	Right eye	Left eye
ℓ	-333.3 mm	-333.3 mm
L	-3.00 D	-3.00 D
F	-5.00 D	-9.00 D
L'	-8.00 D	-12.00 D
ℓ'	-125 mm	-83.33 mm
z	$+25$ mm	$+25$ mm
Z	$+40$ D	$+40$ D
h	-120 mm	-120 mm
h'	-45 mm	-30 mm
θ_0	-33.49Δ (downwards)	-33.49Δ (downwards)
θ	-30.00Δ (downwards)	-27.69Δ (downwards)
c	-0.75 cm	-0.692 cm
P	3.75Δ (base down)	6.23Δ (base down)
$\theta - \theta_0$	3.49Δ	5.80Δ

It can be verified that $(\theta - \theta_0)$ for each eye is equal to P multiplied by the factor $Z/(Z - L)$, as indicated in equation (13.47).

The difference between the right and left ocular rotations is nominally $30 - 27.69$ or 2.31Δ. It should be remembered, however, that the prism dioptre is not a strictly additive unit. If the two values of θ are converted into degrees, they become $16.70°$ and $15.48°$, the difference being $1.22°$ which is equivalent to 2.13Δ. The same procedure should really be adopted to evaluate $(\theta - \theta_0)$ when these angles are large.

It will be noted that the two values of c differ by about 0.6 mm. The larger value is always associated with the lower minus or higher plus power.

The conventional approach would be to assume that both visual points were at the same distance from the optical centre. It would be argued, for example, that at 0.75 cm below the optical centres, the prismatic effects

would be R 3.75Δ base down and L 6.75Δ base down, the relative prismatic effect thus being 3.00Δ base down L. This is appreciably greater than the actual difference between the necessary ocular rotations, but the error can at least be said to be on the safe side.

General expression for ocular rotations

This has already been discussed in relation to spherical lenses. The same simple treatment can be extended to astigmatic lenses when the cylinder axis is horizontal or vertical, in which case the horizontal and vertical components of ocular rotations are calculated separately by applying equation (13.42) to each of the two principal meridians in turn.

When the cylinder axis is oblique, the solution becomes more complicated. In *Figure 13.15*, Z is the eye's centre of rotation and O the optical centre of the lens, its optical axis coinciding with the primary line of the eye. The object of regard is the point $Q(x_0, y_0)$, lying in a vertical plane containing the axial point B at a distance ℓ from the lens. The chief ray path by which a retinal image of Q is formed on the fovea is QVZ, V being the visual point.

To determine the necessary ocular rotation, resolved into horizontal and vertical components, the co-ordinates (x, y) of the visual point must be found. The direction ZV of the visual axis can be considered as the resultant of a horizontal rotation θ_H defined by

$$\theta_H = x/OZ = x/z = xZ \qquad (13.48)$$

and a vertical rotation θ_V, defined by

$$\theta_V = y/OZ = y/z = yZ \qquad (13.49)$$

The required relationship between the co-ordinates (x_0, y_0) and (x, y) can be found by treating ZV as an incident ray to be traced backwards through the lens regarding (x, y) as the known and (x_0, y_0) as the unknown quantities.

But for the prismatic effect of the lens at V, the ray ZV would continue undeviated to meet the object plane at the point $V'(x', y')$ such that

$$\frac{x'}{x} = \frac{y'}{y} = \frac{BZ}{OZ} = \frac{-\ell + z}{z} = \frac{Z - L}{-L}$$

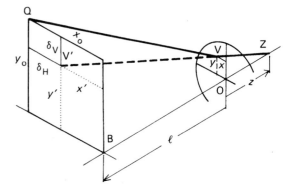

Figure 13.15. Prismatic effect of an astigmatic lens at a given visual point V: three-dimensional representation of the general case.

In fact, the prismatic effect of the lens displaces V' to Q by a horizontal shift δ_H and a vertical shift δ_V, in accordance with equation (13.31). Since the displacement is being measured in the refracted ray path, the distance q in this expression must be regarded as positive and must be replaced by $-\ell$. Thus

$$\delta_H = \ell H = H/L \quad \text{and} \quad \delta_V = \ell V = V/L$$

in which H and V are respectively the horizontal and vertical components of the prismatic effect at the visual point. From the diagram it can be seen that

$$x_o = x' + \delta_H = \frac{x(Z - L)}{-L} + \frac{H}{L}$$

and

$$y_o = y' + \delta_V = \frac{y(Z - L)}{-L} + \frac{V}{L}$$

which gives

$$x = \frac{H - x_o L}{Z - L} \quad \text{and} \quad y = \frac{V - y_o L}{Z - L}$$

In these expressions, H and V can be replaced, using equations (13.35) and (13.36) to give

$$x = \frac{Ax + By - x_o L}{Z - L}$$

and

$$y = \frac{Bx + Dy - y_o L}{Z - L}$$

which gives

$$(Z - L - A)x - By = -x_o L$$

and

$$Bx - (Z - L - D)y = y_o L$$

The solution of these as a simultaneous equation is

$$x = \frac{-L\{(Z - L - D)x_o + By_o\}}{(Z - L - A)(Z - L - D) - B^2}$$

and

$$y = \frac{-L\{Bx_o + (Z - L - A)y_o\}}{(Z - L - A)(Z - L - D) - B^2}$$

These expressions become lengthier when the coefficients A, B and D are written out in full. On the other hand, a useful piece of simplification can be introduced by putting

$$J = Z - L - S$$

which enables the expressions for x and y to be reduced to

$$x = \frac{-L\{(J - C\cos^2\phi)x_o + (C\sin\phi\cos\phi)y_o\}}{J(J - C)}$$

(13.50)

and

$$y = \frac{-L\{(C\sin\phi\cos\phi)x_o + (J - C\sin^2\phi)y_o\}}{J(J - C)}$$

(13.51)

Finally, when these expressions for x and y are inserted

in equations (13.48) and (13.49), these equations become

$$\theta_H = \frac{-LZ\{(J - C\cos^2\phi)x_o + (C\sin\phi\cos\phi)y_o\}}{J(J - C)}$$

(13.52)

and

$$\theta_V = \frac{-LZ\{(C\sin\phi\cos\phi)x_o + (J - C\sin^2\phi)y_o\}}{J(J - C)}$$

(13.53)

Example (5)

The correction for the right eye is

+2.00 DS/ + 4.00 DC axis 150

The co-ordinates of the point of fixation in a plane 250 mm from the lens are $x_o = +6$ cm, $y_o = -15$ cm, the distance z being 25 mm. Find the horizontal and vertical components of the necessary ocular rotation.

We have $S = +2$, $C = +4$, $\phi = 30°$, $Z = +40$ and $J = +42$.

Thus

$$\theta_H = \frac{4 \times 40\{(39 \times 6) + (1.732 \times -15)\}}{42 \times 38}$$

$$= +20.85\Delta \text{ (inwards)}$$

and

$$\theta_V = \frac{4 \times 40\{(1.732 \times 6) + (41 \times -15)\}}{42 \times 38}$$

$$= -60.61\Delta \text{ (downwards)}$$

(The sign convention for ocular rotations was given on page 237.)

Binocular vision through spectacle lenses or prisms

The effective binocular object

In *Figure 13.16*, a horizontal line object GH is viewed through base-out prisms of equal power. The right prism forms an image $G'_R H'_R$ of the same size and in the same plane as the object but displaced towards the apex of the prism. In a similar manner, the left prism forms the image $G'_L H'_L$. In order that the image of G should fall on the fovea of each eye, the right visual axis must be directed so as to pass through G'_R and the left visual axis through G'_L. These two axes intersect at the point G_B. A similar construction determines the point H_B. Thus, corresponding to the real object GH there is a hypothetical object $G_B H_B$ which, if viewed by the unaided eyes, would require the same ocular rotations for binocular fixation. It has been called the 'effective binocular object', defined by Bennett (1977/8) as the hypothetical object corresponding to a real object of regard, that would require, at all points, the same ocular

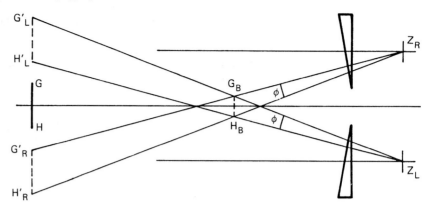

Figure 13.16. The effective binocular object $G_B H_B$ corresponding to the real object GH viewed through equal-powered base-out prisms.

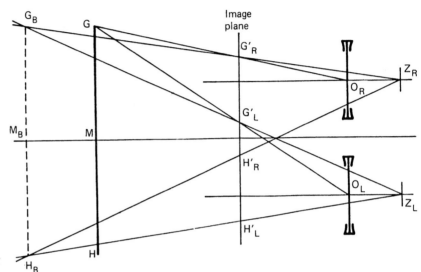

Figure 13.17. The effective binocular object $G_B H_B$ corresponding to the real object GH viewed through equal powered minus lenses centred for distance vision.

rotations for binocular fixation by the unaided eyes as the real object viewed through spectacle lenses or prisms.

The importance of this concept is that it provides a valuable clue to the probable appearance of the real object seen binocularly. For example, it has already been used in Chapter 11 to explain the theory of the prism stereoscope. The principal conclusions reached by Bennett can be summarized as follows.

Horizontal prisms

The effective binocular object is formed at a distance ℓ_B from the spectacle plane such that

$$\ell_B = \frac{2p - z}{2pL - \Delta} \quad (\ell_B \text{ and } z \text{ in m, } p \text{ in cm}) \quad (13.54)$$

where L denotes the dioptric distance of the real object, p the semi-interocular distance and Δ the total prism power, positive if base out and negative if base in.

The effective object subtends at each eye the same angle as the real object viewed directly, but is not at the same distance. In the case of base-out prisms it is at a nearer position where the real object would subtend a larger angle. Since, however, the visual angle is not increased, the subjective impression is an apparent reduction in size. The opposite occurs in the case of base-in

prisms. If the prisms are of unequal power, an additional effect occurs: the effective binocular object is displaced laterally towards the primary line of the eye wearing the stronger base-in or weaker base-out prism.

Lenses

Figure 13.17 illustrates the principle of the construction applied to the particular case in which minus lenses, centred for distance vision, are of the same power. As before, GH is a horizontal line object. The image distance and size, the same for both lenses, are determined from the basic conjugate foci relationships. In this case, the effective binocular object is the same size as the real object but at a greater distance from the eyes. These properties are characteristic of all corrections of equal minus power, whatever that power might be, provided that the lenses are centred for distance vision. With similar centration, plus lenses of equal power give rise to an effective binocular object of the same size as the real object but situated nearer to the eyes.

The effect of horizontal decentration with lenses of equal power is an equal lateral displacement of the images formed by the right and left lenses. In consequence, both the distance and size of the effective binocular object are altered, though it retains the same angular subtense. If the decentration produces base-in prismatic effect, the binocular object moves away from the eyes while increasing in size. The opposite effects arise from decentration producing base-out prism. An interesting case arises when the lenses are decentred inwards to suit a given working distance. The effective binocular object corresponding to a real object in this plane is then formed in the same plane, but is larger if the lenses are of plus power and smaller if of minus power.

Limitations on the construction

If the eyes' centres of rotation are regarded as lying in a horizontal plane, the visual axes are bound to intersect when the ocular rotations needed for binocular fixation are purely horizontal. If, however, the necessary rotations include a vertical component, the visual axes cannot intersect unless this component is the same for each eye.

In spherical anisometropia, for example, the effective binocular object can be constructed for any point or line lying in the horizontal plane containing the optical centres of the two lenses. A line such as GH in *Figure 13.17* can then be shown to give rise to an effective binocular object that is tilted towards the eye wearing the higher minus or lower plus correction. A typical value of this tilt would be approximately 8° for every dioptre of anisometropia. For any object point lying above or below the horizontal plane just specified, the images formed by the right and left lenses would be of different heights and require unequal vertical components of rotation to obtain binocular fixation. The visual axes would consequently fail to intersect, in which case the effective binocular object cannot be constructed. Unequal vertical rotations would also be required with a large number of astigmatic prescriptions and in all prescriptions incorporating vertical prism. The possibilities of constructing extended effective binocular objects are thus severely limited.

In some cases the effective binocular object is found to be behind the subject's head. This would occur, for example, when a distant object is viewed through base-in prisms, requiring the visual axes to diverge.

These various limitations illustrate the fact that spectacle-corrected eyes are frequently required to make co-ordinated ocular rotations that no real object could demand of the unaided eyes.

Further details are given in the paper by Bennett already mentioned. It includes mathematical expressions enabling the effective binocular object to be located by calculation instead of by graphical construction.

Apparent field curvature

The geometrical construction of the equivalent binocular object as shown in *Figures 13.16* and *13.17* assumes the lenses and prisms to be free from aberrations. On this basis, the equivalent binocular object of a plane surface is another plane surface. Experiment shows this to be an over-simplification. If a plane surface is viewed through a pair of centred plus lenses of equal power, it appears concave to the normal observer. A

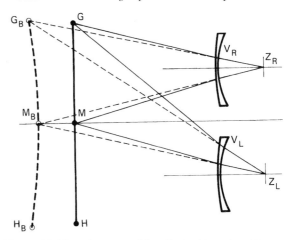

Figure 13.18. Curvature of the effective binocular object $G_B H_B$ constructed from accurate ray tracing as opposed to paraxial approximations.

similar effect is produced by base-out prisms. With minus lenses and base-in prisms, a convex appearance is normally seen.

The explanation is that the deviation undergone by a ray on refraction is always greater than that given by the simplified 'paraxial' law of refraction ($n'i' = ni$). Moreover, the excess deviation increases at a faster rate than the angle of incidence. This is the basic cause of image defects such as spherical aberration and distortion.

When exact ray-tracing methods are employed, the equivalent binocular object for a plane surface is found to be curved in accordance with observations. The procedure is shown in *Figure 13.18*, in which M is a point on the median line and G and H, equidistant from M, are points on the horizontal perpendicular through M. By a process of iteration (successive approximations), the position of the visual point V_R is determined such that the reverse ray $Z_R V_R$ passes through the point G after refraction by the right lens. The visual point V_L for the left lens is located in the same way. By definition, the intersection G_B of the visual lines $Z_R V_R$ and $Z_L V_L$ is the equivalent binocular object point corresponding to the real point G. By the same procedure, the equivalent binocular object point M_B can be located, while H_B is symmetrically placed with respect to G_B. The curved line through these three points is not necessarily circular, but when additional points on it are plotted by the same method it is found to be very nearly circular for lenses of moderate power.

The pioneer work in this field of Whitwell (1921/22) is worthy of mention. To reduce the amount of ray-tracing required – then an extremely laborious procedure – Whitwell assumed the equivalent binocular object to be a plane surface and determined the curvature of the corresponding real object plane. He also described a simple but ingenious method of calculating the vertical curvature from the results obtained in the horizontal meridian. For a +4.00 D lens he found the vertical curvature to be approximately one-third of the horizontal, irrespective of the lens form. This is also the case for a −4.00 D lens. Thus, a real plane surface viewed through lenses of equal power gives rise to an equivalent bin-

Table 13.3   Typical binocular field curvatures (m^{-1})

	Horizontal	Vertical
+4.00 DS each eye		
Plano-convex	+3.0	+1.0
Meniscus: base −6.00 D	+2.0	+0.7
−4.00 DS each eye		
Plano-concave	−2.3	−0.8
Meniscus: base +6.00 D	−1.4	−0.5
5Δ base-in each eye	−4.9	−2.3
5Δ base-out each eye	+5.1	+2.4

Field curvatures computed for a near object plane at −350 mm from the lenses and for $n = 1.523$, average centre thicknesses, $z = 27$ mm and inter-ocular distance 64 mm.

Plus curvatures denote a surface concave towards the observer, minus curvatures the opposite effect.

ocular surface of approximately toroidal formation, with its shallower principal meridian vertical. Whitwell also showed that the horizontal field curvature produced by lenses is affected by inward or outward decentration. He did not investigate the behaviour of plano prisms.

Binocular field curvatures in reciprocal metres (m^{-1}) for typical plus and minus spectacle lenses and for flat plano base-in and base-out prisms have been calculated by the authors. An indication of the trend can be gleaned from *Table 13.3*.

Unlike other aberrations of spectacle lenses such as oblique astigmatism and distortion, binocular field curvature is not a property of the lens or lenses alone. Nevertheless, it is affected by the lens form and, like distortion, diminishes as the base curve becomes increasingly steep.

Fields of view

Definitions

A distinction must be made between the macular field of view, within which objects can be imaged on the fovea of the rotating eye, and the peripheral field (of indirect vision) with the stationary eye in its primary position. The term field of fixation is sometimes applied to the macular field, though its meaning is not as precise. The expression field of view implies that the eye is viewing through an optical appliance, whereas field of fixation is also applied to the naked eye.

In addition to the field of corrected vision through a lens, there is also an uncorrected peripheral and possibly an uncorrected macular field of view outside the lens periphery, especially in the temporal region.

The following definitions of the corrected fields, illustrated in *Figure 13.19*, apply to any specified meridian of a spectacle lens. In this diagram, the upper half shows the macular and the lower half the peripheral fields when the eye is in its primary position.

Apparent macular field of view

The angle subtended by the lens periphery at the eye's centre of rotation Z. This may also be termed the apparent field of fixation.

Real macular field of view

The object space contained within the angle subtended by the lens periphery at the virtual image Z′ of the eye's centre of rotation formed by the lens.

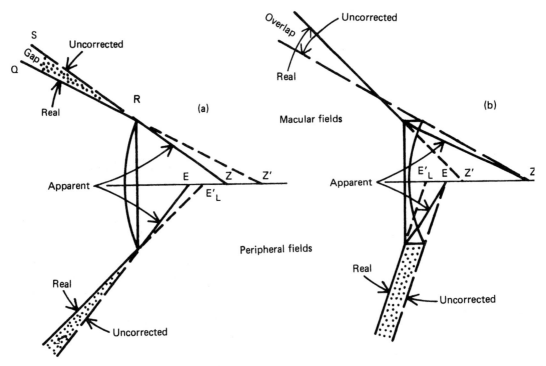

Figure 13.19.   The fields of view through (a) plus and (b) minus lenses. The upper part of the diagram illustrates the macular fields of view with the rotating eye, the lower part the peripheral field with the static eye. E is the centre of the eye's entrance pupil, Z its centre of rotation. The corrected fields apply to the most oblique peripheral ray path through the lens, the uncorrected fields to the least oblique ray passing outside the lens. The stippled area is not seen.

Apparent peripheral field of view

The angle subtended by the lens periphery at the centre E of the eye's entrance pupil.

Real peripheral field of view

The object space contained within the angle subtended by the lens periphery at the virtual image E'_L of the centre of the eye's entrance pupil formed by the lens.

Linear extent of field

The height or width of the real field of view, generally the macular field, measured at a specified distance from the lens.

Semi-field of view

Applicable to any of the above, that part of the total field from the optical axis of the lens outwards.

The field of view provided by a lens of given power depends mainly on its diameter, but is maximized by fitting it as close to the eye as possible. A third factor is the back surface curvature; the more concave this is made, all other things being equal, the larger the field of view. Hence, high-powered lenses, if made in bi-convex or bi-concave form, perform poorly even if they are thinner.

Boundary effects

Because of the finite size of the pupil, the sharp boundaries between the various fields are, in fact, blurred and show some overlapping. As a result, the effects about to be described may be masked or modified to some extent.

Plus lenses

It will be seen from *Figure 13.19(a)* that the incident ray QR aimed at Z' enters the rotated eye in the changed direction RZ. Consequently, an object point situated along QR will be seen in the direction ZRS. There is thus, in object space, an angular gap surrounding the lens periphery. Objects within this gap, indicated by the stippled area in the diagram, cannot be seen in direct vision either through or outside the lens. A similar gap surrounds the segment of an 'invisible' fused or solid (one-piece) bifocal and the effective aperture of a lenticular lens. As shown in the diagram, the peripheral field is affected in precisely the same way.

The angular width of the gap, being equal to the prismatic effect of the lens at its periphery, can be found to a first approximation from Prentice's rule.

Jack-in-the-box effect

This term, given currency by Welsh (1961), describes a phenomenon particularly noticeable to aphakics wearing high-powered spectacle lenses. Suppose an object is moving from right to left across the field of view, the subject originally looking approximately straight ahead. The object, first seen in the uncorrected peripheral field, disappears from view while crossing the gap in this field. It then reappears on entering the corrected portion of the peripheral field. If it has now engaged the subject's attention and he turns his eye to view it directly, it will again disappear and reappear on crossing the gap in the macular field of view.

Minus lenses

The real field of view of a minus lens is larger than the apparent field, resulting in a band of diplopia. Objects within this area can be seen doubly, both through and outside the lens. The macular band of diplopia is shown in the upper part of *Figure 13.19(b)*. In some cases, the obstruction caused by the edge of the lens or rim of the frame may prevent the formation of a diplopic band, as shown in the lower part of this diagram.

Vignetting

The area of a lens transmitting pencils filling the pupil does not extend to the extreme edge. There is a peripheral zone within which the width of those pencils entering the pupil gradually diminishes to zero. There is thus a progressive loss of illumination called 'vignetting'. This word originally meant the artistic border of vine leaves round the title page of a book and then, by extension, the variably shaded border that used to be put round photographic portraits.

Spectacle frame obstruction

Depending on the pupil size in relation to other dimensions, the rims and sides (temples) of a spectacle frame may cause either a partial or total occlusion (Swaine, 1933). In the former case there is merely a penumbra effect of which the wearer is conscious, though he can see through it. Wide temples, which are totally occluding, create potentially dangerous scotomata in the temporal fields of vision, especially when the frame is not of 'high joint' construction.

Optics of magnifying devices

Definition

The definition of magnification given in the draft International Standard is 'the ratio between any linear dimension of the retinal image when the magnifying device is in use and the corresponding dimension when the object is viewed without the magnifier'. Although the phrase 'retinal image size' is included, it is usually only necessary to calculate the change in angular subtense at the entrance pupil of the eye. The small change in image size caused by changes in the principal power of the eye with accommodation can generally be ignored.

Because the magnification given by a lens varies with the manner in which it is used, any numerical value for magnification needs clarification.

Angular magnification

Applicable to telescopic devices for distance vision, this term denotes the ratio of the angle subtended by the image to that subtended by the object. The system is assumed to be in 'normal adjustment', both object and image then lying at infinity.

The following terms relate to near-vision devices.

Conventional magnification

The traditional formula for determining the 'magnification' of magnifiers and eyepieces for optical instruments is $F/4$, where F is the equivalent power of the lens or system. We shall call this the 'conventional magnification'.

Note should be taken of the assumptions made in deriving the formula quoted. The first is that the eye is emmetropic or corrected for distance vision. The second is that when the object is viewed by the naked eye it will be held at what used to be termed the 'least distance of distinct vision'. This depends on the amplitude of accommodation but the traditional distance of 10 in or 250 mm, requiring 4 D of accommodation, is now better termed the 'reference seeing distance'. The third assumption is that when the magnifier is in use, the object will be held in its anterior focal plane. Since the image will then be formed at infinity it can be viewed without accommodation.

In *Figure 13.20*, an object BQ of height h is placed at a distance p from an eye at E, thus subtending a positive visual angle u_o given by

$$u_o = -h/p = -hP$$

If placed at the anterior focus of a magnifier of equivalent power F, the same object would subtend a larger angle u at the optical centre (or first principal point) of the lens defined by

$$u = -h/f = hF$$

The image, formed at infinity, would subtend the same angle u at the eye because all the rays from Q are parallel after refraction. The magnification m is thus given by

$$m = u/u_o = F/-P$$

If, following the accepted convention, P is taken as -4 D, then

$$m = F/4 \qquad (13.55)$$

In the assumed condition of use, the distance of the lens from the eye does not affect the magnification, though it does affect the field of view. Thus, if the eye were placed at E′ instead of E, the raypath from Q would pass nearer to the edge of the lens, but the image Q′ at infinity would still subtend the same angle u' at the eye.

Although the front or back vertex powers of the magnifier are frequently easier to measure than the equivalent power, they are numerically larger and give a false indication of the magnification. Hence both the draft International and the current British Standard (BS 7522: 1992: Low Vision Aids: Part 1: *Specification for hand and stand magnifiers, including magnifiers with an integral source of illumination*) stipulate that equivalent power shall be used in determining the magnification and in labelling on the magnifier or its packaging.

Magnifiers and the accommodating eye or near addition

It is unrealistic to expect a magnifier to be used with its image at infinity – a young observer will accommodate, while the presbyopic patient will probably be wearing near-vision spectacles or bifocals. If the accommodating eye or an eye corrected for near vision is regarded as a relaxed emmetropic eye with a supplementary positive power A, then the equivalent power entered in the equation is that of the combination of the magnifier's power, F, and A, thus giving:

$$F_{eq} = F + A - dFA \qquad (13.56)$$

where d is the separation between magnifier and eye. For example, a $+20$ D equivalent power magnifier held 200 mm in front of spectacles incorporating a $+2.50$ D near addition gives a total equivalent power of:

$$F_{eq} = +20 + 2.50 - 0.2 \times 20 \times 2.5 = +12.50 \text{ D}$$

Hence, provided that the object is held in the anterior focal plane of the combination so that it is seen in focus, the magnification will be $+12.50/4$ or 3.25.

The magnification is now seen to depend upon the separation of magnifier and eye. If the magnifier is brought closer, to say 100 mm from the spectacles, the equivalent power becomes $+17.50$ D, whereas it falls to only $+7.50$ D if it is held further away at 300 mm. As pointed out by Rumney (1992), the equivalent power formula reduces to $F_{eq} = F_m$ when the separation d approximates to the focal length of the magnifier – see Exercise 13.19. Also, when the magnifier is held in this position, the field of view equals the diameter of the lens.

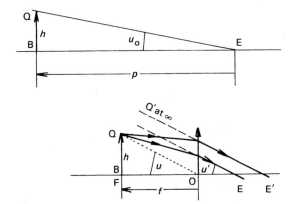

Figure 13.20. Conventional magnification formula. Without the magnifier, the object is held at a specified distance p from the eye, at which it subtends an angle u_o. With the magnifier in use, the object is placed at its anterior focal point, where it subtends the increased angle u, equal to the angular subtence u' of the image.

Trade magnification

If the separation between the magnifier and spectacle plane reduces to nil, $F_{eq} = F + A$. If A is assumed to take the relatively high value of $+4.00\,\text{D}$, then $F_{eq} = F + 4$, whence the magnification becomes

$$m = 1 + F/4 \qquad (13.57)$$

This formula increases the conventional magnification of a lens by one. It has been promoted by manufacturers in several countries, and perhaps could be termed 'trade magnification'. Because it assumes the user to have a high level of accommodation or a near addition, together with minimal vertex distance, this amount of magnification is unlikely to be realized in practice. For this reason, this formula is no longer used in the draft International Standard.

Conversely, the conventional formula would suggest that a $+4\,\text{D}$ lens does not give a magnified image. Depending upon the conditions of use, equation (13.56) shows that it does. Thus, if held 15 cm from an eye accommodating 2 D, F_{eq} is $+5.88\,\text{D}$, giving a magnification of 1.47.

Iso-accommodative magnification

To overcome the objection that magnifiers are rarely held very close to the eye or with the image at the reference seeing distance, Bennett (1977) introduced the concept of iso-accommodative magnification. This denotes the magnification achieved if the observer has the same amount of accommodation or the same near addition, both with and without the magnifier in use. In *Figure 13.21*, q denotes the subject's normal reading distance, taken to equal $1/A$. If no reading correction is worn, q is measured from E, the centre of the eye's entrance pupil; otherwise it is measured from the spectacle point S. The magnification is then

$$m = F_{eq}/A \qquad (13.58)$$

An early British Standard on magnifiers (BS 5043 : 1973: *Bookholders, magnifiers and prismatic spectacles for use as reading aids in hospitals and the home*) adopted a separation d of 100 mm and A as 4 D, whence the iso-accommodative magnification is $1 + 0.15\,F$.

A more general expression is given if the magnifier is used with accommodation A, but compared with unaided viewing of the object at any arbitrary dioptric distance P. The magnification is now given by

$$m = F_{eq}/-P \qquad (13.59)$$

The reader is directed to Exercise 13.18 for an alternative derivation and formula.

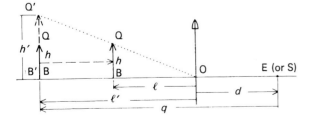

Figure 13.21. Iso-accommodative magnification. Without the magnifier, the object is placed at a distance $q \ (= 1/A)$ from the eye E (or spectacle plane S). With the lens at O, the object is moved until its image lies in the original object position.

Equivalent viewing distance and power

These terms were introduced by Bailey (see, for example, Bullimore and Bailey, 1989) as an aid to low-vision work and to break away from the concept of magnification linked to the reference seeing distance. If, for example, a patient can read N10 print with a spectacle correction at $-\frac{1}{3}\,\text{m}$, then N5 print should then, in theory, be legible at half the distance. Rather than hold print this close with a $+6.00\,\text{D}$ addition, or using a $+6.00\,\text{D}$ magnifier with the image at infinity, a combination of a magnifier and near addition having an equivalent focal length, f_{eq}, of $-167\,\text{mm}$ may allow a more comfortable posture.

The equivalent focal length can be shown to be identical to Bailey's equivalent viewing distance, EVD. He defined this as the actual viewing distance, a, to the virtual image formed by the magnifier divided by the magnification ($m_t = L/L'$). Bailey termed this magnification the 'enlargement ratio'. Ignoring signs, and assuming that the image is placed in the anterior focal plane of the spectacles so that $f_{eq} = a$,

$$\text{EVD} = a/m_t \qquad (13.60)$$

Thus, in the above example, a magnifier giving a linear magnification of 2.5 will give an EVD of 167 mm if the image is viewed at $167 \times 2.5 = 415\,\text{mm}$ from the spectacle plane.

If, for example, the patient holds the magnifier too far away so that the virtual image is not in the anterior focal plane of the spectacle addition, the final image will be out of focus on the retina. The equivalent power formula should not be applied, but the EVD can still give an idea of the magnification. In general, the present authors prefer the equivalent power formulation since it is such a fundamental optical principle.

The equivalent viewing distance concept can also be applied to closed circuit television systems. If such a system gives an image on the screen which is ten times larger than the original, but is viewed from 0.5 m, then the EVD is $0.5/10$ m or 50 mm.

Equivalent viewing power is defined as the reciprocal of the EVD, and may be shown as follows to be the equivalent power of the system. Thus, for the magnifier:

$$m_t = \frac{L}{L'} = \frac{L' - F}{L'}$$

Then, equivalent viewing power, from equation (13.60) is given by

$$\text{EVP} = \frac{1}{\text{EVD}} = \frac{m_t}{a} = \frac{L' - F}{aL'}$$

but, from *Figure 13.21*, and writing a instead of q,

$$\ell' = \text{OB}' = \text{OE} + \text{EB}' = d - a$$

so, therefore

$$L' = \frac{1}{d - a} = \frac{A}{Ad - 1}$$

and substituting for L' gives

$$\text{EVP} = \frac{A - F(Ad - 1)}{Aa} = F + A - dFA$$

From equation (13.60), EVP may also be expressed as:

$$EVP = m_t A \qquad (13.61)$$

The identity of the EVP and the equivalent power of the system was demonstrated by Bailey (1981a).

Spectacle magnifiers

Spectacle magnifiers* are high-powered plus lenses mounted close to the eye, either in a spectacle frame or as a clip-on. They are limited to monocular use, the other eye being occluded if necessary.

Despite the fact that iso-accommodative magnification is a more appropriate basis of numbering in all clinical applications, it has become customary for manufacturers to specify spectacle magnifiers by their conventional magnification.

One of the drawbacks of spectacle magnifiers is that since the object has to be held close to the anterior focal plane of the lens, the working distance is often uncomfortably short. A further difficulty is the extremely restricted depth of field, requiring the reading matter to be positioned very accurately. When the object is held in the anterior focal plane of the lens, $L = -F$ and $L' = 0$. Suppose that L' may vary up to $\pm E$ dioptres before acuity is noticeably impaired by out-of-focus blurring. Then L in turn may vary by $\pm E$ dioptres. The corresponding variation in the object distance may be found by differentiating the expression $\ell = 1/L$, giving

$$d\ell/dL = -1/L^2 = -1/F^2$$

In this context, dL represents the permitted tolerance $\pm E$ in the value of L, while $d\ell$ is the depth of field or permissible variation in the object distance. By substitution in the previous expression, we therefore obtain

$$\text{Depth of field (in mm)} = \pm 1000\, E/F^2 \qquad (13.62)$$

It can be found from this that if E is taken as ± 1.00 D, the depth of field is about ± 7 mm on a $3\times$ spectacle magnifier, reducing to as little as ± 1 mm with an $8\times$ and ± 0.6 mm with a $10\times$ lens.

As the magnification increases, the field of view contracts, reducing to approximately the diameter of the lens itself when the magnification reaches $10\times$.

Hand readers

Hand readers are used mainly by elderly people whose visual acuity has declined and whose accommodation is very limited. In most cases a reading correction is worn. This enables the patient to look at large print, for example, the headlines in the paper, and then use the hand reader as an adjunct for the smaller print. Magnification is greater with the near addition in use than with the distance correction. A typical hand reader consists of a single lens of relatively large diameter and of power between $+3.50$ D and $+2.00$ D. Although the maximum monocular field of view and magnification are obtained when the reader is held close to the eye

like a spectacle magnifier, this is not the way such magnifiers are commonly used. Despite the reduction in magnification, they are usually held at about 10 cm from the eye in order to increase the working distance.

If one of the patient's eyes is significantly poorer than the other, it may be advantageous to close or occlude the weak eye. If the two eyes are equally good, one would expect a better performance if they could both view through the same magnifier. This is termed bi-ocular viewing, as opposed to binocular viewing when a separate lens is used for each eye, as in the prismatic binocular loupes discussed below. Unfortunately, there are two possible disadvantages in bi-ocular use. First, the magnifier restricts both monocular fields, generally allowing each eye to see only a portion of a line of print. If so, only the overlapping area in the centre can be seen simultaneously by the two eyes. This area increases with longer working distances, but to the disadvantage of magnification. Increasing the power of the lens to compensate is counter-productive as it usually entails a smaller size. A second disadvantage is that the magnification across the lens is not uniform, so there may be discomfort in fusing the two images. These objections do not apply to large aspherical magnifiers of low power specially designed for bi-ocular use.

Galilean-type magnifiers[†]

The short working distance of a spectacle magnifier can be increased, perhaps more than doubled, by using a Galilean system comprising a positive front lens of power F_1 and an eye lens of power F_2. The conventional magnification of the system is $F/4$, where F is its equivalent power calculated from

$$F = F_1 + F_2 - dF_1F_2$$

In this expression d represents the optical separation in metres between the components, measured from the second principal point of the first to the first principal point of the second lens. Very high lens powers are needed to keep d below 30 mm while doubling the working distance.

By comparison with spectacle magnifiers of the same power, Galilean magnifiers have a smaller field of view and the same restricted depth of field. On the other hand, the longer working distance has the further great advantage of making possible a binocular construction.

Prismatic binocular loupes

Another method of adapting spectacle magnifiers to binocular use is to add strong base-in prisms. An empirical rule which has been found generally successful is to incorporate in each lens one prism dioptre base in for every dioptre of lens power.

A theoretical basis of design for a standard range is shown in *Figure 13.22*. The eyes' centres of rotation are at Z_R and Z_L. First, the lens power for a given conventional magnification is determined from the formula $m = F/4$. Next, the image plane is fixed at a suitable dis-

---

* Occasionally called 'microscopic lenses', following the obsolete term 'simple microscope' for a single magnifying lens.
[†] Occasionally called 'telemicroscopes'.

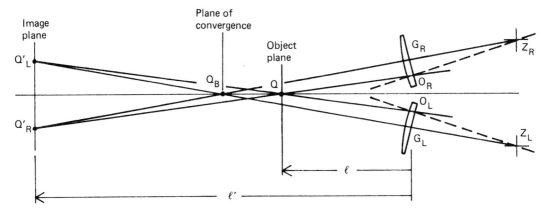

Figure 13.22. Scheme for designing a prismatic binocular loupe. Q_B represents the axial position of the effective binocular object to which the eyes converge.

tance ℓ' from the lens, which in turn determines the object distance. One further arbitrary distance remains to be fixed – from the lens to the plane of convergence in which the effective binocular object (EBO) is situated. Let Q, lying on the median line, denote the mid-point of the object and Q_B the corresponding EBO at the predetermined distance from the lens. Lines drawn from Z_R and Z_L through Q_B meet the image plane at Q'_R and Q'_L, the images of Q formed by the right and left lenses respectively. It thus follows that lines then drawn from Q'_R and Q'_L through the object point Q will determine the required positions of the respective optical centres, O_R and O_L. Finally, to obtain coincident fields of view, the geometrical centres of the lenses, G_R and G_L should be located on $Z_R Q_B$ and $Z_L Q_B$ respectively.

From drawings such as *Figure 13.22* the essential lens and frame dimensions could be obtained for a range of conventional magnification and inter-ocular distances. The optical performance of the lenses is improved by angling them, as shown, so that the optical axis (represented by the broken line) passes through the eye's centre of rotation.

A more flexible design procedure enabling prescribers to draw up specifications to suit patients' individual requirements has been described by Westheimer (1954).

In another type of prismatic binocular loupe, the lenses are held at a distance of some 40–60 mm from the eyes, thus permitting a longer working distance with moderate magnification. Headband magnifiers for industrial and general use are in this category. The user is able to wear spectacles if necessary and to look below as well as through the prismatic magnifying lenses.

Telescopic spectacles

Magnification in distance vision requires some form of telescopic system, the choice of a Galilean design being dictated by the need for compactness and an erect image. When the system is in normal adjustment, the angu-

lar magnification is $f'_1/-f'_2$, while the optical separation d between the lenses is $f'_1 + f'_2$. Thus

$$m = \frac{f'_1}{-f'_2} = \frac{f'_1}{f'_1 - d} = \frac{1}{1 - dF_1} \qquad (13.63)$$

where d is in metres. This is the basic design formula.

Correction of any ametropia is essential. In the original design introduced by Carl Zeiss of Jena, a separate correcting lens was mounted immediately behind the eye lens. In the design produced by Stigmat Ltd in 1951 – the first to use an aspherical object glass – every eye lens was worked individually so as to incorporate the correction needed.

According to a well-known theorem in geometrical optics, if light of vergence L is incident on a telescopic system of magnification m, the vergence of the emergent light is approximately $m^2 L$. Thus if $m = 2\times$, four dioptres of accommodation would be needed to focus an object at one metre. For this reason, an auxiliary lens of power $-L$ needs to be fitted in front of the object glass to adapt the basic unit to vision at a dioptric distance L.

By decreasing the working distance and fitting a 'reading cap' of high plus power over the objective, the magnification in near vision can be increased. If the power of the auxiliary lens is F_{cap}, the total magnification becomes $m \times (F_{cap}/4)$. Thus, a basic unit of magnification 1.8 used with a +12 D reading cap would have a conventional magnification of 1.8×3 or $5.4\times$.

An alternative method to focus for near vision is to increase the separation between the components of the system. If the increase in the separation from that for a distant object is Δ, then the equivalent power in near vision is $-\Delta F_1 F_2$, which can be shown to equal $\Delta m F_1^2$ or $(L_1/L'_1)F_2$ or $m/(\ell_1 + f'_1)$, where m is given by equation (13.61) above. For an ametropic observer, the effective eyepiece power to be inserted is $(F_2 - K)$.

For Keplerian systems similarly adjusted, the equivalent power is negative, but because the object is situated closer to the instrument than the first principal plane, the object vergence for the system as a whole is positive. The image would, of course, be erected by a compact prism system.

For further discussion on the optics of telescopic aids, the reader is referred to Bailey (1978, 1979, 1981b), Long and Woo (1986) and Woo *et al.* (1995).

Helping the partially sighted patient

Some guiding principles

For occasional use in distance vision, high-powered telescopes may be of use for identifying bus numbers, train indicator boards, etc. For prolonged use in distance and intermediate vision, the only help available is limited to telescopic systems with a magnification seldom exceeding 2.5×. Otherwise, the normal refractive correction must suffice. Patients with cloudy media may be further helped by tinted lenses, especially prescription sunglasses when out of doors, since these reduce pupil miosis. For television viewing, sitting nearer to the screen will make the picture appear larger.

For near vision much higher magnifications can be provided. Nevertheless, the lowest magnification that meets the patient's needs should normally be prescribed. Inherent drawbacks and difficulties – in particular, a reduced field of view and shorter working distance – are then minimized. Patients with a strong desire not to lose their ability to read have a good chance of adapting themselves to these limitations. Unfortunately, some elderly patients in particular may be unable or lack sufficient motivation to do so.

Improving the near acuity to N5 (or J2) should not necessarily be the aim. Although the most common size of newsprint is equivalent to N8 (J6), the contrast is poorer than in test types. An improvement to N6 (J3) may be necessary to enable a newspaper to be read satisfactorily. The use of a typical newspaper for test purposes is both practically and psychologically beneficial. Large-print books have already been mentioned on page 44, while a large print newpaper is available weekly in the UK.* For patients with poor vision, the ability to read newsprint is a grossly optimistic aim: it is better to concentrate on achieving 'survival reading' to enable the patient to read cooker settings, instructions or correspondence. Rumney (1995) points out that contrast sensitivity is also an important factor in reading. Apart from CCTV systems, described on pages 44 and 249, magnifiers cannot enhance the contrast of an object. Increased illumination, however, often improves the contrast sensitivity of the eye, thus effectively improving the contrast. Whittaker and Lovie-Kitchen (1993) emphasize that a reserve of magnification and contrast sensitivity are required to provide a reserve for comfortable reading.

A difficulty may arise if there is a field defect immediately to one side of fixation, as shown by the Amsler chart (usually a chart with a grid of white lines on a black ground). In this case the patient may benefit by a magnifier which is more powerful in the vertical than in the horizontal meridian. A number of simple stand magnifiers, generally of elongated or rectangular shape, are designed in this way. Patients with a homonymous hemianopia or bilateral loss of field to the right of fixation may be helped by learning to read with the print held diagonally, or even upside down, so as not to be reading into the blind area.

It is not easy to keep on track of a line of print when reading with a high-powered magnifier. With small stand magnifiers, a thin narrow strip of suitable material may be fixed across the bottom of the stand to provide a reference line. Alternatively, a ruler may be placed across the page and the magnifier slid along it. A simple device with added advantages was introduced by Charles F. Prentice, who called it a typoscope. It consists of a rectangular piece of matt black material with a long but narrow horizontal slit exposing just one or two lines of print. The patient slides the device down the page as he reads. Light from above and below the line of regard is absorbed by the black material and cannot be scattered within the eye by hazy media. A rigid clipboard to hold the paper flat and still may be helpful.

Refraction; high reading additions

Refraction of the partially sighted patient begins in the normal manner with retinoscopy or some other objective technique. If the patient is aphakic and the vitreous cloudy, keratometry will give a good indication of the ocular astigmatism. In this case the correcting cylinder in the spectacle plane should be of somewhat lower power, as indicated by the approximate expression (20.5). When necessary, the subjective refraction can be carried out at the reduced distance of 3, 2 or even 1 m, with lens powers changed in 1 or 2 D steps as indicated by the acuity.

In near-vision testing, a trial frame is preferable to a refracting unit because it allows normal head posture and movements. When the unaided acuity is very low, standard reading test types are unsuitable for assessing the magnification required. A specially designed set of types such as the Keeler A Series, described on page 29, makes this task much simpler.

With about a +2.50 D addition in place, the near acuity should be measured both monocularly and binocularly. The first line of approach is to determine whether the acuity can be raised to the desired level by increasing the reading addition. If, for example, N12 (or J10) can be read at the patient's normal working distance, a magnification of 2× should give N6 (J4). This may be obtained by halving the normal working distance, which will require the near addition to be increased by the dioptric change in the working distance. Thus, a change from 35 cm (−2.86 D) to 17.5 cm (−5.70 D) would require an extra addition of about +2.75 or possibly +3.00 D.

With the stronger reading addition in place, the patient is encouraged to read smaller and smaller print, shortening and adjusting the working distance to find the clearest position. The effect of increasing or decreasing the addition by 0.50 or 1.00 D should also be tried. If a reduced addition does not noticeably impair the per-

---

* Big Print, PO Box 308, Warrington WA1 1JE.

formance, it should be prescribed. In addition to giving a more comfortable reading position, it will also reduce the effort of convergence required.

Relatively high binocular additions often require the help of base-in prisms. The amount can be based on the cover and fixation disparity tests, with a check on the 'better with or without?' basis. For this purpose, the trial frame should be correctly centred for the near PD at the given working distance. Even when base-in prisms appear to give little subjective improvement in comfort, it is a good idea to prescribe them when prolonged reading is likely. In this case the empirical rule normally adopted for binocular loupes (1Δ base-in each eye for each dioptre of near addition) can be taken as a guide.

If binocular vision is poorly sustained or one eye has a much lower acuity, it is probably wiser to concentrate on the better eye. The poorer eye can be occluded or possibly furnished with a distance correction or much weaker addition for looking at headlines. Many elderly patients appear to be exotropic in near vision without noticing diplopia.

Other magnifying devices

Spectacle magnifiers

If a binocular addition as high as +6.00 D is still insufficient, a higher monocular addition may be given, the other eye being occluded. When the total lens power for reading reaches about +10 D or more, a lens designed as a spectacle magnifier is indicated. If the curves are specially calculated to minimize aberrations for the appropriate working distance, spectacle magnifiers with spherical surfaces will give quite acceptable results in magnifications up to about 5×. One such series is the Stigmagna range (3×, 4× and 5×). For higher magnifications aspherical surfaces are required, as in the Igard Hyperocular range (4×, 5×, 6×, 8×, 10× and 12×). Compound magnifiers, each comprising two lenses (preferably both aspheric) with magnifications up to 20× are also available.

No correction for spherical ametropia need normally be considered, because a small adjustment of the working distance will suitably modify the vergence of the pencils reaching the eye. A troublesome degree of astigmatism can be overcome by incorporating a prescribed cylinder in a specially worked lens of the same basic design as the standard range.

To enable a very short working distance to be correctly maintained, the lens may be surrounded by an adjustable transparent collar against which the reading matter is held. Another method is to attach an adjustable post to the spectacle frame. It is generally easier to pass a book across the face than to scan it by head and eye movements. The book should be moved in a series of steps like the saccades of the normally sighted. By this means, the advantage of a stationary field is obtained. The same principle applies when a hand-held magnifier is moved across the reading matter. With weaker additions, a plank may be placed across the arms of a chair to support the reading matter, or a piece of tape passed behind the neck with loops to support the wrists. Alternatively, a reading stand to be placed on a table may be formed by upturning a cardboard box cut diagonally.

With a short working distance, illumination of the reading matter may require special attention. Built-in illumination is provided for magnifiers of very high power in some manufacturers' ranges.

Hand magnifiers (hand readers)

While a younger patient can learn to master a very short reading distance, the older patient is rarely able to change the habits of a lifetime. Provided the acuity is not too poor, the familiar hand reader may prove helpful. It enables the reading matter to be held at nearly the normal distance. Moreover, the ordinary reading spectacles may enable headlines and pictures to be discerned, with resort to the magnifier only when needed.

The weakest (also, generally the largest) lens consistent with adequate vision should be advised, so as to obtain the additional advantage of less critical positioning. A plastics lens reduces weight considerably, though demanding more care to prevent scratching. An aspheric lens with its larger field of good definition is worth the extra cost if more than minimal use is contemplated.

Though Fresnel sheet magnifiers appear attractive because of their thinness and weight saving, it is rarely understood by the layman that, like conventional magnifiers, they have to be held off the page. In general, the image contrast and quality are relatively poor while the magnification of the large ones is limited.

It is useful to demonstrate to the patient that the field of view of a hand reader is increased if the lens and print are held closer to the eye, though they need not be as close as with a spectacle magnifier.

Stand magnifiers

A hand tremor or poor dexterity caused by arthritis, for example, may rule out a hand reader. In such cases a stand magnifier may be helpful because it rests directly on the object to be viewed. This then fixes the object and image conjugates, thus determining the magnification of the virtual image. Provided that the distance or vergence of this image from the surface of the magnifier nearer the eye is known (a requirement of the draft International Standard on magnifiers), the separation between lens and eye or spectacles can be determined, and hence the equivalent power. Expression (13.61) also shows that the transverse magnification m_t would usefully be marked on the device.

One type, designed specifically for low visual acuity, consists of an aspheric lens of about 44 mm diameter and equivalent power about +15 D. The image is formed about 250 mm behind the object plane, enabling the magnifier to be used in conjunction with ordinary reading spectacles. If these incorporated a +3.00 addition, then the distance between magnifier and spectacles will need to be about 80 mm, giving an equivalent power of about +14.5 D and hence magnification about

3.5. This will vary with the near addition and separation. Another convenient form of stand magnifier is the 'bright field' lens formed from a hyper-hemisphere of glass or plastic, the flat face resting on the paper, or with a shallow rim on the underside to lift it slightly to prevent scratching.

A large number of bulkier but adjustable stand magnifiers have been produced with normally sighted users in mind. In suitable cases they could be equally useful to partially sighted patients.

Fibreoptic magnifiers

A promising innovation is to employ fibreoptic bundles (Peli and Siegmund, 1995) to act as a magnifier. Each individual fibre is tapered, with the narrow end resting on the paper. Provided that the mosaic of the fibre ends is fine enough to resolve the print, an enlarged view is seen on the upper face of the magnifier, the magnification simply being the ratio of the diameters of the two ends of the fibre. As Peli and Siegmund point out, the optics of fibre bundles means that the patient does not have to align the eye with the magnifier, while illumination is provided by light passing down the tapered fibres.

Telescopic systems

The Galilean telescopic system can be adapted for use as a spectacle magnifier at near or intermediate distances. It has the big advantage of giving a longer working distance. When such a system is used binocularly, the optical axes of the right and left halves must be aligned very accurately so as to intersect on the median line at the intended working distance. It is therefore impracticable to adapt the same unit for use at different distances. On the other hand, a monocular Galilean unit designed for near vision can easily be converted for distance use, or vice versa, by means of an auxiliary lens fitted over the objective. In fact, a bifocal lens allows simultaneous use at two different distances.

A telescopic spectacle designed for distance vision should incorporate the patient's distance correction. A suggested routine is to put up this correction in a trial frame with an afocal telescopic unit in front of it. The resulting improved acuity may enable the refraction to be further refined.

For magnification in outdoor situations – for example, to distinguish bus numbers or street names across the road – a small Galilean telescope mounted on a finger ring can be of great assistance. A miniature prismatic monocular or binoculars will provide even greater magnification and a bigger field of view. Binoculars of the roof prism type are smaller and neater than those of the Porro prism type.

The use of auxiliary plus lenses to increase the magnification of a telescopic unit for near vision has already been discussed in the previous section on page 251. Compared with a spectacle magnifier giving the same magnification, the telescopic system gives a useful increase in the working distance but a smaller field of view. For example, the Stigmat telescopic unit with a reading cap giving a total magnification of 5.25× has a working distance of about 11 cm compared with the 5 cm working distance of the 5× hyperocular. On the other hand, the respective fields of view are approximately 5 cm and 7 cm.

In theory, a much less conspicuous telescopic system can be provided by mounting the object glass in a spectacle frame and using a high-powered minus contact lens as the eyepiece. The magnification obtainable is limited by the relatively small optical separation, 16–18 mm at the most. To avoid disconcerting prismatic effects, the contact lens must be fitted so that it moves relatively little in relation to the eye. Unlike a spectacle-mounted telescope which can be removed for walking about, the contact-lens device would have to be worn constantly.

Television magnifiers

These devices have been described on page 44.

A more detailed treatment of the whole subject of low-vision aids can be found in one of the specialized textbooks, such as those by Mehr and Freid (1975), Faye (1976) and Dowie (1988).

Field expanders

The opposite principle of minifying the external scene to increase the effective field of patients with severely restricted or tunnel vision has been suggested in the form of a field expander (Drasdo and Murray, 1978). A reverse Galilean system is used, the object glass being of negative and the eye lens of positive power. The suggested magnification is of the order of 0.2×. Unfortunately, the reduced size of the retinal image results in a corresponding reduction in visual acuity.

Aberrations of correcting lenses

General considerations

Spectacle lenses are subject to various 'geometrical' aberrations which should be noted in prescribing or dispensing.

Monochromatic aberrations

This term is given to those aberrations which would be present even if light of only one wavelength were considered, though the amount may differ with wavelength. Spherical aberration and coma come into this category, but in general are disregarded in spectacle lenses because the pupil admits only relatively narrow pencils of rays. Oblique astigmatism and distortion are the monochromatic aberrations that need to be taken seriously.

Chromatic aberration

This takes two forms. Axial chromatic aberration (ACA) refers to the variation with wavelength in the paraxial power or focal length of an optical surface or lens. The power variation over a given spectral range is proportional to the paraxial power itself but is basically dependent on the dispersive properties of the lens material (*see also* pages 275–281).

Transverse chromatic aberration (TCA) arises from the variation with wavelength in the prismatic effect at given distance from the optical centre or axis. As a result, blue or orange–red colour fringes may sometimes be noticed when the gaze is directed through a peripheral part of the lens, though transverse chromatic aberration is more often noticed as a reduction in sharpness.

Common properties

With the exception of axial chromatic aberration, all the significant aberrations mentioned have certain properties in common:

(1) They apply only to pencils passing obliquely through the lens and entering the rotated eye.
(2) They are approximately proportional to the square of the distance y from the optical axis at which the incident pencil meets the lens.
(3) They are affected by the form of the lens, defined by the value given to one of its surface powers. Unfortunately, the form needed for optimum correction differs from one aberration to another. Moreover, the lens form best for distance vision is generally not the best for vision at intermediate and near ranges.

Oblique astigmatism

Oblique astigmatism is an important defect because it impairs the sharpness of the images presented to the eye. It is essentially a defect of narrow pencils obliquely incident on a reflecting or refracting surface. The reflected or refracted pencil then forms two separate focal 'lines', characteristic of astigmatism, in two principal meridians called tangential and sagittal. The tangential meridian contains the incident and reflected or refracted rays, together with the optical axis, while the sagittal meridian is perpendicular to the tangential.

Figure 13.23(a) shows a parallel pencil of rays obliquely incident on a plus spectacle lens, the eye having pivoted about its assumed centre of rotation Z so that the refracted pencil falls on the fovea. Though the pupil moves with the eye, all the oblique pencils entering the eye in direct vision must necessarily pass through Z. In effect, the real pupil is replaced by an imaginary diaphragm situated at Z.

To correct the eye for distance, the second principal focus F' of the lens must coincide with the eye's far point M_R. As the eye rotates, the far point travels along a curved surface, with its centre of curvature at Z, known as the far point sphere. Ideally, all the refracted pencils should focus on this surface but generally exhibit oblique astigmatism. In *Figure 13.23(a)*, rays in the tangential meridian of the pencil illustrated form a short line focus at T_2' and in the sagittal meridian at S_2'. For a given object distance, these separate foci of pencils from all possible directions lie on two curved surfaces known as image shells. Their sections are represented in the diagram by the solid lines. When the defect is very marked, they resemble a teacup (tangential) and saucer (sagittal) – a useful mnemonic.

As with astigmatic refraction in general, the focal lines are each perpendicular to the associated principal meridian. Thus, if the pencil is incident immediately above the optical centre, making the tangential meridian the vertical one, the focal line at T_2' is horizontal while the line at S_2' is vertical. In *Figure 13.23(b)*, the directions of the focal lines are shown in various meridional sections of the image shells taken at regular intervals round the circle. The tangential line foci lie along the tyre, and the sagittal foci form the spokes of a wheel – another useful mnemonic.

The elimination of oblique astigmatism requires the two image shells to coincide. Within limits, but over a wide range of lens powers, this aim can be achieved by a correct choice of lens form. A lens free from oblique astigmatism for a stated object distance and centre of rotation distance A_2Z is called point-focal. A valid equation for determining the necessary lens form was first derived by Airy (1830). It was also shown by Airy in the same paper – and later, independently, by Petzval – that if oblique astigmatism is eliminated, the single image shell (generally known as the Petzval surface) remains curved. For a thin lens, its radius of curvature was correctly given by Airy as $-nf'$. As indicated by *Figure 13.23*, this is generally longer than the radius of the far point sphere, both for plus and minus lenses. A hypermetrope would accordingly have to accommodate a little to place the image on the retina in oblique directions of the gaze. A myope would be slightly blurred and not helped by accommodating.

Although the foregoing discussion has been limited to spherical lenses, the same considerations apply separately to the two principal meridians of an astigmatic

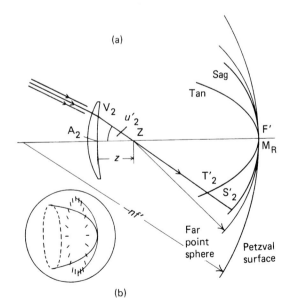

Figure 13.23. Oblique astigmatism of a plus spherical lens in distance vision. (a) Tangential and sagittal image shells, the Petzval surface and the far-point sphere. (b) A three-dimensional view of the 'teacup and saucer' formation of the image shells is outlined in the inset figure.

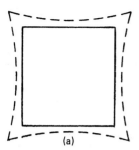
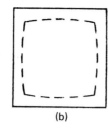

Figure 13.24. (a) Pincushion and (b) barrel distortion caused by plus and minus lenses.

lens. If a point is selected on one of these meridians and a second point on the other, both at the same distance from the optical centre, the main effect of oblique astigmatism is generally to change the prescribed cylinder power at the two given points by different amounts. Nevertheless, a lens form can often be found in which the effective cylinder power is the same at both points, though slightly different from the prescribed power.

Distortion and transverse chromatic aberration

In an optical context, distortion means a lack of correspondence between the shapes of object and conjugate image. In general, rays incident at increasing distances from the optical centre of a lens are deviated more and more in excess of the paraxial value expressed by Prentice's rule. Consequently, the magnification of a plus lens increases from the centre outwards and the image of a square exhibits the 'pincushion' distortion shown in *Figure 13.24(a)*. Conversely, a minus lens gives rise to the 'barrel' distortion shown in *Figure 13.24(b)*. As in a plano prism, an oblique ray passing through a lens undergoes the minimum deviation when the total is equally divided between the two surfaces. This requirement when applied to spectacle lenses leads to an unacceptably bulbous appearance if spherical surfaces are used.

Similarly, since dispersion is approximately proportional to the mean deviation, the lens forms for minimum transverse chromatic aberration are far too steeply curved to be practicable.

Spectacle-lens design

There has been a long history of controversy in the field of spectacle-lens design, principally about what its aims should be, particularly in relation to oblique astigmatism. One school of thought favoured its elimination whenever possible by means of point-focal lenses. An opposing view first advocated in 1901 by the English ophthalmologist Percival and later in 1928 with some corrections in matters of detail, was that the tangential and sagittal image shells should be made to straddle the far (or near) point sphere as the case may be. The circles of least confusion would then be focused on the retina, thus avoiding the marginal loss of power of point-focal lenses at the expense of a small amount of residual astigmatism.

Ideally there should be two different ranges of 'best form' or 'corrected curve' lenses, one designed specifically for distance and the other for near vision. Since this is neither commercially nor otherwise feasible, most designs are now based on a compromise between the conflicting requirements of distance and near vision.

The introduction of several new glasses of high mean refractive index (1.7 or over) and mid-index resins (of index over 1.55) but also of greater dispersive power has raised an interesting question. Because of these materials, high-powered lenses, both plus and minus, can be made much thinner and often lighter in weight than is possible in the traditional hard crown glass. However, the higher dispersion means a substantial increase in both axial and transverse chromatic aberrations. The axial aberration of plus lenses is additive to the eye's own appreciable error, whereas that of minus lenses helps to counteract the eye's. There is some evidence to suggest that the increased chromatic aberration of high-index lenses of high powers is less acceptable to hypermetropic and aphakic patients than to myopes.

Even the most favourable form of plus lenses in the cataract range of powers leaves large amounts of uncorrected oblique astigmatism and distortion, if spherical surfaces are used. Both defects can be greatly reduced simultaneously by the use of one aspheric surface of substantially ellipsoidal form. Though lenses of this type were introduced by Carl Zeiss of Jena as long ago as 1909, their mass production in both single vision and bifocal forms has only become possible by plastics lens technology in the late 1970s. Aspheric surfaces are now employed in low power lenses, both to improve appearance and optical performance in large lens sizes.

For a more detailed treatment of spectacle lens design, including many tables of the various aberrations present over a wide range of lens forms, see Bennett and Edgar (1979/80). The last one of these papers summarizes the entire series.

Contact lenses

Because contact lenses move with the eye, at least to a great extent, they do not give rise to the oblique aberrations of spectacle lenses. Their principal effect is on the eye's spherical aberration. The liquid meniscus formed by hard contact lenses largely neutralizes the front surface of the cornea and replaces it with a convex spherical surface. Since the peripheral flattening of the cornea has been rendered ineffective, the spherical aberration of the corrected eye must show a substantial increase. Contact lenses with aspheric front surfaces are designed to remedy this drawback – *see* Chapter 15.

Exercises

13.1 A meniscus lens ($n = 1.523$) of power +4.00 D, centre thickness 3.8 mm and front surface power +10.50 D, is placed 16 mm from the entrance pupil of the subject's eye. Find the spectacle magnification: (a) ignoring lens form and thickness, (b) taking these factors into account.

13.2 (a) Define spectacle magnification and relative spectacle magnification. (b) An eye is corrected for distance by a thin –4.00 D lens placed 16 mm from the entrance pupil. What is the spectacle magnification? (c) A hypermetropic eye is corrected for distance by a thin $+5.50$ D lens. Find the relative spectacle magnification assuming (i) axial ametropia, (ii) refractive ametropia, (iii) an axial length of 21 mm. Use the reduced eye as the basis of calculation, the reduced surface being 14 mm behind the spectacle plane.

13.3 A thin correcting lens of power -12.00 DS$/-4.00$ DC axis 150 is placed at 15 mm from the principal point of a reduced eye. Find the relative spectacle magnification, given that the axial length of this eye is 26.0 mm and the power of the reference eye $+60.0$ D.

13.4 In a certain eye, the size of the retinal image of a distant object is 10% larger when the eye is corrected by a spherical lens placed in contact with the reduced surface than when a correction is worn in its anterior focal plane. Find the spectacle refraction and ocular refraction on the assumption that the power of the eye is $+60.0$ D.

13.5 A subject's right eye is corrected for distance by the thin lens -10.00 DS$/-4.00$ DC axis 45 placed 14 mm from the reduced surface. Find the dimensions of the retinal image of a circular object 6 m in diameter at a distance of 300 m, assuming the eye to have an axial length of 26.00 mm.

13.6 By means of a backwards ray trace from the ocular entrance pupil, and using effectivity relationships, show that pupil magnification by the correcting lens may be expressed as $S \times P$, where S and P are the shape and power factors of the lens.

13.7 A myope is corrected by a -5.00 DS thin lens at 18 mm distance from the ocular entrance pupil which is 4 mm in diameter. Compare the effective entrance pupil areas when corrected by a spectacle lens and a contact lens. Take the entrance pupil as 3 mm behind the corneal pole.

13.8 An aphakic with an originally emmetropic Bennett–Rabbetts schematic eye is corrected by a plastics lenticular lens of thickness 6 mm, refractive index 1.500 and back surface power -5.00 D at a vertex distance of 14 mm from the cornea. Compare the effective entrance pupil diameters in the pre-aphakic and corrected post-aphakic state, given a 3 mm ocular entrance pupil diameter in both cases and $K = +12.38$ D in the aphakic state. Also, compare the illuminances of the retinal image of an extended object in the two states.

13.9 (a) Find the apparent inclination of: (i) a distant vertical line, (ii) a distant horizontal line viewed through the plano-cylinder -3.00 DC axis 45 placed 15 mm from the cornea. Assume the entrance pupil to be 3 mm behind the cornea. (b) Find the apparent inclination of the same lines viewed directly by an eye with -3.00 D of corneal astigmatism at axis 45. Assume the corneal power to be $+40$ D in the weaker principal meridian and the real pupil to be 3.6 mm behind the corneal vertex.

13.10 At what distance should a lens $+5.00$ DS$/-2.00$ DC be held from the eye so that the lines on a cross-line chart at -1.0 m from the eye appear to rotate without scissors distortion?

13.11 A cross-line chart at -1 m from the eye is viewed through a $+3.00$ DS$/+2.00$ DC lens held at 40 cm from the eye. What type of image movement will be seen on rotating the lens?

13.12 An eye views an object point at a distance of 350 mm from its centre of rotation. A 10Δ prism base up is now interposed at a distance of 320 mm from the object. Through what angle would the eye need to rotate in order to keep the retinal image on the fovea?

13.13 A patient wearing: RE $+1.00$ DS, LE $+1.50$ DS$/+1.50$ DC axis 90 views a point on the median line 500 mm from the spectacle plane. Both lenses are decentred 5 mm outwards with respect to the subject's inter-ocular distance of 65 mm. Assuming the centres of rotation to lie 27 mm behind the spectacle plane, find the necessary convergence of the visual axes for binocular fixation of the given point.

13.14 A patient wearing R $+5.00$ DS and L $+9.00$ DS fixates an object point 120 mm below the level of the primary line of sight in a plane at one-third of a metre from the lenses. The centre of rotation of the eye is 25 mm from the lens. Calculate the vertical rotation of each eye to view the object, and compare with Example (4) in the text on page 242.

13.15 Tabulate the effective power in near vision at

$L = -2.50$ D of a 1Δ prism associated with lens powers of $+10.0$, $+5.0$, $+2.5$, 0, -2.5, -5.0 and -10.0 D, taking the centre of rotation distance as 25 mm.

13.16 Construct a diagram to half scale showing the position of the effective binocular object for: $L = -4.00$ D, $F_{sp} = +7.00$ D, $z = 25$ mm and PD $= 64$ mm, the lenses being centred for distance vision.

13.17 A 38 mm diameter spherical lens of power $+12.00$ D is mounted 15 mm from the entrance pupil and 25 mm from the centre of rotation of an aphakic eye. On an accurate drawing twice actual size, show the angular extent of: (a) the real macular field of view, (b) the real peripheral field of view with the eye in its primary position. Include the fields seen both through and outside the lens. Ignore the effects of pupil diameter and lens thickness.

13.18 Derive from first principles the expression $m = 1 - F/L'$ for the iso-accommodative magnification of a lens held close to the eye. Compare the effects of taking the dioptric distance of the image L' as -3.00 and -4.00 D.

13.19 Using equations (13.56) and (13.59), tabulate the magnifications given by a $+8$ D lens when $d = 0$, 5, 10, and 20 cm, with the eye in focus for each of the following dioptric distances (A): 4 D, 2 D, 1 D and 0. The value of P is to be taken as -4 D, as in the expression for conventional magnification. Why is the combination of $d = 30$ cm and $A = 4$ D not a practical possibility?

13.20 Compare the magnification produced by a thin $+3.00$ DS lens when used as: (a) a spectacle lens at an entrance pupil distance of 17 mm correcting an eye for distance vision, (b) its conventional magnification and (c) its iso-accommodative magnification, the eye being in focus for vergence -4.00 D with (i) the lens held close to the eye and (ii) the lens held 100 mm in front of the eye.

13.21 An absolute presbyope with poor vision can just read N10 print with a $+2.50$ D addition. What power addition should be chosen initially for trial in attempting to read N5?

13.22 A patient wears a telescopic unit adjusted for near vision at 20 cm from the objective. What power of end cap is required to enable him to focus on a television screen at $1\frac{1}{3}$ m?

13.23 A patient wears a telescopic unit adjusted for near vision at 25 cm. What power of end cap is needed to increase the magnification by: (a) 50%, (b) 100%?

13.24 A presbyopic, emmetropic patient's eye has a depth of focus of ± 1.00 D. What is the range of clear vision when: (a) wearing a thin lens spectacle magnifier of $4\times$ conventional magnification and (b) wearing a Galilean telescope also giving a $4\times$ conventional magnification with a working distance of $-\frac{1}{6}$ m from the objective lens and a lens separation of 25 mm? (Assume the objective lens to be composed of a collimating lens and an objective for a distance telescope.)

13.25 The angular field of half illumination of a Galilean telescope is limited by the ray passing through the extremity of the objective and the centre of the eye's entrance pupil. Determine this field for: (a) a $1.5\times$ telescopic spectacle with a component separation of $16\frac{2}{3}$ mm and vertex distance 12 mm, (b) a $1.5\times$ system comprising a spectacle-lens objective at a distance of $16\frac{2}{3}$ mm from a contact-lens eyepiece. Assume all elements thin, the objective aperture 34 mm, and entrance pupil 3 mm behind the corneal vertex.

13.26 A fixed-focus stand magnifier is designed for an object distance ℓ_1 of $-33\frac{1}{3}$ mm from the front surface. The lens ($n = 1.490$) has surface powers of $+4.50$ D (front) and $+13.50$ D (back) and its centre thickness is 13 mm. Calculate: (a) the conventional magnification, (b) the actual magnification when the eye is placed at the following distances from the object: (i) 150 mm, (ii) 250 mm, (iii) 350 mm.

13.27 A -6.00 D myope uses a $+20.0$ D lens close to the unaccommodated eye as a magnifier. Is the magnification greater when wearing spectacles or without?

13.28 Both by algebraical manipulation of equation (13.5), and by regarding the spectacle corrected eye as a telescope of objective power F_{sp} and eyepiece power K, show that the power factor of spectacle magnification is $P = K/F_{sp}$. Discuss the errors or assumptions inherent in this expression. Show also that the power factor may be expressed as $(1 + aK)$.

13.29 Calculate the power factor of the spectacle magnification in each principal meridian of a ± 0.25 D and a ± 0.50 D cross cylinder used at a vertex distance (a) 25 mm (typical for a trial frame) and (b) 60 mm (typical for a refracting unit).

References

ADAMS, A.J., KAPASH, R.J. and BARKAN, E. (1971) Visual performance and optical properties of Fresnel membrane prisms. *Am. J. Optom.*, **48**, 289–297

AIRY, G.B. (1830) On the spherical aberration of the eye-pieces of telescopes. *Trans. Camb. Phil. Soc.*, **3**, 1–63, 18

BAILEY, I.L. (1978) Measuring the magnifying power of Keplerian telescopes. *Appl. Optics*, **17**, 3520–3521

BAILEY, I.L. (1979) A lensometer method for checking telescopes. *Optom. Monthly*, **70**, 94–97

BAILEY, I.L. (1981a) The use of fixed-focus stand magnifiers. *Optom. Monthly*, **72**, 37–39

BAILEY, I.L. (1981b) New method for determining the magnifying power of telescopes. *Am. J. Optom. Physiol. Opt.*, **55**, 203–207

BENNETT, A.G. (1951) Some curious optical systems. IV: prism magnification. *Optician*, **121**, 37–39

BENNETT, A.G. (1977) Review of ophthalmic standards. Part 11: Hand and stand magnifiers. *Manufact. Opt. Internat.*, Feb, 67–73

BENNETT, A.G. (1977/78) Binocular vision through lenses and prisms. *Optician*, **174**(4511), 7–11; (4512), 7–12; **176**(4560), 8

BENNETT, A.G. (1986) Two simple calculating schemes for use in ophthalmic optics – I. Tracing oblique rays through systems including astigmatic surfaces. II. Tracing axial pencils through systems including astigmatic surfaces at random axes. *Ophthal. Physiol. Opt.*, **6**, 325–331, 419–429

BENNETT, A.G. and EDGAR, D.F. (1979/80) Spectacle lens design and performance. *Optician*, **178**(4597), 9–13; (4602), 9–13; (4606), 21–26; (4610), 13–15, 20; (4615), 9–11, 15–17; **179**(4), 20–22, 28–30; (9), 13–16, 20–23; (13), 10–11, 15–18; (17), 10–11, 15–18; (23), 30–35; **180**(4653), 18–25; (4659), 25–28; (4666), 28–31; (4669), 14–22, 42

BREWSTER, D. (1813) *A Treatise on New Philosophical Instruments*. Edinburgh: W. Blackwood, and London: J. Murray

BULLIMORE, M.A. and BAILEY, I.L. (1989) Stand magnifiers: an evaluation of new optical aids from COIL. *Am. J. Optom. Physiol. Opt.*, **66**, 766

DOWIE, A.T. (1988) *Management and Practice of Low Visual Acuity*. London: Association of British Dispensing Opticians

DRASDO, N. and MURRAY, I.J. (1978) A pilot study on the use of visual field expanders. *Br. J. Physiol. Optics*, **32**, 22–29

FAYE, E.E. (1976) *Clinical Low Vision*. Boston: Little, Brown

GARCÍA, M., GONZÁLEZ, C. and PASCUAL, I. (1995) New matrix formulation of spectacle magnification using pupil magnification. 1. High myopia corrected with ophthalmic lenses. *Ophthal. Physiol. Opt.*, **15**, 195–205

KEATING, M.P. (1982) A matrix formulation of spectacle magnification. *Ophthal. Physiol. Opt.*, **2**, 145–158

LONG, W. and WOO, G. (1986) The spectacle magnification of focal telescopes. *Ophthal. Physiol. Opt.*, **6**, 101–112

MEHR, E.B. and FREID, A.N. (1975) *Low Vision Care*. Chicago: Professional Press

OGLE, K.N. (1936) Correction of aniseikonia with ophthalmic lenses. *J. Am. Opt. Soc.*, **26**, 323–337

OGLE, K.N. (1951) Distortion of the image by prisms. *J. Opt. Soc. Am.*, **41**, 1023–1028

OGLE, K.N. (1952) Distortion of the image by ophthalmic prisms. *AMA Archs. Ophthal.*, **47**, 121–131

PELI, E. and SIEGMUND, W.P. (1995) Fiber-optic reading magnifiers for the visually impaired. *J. Opt. Soc. Am. A.*, **12**, 2274–2285

PERCIVAL, A.S. (1928) *The Prescribing of Spectacles*, 3rd edn. Bristol: John Wright

RUMNEY, N.J. (1992) Low vision aids in practice. *Optom. Today*, 21 Sept., 22–27

RUMNEY, N.J. (1995) Contrast thresholds in low-vision practice. *Optician*, **210**(5531), 24–27

SWAINE, W. (1933) Some difficulties of ophthalmic lens fitting. In *Proceedings of the Optical Congress*. London: Hatton Press

WELSH, R.C. (1961) *Postoperative-Cataract Spectacle Lenses*. Miami: Miami Educational Press

WESTHEIMER, G. (1954) The design and ophthalmic properties of binocular magnification devices. *Am. J. Optom.*, **31**, 578–584

WHITTAKER, S.G. and LOVIE-KITCHEN, J.E. (1993) Visual requirements for reading. *Optom. Vis. Sci.*, **70**, 154–165

WHITWELL, A. (1921/22) On the best form of spectacle lenses – XX to XXV. *Optn Scient. Instrum. Mkr*, **62**, 209–213, 311–313, 387–389; **63**, 19–21, 143–148, 331–332

WOO, G.C., LU, C. and WESSEL, J.A. (1995) Estimation of back vertex power and magnification of variable focus telescopes. *Ophthal. Physiol. Opt.*, **15**, 319–325

Anisometropia and aniseikonia

Anisometropia: optical difficulties

Anisometropia is a difference in the refractive state of the right and left eyes. Trivial amounts excepted, the condition is not common because the two eyes of a pair tend to be generally similar. There is even a tendency, when astigmatism is present, for the right and left cylinder axes to be symmetrically orientated.

Prescribing for anisometropia of moderate and high degree presents problems of its own which are made worse by the unwanted side-effects of correcting lenses discussed in Chapter 13. Those with particular relevance to anisometropia are:

(1) unequal prismatic effects of the right and left lenses,
(2) unequal amounts of ocular accommodation theoretically required,
(3) unequal relative spectacle magnifications.

The first two of these need not be considered when contact lenses are worn.

Relative prismatic effects

In any given direction of gaze, the intersection of the visual axis with the back surface of the lens is called the visual point. The difference between the prismatic effects at the right and left visual points is the relative prismatic effect. To obtain single vision, this unwanted prismatic difference must be overcome by adjustments to the ocular rotations.

For the purposes of discussion, relative prismatic effects are usually resolved into horizontal and vertical components. The latter is the more troublesome one. Few subjects can maintain single vision with a plano prism over 4 base down placed before one eye or tolerate half this amount for a prolonged period.

For spherical lens or surface powers, the approximate prismatic effects can be found from Prentice's rule. The prismatic effect of a cylinder is invariably exerted in a direction perpendicular to its axis. If this is oblique, the prismatic effect has both horizontal and vertical components.

Prismatic effects over the whole area of a lens can be depicted graphically by iso-prism lines. These are lines joining all the points on a lens at which the prismatic effect has a given value, its direction being ignored. In spherical lenses, iso-prism lines are concentric circles surrounding the optical centre. For example, with a 4.00 D lens the iso-prism lines for 1Δ and 2Δ would be circles of radius 2.5 and 5 mm respectively. In all astigmatic lenses, the iso-prism lines are concentric ellipses, degenerating into straight lines parallel to the axis in the case of a plano-cylinder. The direction of the prismatic effect at any point on an elliptical iso-prism line can be found by a simple graphical construction due to Bennett (1968).

For spherical lens or surface powers, the concept is that of iso-V-prism lines, which join all the points on a lens at which the vertical component of the prismatic effect has a given value. As shown by Bennett, they are parallel straight lines, obliquely orientated in the presence of an oblique cylinder, though not necessarily parallel to its axis. If such a map is constructed for the two lenses of a pair, inspection will show the extent of common field within which vertical relative prismatic effects remain within a specified limit.

Unequal demand on accommodation

The relationship between ocular and spectacle accommodation when a distance correcting lens is used in near vision was discussed in Chapter 7. It was shown that the ocular accommodation demanded varies with the spectacle refraction, other factors remaining equal. In cases of anisometropia, it follows that the ocular accommodation theoretically required is different for the two eyes.

A good idea of the magnitude of this effect can be obtained from a study of *Figure 7.6*. The change in ocular accommodation per dioptre of anisometropia is seen to vary between extremes of 0.05 D in high myopia to about 0.12 D in high hypermetropia. A typical value is in the neighbourhood of 0.07–0.08 D. It would thus take about 3 D of anisometropia to make a difference of 0.25 D in the accommodative demand on the two eyes.

Unequal retinal image sizes

The sharp retinal images in a corrected pair of eyes will be of equal size if the relative spectacle magnification is the same for each. Unfortunately, as pointed out on page 236, this quantity cannot be determined without a knowledge of the eye's equivalent power or its axial length.

Some useful generalizations can nevertheless be deduced from the analysis of 67 cases of anisometropia ranging from 2 to over 15 D, made by Sorsby *et al.* (1962). The ocular dimensions of each subject were measured and separate tabulations made of the difference between the right and left corneal power, depth of anterior chamber, crystalline lens power and axial length – the last of these both in millimetres and dioptres. From these data it emerged that axial length was the predominant causative factor. There was no substantial difference between hypermetropic and myopic anisometropia. In 49 cases it contributed at least 70% to the total anisometropia and at least 90% in 23 cases. In only two cases did it make no significant contribution whatever. No differences greater than 2.0 D in corneal power were found and only 10 greater than 1.0 D. In 45 of the cases, the difference ranged from zero to 0.5 D. Differences in the crystalline lens power covered a wider range, up to approximately 4 D, but even so the difference did not exceed 1.0 D in 50 of the subjects. In the 53 subjects with anisometropia between 2.0 and 5.0 D, differences in lenticular or corneal power were the main cause in only four cases each. Similar findings were reported by Garner *et al.* (1992) for Malay children, the 2 D weaker lens partially compensating for the 3 mm longer axial length in their myopic sample (mean refractive error $-6\,D \pm 1.8\,D$). The myopes also showed a slightly flatter corneal radius than the emmetropes but this was not statistically significant.

Differences in corneal and lens powers are the main components of refractive anisometropia, since the anterior chamber depth plays only a negligible part in this context. In routine ophthalmic practice, the corneal powers can readily be determined by keratometry, but the contribution of the lens can only be conjectured within the guidelines already indicated. Thus most cases of natural anisometropia are axial. Surgically induced anisometropia, however, will be refractive. Unilateral aphakia was both the most common cause and gave the greatest amount of difference, but the use of intraocular lenses has minimized its occurrence, though it may still arise as a result of trauma. Smaller amounts of refractive anisometropia may be met when intra-ocular implants are of the incorrect power, or after refractive surgery (*see* page 417), especially in the period between the operations on the first and second eyes. Applegate and Howland (1993) discuss the implications of the change in retinal image size after refractive surgery on visual acuity.

In cases where both axial and refractive elements are operative, the percentage size difference can be calculated from each of the two expressions (14.4) and (14.6). The correct value can reasonably be assumed to lie within these limits at a point corresponding to the relative weight of the axial and refractive elements.

Although the division is too schematic, it is helpful in this context to consider ametropia as either axial or refractive, so that the range of possibilities can be explored. In the following discussion, the spectacle lenses

will initially be assumed to be thin, so that the shape factor of magnification becomes unity.

There are two approaches to evaluating the difference in image sizes between two eyes. The first is based on deriving useful approximations from the formula for relative spectacle magnification. The second is based on the retinal image size ratio (RISR), a term introduced by Obstfeldt (1978).

Axial anisometropia

In axial ametropia the eye is assumed to have the 'standard' power F_o. Hence, when F_o is substituted for F_e in equation (13.24) for relative spectacle magnification, it becomes

$$\text{RSM} = \frac{F_o}{F_v' + F_o - dF_v'F_o}$$
$$= \frac{F_o}{F_o + F_v'(1 - dF_o)} \qquad (14.1)$$

This expression can be simplified if the position of the spectacle point is now defined by its distance x from the anterior focal plane of the eye, so that

$$x = -f_o - d = 1/F_o - d = \frac{1 - dF_o}{F_o} \qquad (14.2)$$

(A similar use of the symbol x is used in Newton's equation.) Hence, by substitution in equation (14.1)

$$\text{RSM} = \frac{F_o}{F_o + xF_oF_v'} = \frac{1}{1 + xF_v'}$$
$$\approx 1 - xF_v' \quad (x \text{ in m}) \qquad (14.3)$$

Thus, given purely axial anisometropia, the difference in relative spectacle magnification between the two eyes is $(-x\Delta F_v')$, where $\Delta F_v'$ is the anisometropia in terms of spectacle refraction. The percentage difference in RSM is therefore, with x now in millimetres,

$$\% \text{ size difference} \approx 0.1x\Delta F_v' \quad (x \text{ in mm}) \qquad (14.4)$$

For example, with the spectacle plane 2 mm closer to the eye than its anterior focal point, the retinal image size difference would be approximately 0.2% per dioptre of anisometropia. The size difference and $\Delta F_v'$ must both be taken as right minus left.

When the spectacle point is in the eye's anterior focal plane, $x = 0$ and the relative spectacle magnification becomes unity for all degrees of axial ametropia (Knapp's law). A graphical demonstration of Knapp's law is given by *Figure 14.1*, showing a hypothetical ray (dotted line) from a distant object Q passing undeviated through the optical centre of a thin correcting lens placed at the eye's anterior principal focus F_o. After refraction by the eye, the ray proceeds parallel to the optical axis, so that the height of the sharp image is independent of the position of the retina. If the eye were emmetropic and no correction in use, the ray RP falling on the eye's principal point would be the one refracted to the image point Q_o' on the retina. If, however, the eye was myopic and had a greater axial length, the ray TU incident on the minus correcting lens would be deviated to the eye's principal point P and from there to the image point Q' on the retina of the myopic eye. All

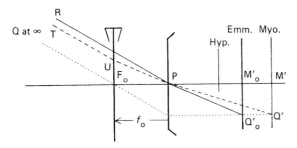

Figure 14.1.   Spectacle magnification and Knapp's law in axial myopia. If the spectacle lens is placed in the anterior focal plane of the eye, the resulting image height is independent of axial length.

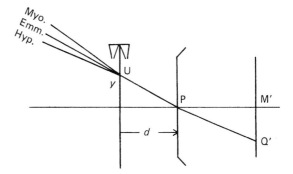

Figure 14.2.   Spectacle magnification in refractive ametropia.

three incident rays in the diagram are parallel because they originate from the same distant object point. A similar ray construction could be drawn for the axially hypermetropic eye.

The shape factor of the actual lenses, given by equation (13.4), should now be taken into account. If they are of minus power, the small centre thickness and rather shallow front surface curvature will in many cases make the shape factor very nearly the same for both. With plus lenses, the difference would tend to be larger. In terms of percentage magnification, the shape factor S is reducible to

$$S\% \approx 0.1(t/n)F_1 \quad (t \text{ in mm}) \tag{14.5}$$

For example, given $t = 4.8$ mm, $n = 1.498$ and $F_1 = +9.00$ D, the value of S would be approximately 2.9% The value would need to be calculated for each lens separately. Small percentage magnifications can simply be added or subtracted without significant error.

To summarize: the right and left retinal images in uncorrected axial anisometropia are unequal in size, being proportional to axial length, but can be made approximately equal by spectacle lenses placed close to the eyes' anterior focal plane. The shape factor may need consideration.

It would be wrong to conclude from this that contact lenses, which make little alteration to retinal image sizes, are necessarily inferior to spectacles in this refractive condition. They have the merit of causing little of the induced prismatic effects in oblique vision associated with spectacles. Moreover, it is open to question whether equality of retinal image sizes is the right aim to pursue. Unequal density or spacing of retinal receptors, which may result from a difference in axial lengths, could partly or wholly offset the effect of unequal image sizes. Thus although in spectacle corrected anisometropia, the image sizes in the two eyes will be physically similar, the possibly increased retinal receptor spacing in the longer, more myopic eye may mean that this eye's image is interpreted as being smaller than the physical dimensions would predict. Contact lens correction would leave the more myopic eye's image physically larger and hence physiologically more similar to that in the less myopic eye. Support for this view is given in the paper by Winn *et al.* (1988). Despite the axial anisometropia of the 18 subjects examined, each showed less aniseikonia with a contact lens correction than with spectacles. A synoptophore was used to measure

the amounts. Laird (1991) showed that a model elliptical scleral contour almost exactly predicted the experimental differences in aniseikonia in spectacle and contact lens corrected anisometropic myopes. It has also been argued in another context (*see* page 272) that image sizes in the uncorrected eyes should be left undisturbed.

Refractive anisometropia

As shown in *Figure 14.2*, the situation in refractive anisometropia is the reverse. In this case the two eyes of a pair are of the same length, so that the retinal image point Q' could be taken to apply to both, irrespective of refractive error. If a ray from Q' were traced backwards through the principal point P, it would emerge from the eye in the direction PU and meet the spectacle plane at the same height y for both lenses. Since they are of different power, however, they exert a different prismatic effect and so the ray paths in object space would differ, as shown in the diagram. It follows, therefore, that the same point in object space cannot give rise to equal retinal images unless the separation d is reduced to zero.

On the assumption of thin lenses, the only component of relative spectacle magnification applying to refractive ametropia is the ametropia factor A, given by equation (13.27) as

$$A \approx 1 + dK \quad (d \text{ in m})$$

which gives

$$\frac{\text{Percentage}}{\text{size difference}} = 0.1d\,\Delta K \quad (d \text{ in mm}) \tag{14.6}$$

where ΔK is the anisometropia in terms of ocular refraction. For example, if $d = 12$ mm, the retinal image size difference is approximately 1.2% per dioptre of ocular anisometropia. The shape factor may again need consideration. As before, the size difference and ΔK must both be taken as right minus left.

Retinal image size ratio

Obstfeld (1978) defined the retinal image size ratio, RISR, as:

$$\text{RISR} = \frac{\text{Relative spectacle magnification for right eye}}{\text{Relative spectacle magnification for left eye}} \tag{14.7}$$

which, from equation (13.24), simplifies to

$$\text{RISR} = \frac{F'_{\text{spL}} + F_{\text{eL}} - d_{\text{L}}F'_{\text{spL}}F_{\text{eL}}}{F'_{\text{spR}} + F_{\text{eR}} - d_{\text{R}}F'_{\text{spR}}F_{\text{eR}}} \times \frac{S_{\text{R}}}{S_{\text{L}}} \qquad (14.8)$$

In axial ametropia, the eye is assumed to have the standard power F_{o}, so if the vertex distance is the same for the two eyes, expression (14.8) reduces to:

$$\text{RISR} = \frac{F'_{\text{spL}} + F_{\text{o}} - dF'_{\text{spL}}F_{\text{o}}}{F'_{\text{spR}} + F_{\text{o}} - dF'_{\text{spR}}F_{\text{o}}} \times \frac{S_{\text{R}}}{S_{\text{L}}} \qquad (14.9)$$

Alternatively, equation (13.26) for RSM may be employed to give the RISR:

$$\text{RISR} = \frac{A_{\text{R}}E_{\text{R}}S_{\text{R}}}{A_{\text{E}}E_{\text{L}}S_{\text{L}}} = \frac{(1 + dK_{\text{R}})k'_{\text{R}}S_{\text{R}}}{(1 + dK_{\text{L}})k'_{\text{L}}S_{\text{L}}}$$

The ametropia factor A can, by substitution and manipulation of the vergence effectivity formula (equation 2.11), be shown to equal the power factor P of spectacle magnification and also the ratio K/F'_{sp} – see Exercise 13.28. Hence

$$\text{RISR} = \frac{P_{\text{R}}S_{\text{R}}k'_{\text{R}}}{P_{\text{L}}S_{\text{L}}k'_{\text{L}}} = \frac{\text{SM}_{\text{R}}}{\text{SM}_{\text{R}}} \times \frac{k'_{\text{R}}}{k'_{\text{L}}} \qquad (14.10)$$

and

$$\frac{K'_{\text{R}}.F'_{\text{spL}}}{K'_{\text{L}}.F'_{\text{spR}}} \times \frac{k'_{\text{R}}}{k'_{\text{L}}} \times \frac{S_{\text{R}}}{S_{\text{L}}} \qquad (14.11)$$

In refractive anisometropia, the eye is of standard length so that the elongation factor $k'_{\text{R}}/k'_{\text{L}}$ is unity, whence equation (14.10) becomes simply the ratio of the spectacle magnifications.

Unilateral aphakia

Unilateral aphakia can be regarded as an extreme form of refractive anisometropia in which single binocular vision is impossible if a spectacle correction is worn. The insuperable obstacle is the great increase in the size of the retinal image in the aphakic eye, often exceeding 30%. When contact lenses are worn, this increase is reduced to the order of 10% in cases where the refractive error of the pre-aphakic eye was small.

A general comparison is shown in *Figure 14.3*, which shows the increase in the retinal image size in the aphakic eye in comparison with its pre-aphakic state with a spectacle correction in use. A typical form and thickness were assumed for each lens so that the shape factor of magnification could be taken into account. The graph is based on calculations covering a wide range of possible combinations of the eye's optical dimensions. Because of these variables there is a surprising spread in the calculated figures for spectacle-lens corrections. The black line near the centre of this band gives the results for eyes with the Gullstrand–Emsley dioptric system. With contact lenses, the effect on the previous retinal image size varies appreciably with the pre-aphakic spectacle refraction, but the possible spread is much narrower. The lowest increase in size occurs when the eye was previously strongly hypermetropic. Within this refractive range, the size difference between

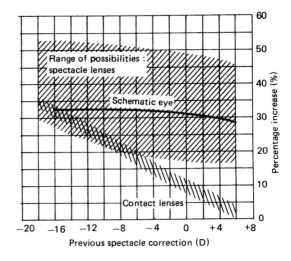

Figure 14.3.   Percentage increase in the retinal image size in the aphakic eye corrected by spectacle and contact lenses. The graph indicates the possible spread of values.

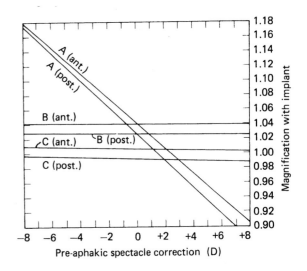

Figure 14.4.   Graphs illustrating the magnification of the retinal image in the pseudophakic eye relative to the pre-aphakic state: A, implant giving full correction; B, implant requiring pre-aphakic spectacle correction; C, implant requiring −2.00 D addition to pre-aphakic spectacle correction. Ant. and Post. refer to anterior and posterior chamber implants.

the two eyes may be small enough to permit single binocular vision.

Intra-ocular lenses, described on pages 224–226, open up wider possibilities for single binocular vision in unilateral aphakia. The relative spectacle magnification RSM compares the image size in the pseudophakic eye with that in the schematic emmetropic eye. Though this is a useful guide, it may be better to know the magnification in comparison with the patient's own pre-aphakic eye, assumed to be corrected when necessary by spectacles. *Figure 14.4* presents a general picture based on theoretical calculations. It covers spherical refractive errors in the pre-aphakic eye ranging from −8.00 to +8.00 D.

Three different aims of correction (denoted by A, B and C) have been considered and two separate graph lines given for each, one relating to anterior-chamber and the other to posterior-chamber implants. The pair marked A refer to implants intended to neutralize any previous spherical ametropia. When this course is followed, it will be seen that the magnification varies considerably with the previous spectacle correction. The lines marked B refer to implants intended to leave the patient requiring the same spherical correction as previously. This course leads to a magnification of about 4% for anterior implants and about 2.5% for posterior implants, irrespective of the previous spectacle correction. The lines marked C refer to implants designed to leave the patient needing a -2.00 D addition to the previous spectacle correction. This technique, aimed at avoiding any appreciable change in the retinal image size, is seen from the graph to be well founded.

All the graphs are based on eyes of average dimensions with a crystalline lens (assumed thin) of power $+20$ D, placed at 6 mm from the corneal vertex, the approximate mean position of the principal points of the real lens. The implant, also regarded as thin, was placed at 3 mm from the corneal vertex if in the anterior chamber and at 5 mm from it if in the posterior chamber. It would need a variation of about ± 5 D in the lens power to alter the magnification by $\pm 1\%$. Corneal power variations have even less significance. Changes in the form of the implant have a slight effect. The magnification may be reduced by up to 1% or so (e.g. from 4 to 3%) by incorporating the whole of the power in the back surface of the implant lens.

For simplicity, the calculations for *Figure 14.4* assumed the corneal radius to be unchanged by surgery. If predictable, any such changes should be taken into account when determining the necessary power of the implant. The magnification indicated by *Figure 14.4* would be little affected.

Prescribing for anisometropia

Refraction of the anisometropic patient

While a cycloplegic refraction may be needed or necessary, a normal routine refractive examination will work satisfactorily with many anisometropic patients, provided that the corrected acuities are similar. The ocular dominance is likely to be strong, so that the Humphriss fogging technique will probably not work for the refraction of the weaker eye. Monocular refraction in a young patient with anisometropic hypermetropia often leads to an under-estimate of the anisometropia because the more ametropic eye is often slightly amblyopic and accommodation goes into spasm in an effort to see more clearly. Prescribing these findings will result in the more hypermetropic eye remaining under-corrected.

Static, Barrett or dynamic retinoscopy should give a good indication of the anisometropia, which can be confirmed subjectively under binocular conditions. Either the Turville infinity balance septum technique or dissociation by polarization may be used. The bichromatic test usually works well since it is independent of a difference in acuity between the two eyes. Slight amblyopia will prevent an acuity balance with black figures on a white ground, though it is possible to confirm that the addition of extra positive power blurs both eyes. Where slight amblyopia is present, the inability to read small letters on a binocularity or suppression test, such as that illustrated in *Figure 10.13(b)*, may indicate insufficient acuity rather than true suppression. Reduction of the anisometropia to that indicated by monocular findings or to equal spherical powers often results in a disappearance of the test characters in the field of view of the worse eye. This may be used to show the patient the benefits of the full refractive correction. The patient should also be told that when the better eye is shut, vision in the poorer eye will seem blurred because of the over-action of the focusing muscles; the idea is to give the maximum benefit with both eyes open.

Prescribing

The amblyopic patient

Anisometropic amblyopia is a type of refractive amblyopia, and has been discussed on page 42. If the child is young enough and the acuity not worse than 6/60 (20/200) so that there is a chance of improving it, a full anisometropic correction should be provided for constant wear, coupled with part-time occlusion of the better eye. The relative prismatic effects when looking through the marginal areas of the lenses may cause suppression, thus preventing stimulation of the weaker eye's macula. This may be avoided if the patient wears a contact-lens correction. Although the practitioner usually cannot ascertain how this affects retinal image sizes, it does appear to assist the improvement in acuity (Edwards, 1980). In general, soft lenses give better results than rigid ones. Once the acuity has improved, the patient will probably prefer to wear the full anisometropic correction, especially for critical vision.

If the patient is over 10 years old, with the acuity less than 6/60 (20/200) or the anisometropia more than about 5 D, it is probably not worth trying to improve the acuity. The amblyopia will cause no symptoms and a refractive correction will be needed only if the better eye requires it. Protective lenses are essential in these circumstances. Even if a spectacle correction is unlikely to be needed in the future, the patient or the parents should be advised of the possible need for eye protection in hazardous situations. They should also be advised that having only one good eye will not cause it to deteriorate through 'having to work harder' or 'extra strain'.

Anisometropia without significant amblyopia

The presence of even several dioptres of anisometropia in later years does not necessarily imply that there was a significant refractive difference in infancy, when the development of vision is at its most rapid and critical stage.

It is thus possible for a patient to have one clinically emmetropic eye, while the other is moderately hypermetropic, myopic or astigmatic. If the patient has merely been referred because of a screening test, there may be no need to prescribe the correction unless the patient feels that it produces a significant improvement in comfort or clarity. If, however, the better eye needs a refractive correction, the anisometropic correction should be tried, especially if the binocularity test shows little suppression. A partial correction of the anisometropia may be more readily accepted by the patient initially.

Anisometropia in the presbyopic patient

Many patients come for their first eye examination with near vision difficulties at the onset of presbyopia. Since the patient has probably relied for several years on one eye, the more ametropic eye being out of focus, some practitioners would advise giving an equal correction to both eyes to avoid upsetting the habitual arrangement. It is generally worth trying to correct the anisometropia if there is only 2–3 D difference of either spherical or astigmatic power, provided that the cylinder axes are close to horizontal or vertical. However, a strong oblique cylinder before one eye will almost certainly cause greater symptoms than benefits and is probably best omitted. Bilateral astigmatic corrections should be tried since they may gradually give improved vision, but a partial prescription would be sensible initially. Again, if the binocularity test shows significant suppression, a balancing lens for the poorer eye is probably advisable. An indication of the value of the full correction may be given by holding the appropriate supplementary lens in front of the poorer eye with the reduced correction in position.

If the anisometropic correction is prescribed, the patient should be told that he will be using his two eyes fully together for the first time for years and consequently it may take a few days or weeks to become accustomed to the lenses and gain the resulting benefits. Should this not occur, a 'balance' lens can then be prescribed.

The occasional patient has one emmetropic and one moderately myopic eye. One eye may therefore be used for distance and the other for near vision. This type of imbalance is sometimes copied for contact-lens wearers to avoid a bifocal correction. In the pre-presbyopic patient, dynamic retinoscopy or the polarized bichromatic test should be used to check which eye is in focus in near vision since, surprisingly, it is occasionally the emmetropic eye. For prolonged viewing, the proper binocular correction is likely to be preferred.

Anisometropia and bifocals

Unlike wearers of single-vision lenses, who can reduce unwanted prismatic effects by head movements to bring the visual points much closer to the optical centres, bifocal wearers cannot take advantage of this manoeuvre in near vision. They are obliged to look through the segments, the near visual points having a mean position some 8–10 mm below and 2 mm inwards from the distance optical centres. With conventional types of bifocals, relative prismatic effects at the near visual points

are the same as those due to single-vision lenses of the same distance prescription. To simplify the determination of these effects, many tables and graphs have been produced by lens manufacturers and writers on ophthalmic lenses. It should be noted that strong cylinders at oblique axes, on their own, can generate an undesirable amount of horizontal prism at the near visual points.

If the patient has worn a correction for several years, he may have adapted to relative prismatic effects. Thus, Allen (1974) found a high degree of compensation for oculo-motor imbalance in a study of 20 anisometropes.[*] Transition from all-purpose single-vision lenses to bifocals should be uneventful, provided that the vertical imbalance in near vision is small or compensated when examined with typically depressed gaze through the existing correction. Neither the refractor head nor reduced-aperture trial case lenses permit a sufficient angle of depression for this purpose.

A patient who has rarely worn spectacles or whose anisometropia is increasing, possibly because of nuclear sclerosis of the crystalline lens, may need vertical prismatic relief in the near portion of bifocals. Several special types of bifocals have been designed to fill this need. Some permit the near optical centres to be placed at any specified position. Others enable the vertical prismatic effects at the near visual points to be equalized by a compensating prism incorporated in the near portion of one or both lenses. The dividing lines of all such lenses are somewhat conspicuous.

In suitable cases, conventional bifocal types can be used. One possibility is to prescribe solid (one-piece) bifocals with different segment diameters, for example, 45 with 38, 38 with 28 or even 38 with 22 mm. The amount of vertical prism compensation in prism dioptres is half the difference in centimetres of the segment diameters multiplied by the reading addition. The smaller segment is prescribed for the eye with the greater myopia or smaller amount of hypermetropia in the vertical meridian.

Another possibility is to use fused or hard resin bifocals with straight-top segments and to work a compensating prism over the entire lower half of one lens by the bi-prism (slab-off) construction. 'Executive'-type solid bifocals can be treated similarly. Alternatively, conventional bifocals to be worn for brief periods of near vision can be supplemented by single vision lenses for prolonged close work.

The effects of vertical centration should be considered when dispensing all anisometropic prescriptions. The distance refraction is normally measured with the lenses centred to the visual axes, but the primary line of sight often passes 2–5 mm above the optical centres of the prescribed spectacle lenses. Thus, a person for whom the refractive findings are

R plano   L +3.00 DS   1Δ base down

---

[*] After as little as $2\frac{1}{2}$ hours of wear, Henson and Dharamshi (1982) found marked oculo-motor adaptations to 3 D of induced anisometropia. Adaptation to induced prismatic effects is further discussed. *See also* page 181.

may well need no prismatic help in the spectacles. The prism indicated during the refraction procedure may have been merely to correct a compensating heterophoria induced by habitually viewing above the optical centres of spectacle lenses.

In general, a prescribed vertical prism has its nominal effect only at the point where it is intended to be measured. In British Standards this is called the centration point and in US Standards the major reference point. At other points above or below it, the effect of the prism is modified by the relative prismatic effect due to the anisometropia.

For example, given the above prescription with the prism included, the actual effect would be approximately 2.5Δ base down L at 5 mm above the centration point and 0.5Δ base up L at 5 mm below it.

With conventional bifocals, another method of reducing the vertical prismatic imbalance at the near visual points is to order the distance optical centres to be placed near the dividing line instead of the usual 5–6 mm above it. Thus, with 3 D of vertical anisometropia the relative prismatic effect at the near visual points would be reduced by 1.5–1.8Δ. Unfortunately, there would now be an opposite imbalance of this same amount at the normal optical centre level, but this expedient is worth consideration in suitable cases.

Aniseikonia

Introduction

Aniseikonia, a term denoting inequality of image sizes, is the name given to anomalies of binocular space perception which can be corrected or alleviated by altering the relative dimensions of the right and left retinal images. Fortunately, no knowledge of their actual dimensions is required and, in any case, aniseikonia may have other causes. For example, the relative distribution of retinal receptors is a possible source. The larger globe of the moderate to high myope may result in a larger spacing between receptors, and the converse may apply to a small hypermetropic eye. Space perception could thereby be affected if interpretation of retinal image size is based on the number of receptors stimulated. Stretching of the retina following treatment for a detachment has been found to result in very marked aniseikonia.

The pioneer work in this field was carried out at the Dartmouth Eye Institute, New Hampshire, USA by a large research team.[*] Basic principles were established and an instrument known as a space eikonometer was developed to facilitate clinical prescribing. On the practical side, the American Optical Company produced a table model of the space eikonometer suitable for clinical use and created facilities for the execution of prescription orders. This service included the computation of the surface powers and lens thicknesses required to

produce the specified magnification, as well as the subsequent manufacture of the lenses. (For a full account of the theoretical and experimental bases, *see* Ogle, 1950.)

Size lenses

Lenses designed for the investigation or correction of aniseikonia are usually called size lenses. Afocal size lenses are of two main types. Those giving overall magnification, that is, the same in all meridians, are of meniscus form, an afocal meniscus lens acting as a solid Galilean telescope. Such a lens possesses spectacle magnification by virtue of its shape factor, even though the power factor is zero. As expected, the use of higher refractive indices than standard crown glass or resin will result in thinner lenses or flatter front surfaces – *see* Exercise 14.8 or Stephens and Polasky (1991) who have published nomograms relating magnification, thickness and front surface power for various refractive indices. If the spherical surfaces are replaced by cylindrical surfaces with their axes parallel, the result is an afocal meridional size lens with its magnification in the direction perpendicular to the cylinder axes.

Great care is required in manufacturing these bi-cylindrical lenses to keep the two axes in register, because the afocal property of the lens depends on their exact alignment. If there is an error, the magnification may not be appreciably affected, but the lens will exhibit an astigmatic effect arising from the obliquely crossed cylinders. Surprisingly enough at first sight, the axis direction of the unwanted cylinder is approximately at $45°$ to the meridian of magnification.

The numbering of afocal size lenses denotes the spectacle magnification expressed as a percentage, either overall or meridional as the case may be. Thus, if m is the percentage magnification and M the corresponding spectacle magnification,

$$m = 100\,(M - 1) \qquad (14.12)$$

and

$$M = 1 + m/100 \qquad (14.13)$$

By convention, the orientation of a meridional magnification is specified as in the example $2\% \times 30°$, indicating that the direction of the magnification is along the $120°$ meridian.

Provided that they are small, percentage magnifications can be regarded as additive. For example, a 2% and a 4% overall size lens in combination could be taken as equivalent to a single 6% lens. Strictly, the spectacle magnifications are 1.02 and 1.04, giving a product of 1.0608 or a magnification of 6.08%.

If an afocal size lens is placed with its convex surface next to the eye, its effect is to diminish the retinal image size. Experiment confirms that increasing the retinal image size in one eye has the same apparent effect as a corresponding reduction in the other eye. The crucial quantity is evidently the ratio of the right and left image sizes.

Because of this it is possible, as well as convenient for calculation, to regard any required magnification as

---

[*] Including (in alphabetical order) Adelbert Ames Jr, R.E. Bannon, P. Boeder, H. Burian, G.H. Gliddon, W.B. Lancaster and K.N. Ogle.

placed before the patient's right eye. Suppose, for example, that the correction found by test is

R 2% × 90   L 1% × 180

The 1% magnification at axis 180° for the left eye is equivalent to a 1% decrease at axis 180° for the right eye. Thus, in terms of spectacle (not percentage) magnification, the aniseikonic correction could be written as

R 1.02 × 90   by   0.99 × 180

This approach leads to the useful concept of the magnification ellipse.

The magnification ellipse

The correction of aniseikonia may require the relative size of one retinal image to be magnified or diminished by two different amounts in mutually perpendicular meridians, the orientation of which must also be specified. There are thus three parameters to be determined.

Figure 14.5, referring to the right eye, represents a circle which has been magnified by approximately 100% at axis 25° and 40% at axis 115°. The resulting figure is the magnification ellipse. Because of the obliquity a scissors effect is introduced: the horizontal and vertical radii of the circle, OH and OV, are transformed into the oblique lines OH′ and OV′ – both tilted towards the meridian of higher magnification (115°).

In practice, a direct determination of oblique magnifications and their orientation is not feasible. It therefore becomes necessary to determine the magnification ellipse by a different set of three parameters. The most amenable to clinical procedures are the horizontal magnification (OH′/OH), the vertical magnification (OV′/OV) and the vertical declination angle (VOV′). All three can normally be measured subjectively with a single piece of apparatus known as an eikonometer.

If only for cosmetic reasons, spectacle lenses for aniseikonia are designed so that, where possible, each lens makes a roughly equal contribution to the required image-size adjustment. The magnification ellipse is the basis for these subsequent computations.

Basis of eikonometry

The test object of the space eikonometer

Eikonometry depends on the observed effect of various afocal size lenses on a specially designed test object (*Figure 14.6a*). It consists of two pairs of vertical cords or narrow rods, each pair lying in a fronto-parallel plane. Between them, in another such plane, is an arrangement of three cords forming a cross with its limbs at 45° and 135° together with a third vertical cord through the centre of the cross. The test object is viewed against a plain black ground through an aperture which masks the extremities of all the cords, thereby eliminating as far as possible extraneous clues to their location. *Figure 14.6(b)–(e)* illustrates the effects produced when an afocal meridional size lens is placed before a normal subject's right eye so as to magnify the retinal image in the meridian stated. In all these diagrams the arrow indicates the direction in which the subject is looking.

(b) *R Overall magnification*
   The right-hand cord of each vertical pair apparently recedes but the appearance of the cross is unchanged.

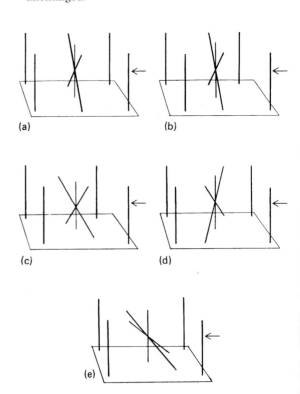

Figure 14.6. The space eikonometer: various appearances of test object when viewed in the direction of the arrow through afocal size lens. (a) Normal appearance, (b) R overall, (c) R horizontal (×90°), (d) R vertical (×180°), (e) R oblique (×45°).

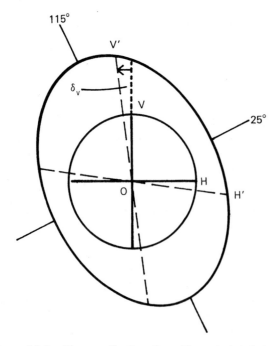

Figure 14.5. The magnification ellipse. The central circle is magnified by 2.0 axis 25 and 1.4 ax 115. δ$_v$ is the declination angle or tilt of the originally vertical meridian.

(c) *R Horizontal magnification (axis 90°)*

The right-hand cord of each vertical pair apparently recedes and the cross appears to have pivoted about a vertical axis, making its right side further away.

(d) *R Vertical magnification (axis 180°)*

The position of the vertical cords appears unchanged but the cross appears to have pivoted about a vertical axis, making its left side farther away.

(e) *R Oblique magnification (axis 45°)*

The cross appears to have rotated about a horizontal axis, its top receding from the observer.

The effects described above are those caused by magnifying the right eye's retinal image. It follows, therefore, that if the patient experiences any such effects without size lenses, the relative size of the right eye's retinal image in the appropriate meridian should be reduced. The same argument applies to any effect seen in reverse, indicating that the relative size of the left retinal image needs to be reduced.

Horizontal and vertical magnifications

For brevity, an apparent rotation of the cross about a vertical axis will be called lateral and rotation about a horizontal axis frontal.

The effect of a horizontal magnification of the right eye's retinal image can be explained using *Figure 14.7*. Suppose two vertical rods are placed obliquely at S and T on the primary lines of the eyes: if the angle they subtend at the left nodal point is θ, a larger angle $M\theta$ will be subtended at the right eye. It can therefore be argued that the effect on a normal subject of increasing the horizontal size of one retinal image is to produce an apparent lateral rotation ϕ of a fronto-parallel plane. From the diagram,

$$\tan M\theta = 2p/d$$

and

$$\tan \theta = 2p(d + e)$$

where $2p$ is the inter-ocular distance, d the distance from T to the left nodal point N_L and $(d + e)$ the distance from S to the right nodal point N_R.

Since θ and M are both small we can put

$$\tan M\theta/\tan \theta = M = (d + e)/d$$

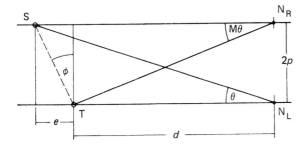

Figure 14.7. The relationship between horizontal image magnification M and apparent tilt ϕ of a fronto-parallel plane.

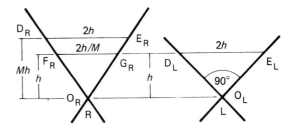

Figure 14.8. Effect of a vertical magnification of the right eye's image of the cross.

The percentage increase m is $100 (M - 1)$, so that

$$m\% = 100 \, e/d \tag{14.14}$$

It can also be seen from the diagram that $e = 2p \tan \phi$. Thus

$$m\% = \frac{200p \tan \phi}{d} \tag{14.15}$$

By considering the effect of a horizontal image-size disparity on the longitudinal horopter, Ogle arrived at a theoretical relationship equivalent to

$$m\% = \frac{200p \tan \phi}{d - p \tan \phi} \tag{14.16}$$

Equations (14.15) and (14.16) yield very similar numerical results, since d is usually large in relation to p.

In the following brief discussion of vertical magnification, consideration is limited to the effect produced when the oblique cross of the eikonometer test object is viewed by a normal observer through afocal size lenses. Other forms of test objects may give rise to different effects.

As already stated, a horizontal magnification of one retinal image makes the cross appear to have rotated about a vertical axis in one direction, whereas a vertical magnification in the same eye will produce an apparent rotation in the opposite direction. In other words, a vertical magnification in one eye has the same effect as a horizontal magnification in the fellow eye.

An explanation on geometrical lines can be given as follows. In *Figure 14.8*, L is the upper part of the cross seen directly by the left eye and R the cross as it would appear to the right eye monocularly when magnified by a factor M in the vertical meridian. D_L and E_L are points on the limbs of cross L at the same height h from the centre line and D_R and E_R are the corresponding points on cross R at a height Mh from the centre line. In the single binocular percept, the two points of intersection O_L and O_R would certainly be fused, but since there is nothing to identify any other points on any of the lines, fusion is most likely to occur between points at the same level. Thus, D_L and E_L would be fused with F_R and G_R at the same height h. From the geometry of the figure it can be seen that $D_L E_L = 2$ and that $F_R G_R = 2h/M$, the ratio of the two widths being $1/M$ for all values of h. The cross thus appears to have rotated laterally so as to present (in this case) a smaller angle to the right eye.

It follows from the above that the respective widths at any height h would subtend angles θ_R and θ_L at the

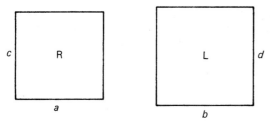

Figure 14.9. Letter symbols denoting the dimensions of the right and left retinal images.

right and left nodal points such that

$$\theta_R/\theta_L = 1/M$$

This is the inverse relationship between the same angles in *Figure 14.7* in which the retinal image of the right eye is magnified by M horizontally. Consequently, equation (14.15) for the magnitude θ of the tilt is equally valid for a vertical magnification, though the apparent tilt is in the opposite direction.

It should be noted that the apparent location of the paired vertical lines of the eikonometer test object is not affected because the effect of vertical magnification is merely to elongate them. Similarly, an overall magnification of one retinal image does not give rise to an apparent lateral tilt of the cross because the magnified image has its limbs in the same orientations as the original.

With certain forms of test objects or scenes, an apparent lateral tilt may still be observed when one retinal image is magnified vertically. Because it cannot be explained in the same simple way as the tilt of the oblique cross, it has been called an induced effect. The following consideration of relative image sizes could, perhaps, suggest a basis for a general explanation.

In *Figure 14.9*, the initial right and left retinal images are represented schematically by rectangles having the dimensions a, b, c and d as shown. The ratio of the two image sizes (right divided by left) in the horizontal meridian will be denoted by H and in the vertical meridian by V. Initially

$$H = a/b \quad \text{and} \quad V = c/d$$

so that

$$H/V = ad/bc$$

If the right eye's retinal image is now magnified by M vertically, dimension c becomes Mc and

$$H/V = ad/Mbc$$

If, instead, the left retinal image is magnified by M horizontally, dimension b becomes Mb and the ratio remains

$$H/V = ad/Mbc$$

Finally, if either retinal image is given an overall magnification, the initial ratio ad/bc is not affected. It will be recalled that an overall magnification of one image does not appear to tilt the cross.

Oblique magnifications

Figure 14.10 shows an initially vertical line BT of height h with its base on the median line, tilted backwards from the observer through the positive (anticlockwise) angle ψ. It is now in the position BT'. The perpendicular dropped from T' meets the median line at G. From the nodal point N_R of the observer's right eye, a line is drawn through B produced to B', the point at which it meets the fronto-parallel plane containing GT'. Thus, B'T' is the apparent position of the tilted line

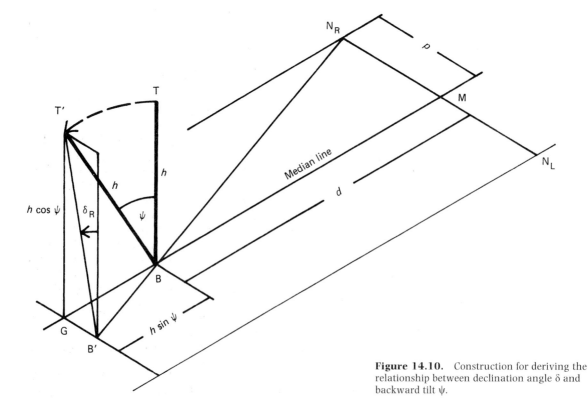

Figure 14.10. Construction for deriving the relationship between declination angle δ and backward tilt ψ.

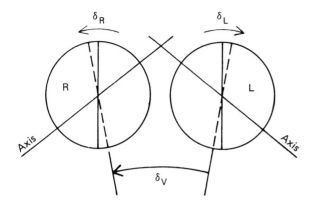

Figure 14.11. Generation of the vertical declination errors δ_R and δ_L by means of magnifying meridional size lenses, axes as shown.

projected on to this plane, as seen by the right eye. From the examiner's standpoint, looking at the patient, it makes a positive angle δ_R with the vertical, which is also the case with its retinal image. In the left eye there would be an equal tilt in the opposite (negative) direction.

If the right and left vertical declination errors, δ_R and δ_L, are in opposite directions – whatever their sizes – their effects are numerically additive. Thus in all cases the vertical declination angle δ_V of the magnification ellipse is found from

$$\delta_V = \delta_R - \delta_L \qquad (14.17)$$

Let us now suppose that the line object BT is in its upright position, giving rise to a vertical line image on each retina. From *Figure 14.5* it is apparent that these images could be made to tilt as before by the declination errors inherent in oblique magnification. In the case under discussion (*Figure 14.10*) the right eye's retinal image (from a front view) was tilted anticlockwise and the left eye's clockwise. This would be the effect produced by a pair of afocal meridional size lenses placed before the eyes, as shown in *Figure 14.11*, with their axes symmetrically orientated and converging upwards. With these lenses, a normal observer would be expected to see a vertical line or plane as though it were frontally tilted with its top away from him. This inference is borne out by experiment, subject to a surprising reservation. A plain expanse of wall does appear to be leaning with its top farther away, and the floor to run downhill. Nevertheless, the test object of the space eikonometer behaves differently. The vertical lines should appear to tilt while the cross should remain unaffected. In fact, the opposite occurs. The mind refuses to accept that the separated vertical lines are tilted. Instead, cyclofusional movements take place, as a result of which the lines appear vertical and the oblique cross frontally tilted in the opposite direction to the wall and the floor. In this case, with the axes of the size lenses converging upwards and δ_R positive, the tilt would be towards the observer.

Whatever the perceived direction of the frontal tilt, the remedy is to counteract the relative vertical declina-

tion error of the patient's own eyes. Thus, a positive error would be corrected by an oblique magnification with axes converging downwards so as to produce a compensating negative error.

From *Figure 14.10*, a simple theoretical relationship can be deduced between the angles ψ and δ. First

$$GT' = h\cos\psi \quad \text{and} \quad GB = h\sin\psi$$

Next, from the similar triangles in the diagram,

$$GB'/h\sin\psi = p/d \qquad (14.18)$$

where p can be taken as half the inter-pupillary distance and d is the distance BM, both regarded as positive. Then

$$\tan\delta_R = GB'/GT' = GB'/h\cos\psi \qquad (14.19)$$

Finally, by eliminating GB' from equations (14.18) and (14.19) we obtain

$$\tan\delta_R = (p/d)\tan\psi \qquad (14.20)$$

It can be seen from this that ψ and δ_R have the same sign and that δ_R would normally be quite small in relation to ψ.

To vary the vertical declination angle produced by a given meridional size lens it merely needs to be rotated. This is the principle of the declination unit used for measurement in the space eikonometer. A pair of afocal lenses of the same meridional magnification, one before each eye, are geared together so as to rotate equally in opposite directions from the zero setting in which both axes are vertical. Symmetry is thus obtained, leaving relative image dimensions in the horizontal and vertical meridians undisturbed. The calibration of the unit follows from the general expression (14.32), giving the relationship between the vertical declination angle of a single meridional size lens and the orientation of its axis in standard axis notation.

Clinical eikonometry

The AO space eikonometer

A direct comparison of the right and left visual images can be made with the aid of a stereoscope or synoptophore or by presenting a test object to each eye alternately in a regular sequence of exposures (Brecher, 1957). A simple test could be constructed by horizontal lines placed equidistant above and below a fixation mark. If the lines for the left eye are placed slightly to the left of fixation, those for the right eye to the right, then any aniseikonia in the vertical meridian should be visible as a misalignment of the images for the two eyes. Fixation disparity and the precision of vernier acuity in peripheral vision limit the success of this method. McCormack *et al.* (1992) found that a similar printed test (the New Aniseikonia Test) employing red/green anaglyphic dissociation grossly underestimated aniseikonia induced with size lenses. A computer screen simulation proved better. Such methods have their uses, but prescribing for aniseikonia requires a sensitive method of measurement.

This need was filled by the AO space eikonometer. It presents the patient with a three-dimensional image of the test object shown in *Figure 14.6(a)*, apparently at a distance of about 3 m (10 ft). A compact optical system for producing variable magnification at axis 90° is positioned in front of the patient's right eye and a similar unit set at axis 180° before the left eye. Each unit has a range from 5% magnification to 5% reduction, but reductions are calibrated to read as relative magnification for the opposite eye. In front of these units is the geared pair of afocal meridional lenses used to determine the vertical declination angle.

In brief outline, the recommended routine proceeds as follows. With all three units set at zero, the patient is asked to say if there is an observable lateral tilt of the two pairs of vertical rods. If so, a horizontal difference is indicated and the unit before the right eye is adjusted until the tilt is corrected. With this horizontal correction left in position, the patient's attention is now directed to the oblique cross. If this, too, appears laterally tilted in either direction, it can only be due to a vertical discrepancy. Accordingly, the unit before the left eye is adjusted so as to correct the tilt. Then, with both corrections in place, the patient is asked to report if there is a frontal tilt of the oblique cross. If so, it denotes that the magnification ellipse is obliquely orientated. The declination unit is then brought into play and the geared lenses rotated to bring the cross into an upright position. The scale reading gives the vertical declination angle of the magnification ellipse.

There are, of course, possible complications and difficulties arising from anomalous appearances of the test object, the presence of heterophoria, poor stereoscopic acuity and other causes. These and other practical points are discussed in the manual issued with the instrument (American Optical Company, 1951) and in the later work by Bannon (1954).

Simple eikonometers

Another method of eikonometry uses a real test object of the classic space eikonometer design, made on a conveniently reduced scale with movable parts. After the test object has been put out of square, the patient is required to re-locate the movable elements in what appears to be their correct position or orientation. Any errors which are made are shown by graduated scales. They are converted into the three parameters of the magnification ellipse by means of the theoretical relationships given by equations (14.16) and (14.20). Conversion tables can easily be prepared from these expressions.

A simple portable eikonometer of this type was designed by Hawkeswell (1975). The oblique cross (without the vertical line through its centre) was mounted in a frame rotatable about horizontal and vertical axes independently. Narrow rods, one fixed and the other movable, replaced the front pair of vertical lines, the rear pair being omitted. A test procedure aided by tables was also described.

A space eikonometer of simpler design than the AO model has been described by Remole (1983). A battery of 11 parallel rods, each separately movable, is viewed by the patient in binocular vision. In the first presentation the rods are vertical and the patient has to position

each one so that the whole array appears to be in a fronto-parallel plane. The angle of any tilt in this array is then recorded. This procedure is repeated with the rods set at 45° and 135° in standard axis notation. From the results of these three settings it is possible to construct the aniseikonic ellipse. In clinical practice, this procedure would have the great advantage of being readily understood and carried out by patients without the need for prior training.

The aniseikonic correction

Iseikonic lenses: translation procedure

Translation of the eikonometer findings into a spectacle correction incorporating a regular prescription as well is an intricate process. One essential step is to determine the magnification ellipse from the given values of the three parameters. In the main, the following outline is based on Ogle's treatment (1950).

Figure 14.12 represents an afocal combination of two meridional magnifications, A at axis θ and B at axis $(90 + \theta)$. As in *Figure 13.8*, the angle measured from the reference axis θ to the vertical meridian is denoted by ϕ_V and the corresponding angle to the horizontal meridian ϕ_H. From any point Q on the vertical meridian a perpendicular is drawn to the reference axis, meeting it at R. The image Q′ of the point Q is found by making OS/OR = B and the perpendicular Q′S/QR = A. The angle from the reference axis to the meridian OQ′ is denoted by ϕ_V'. In the vertical meridian, the magnification M_V is defined by the ratio OQ′/OQ, which is seen from the

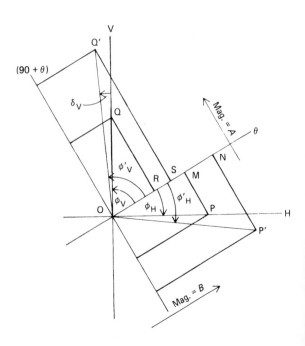

Figure 14.12. Derivation of the parameters of the magnification ellipse A, B and θ from the horizontal and vertical magnifications and vertical declination δ_V.

triangle OSQ' to be

$$M_V = \frac{OS/\cos \phi'_V}{OR/\cos \phi_V}$$

$$= B \cos \phi_V/\cos \phi'_V$$

so that

$$M_V^2 \cos^2 \phi'_V = B^2 \cos^2 \phi_V \qquad (14.21)$$

also

$$M_V = \frac{Q'S/\sin \phi'_V}{QR/\sin \phi_V}$$

$$= A \sin \phi_V/\sin \phi'_V$$

so that

$$M_V^2 \sin^2 \phi'_V = A^2 \sin^2 \phi_V \qquad (14.22)$$

Adding equations (14.21) and (14.22) we obtain

$$M_V^2 = A^2 \sin^2 \phi_V + B^2 \cos^2 \phi_V \qquad (14.23)$$

The percentage magnification v is now substituted for M_V, as indicated by equation (14.13), while A and B are similarly replaced by the percentage magnifications a and b. As a result, M_V^2 becomes $(1 + 0.01v)^2$ which can be taken as $(1 + 0.02v)$. When the other quantities are similarly treated, the modified equation (14.23) can be reduced to

$$v = b + (a - b) \sin^2 \phi_v \qquad (14.24)$$

Similarly, the horizontal percentage magnification is given by

$$h = b + (a - b) \sin^2 \phi_H \qquad (14.25)$$

From *Figure 14.12* it can be seen that $\phi_V = (90 - \theta)$ and $\phi_H = -\theta$. Then, if these substitutions are made and $(a - b)$ is replaced, following Ogle, by the symbol f, equations (14.24) and (14.25) become

$$v = b + f \cos^2 \theta \qquad (14.26)$$

and

$$h = b + f \sin^2 \theta \qquad (14.27)$$

Adding these last two equations gives

$$v + h = 2b + f = a + b \qquad (14.28)$$

while subtraction gives

$$v - h = f(\cos^2 \theta - \sin^2 \theta) = f \cos 2\theta \qquad (14.29)$$

The vertical declination angle δ_V is defined by

$$\delta_V = \phi'_V - \phi_V \qquad (14.30)$$

To eliminate ϕ'_V we can see from the diagram that

$$\tan \phi'_V = (Q'S/OS) \text{ and } \tan \phi_v = QR/OR$$

so that

$$\tan \phi'_V = \left(\frac{Q'S/QR}{OR/OS} \right) \tan \phi_V$$

$$= (A/B) \tan \phi_V \qquad (14.31)$$

From a well-known identity, equation (14.30) leads to

$$\tan \delta_V = \frac{\tan \phi'_V - \tan \phi_V}{1 + \tan \phi'_V \tan \phi_V}$$

which, using equation (14.31), reduces to

$$\tan \delta_V = \frac{(A - B) \tan \phi_V}{B + A \tan^2 \phi_V}$$

Multiplying throughout by $\cos^2 \phi_V$ then gives

$$\tan \delta_V = \frac{(A - B) \sin \phi_V \cos \phi_V}{A \sin^2 \phi_V + B \cos^2 \phi_V}$$

Since the denominator differs little from unity, it can be ignored without serious error, leading to

$$\tan \delta_V = (0.01a - 0.01b) \sin \phi_V \cos \phi_V$$

$$= 0.005 (a - b) \sin 2\phi_V$$

$$= 0.005f \sin (180 - 2\theta)$$

$$= 0.005f \sin 2\theta \qquad (14.32)$$

Since for small angles

$$\tan \delta_V = \delta_V \text{ rad} = \delta_V/57.3°$$

equation (14.32) may be written as

$$\delta_V° = 0.29f \sin 2\theta \qquad (14.33)$$

Division by equation (14.29) then gives

$$\tan 2\theta = \frac{3.5\delta_V}{v - h} \qquad (14.34)$$

The effect of magnifying the image in the right eye by $x\%$ in any given meridian is the same as reducing the left eye's image by $x\%$ in the same meridian. Hence, a meridional magnification is regarded as positive if placed before the right eye but negative if placed before the left eye.

The eikonometer gives δ_V, together with the horizontal magnification h and vertical magnification v expressed as

> h R or L% $\times$ 90
>
> v R or L% $\times$ 180

These three readings can then be converted as follows into the required mutually perpendicular meridional magnifications, together with the *axis* direction θ appropriate to a. First, θ is determined from equation (14.34). If 2θ is found to have a negative value, it is converted into standard axis notation by adding 180°; for example, $-124°$ would become 56°.

The quantity f can now be found by rewriting equation (14.29) in the form

$$f = (v - h)/\cos 2\theta \qquad (14.35)$$

Then, from equation (14.28)

$$b = \tfrac{1}{2}(v + h - f) \text{ at axis } \theta \pm 90 \qquad (14.36)$$

and

$$a = \tfrac{1}{2}(v + h + f) \text{ at axis } \theta \qquad (14.37)$$

As with h and v, positive values of a or b denote magnification for the right eye, negative values for the left eye.

Example (1)

$$\text{Axis } 90: \quad \text{R } 2\% \quad (h = 2)$$
$$\text{Axis } 180: \quad \text{L } 1.5\% \quad (v = -1.5)$$
$$\delta_V : \quad +0.50$$

From equation (14.34)

$$2\theta = -26.6° = 153.4°$$

which gives

$$\theta = 76.7°$$

From equation (14.35) $\quad f = 3.91$
From equation (14.36) $\quad b = -1.71 \times 166.7°$
From equation (14.37) $\quad a = 2.20 \times 76.7°$

Rounded off, the required magnification would be

$$\text{R } 2.25\% \times 77, \text{L} - 1.75\% \times 167$$

If $v = h$, equation (14.34) gives $2\theta = 90°$, thus $\cos 2\theta = 0$ and equation (14.35) becomes indeterminate. In this case, f can be obtained by eliminating 2θ from equations (14.29) and (14.33), giving

$$f^2 = (v - h)^2 + (3.5\delta_V)^2 \qquad (14.38)$$

A graphical method of solution is explained in the comprehensive set of magnification tables issued by American Optical Company (1957).

Before carrying out the above procedure, it may be necessary to modify the eikonometer readings. In general, any refractive correction worn during the test will affect the magnification of the retinal images. Therefore, if there is any difference between the spectacle magnifications of the right and left trial lens combinations, it must be added to the eikonometer readings. To calculate this so-called 'spurious' magnification, the form, thickness and separations of the trial lenses must be known.

In the case of astigmatism at oblique axes, a further complication arises because the axes of the spurious magnification will also be oblique. However, by following a procedure based on equations (14.28) and (14.30), spurious magnification can be expressed in terms of the eikonometer parameters, thus permitting a simple summation. The magnification ellipse is then determined from these new values of v, h and δ_V.

In designing a pair of iseikonic lenses, the essential requirement is to control the spectacle magnification of each lens so that, in conjunction, they conform to the specified magnification ellipse. As shown on pages 229–231, spectacle magnification has two components. The power factor contains the distance a from the back vertex of the lens to the eye's entrance pupil. Altering this distance may, in suitable cases, make a useful contribution. In general, the shape factor affords more scope for manipulation because it contains two variables: the front surface power and the centre thickness of the lens. Since an increase in either increases the spectacle magnification, cosmetic considerations can be borne in mind to some extent. Once again, complications arise if the axes of the magnification do not coincide with the axes of astigmatism. Two possibilities then arise. One is based on the theorem that a meridional magnification at a given axis can be replaced by two meridional magnifications at any axes desired. By

this means, the two sets of axes can be reconciled. Both lenses could in theory then be made in bi-toroidal form, with the mechanical axes of front and rear surfaces in alignment. If this expedient should lead to a cosmetically unacceptable solution, the lenses could be made in bi-toroidal form with the mechanical axes obliquely crossed. In either case, even a small error in axis alignment could give rise to unacceptable errors of effective lens power.

A fully detailed exposition of the entire translation procedure, with many worked examples, is given in a publication by American Optical Company (1967). Solution by matrix methods of magnification problems relating to aniseikonia and its correction have been formulated by Keating (1982).

Before prescribing iseikonic lenses, it is often considered advisable to make a preliminary trial by mounting an afocal size lens in a clip-over fitted to one rim of the patient's spectacles. If this is apparently successful, the clip-over is transferred to the opposite rim and the correction is not prescribed unless decisively rejected when over the wrong eye.

Isogonal lenses

The idea of isogonal lenses was put forward by Halass (1959). They are based on the proposition that since aniseikonia is significantly related to anisometropia, it may well be caused in such cases by the unequal spectacle magnifications of the subject's spectacle lenses. If this is so, the remedy is to disturb the basic retinal image sizes in the naked eyes as little as possible. Contact lenses would thus be the ideal form of correction. If contact lenses are ruled out, an alternative solution would be to design a pair of isogonal spectacle lenses such that the spectacle magnification is the same for each one and for both principal meridians as well if the lens incorporates a prescribed cylinder.

A computer program for the design of isogonal lenses has been devised by Lang and Lederer (1972). Astigmatic isogonal lenses are bi-cylindrical or bi-toroidal in form. Like iseikonic lenses, they are usually very thick and steeply curved, at least in one of the principal meridians.

Various compromise lens designs known as non-symmetrical isogonal, semi-isogonal and semi-iseikonic have also been proposed, based on different principles of correction (Halass, 1960).

Incidence and importance of aniseikonia

The predominant symptoms of aniseikonia – asthenopia, headaches, photophobia and reading difficulty – are not distinctive and anomalies of space perception are reported in only a small percentage of cases. Because of this, eikonometry has generally been regarded as a last resort in difficult cases when other attempts to relieve ocular discomfort have failed.

Image-size disparities up to 1% are not uncommon and generally cause no problems. Nevertheless, amounts as low as 0.75% can be clinically significant if accompanied by severe symptoms (Bannon, 1954). Estimates of the number of cases in which an iseikonic correction would prove beneficial are necessarily tentative but generally in the region of 3–5% of the population. Some 70% of prescribed corrections are believed to have been successful.

Nevertheless, after an initial burst, interest in aniseikonia has now waned to the point where investigation and prescribing are now almost confined to a few specialist clinics and university optometry departments. The special facilities originally provided by American Optical Company are no longer available. As possible reasons for this decline, Burian suggested inertia, the need for simpler instruments, the complications of lens design and unsatisfactory economic return (Neumueller *et al.*, 1970).

It is understandable that few practitioners would have the confidence to undertake themselves the translation procedure in its full rigour

Recognizing this fact, Berens and Bannon in an earlier paper (1963) had summarized a number of methods whereby an estimate can be made of the probable amount of aniseikonia and an approximate correction provided by altering the base curves and centre thickness of the patient's existing spectacle lenses. Further contributions to this approach were made by Rayner (1966) and Brown and Enoch (1970). It is possible that a number of cases are successfully treated in this way.

Another practical problem is the difficulty in getting iseikonic prescriptions manufactured. Paradoxically, the revolution in lens production methods in recent decades has made it increasingly uneconomic to make special lenses of complicated design.

There is no doubt whatever that aniseikonia is the cause of curable ocular discomfort suffered by a relatively small but not insignificant number of people. It would be highly regrettable if this branch of optometry were allowed to wither away completely.

Exercises

14.1 Suggest cosmetically acceptable front surface powers and thicknesses for the lenses in the following anisometropic prescriptions, the object being to reduce the difference in the spectacle magnifications between right and left:

(a) R +4.00 DS L +1.00 DS
(b) R −6.00 DS L −2.00 DS

State the spectacle magnifications of the lenses proposed.

14.2 Draw a diagram similar to *Figure 14.1* showing the ray paths for a corrected and uncorrected hypermetropic eye.

14.3 A patient requires a near addition of +2.00 DS. What compensating prismatic effect could be obtained by using invisible solid (one-piece) bifocals with a 45 mm diameter segment for the right eye and a 30 mm diameter for the left eye? Assume the near visual points to be: (a) 5 mm, (b) 8 mm below the segment tops.

14.4 A patient with the distance correction

R   −3.00
L   −5.00/−2.00×180

shows no hyperphoria when looking through the optical centres of the trial lenses. Discuss the vertical optical centration desirable for (a) single-vision lenses, the horizontal centre line

(HCL) of the frame being 6 mm below the primary line of sight, and (b) executive-type bifocals with a +1.50 D addition, the HCL of the frame being 3 mm below the primary line of sight and the segment tops 3 mm below HCL. Assume the near visual points to be 10 mm below the primary line of sight.

14.5 A test for cyclophoria due to Meissner (1858) is based on the principle of *Figure 14.10*. A string in the median plane is viewed in crossed diplopia. If the string is placed at 400 mm from the eyes, and its top has to be tilted 8° away from the vertical (and patient) for the diplopic images to appear parallel, what is the cyclophoria given a PD of 66 mm? (The cyclophoria measured is that present for the actual fixation distance, but the declination equation applies to the distance of the string.)

14.6 A patient's vision was investigated with a space eikonometer, and the settings for the correct appearance of the display were found to be:

$$\times 90: \text{R } 3\% \text{ (i.e. } h = +3)$$
$$\times 180: \text{L } 2\% \text{ (i.e. } v = -2)$$
$$\delta: +0.4$$

What are the parameters of the magnification ellipse?

14.7 Compare (a) the basic retinal image heights for distance vision in two 60 D reduced eyes, one of which is emmetropic and the other axially myopic by −6.00 D, and (b) the number of retinal receptors per unit length, assuming the posterior hemisphere to contain the same number of retinal receptors and the globe to have a radius of curvature equal to 45% of the axial length. Also discuss the implications for aniseikonia when corrected by spectacles and contact lenses.

14.8 A size lens of 5% magnification has a front surface radius of curvature of 70 mm. What thickness is required if made (a) in resin with $n = 1.498$, (b) in high-index glass with $n = 1.700$?

14.9 Show that the power factor of spectacle magnification of a lens of the required power at a vertex distance d of an eye showing ocular refraction K, assumed to be measured at the cornea, can be expressed as $P = 1 + aK$.

References

ALLEN, D.C. (1974) Vertical prism adaptation in anisometropes. *Am. J. Optom.*, **51**, 252–259

AMERICAN OPTICAL COMPANY (1951) *The AO Space Eikonometer and the Measurement and Correction of Aniseikonia.* Southbridge, Mass.: AO Co Bureau of Visual Science

AMERICAN OPTICAL COMPANY (1957) *Magnification Tables for Use with the Space Eikonometer.* Buffalo, NY: AO Co Instrument Division

AMERICAN OPTICAL COMPANY (1967) *How to Design Iseikonic Lenses.* Southbridge, Mass: AO Co Lens Development Dept.

APPLEGATE, R.E. and HOWLAND, H.C. (1993) Magnification and visual acuity in refractive surgery. *Arch. Ophthalmol.*, **111**, 1335–1342

BANNON, R.E. (1954) *Clinical Manual on Aniseikonia.* Buffalo, NY: AO Co Instrument Division

BENNETT, A.G. (1968) *Emsley and Swaine's Ophthalmic Lenses*, pp. 213–223. London: Hatton Press

BERENS, C. and BANNON, R.E. (1963) Aniseikonia: a present appraisal and some practical considerations. *Archs. Ophthal.*, NY, **70**, 181–188

BRECHER, G.A. (1957) Image aberrations as a method for aniseikonia measurement. *Am. J. Ophthal.*, **43**, 464–465

BROWN, R.M. and ENOCH, J.M. (1970) Combined rules of thumb in aniseikonic prescriptions. *Am. J. Ophthal.*, **69**, 118–126

EDWARDS, K.H. (1980) The management of ametropic and anisometropic amblyopia with contact lenses. *Ophthal. Optn*, **19**, 925–929

GARNER, L.F., YAP, M. and SCOTT, R. (1992) Crystalline lens power in myopia. *Optom. Vision Sci.*, **69**, 863–865

HALASS, S. (1959) Aniseikonic lenses of improved design and their application. *Aust. J. Optom.*, **42**, 387–393

HALASS, S. (1960) Special lenses in anisometropia and aniseikonia. *Aust. J. Optom.*, **43**, 417–420, 469–471

HAWKESWELL, A. (1975) The development of a portable space eikonometer. *Br. J. Physiol. Optics*, **30**, 25–33

HENSON, D.B. and DHARAMASHI, B.G. (1982) Oculomotor adaptation to induced heterophoria and anisometropia. *Invest. Ophthalmol. Vis. Sci.*, **22**, 234–240

KEATING, M.P. (1982) The aniseikonic matrix. *Ophthal. Physiol. Opt.*, **2**, 193–204

LAIRD, I.K. (1991) Anisometropia. In *Refractive Anomalies, Research and Clinical Applications* (Grosvenor, T. and Flom, M. C., eds), pp. 174–198. Boston, Mass.: Butterworth-Heinemann

LANG, M.MCN. and LEDERER, J. (1972) Computerised optometry. *Aust. J. Optom.*, **55**, 373–399

MCCORMACK, G., PELI, E. and STONE, P. (1992) Differences in tests of aniseikonia. *Invest. Ophthalmol. Vis. Sci.*, **33**, 2063–2067

MEISSNER (1851) *Beiträge zur Physiologicedes Sehorgans.* Cited by Helmholtz, H. Von, *Physiological Optics*, Vol.3, p.114. English translation ed. J.P.C. Southall, N. Y.: Optical Society of America. (Reprinted 1962 by Dover Publications, N. Y.)

NEUMUELLER, J., BANNON, R.E., BOEDER, P. and BURIAN, H.M. (1970) Aniseikonia and space perception – after 50 years. *Am. J. Optom.*, **47**, 423–441

OBSTFELD, H. (1978) *Optics in Vision*, pp. 132–134. London: Butterworths

OGLE, K. (1950) *Researches in Binocular Vision*. Philadelphia: W.B. Saunders Co.

RAYNER, A.W. (1966) Aniseikonia and magnification in ophthalmic lenses. Problems and solutions. *Am. J. Optom.*, **43**, 617–632

REMOLE, A. (1983) A new eikonometer: the multimeridional apparent frontoparallel plane. *Am. J. Optom.*, **60**, 519–529

SORSBY, A., LEARY, G.A. and RICHARDS, M.J. (1962) The optical components of anisometropia. *Vision Res.*, **2**, 43–51

STEPHENS, G.L. and POLASKY, M. (1991) New options for aniseikonic correction: the use of high index material. *Optom. Vis. Sci.*, **68**, 899–906

WINN, B., ACKERLEY, R.G., BROWN, C.A., MURRAY, F.K., PRAIS, J. and ST. JOHN, M.F. (1988) Reduced aniseikonia in axial anisometropia with contact lens correction. *Ophthal. Physiol. Opt.*, **8**, 341–344

15

Ocular aberrations

General considerations

The eye, in common with many other refracting systems, is subject to a number of aberrations affecting the resolution and fidelity of the image. A partial correction for spherical aberration is provided by the peripheral flattening of the cornea and probably of the crystalline lens, especially in its accommodated state. On the other hand, the eye's optical system is virtually uncorrected for chromatic aberration. Despite these imperfections, the overall performance of the eye is little short of astonishing.

Traditional methods of examining the resolution of the image and measuring its various aberrations cannot be applied to the eye because its interior is inaccessible for this purpose. Consequently, objective measurement of ocular aberrations must be made in object space on pencils of light originating from the retina. Despite its limitations, this method at least has the advantage of expressing spherical and chromatic aberration in terms of refractive errors relative to a definable norm.

Chromatic aberration

Basic concepts and data

Chromatic aberration arises from the fact that the refractive index of the optical media decreases as the wavelength increases. The shorter wavelengths at the blue end of the visible spectrum are thus more strongly refracted than the longer ones at the red end.

For practical purposes, it is necessary to choose a wavelength to which the 'mean refractive index' of optical materials is to be related. Dioptric powers and focal lengths are then understood to refer to this wavelength unless otherwise indicated. The mean wavelength ($\lambda = 589.3$ nm) of the two adjacent D-lines of the sodium spectrum used to be the accepted standard, but this has been replaced in some countries by the d-line of the helium spectrum ($\lambda = 587.6$ nm). More recently there has been a move in some countries to replace the d-line by the mercury e-line ($\lambda = 546.1$ nm), but no general agreement on such a change is in prospect. The wavelength 587.6 nm will accordingly be taken as the norm for the determination of chromatic aberration.

The International Commission on Illumination (ICI),

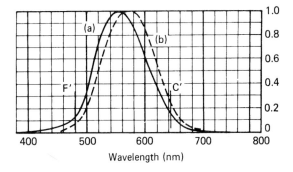

Figure 15.1. Graph of the spectral luminous efficiency function $V(\lambda)$. (a) The photopic curve for an equi-energy spectrum. (b) The curve when weighted for the redder light of a tungsten lamp, Standard Illuminant A.

known in Great Britain by the initials CIE of its French name (Commission Internationale de l'Eclairage), is the accepted international organization concerned with photometry and colorimetry. Its various published tables, reproduced in most textbooks on these subjects, are of fundamental importance in quantitative work. They relate, in part, to the properties of a number of 'standard illuminants' and to certain characteristics of the eye of a 'standard observer'.

The normal human eye perceives as 'light' the range of electromagnetic radiations between wavelengths of approximately 380–780 nm. The relative luminosity at different wavelengths is called the spectral luminous efficiency, also known as the '$V(\lambda)$ function'. The two curves in *Figure 15.1* are plotted from the CIE tables and show the $V(\lambda)$ function under different conditions. Curve (a) shows the relative luminosity at different wavelengths when the physical energy has been adjusted to remain at the same level throughout, the wavelength of peak luminosity then being at approximately 555 nm.

Although the energy distribution of sunlight is approximately uniform within the visible spectrum, this is not characteristic of light sources in general. In particular, the energy emitted by the CIE Standard Illuminant A, which typifies the familiar tungsten-filament electric lamp, increases at an almost uniform rate with wavelength. Curve (b) in *Figure 15.1* shows the effect of this type of illumination on the $V(\lambda)$ function.

It was plotted by taking the figures for the equi-energy

Table 15.1   Notional refractive indices at selected wavelengths of the ocular media

Spectral line Wavelength (nm)	380	F' 480.0	d 587.6	C' 643.8	780	Abbe number (v)
Humours	1.3488	1.3407	1.3360	1.3343	1.3314	52.9
Crystalline lens						
Relaxed eye	1.4389	1.4282	1.4220	1.4198	1.4159	50.1
Eye accommodated*	1.4389	1.4282	1.4220	1.4198	1.4159	
Elderly eye	1.4223	1.4120	1.4060	1.4039	1.4001	

* On the provisional basis that the accommodated lens has the same refractive index as the unaccommodated lens (*see* page 212), these values are the same as in the row above.

spectrum, represented by curve (a), and weighting them by the relative energy of Standard Illuminant A, the amended figures then being re-scaled to make the maximum equal to unity. This has the effect of shifting the wavelength of peak luminosity towards the red end of the spectrum, to approximately 570 nm. This has an important bearing of the theory of bichromatic tests, discussed later in this chapter.

In designing achromatic lenses and optical instruments for visual use, consideration has traditionally been limited to that part of the visible spectrum bounded by the hydrogen F-line ($\lambda = 486.1$ nm) and the hydrogen C-line ($\lambda = 656.3$ nm). *Figure 15.1* shows that beyond these limits the relative luminous efficiency becomes very low. In 1962, the International Commission for Optics decided to adopt a revised list of wavelengths for refractive index determination, the main consideration being experimental convenience. As a result, the F and C lines were both discarded and replaced by the neighbouring F' and C' lines ($\lambda = 480.0$ and 643.8 nm respectively) of the cadmium spectrum. Despite this, the 1984 version of ISO 7944: *Reference wavelengths* defines the Abbe number or constringence v of an optical material as

$$v_d = \frac{n_d - 1}{n_F - n_C} \quad \text{or} \quad v_e = \frac{n_e - 1}{n_{F'} - n_{C'}} \quad (15.1)$$

in which the subscripts denote the spectral line to which the refractive index refers. If F is the mean power (for the d-line) of a thin lens or surface in air, its axial chromatic aberration, or difference in power over the spectral interval F' to C', is the fraction F/v.

The ocular humours are largely composed of water, which has an Abbe number of approximately 55. Thus the axial chromatic aberration of the single-surface reduced eye of power +60 D would be about 60/55 or just over 1.00 D. In the accommodated state when the power of the eye is increased, the chromatic aberration would increase proportionately.

Chromatic aberration of the schematic eye

It is useful to study chromatic aberration in the schematic eye as it provides a valuable guide to the performance of the living eye. Initially, a set of values must be decided upon for the refractive indices of the ocular media over the visible spectrum. Another requirement is to distinguish between three different aspects of chromatic aberration, since the term is too vague to be used in a quantitative sense.

Refractive indices of the ocular media

The values adopted by Le Grand (1956) for the humours are undoubtedly typical of the human eye, while his figures for the crystalline lens necessarily relate to a simplified hypothetical substitute.

In determining a set of values for the Bennett–Rabbetts schematic eye, the authors have adopted the d-line values of 1.336 for the humours and 1.422 for the unaccommodated lens. Values for the F' and C' wavelengths were calculated in the light of Le Grand's figures for constringencies and partial dispersions, for example $(n_{F'} - n_d)/(n_{F'} - n_{C'})$. Finally, the values for wavelengths 380 and 780 nm – the limits of the visible spectrum – were calculated from Schmidt's dispersion formula $(n = n_o + A\lambda^{-1} + B\lambda^{-4})$. The complete list is set out in *Table 15.1*. A detailed discussion of this topic can be found in Le Grand (1956).

Chromatic difference of equivalent power

Aberration implies departure from a norm. In this case, the norm is the equivalent power of the eye for a given reference wavelength. Thus if λ_o is the reference wavelength, n'_o the refractive index of the vitreous humour and F_o the equivalent power of eye for this wavelength, n'_λ the refractive index of the vitreous humour and F_λ the equivalent power of the eye for the new wavelength λ and ΔF_e the chromatic difference of equivalent power, then

$$\Delta F_e = F_\lambda - F_o \quad (15.2)$$

Table 15.2 gives values of F_λ and ΔF_e for the Bennett–Rabbetts schematic eye, both in its relaxed state and accommodated 2.50 D. As expected, the aberration is slightly greater in the accommodated state because the mean power of the eye is greater. It can be seen that the total variation in the equivalent power of the relaxed eye over the entire visible spectrum is very nearly 3.25 D. Over the central band between the F' and C' wavelengths it is 1.20 D.

Table 15.2 also gives the positions of the principal points and entrance and exit pupils. The variation with wavelength is very small and can be ignored over the F'–C' interval.

Chromatic difference of refraction

It is not feasible to determine values of F_λ by experiment on the living eye. A related but clinically more signifi-

Table 15.2 Chromatic aberration of the Bennett–Rabbetts schematic eye

(a) Unaccommodated

Spectral line Wavelength (nm)		380	F′ 480.0	d 587.6	C′ 643.8	780
Equivalent power of eye (D)	F_λ	62.33	60.85	60.00	59.70	59.16
Position of principal points (mm)	A_1P	1.51	1.51	1.51	1.51	1.51
	A_1P'	1.83	1.82	1.82	1.82	1.82
Position of entrance and exit pupils (mm)	A_1E	3.03	3.04	3.05	3.05	3.05
	A_1E'	3.70	3.70	3.70	3.70	3.70
Chromatic difference of power (D)	ΔF_e	+2.33	+0.85	0.00	−0.30	−0.84
Chromatic difference of refraction (D)	ΔK	−1.73	−0.64	0.00	+0.22	+0.63
Chromatic difference of magnification	y_λ/y_o	0.9928	0.9974	1	1.0010	1.0027

(b) Accommodated 2.50 D*

Spectral line Wavelength (nm)		380	F′ 480.0	d 587.6	C′ 643.8	780
Equivalent power of eye (D)	F_λ	65.29	63.75	62.84	62.53	61.96
Position of principal points (mm)	A_1P	1.62	1.62	1.62	1.62	1.62
	A_1P'	1.96	1.95	1.95	1.95	1.94
Position of entrance and exit pupils (mm)	A_1E	2.96	2.92	2.93	2.93	2.94
	A_1E'	3.56	3.56	3.56	3.56	3.56
Chromatic difference of power (D)	ΔF_e	+2.45	+0.90	0.00	−0.32	−0.89
Chromatic difference of refraction (D)	ΔK	−1.73	−0.68	0.00	+0.24	+0.67
Chromatic difference of magnification	y_λ/y_o	0.9923	0.9972	1	1.0010	1.0027

* That is, for an object plane −400 mm from the first principal plane. The author (R.B.R.) has data for the other levels of accommodation.

cant quantity is the chromatic difference of refraction ΔK measured at the first principal point. In simple terms, this quantity is the variation in refractive error with wavelength and can easily be determined experimentally.

It might be natural to suppose that a given chromatic difference of equivalent power would result in a refractive change of equal magnitude but opposite in sign. For example, an increase in power of 0.30 D ($\Delta F_e = +0.30$ D) could be expected to result in relative myopia of the same amount ($\Delta K = -0.30$ D). In fact, this is not so. In the schematic eye, the distance k' to the retina is measured from the second principal point, the position of which varies very little with wavelength. Nevertheless, its dioptric equivalent K', being equal to n'/k', is affected. Since the basic relationship

$$K = K' - F_e \qquad (4.3)$$

holds good for all wavelengths and since K' and F_e are both affected, it follows that ΔK cannot be equal to $-\Delta F_e$.

If $k'_o = k'$ for a reference wavelength λ_o and $K'_o = n'_o/k'_o, k'_\lambda = k'$ for wavelength λ and $K'_\lambda = n'_\lambda/k'_\lambda$, K_o is the ocular error of refraction for wavelength

λ_o, K_λ the ocular error of refraction for wavelength λ and ΔK the chromatic difference of refraction, then

$$\Delta K = K_\lambda - K_o \qquad (15.3)$$

which, from equation (4.3), can be put in the form

$$\begin{aligned} \Delta K &= (K'_\lambda - F_\lambda) - (K'_o - F_o) \\ &= (F_o - F_\lambda) + (K'_\lambda - K'_o) \\ &= -\Delta F_e + (K'_\lambda - K'_o) \end{aligned} \qquad (15.4)$$

If the second principal point is regarded as stationary, $k'_\lambda = k'_o$ and equation (15.4) can be written as

$$\Delta K = -\Delta F_e + \left(\frac{n'_\lambda - n'_o}{n'_o}\right) K'_o \qquad (15.5)$$

Values of ΔK and ΔF_e are given in *Table 15.2*, and shown graphically in *Figure 15.2*. Following Pease and Barbeito (1989) and Koczorowski (1990), these results have been plotted against reciprocal wavelength or wavenumber ω. As the above authors point out, the graphs in *Figure 15.2* are nearly linear when plotted against wavenumber ω, whereas they are significantly curved when plotted against the more traditional wavelength. The theoretical justifications for this choice of abscissa are that the frequency of light (its

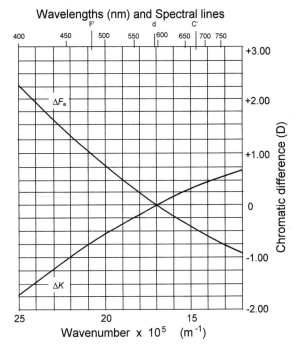

Figure 15.2. The chromatic difference of equivalent power ΔF_e and the chromatic difference of refraction ΔK plotted as a function of wavenumber. The reference wavenumber corresponds to a wavelength of 587.6 nm (the helium d-line).

velocity in vacuum divided by wavelength) is unaltered on passage from one medium to another and that the energy of radiation is proportional to its frequency. Moreover, inspection of Schmidt's equation (page 276) shows that the refractive index may be expressed as $n = n_0 + A\omega + B\omega^4$, and as the last term is about one-twentieth of the second, refractive index is almost a linear function of wavenumber.

Chromatic variation of magnification

The two aspects of chromatic aberration already discussed refer to axial effects, but transverse effects are caused by chromatic aberration. In *Figure 15.3*, E and E′ are the respective centres of the entrance and exit pupils and B′ the posterior pole of a schematic eye, all three of these points lying on the optical axis. QE is the chief ray of an incident pencil filling the pupil and makes an angle u with the optical axis. The conjugate refracted ray, E′Q′, makes an angle u' with the axis, meeting the retina at a height y from this axis. Even if the refracted pencil does not focus on the retina, the point Q′ nevertheless determines the centre of the blurred retinal image of the given object point.

It can be seen from equation (12.10) that if u remains

constant, u' varies with refractive index and hence with wavelength. As a result, even though the position of E′ and hence the distance E′M′ remain practically unchanged, the image height y is affected by wavelength. The change in y for a given angle u can be regarded as a change in magnification. If y_o and y_λ denote the respective values of y for the reference wavelength λ_o and another wavelength λ, the chromatic variation of magnification can be expressed as the ratio y_λ/y_o. Values of this ratio are included in *Table 15.2*.

For a small object at Q, it is not the chromatic variation in magnification at Q′ that is important but the chromatic variation in position or transverse chromatic aberration (TCA). Because the fovea is not situated on the optical axis of the eye, TCA here gives rise to chromatic stereopsis, discussed on pages 290–293. In the retinal periphery, values of TCA will be much larger, but the lower resolution of the retina and reduced spectral sensitivity render TCA unimportant.

Experimental determinations

In experimental determinations, the quantity measured is ΔK, the chromatic difference of refraction. One technique, used by Wald and Griffin (1947), Howarth and Bradley (1986) and Kruger *et al.* (1993) is to determine the ocular refraction for different wavelengths with a Badal optometer system, the optometer lens being well corrected for chromatic aberration. To help keep the accommodation relaxed, a distant fixation object is arranged so that it is visible to both eyes while only one eye sees the optometer test object. Cooper and Pease (1988) similarly used a Badal optometer but combined it with a Scheiner disc to improve precision.

The basis of another method is shown in *Figure 15.4*. A pencil of composite light diverging from the fovea M′ is able to leave the eye only through a small area G of the pupil at a distance y from the axis. If the emergent ray corresponding to the reference wavelength λ_o intersects the axis at a distance k_o, the ray corresponding to some other wavelength λ will intersect the axis at a different distance k_λ. Since ray paths are reversible, it follows that two small or narrow test objects placed at T_1 and T_2 and illuminated by light of wavelength λ_o and λ respectively, would both be imaged on the fovea. To the observer, they would thus appear to be coincident.

This arrangement has been used by several teams. Thibos *et al.* (1990) used a pinhole in front of the eye in order to isolate the required zone of the pupil. The vertical test objects T_1 and T_2 are seen in silhouette against the two different colour backgrounds. Ivanoff (1953) employed a Maxwellian view system in which a pinhole disc is imaged by the upper half of an achromatic doub-

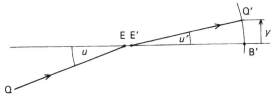

Figure 15.3. Chromatic variation of magnification: angle u' and intercept height y vary with wavelength.

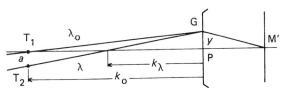

Figure 15.4. Optical arrangement for measuring chromatic difference of refraction by means of light leaving or entering the pupil through a restricted zone at G.

let in the subject's pupillary plane. After reflection by a mirror, a second pinhole is imaged by the lower half of the doublet at the same quasi-point focus G in the subject's pupillary plane. With T_1 and T_2 in actual coincidence, the position of the subject's eye is adjusted until they appear to him coincident. This establishes the 'achromatic axis'[*] of his eye. The subject's head is supported on a carriage and then moved laterally through a predetermined distance y. As a result, the two test objects now appear to be separated. To restore apparent coincidence, T_2 has to be moved through a distance a which is measured.

The distances a and y in *Figure 15.4* are considered opposite in sign if they are on opposite sides of the axis. It can then be seen that

$$\frac{-a}{y} = \frac{k_o - k_\lambda}{k_\lambda} = \frac{K_\lambda - K_o}{K_o} = \frac{\Delta K}{K_o}$$

which gives

$$\Delta K = -aK_o/y \qquad (15.6a)$$

or, rearranging,

$$a/k_o = -y\Delta K \qquad (15.6b)$$

Equation (15.6b) shows that a graph of a/k_o plotted against y has a slope ΔK, the chromatic difference of refraction. This is the technique used by Thibos *et al.* (1990) and Simonet and Campbell (1990).

Published results of experimental determinations are not always based on the same zero-point wavelength. The best choice for this would probably be 587.6 nm, the reference wavelength chosen for the schematic eye and the determination of lens power. When necessary adjustments have been made to put the zero point at 587.6 nm, a remarkable compatibility emerges despite differences in experimental techniques. This is shown by *Figure 15.5*, in which three different sets of results – by Wald and Griffin (1947), Ivanoff (1953) and Bedford and Wyszecki (1957) – have been plotted on the same graph. The curved line represents the mean. The results of Jenkins (1963) for 32 eyes fit the curve well, though showing slightly higher values for wavelengths over 600 nm.

Figure 15.5 also shows some calculated values of ΔK for the Bennett–Rabbetts schematic eye. A number of writers have commented on the difference between the calculated and experimental values in the blue region, but the same trend appears at the other end of the spectrum. A possible explanation is that the dispersions of the ocular media – probably of the crystalline lens in particular – is higher than the values generally adopted.

Since the eye's power increases with accommodation, so should its chromatic aberration. The experimental results of Nutting in 1914 showed such an increase, as pointed out by Jenkins (1963). Over the interval F' to C', *Table 15.2* shows ΔK of the schematic eye to increase from 0.86 D for the relaxed eye to 0.93 D with 2.5 D of

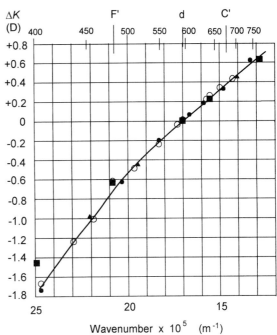

Figure 15.5. Chromatic difference of refraction. Experimental results adjusted for $\lambda_o = 587.6$ nm or wavenumber 1.702×10^6. Results of ● Wald and Griffin (1947), △ Ivanoff (1953), ○ Bedford and Wyszecki (1957). The curved line represents the mean. ■ indicates calculated results for the schematic eye.

accommodation in play, the value of F_o having increased by 2.83 D. In percentage terms, this amounts to an increase in ΔK of about 2.5% per dioptre of ΔF_o. A similar result was obtained experimentally by Charman and Tucker (1978) over the spectral interval 442–633 nm. Similarly, Sivak and Millodot (1974) found the residual longitudinal chromatic aberration with an achromatizing lens (*see* below) to increase from a minimal amount in the unaccommodated state to about 0.75 D at 7 D of accommodation. Cooper and Pease (1988), however, found very little difference in ΔK over the interval 400–700 nm for both all their 14 subjects or for the eight aged less than 30 when changing fixation from a distant object to one at 0.4 m.

An objective method of measurement, devised by Charman and Jennings (1976a) and giving good results, makes use of the double-pass photoelectric scanning technique described on page 49.

Achromatizing lenses

The purpose of an achromatizing lens is to counteract, as far as possible, the eye's chromatic difference of refraction. It requires at least two components made of materials having different dispersions. One such lens (Thomson and Wright, 1947) is a cemented doublet similar in construction to a telescope objective, but with the chromatic aberration greatly over-corrected so as to neutralize the eye's.

An improved design by Carman, described by Bedford

---

[*] This term, used by Ivanoff, denotes the ray path for incident light such that, despite dispersion at the various ocular refracting surfaces, rays of different wavelengths reunite at the fovea. A more detailed explanation is given on pages 290–293 about chromatic stereopsis.

Table 15.3 Details of an achromatizing lens of the Carman design

Spectral line Wavelength (nm)	h 404.7	d 587.6	750
Refractive indices			
Positive component	1.63776	1.62041	1.61417
Negative components	1.65120	1.62049	1.61076
Back vertex power	−1.86 D	−0.01 D	+0.47 D
Effective power at cornea ($d = 12$ mm)	−1.82 D	−0.01 D	+0.48 D
Eye's ΔK (experimental)	−1.70 D	0	+0.58 D
Residual ΔK	+0.12 D	+0.01 D	+0.10 D
Chromatic difference of magnification	0.963 (−3.7%)	1	1.011 (+1.1%)

Radius of curvature of curved surfaces ±14.4 mm. Centre thickness: 1.0 mm (negative components), 5.0 mm (positive component).

and Wyszecki (1957), takes the form of a symmetrical cemented triplet with plane outer surfaces, the central element being equi-convex and the outer ones plano-concave. Ideally, the materials used for the positive and negative components should have the same refractive index for the reference wavelength – usually the helium d-line or the mean sodium D-line. At this wavelength the lens will then act as a flat parallel plate of zero power. Two suitable main-type glasses from Chance–Pilkington's catalogue would be DBC 620603 ($n_d = 1.62041$, $v = 60.3$) for the positive component and DF 620362 ($n_d = 1.62049$, $v = 36.2$) for the negative.

Details of an achromatizing lens made from these materials are given in *Table 15.3*. Its back vertex is assumed to be 12 mm from the Bennett–Rabbetts emmetropic schematic eye. Over the range of wavelengths from the h-line (404.7 nm) to 750 nm, the eye's experimentally determined chromatic difference of refraction ΔK is substantially corrected. The residual errors all lie between zero and +0.12 D of hypermetropia.

Because of the lens–eye separation, an achromatizing lens produces an effect similar to spectacle magnification. Since the lens has negative power at the short-wavelength end of the spectrum and positive power at the other end, the retinal image size increases with wavelength. *Table 15.3* shows that the variation is small – less than 5% over the range of wavelengths considered. Without the achromatizing lens, the blurred retinal images at out-of-focus wavelengths would show a very much larger size difference. Consider, for example, a distant test object of 5 minutes of arc angular subtense viewed by the unaccommodated schematic eye and in focus for the reference wavelength (587.6 nm). The diameter of the sharp retinal image would be 0.024 mm, but the overall sizes of the blurred retinal images at other wavelengths would be 0.056 mm at 480.0 nm (F′) and 0.035 mm at 643.8 nm (C′). These figures refer to a 3 mm entrance pupil.

To make the Carman lens commercially available in

the USA, it has been slightly modified by Lewis *et al.* (1982), using Schott glasses F3 613370 and SK4 613586. The surface radii are unchanged at 14 mm, but the centre thickness of the equi-convex element has been increased to 5.2 mm and that of the outer components reduced to 0.9 mm. The lens diameter is 14.5 mm.

An air-spaced achromatizing lens system, comprising a cemented triplet and a cemented doublet, has been described by Powell (1981). It has the advantage of reducing residual transverse as well as axial chromatic aberration to negligible proportions over a wider field of view than simpler designs.

Two current controversies

The first concerns the eye's chromatic difference of refraction, usually referred to in the literature as LCA (longitudinal chromatic aberration). Despite the close agreement of earlier studies, as indicated by *Figure 15.5*, doubt has been cast on the validity of these findings at the blue end of the spectrum. Measurements of the dispersion of the crystalline lens and cornea by Sivak and Mandelbaum (1982) suggest that their dispersions at short wavelengths are greater than expected, especially that of the lens. As a result, the eye's calculated LCA between wavelengths 440 and 660 nm would become 2.73 D (Mandelbaum and Sivak, 1983). This is considerably higher than the previously accepted value in the neighbourhood of 1.50 D.

Despite this prediction, experimental results for the LCA continue to show results similar to the earlier findings. Thus Howarth and Bradley (1986) measured the right eye of 20 approximately emmetropic subjects, under cycloplegia, to determine the LCA over the spectral range 420–660 nm. The residual chromatic error was also measured with each of two commercially available achromatizing lenses placed before the eye. The mean value of the LCA was found to be 1.82 D, very close to the earlier results, with only small inter-subject differences. Both achromatizing lenses performed satisfactorily, giving a mean under-correction of 0.11 D (Powell) and 0.17 D (Lewis) at the extreme blue end of the spectral range investigated.

Similar results have been obtained by Cooper and Pease (1988) using a Badal optometer combined with a Scheiner disc (2.17 D between 488 and 633 nm), Howarth *et al.* (1988), also using a Badal optometer (0.97 D between 466 and 615 nm, 2 D between 420 and 645 nm), Morrell *et al.* (1991) using a laser speckle technique (1.05 D between 488 and 633 nm) and Kruger *et al.* (1993) with an infra-red optometer (1.7 D between 450 and 670 nm).

The second controversy relates to the possibility of a reduction in LCA of the eye with increasing age. Although this was suggested by Millodot (1976), both Howarth *et al.* (1988) and Morrell *et al.* (1991) found no significant difference between their two age groups. There is no obvious mechanism why the dispersion of the ocular media should vary with age, though the increased absorption and scattering of short wavelengths may have influenced Millodot's work.

Chromatic aberration and visual acuity

Because of the eye's consideration chromatic aberration, there should be an improvement in visual acuity when monochromatic illumination is used. Campbell and Gubisch (1967) showed that this improvement is much more marked and theoretically predictable when expressed in terms of contrast sensitivity. This quantity is the reciprocal of the luminance contrast threshold (*see* pages 46–52). Using a sinusoidal grating with a spatial frequency of 30 cycles per degree, they measured the contrast threshold with white light, monochromatic green (= 546 nm) and monochromatic yellow (= 578nm). Separate readings were taken with artificial pupils of 1.5, 2.5 and 4 mm diameter in use. The mean results, nearly identical for the two monochromatic lights, showed the contrast sensitivity to be increased by 55–57% with the accommodation paralysed and by 31–35% with normal accommodation.

On the other hand, experiments made by various researchers have shown that an achromatizing lens does not improve the visual acuity. The team of researchers at Indiana University have put forward several possible reasons for this, the most important being (a) that longitudinal chromatic aberration has less effect on visual acuity than might be expected, and (b) that unless very carefully centred, an achromatizing lens causes blur because the various coloured images are separated on the retina.

Thus Bradley (1992), expanding on the argument first put forward by Helmholtz in his *Physiological Optics*, argued that although the total LCA in the eye may be around 2 D, the effect of the spectral luminosity function $V(\lambda)$, as shown in *Figure 15.1*, is to diminish the luminosity at the ends of the spectrum where the dioptric error is largest. Moreover, assuming the eye is in focus for the wavelength at the peak of the luminosity curve, the wavelengths at half the luminous intensity will be only about 0.3 D out of focus – well within the depth of focus of the eye, while only the relatively dim ends of the spectrum will be more than 0.5 D out of focus.

In terms of the ocular Modulation Transfer Function (page 46), the same team argue (Thibos *et al.*, 1991) that for a white visual display unit phosphor and a 2.5 mm pupil, the MTF is reduced approximately equally because of diffraction and LCA, the LCA being equivalent to about 0.2 D of spherical defocus. If the LCA were eliminated, they predict that the foveal visual acuity cut-off given by the intersection of the MTF and the retinal contrast threshold curve would improve by only about 5 cycles per degree, i.e. from 50 to 55 cpd. This would predict only a marginal change in acuity.

Their second argument is illustrated by *Figure 15.6*, which is derived from *Figure 15.4*. The upper diagram shows the achromatizing lens aligned with the eye's achromatic axis, a real object B being imaged closer to the lens and eye at B'_b for a short wavelength, and further from the eye at B'_r for a long wavelength. If the lens is decentred, either by a head movement or by faulty positioning, the two images will no longer lie on the achromatic axis, and will be imaged adjacent to each other on the retina giving a blurred image.

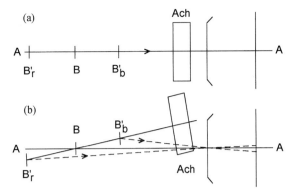

Figure 15.6. Induced transverse chromatic aberration when an achromatizing lens is misaligned with the eye's achromatic axis, AA. (a) When aligned, the images B'_b and B'_r lie on the achromatic axis. (b) When displaced, a transverse spectrum is formed on the retina.

Zhang *et al.* (1991) showed that the angular separation θ between the two images is given by

$$\theta = y(F_R - F_B)$$

where F_R and F_B are the powers of the achromatizing lens for the long and short wavelengths and y the misalignment (in metres). They suggested that only 0.4 mm of misalignment was enough to cancel out any improvement from correcting the LCA.

Other possible causes discussed by the team (Bradley *et al.*, 1991) are that the achromatizing lens inadequately corrects the LCA of the eye, but as *Table 15.3* shows, a Carman lens provides excellent neutralization of the eye's LCA. Also, experimental determination by Howarth and Bradley (1986) and Kruger *et al.* (1993) of the residual LCA of eyes corrected by achromatizing lenses have shown negligible aberration.

Spherical aberration

General characteristics and definitions

The study of spherical aberration can be simplified by initially considering only monochromatic light of the chosen 'mean' wavelength, in this case 587.6 nm.

Spherical aberration of the wavefront can be exhibited by all surfaces of revolution and is a defect of axial pencils. In its classical form, rays become excessively deviated as the point of incidence gets further from the optical axis. Thus, in the case of a converging lens or surface forming a real image, rays passing through zones of increasing diameter are converged to axial points nearer and nearer to the surface. This type of spherical aberration is called 'uncorrected'. If, by some means, the reverse condition applies – the marginal zones becoming progressively weaker than the paraxial region – the aberration is called 'over-corrected'.

In general, a single refracting surface can be made free from spherical aberration for a given pair of conjugate axial points if its section is a Cartesian oval. This is a curve of the fourth degree, not an ellipse but a true oval, named after Descartes who deduced its properties in 1637. For certain special pairs of conjugates, the curve degenerates into various conic sections including a circle, hence the 'aplanatic points' of a sphere. Unfortunately, a surface free from spherical aberration for a specified pair of conjugates will exhibit some aberration for all other pairs.

Spherical aberration of the eye affects both ingoing pencils and pencils diverging from the retina. In numerical terms, the internal spherical aberration (ISA) is the difference between the dioptric distances of the paraxial and marginal foci, measured from the eye's second principal point. Thus, if these distances (in metres) are ℓ'_o for paraxial rays and ℓ'_y for rays incident at a distance y from the axis, the internal aberration in dioptres is

$$\text{ISA} = n'/\ell'_y - n'/\ell'_o \qquad (15.7)$$

where n' is the refractive index of the vitreous humour. A positive value of the ISA denotes uncorrected aberration and relative myopia. For the unaccommodated eye, this amounts to the difference in equivalent power.

Similarly, the external spherical aberration (ESA) – referring to pencils diverging from the retina – is the difference between the dioptric distances of the paraxial and marginal foci, measured from the eye's first principal point. This is the quantity measured in experimental determinations. Hence, for the unaccommodated eye,

$$\text{ESA} = K_y - K_o \qquad (15.8)$$

where K_y and K_o are the respective refractive errors for marginal and paraxial rays. A negative value of the ESA denotes uncorrected aberration and relative myopia. For example, if K_o is $-0.75\,\text{D}$ and K_y is $-1.25\,\text{D}$,

$$\text{ESA} = -1.25 - (-0.75) = -0.50\,\text{D}$$

Spherical aberration exerts its separate effect on light of every wavelength in the incident pencils. The structure of refracted pencils of composite light within the eye is thus extremely complex.

Spherical aberration of the schematic eye

The spherical aberration of the schematic eye is easily determined by accurate ray tracing. This has the value of revealing the great superiority of the real eye. In brief, the results show that

(1) The pattern and amount of the aberration is very nearly the same for all wavelengths.
(2) For any given wavelength and incidence height, there is very little difference between the internal and external values. In practice, it is the external value which is measured, as with chromatic aberration.
(3) For the Bennett–Rabbetts unaccommodated eye, the internal aberration is closely fitted by the approximation

$$\text{ISA} = 0.38y^2 \quad (y \text{ in mm}) \qquad (15.9)$$

(4) For the fully accommodated Bennett–Rabbetts eye, the internal aberration is reasonably fitted for small values of y by the approximation

$$\text{ISA} = 0.61y^2 \quad (y \text{ in mm}) \qquad (15.10)$$

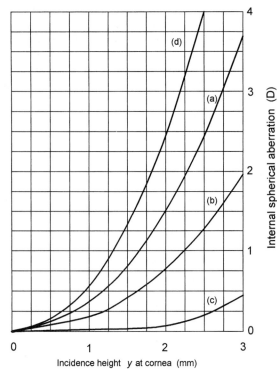

Figure 15.7. Internal spherical aberration of the Bennett–Rabbetts schematic eye in: (a) its unaccommodated and (d) its fully accommodated state. The reduction of the aberration in the relaxed state by a cornea with peripheral flattening is shown by (b) an ellipsoidal cornea ($p = 0.5$) and (c) a paraboloidal cornea.

The spherical aberration of the schematic eye is greatly reduced by making the corneal profile a conic section (the simplest class of curves showing peripheral flattening). As explained on page 208, all its various forms can be defined by the single Cartesian equation

$$y^2 = 2r_o x - px^2 \qquad (15.11)$$

in which they are distinguished by the value given to the parameter p.

In *Figure 15.7*, the internal spherical aberration of the unaccommodated Bennett–Rabbetts schematic eye is plotted for three different corneal forms: (a) spherical, (b) ellipsoidal ($p = 0.5$) and (c) paraboloidal. The calculated figures on which these graphs are based are shown in *Table 15.4*. For any particular incident height, the ISA varies almost linearly with corneal p-value over the range $p = 0$ to $p = 1$. Small changes in the parameters of the eye, for example anterior chamber depth, make a noticeable difference to the aberration.

Table 15.4 Internal spherical aberration in dioptres of the unaccommodated Bennett–Rabbetts schematic eye with various corneal forms

Distance from axis (mm)	Corneal form		
	Spherical	Ellipsoidal ($p = 0.5$)	Paraboloidal
1	+0.36	+0.18	+0.02
2	+1.51	+0.77	+0.08
3	+3.69	+1.96	+0.42

Since accommodation increases the power of the eye, the fully accommodated schematic eye with a spherical cornea shows a marked increase in spherical aberration, as shown by equations (15.9) and (15.10). The figures given by ray-tracing are represented by graph (d) in *Figure 15.7*. As pointed out in Chapter 12, spherical aberration in schematic eyes can be eliminated by making all the surfaces aspheric.

Experimental determinations

Experimental investigations of the eye's spherical aberration have been made by a variety of methods over a long period of time. Perhaps the earliest was made by Thomas Young (1801), using the optometer described on page 75. He replaced the double-slit aperture by four narrowly spaced slits so that he could compare the position of focus for the inner pair with that for the outer pair. With accommodation relaxed and with himself as subject, the two foci coincided, but when accommodating he found his eye to exhibit spherical aberration of the over-corrected type.

Since the reflex locates the exact area of the subject's pupil transmitting rays from his retina into the observer's eye, retinoscopy (*see* Chapter 17) affords a simple means of investigating differences of refraction in different pupillary areas. The pioneer of this method was Edward Jackson (1888). Out of 100 subjects he found the great majority to have uncorrected spherical aberration: 44 with 0.50 D at the pupillary margin and 19 with 1.0 D. Only 6 had 2.0 D or over. Nine subjects exhibited over-corrected aberration, varying from 1.0 to 2.0 D, while another group of 13 were listed as having 0.25 D 'either way'.

Later determinations have attempted a more precise measurement showing the dioptric variation with incidence height. Ames and Proctor (1921) used a series of rotatable double-slit apertures with a range of separations, thus isolating a central and small off-axis area of the pupil. Measurements could then be taken along any desired meridian on both sides of the corneal vertex separately. The far-point distance determined by the intersection of the axial and off-axis pencils emerging from the subject's eye was measured by a Badal-type optometer with a concave mirror instead of a lens. No measurements were taken on the accommodated eye.

Koomen *et al.* (1949) isolated a series of narrow annular zones of the pupil and measured the spectacle refraction for each zone in turn with a refracting unit. By means of a beam-splitting cube placed close to the eye, a subsidiary ray path to a distant fixation object was provided. Lenses of minus power could be placed on this ray path to stimulate various amounts of accommodation.

Because of various experimental difficulties, particularly that of aligning the visual axis with sufficient accuracy, both these teams found it possible to make reliable measurements only on themselves. Using retinoscopy in four pupillary quadrants, Jenkins (1963) recorded the type and mean amount of spherical aberra-

tion in 164 eyes of subjects aged 2–60 years. He found over-corrected aberration in 25 of the 31 children aged under 6, but above that age he found preponderance of the uncorrected type. Of the 42 subjects aged over 8, only one was found with over-corrected aberration. Cornsweet and Crane (1970) also reported on such an eye.

By a method similar to that shown in *Figure 15.4*, Jenkins proceeded to measure the semi-meridional spherical aberration of 12 eyes of subjects aged 18–34. Measurements were made not only on the relaxed eye, but also with −1.50 D and −2.50 D lenses in the spectacle plane to stimulate accommodation. His mean results for both halves of the vertical meridian are plotted in *Figure 15.8(d)*. Results for the horizontal meridian showed less asymmetry, both nasal and temporal sides generally resembling the upper semi-meridian. With the 2.50 D stimulus to accommodation, all semi-meridians were found to have become over-corrected.

For ease of comparison, three results from these investigations have been redrawn on identical grids (*Figure 15.8*), together with the curve for the unaccommodated schematic eye. A different grid was necessary to show the results of Jenkins.

A few generalizations can be ventured on the basis of the limited data available:

(1) Unlike chromatic aberration, ocular spherical aberration varies considerably from person to person.
(2) It rarely shows axial symmetry. The findings of Ames and Proctor are, in general, supported by the results of retinoscopic and other objective measurements of ocular refraction in different pupillary areas of the same eye.
(3) Within a central pupillary area of about 1 mm diameter, the aberration is of the uncorrected type in the relaxed eye and slightly less than that of the schematic eye. As the diameter of the zone increases, the spherical aberration continues to increase but at a much slower rate.
(4) The effect of accommodation is to reduce the amount of uncorrected spherical aberration and occasionally to convert it into the over-corrected type.

In general, the corneal profile is closer in form to an ellipse than a circle. There is little doubt that its peripheral flattening contributes to reducing the eye's spherical aberration, though the mean *p*-values of 0.7 (see pages 391–394) would still leave a schematic eye with considerable aberration (a curve almost midway between (a) and (b) of *Figure 15.7*. The crystalline lens, either by way of its flattening or its refractive index gradient, may also contribute to the reduction in spherical aberration. Although the experiments of Millodot and Sivak (1974) indicate that the crystalline lens plays no role in reducing the aberration of the unaccommodated eye, the reduction which accompanies accommodation can be explained by the reasonable assumption that the front surface (especially) of the lens assumes a shape of relative peripheral flattening as its curvature increases.

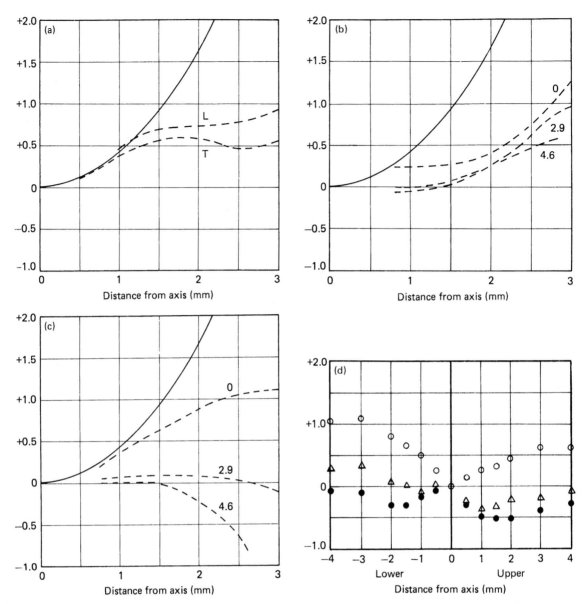

Figure 15.8. Experimental results of the external spherical aberration of the eye. In graphs (a) to (c) the solid line shows the aberration of the relaxed schematic eye. (a) After Ames and Proctor (1921). L: lower quadrant, T: temporal quadrant. (b) and (c) after Koomen *et al.* (1949). Numbers on curves denote stimulus to accommodation. (d) After Jenkins (1963). ○ accommodation relaxed, ● 2.5 D stimulus to accommodation.

Other monochromatic aberrations

The centred optical system of the schematic eye together with the assumption that the image lies on the optical axis means that only spherical aberration is important, coma and other asymmetric aberrations being irrelevant. *Figures 15.7 (a)* and (*b*) show that the aberration of real eyes differs in various quadrants. Possible causes are asymmetry in any of the refracting surfaces, with, for example, steeper curves on one side of the optical axis than the other, lack of centration of the ocular surfaces, a decentred pupil and the fact that the fovea lies some 5° to the side of the optical axis.

The experimental techniques of Koomen *et al.* (1949) using annular apertures meant that only a mean value for spherical aberration could be investigated. They later suggested (Koomen *et al.*, (1956) that the asym-

metrical results of other techniques could be a result of choosing an incorrect position for the reference axis. Although Ivanoff (1953, 1956) used the achromatic axis as his reference, both Jenkins (1963) and Campbell *et al.* (1990) used the centre of the pupil. Campbell and colleagues used a modified version of Ivanoff's technique (*Figure 15.4*), the decentred beam entering the pupil through a Maxwellian view system, the reference beam through the whole pupil area.

Figure 15.9(a) shows an eye with positive spherical aberration, the paraxial conjugates being at B and B′. A ray leaving the fovea through the top of the pupil intercepts the object plane below B at U, while a ray through the bottom of the pupil passes above B. A plot of the intercept height, *a*, against pupil locus *y* is, as shown in the inset, an odd-powered function of *y*. First-order spherical aberration, in these terms, would be

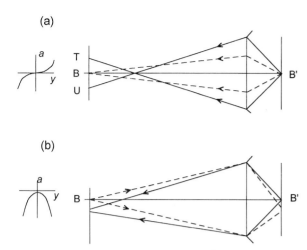

Figure 15.9.   Effects of (a) spherical and (b) comatic aberration on rays emerging from the eye from the top and bottom of the pupil. The inset figures show a plot of deviation *a* in the object plane against emerging height *y* in the pupil.

proportional to y^3. *Figure 15.9(b)* shows an eye with a coma-like aberration. Although a paraxial bundle leaving B would be imaged at B', peripheral rays might intercept the retina below B', giving an asymmetric blurred image. Conversely, rays leaving B' through the top and bottom of the pupil would both pass below B. A plot of *a* against *y* would now be an even-powered function of *y*, for example $a \propto y^2$.

Campbell and colleagues' results show some subjects with mostly spherical aberration, and others with mostly comatic aberration, while another showed virtually no aberration.

Wave-front aberrations

A subjective method of measuring the eye's monochromatic aberrations has been described by Howland and Howland (1977), while Charman (1991) provides a more recent review. Like the 'aberroscope' described by Tscherning (1924), it depends on projecting the shadow of a grating on to the subject's retina, but it uses a more sensitive means of doing so. From a drawing made by the subject of the distorted grid pattern as observed, it is possible to construct and interpret a numerical equation to the wave aberration surface at the pupil. One of the conclusions reached is that spherical aberration is often of a largely meridional character. Another is that coma, an aberration hitherto regarded as unimportant in the eye, plays a dominant role in the wave equation at all pupil sizes.

A notable advance in this method was announced in a paper by Walsh and Charman (1985). By means of an ophthalmoscopic arrangement, the distorted retinal image of the square grid can be photographed. The results obtained from the 10 subjects examined are reproduced, together with computer-generated contour maps of the wave-front departures from the ideal plane surface. From these, in turn, drawings giving a three-dimensional impression of the wave-front surface were produced and are displayed in the paper.

The results indicate that when the pupil diameter exceeds about 3 mm, marked differences between individual eyes are revealed. They also show that the wave-front is rarely symmetrical about the pupil centre. This is further demonstrated in a subsequent paper (1988) in which the wave-front aberrations of two eyes are expressed in sphero-cylindrical notation for small isolated regions, decentred 1, 2 or 3 mm along meridians at 15° intervals. This asymmetry was also shown to give different results for the modulation transfer functions when calculated for 2 and 3 mm artificial pupils decentred horizontally in each direction. Atchison *et al.* (1995) measured the variation in aberrations with accommodation in 15 subjects. They found two subjects showing increased wave-front aberration with increasing accommodation, three with decreasing aberration, eight with maximum aberration at 1.5 D of accommodation, and the remaining two with minimum aberration at this level. Comatic aberrations were four times as pronounced as spherical aberration.

The most recent development (Walsh and Cox, 1995) is to replace the photographic camera with a video device, thus recording the image in a form allowing immediate computer calculation of the wave-front. While the wave-front aberration is more difficult to understand than a refractive error, it enables the optical performance of the eye to be determined in the form of the MTF. The MTF may also be calculated from the point spread function. Thus Santamaria *et al.* (1987) used a video-computer analysing system to record the image of a point light source after the double passage of light in and out of the eye. This, however, again normally gives a radially symmetrical pattern to the apparent aberrations. Artal *et al.* (1995) pointed out that coma could be demonstrated if the diameters of the beams entering and leaving the eye were of unequal size.

A promising objective technique for the measurement of wave aberrations is the use of a Hartmann–Shack wave-front sensor (Liang *et al.*, 1994). In this, a point source of light is focused on the retina to form a secondary source. The emerging wave-front passes through a cylindrical lens array which is formed by two rows of cylindrical lenses placed at right-angles, rather like two trial case Maddox rods superimposed. This gives an array of 1 mm square lenses, each of focal length 170 mm. A perfect wave-front emerging from an emmetropic eye would give a regular grid of spots on the CCD photodetector, just as the aberroscope would give a regular grid pattern on the retina of a perfect eye. The computer linked to the CCD calculates the wave-front aberration. The published data of the two eyes that were measured again shows coma to be as or more important than spherical aberration. Cox and Merino (1996) found the method to give repeatable results on the 10 eyes examined, while Smith *et al.* (1996) give a mathematical analysis.

Hemenger *et al.* (1996) converted the corneal shape data given by a video-keratoscope (*see* Chapter 20) to the wave-front aberrations produced by refraction at the cornea alone. As shown by the eye chosen for illustration, the typical asymmetry of corneal curvature produces comatic aberration.

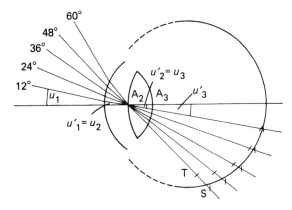

Figure 15.10.   The tangential and sagittal foci of the relaxed Bennett–Rabbetts schematic eye for a distant object and various angles of incidence. The image shells straddle the retina, with the tangential in front of the sagittal as in *Figure 13.23*.

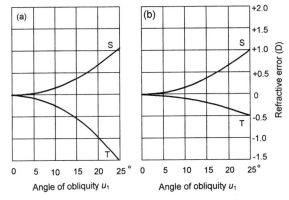

Figure 15.11.   Refractive errors in the sagittal (S) and tangential (T) meridians caused by oblique astigmatism of the ray bundles emerging from the relaxed Bennett–Rabbetts schematic eye: (a) spherical cornea, (b) paraboloidal cornea. Note the reduced astigmatism in (b).

Oblique aberrations

Pencils entering the eye

Objects in the peripheral field are seen by virtue of obliquely incident narrow pencils of rays which are limited by the pupil. Because of this, the refracted pencils show oblique astigmatism. Each one has two principal sections. The tangential (meridional) one lies in the plane containing the chief ray of the pencil and the eye's optical axis; the sagittal (radial) one is perpendicular to the tangential. Thus, a pencil incident on the cornea directly above its centre has its tangential section vertical and its sagittal section horizontal. As with all astigmatic pencils, the two focal lines are each perpendicular to the meridian to which they are related. In this instance, the tangential focal line would be horizontal and the sagittal line vertical.

For a given object distance, the centres of the focal lines formed by pencils entering the eye from all directions lie on two curved surfaces known as the tangential and sagittal image shells. Thomas Young calculated their curvatures for a typical human eye as long ago as 1800, showing that they straddled the retina. Similar results are found by calculation on modern schematic eyes. For example, *Figure 15.10* shows, to scale, the positions of the tangential and sagittal focal lines of five pencils from a distant object plane, incident at different obliquities u_1, on the relaxed Bennett–Rabbetts eye. If the spherical cornea of this eye were replaced by an ellipsoidal or even a paraboloidal surface, the effect on the curvature of the image shells would be relatively slight. Although becoming flatter they would continue to straddle the retina, so that the circles of least confusion would remain very close to it. There is no doubt that the curvature of the retina is admirably adapted to the eye's optical system.

Pencils emerging from the eye (peripheral astigmatism)

Emergent pencils from the peripheral retina are also afflicted with oblique astigmatism. With a reversal of

sign, their sagittal and tangential vergences express the eye's refractive error in these two meridians at the given obliquity or field angle (u_1 in *Figure 15.9*). The algebraic difference between the two vergences has been termed the eye's peripheral astigmatism. *Figure 15.11* shows the results of two sets of calculations on the unaccommodated Bennett–Rabbetts schematic eye, with a spherical cornea ($p = 1$) and with a paraboloidal cornea ($p = 0$) (*see* page 282). Ellipsoidal corneas would give results intermediate between these two.

The differences between graphs (a) and (b) arise from one of the properties of conicoidal surfaces. As conic sections with the same vertex radius progress from the circular through the ellipses to the parabolic and hyperbolic forms, the sagittal[*] radius of curvature at a given distance from the axis becomes longer. At the same time, the tangential radius of curvature increases at an appreciably faster rate. As a result, the oblique errors, as plotted in *Figure 15.11*, both move in the direction of hypermetropia, but the tangential approximately twice as much as the sagittal.

Experimental determinations of the ocular refraction at various angles of obliquity can be made with an objective optometer. In one such study, Ferree and Rand (1932) reported on 21 eyes examined with a Zeiss parallax optometer (*see* previous editions of this text). The refraction was measured at various angles of horizontal obliquity up to 60° on each side of the fixation axis. The eyes had been selected to include pronounced as well as slight errors of central refraction. Three of them exhibited marked asymmetry between the nasal and temporal fields. The others fell into two recognizable categories. Twelve, designated as type A, were found to have oblique errors in general conformity with the pattern of the graph in *Figure 15.11(a)*, while the remaining six (type B) presented the essential features of the graph in *Figure 15.11(b)*.

Though it is reasonable to assume that type B could result from a greater than usual degree of peripheral

---

[*] The sagittal meridian is perpendicular to the tangential, which contains the incident ray and the optimal axis.

corneal flattening, there is another contributory factor. According to Gliddon (1929), it is generally accepted that the retinal radius of curvature is one-half of the overall length of the eye and the calculations for *Figure 15.11* were made on this basis. Any shortening of this radius, with all other dimensions remaining unchanged, would make both principal meridians of the emergent pencil less convergent or more divergent. As a result, the corresponding refractive errors would move in the direction of hypermetropia, towards type B.

Conversely, a lengthening of the retinal radius would make the emergent pencil less divergent or more convergent. The result could be to produce a third type (C) in which the refraction is myopic in both principal meridians, the tangential one having the greater error. Plotted as in *Figure 15.11*, both curves would lie below the horizontal zero line. Obviously an uncorrected myopic eye would be expected to show myopia in the periphery: it is the relative change between the central and peripheral refraction that is of interest.

Variation with ametropia

Figure 15.11 applies to the emmetropic eye. The effect of axial ametropia was briefly considered by Bennett (1951), whose calculated values of peripheral astigmatism were mainly for emmetropic eyes. He assumed the retina to remain spherical and of radius half the axial length. Although the amount of peripheral astigmatism was found to increase in myopia and decrease in hypermetropia, its pattern remained in the type A category over the ametropic range from $-10\,D$ to $+5\,D$.

Measurements by Millodot (1981) on 62 eyes (32 subjects) showed a more fundamental difference between the results in the three main refractive groups. The peripheral astigmatism of the emmetropes was found to be generally of type A, with the hypermetropes in type B and the myopes in type C. These results clearly point to a discernible pattern of change in retinal curvature in relation to ametropia.

A possible basis for such a variation has been advanced by Dunne *et al.* (1987). It assumes the ametropia to be axial, and all such eyes to have a retina of the same equatorial radius. The retina is then envisaged as a semi-ellipsoid in which the semi-minor axis *b* is invariable, while the semi-major axis *a* varies according to the given eye's refractive error. Calculations on this basis showed values of tangential and sagittal errors in conformity with the classifications found by Millodot. This would also agree with the present author's (RBR) observations that the periphery of many medium to high myopes' fundi are less myopic in ophthalmoscopy than the posterior pole.

General agreement with Ferree and Rand's results was shown by Jenkins (1963) for the horizontal and vertical semi-meridians of 10 eyes. Except for one eye, the tangential foci were always in front of the retina, but the position of the sagittal foci varied. Five of the eyes conformed substantially to type A and one to type B, while the others fluctuated between the two at different angles of obliquity or in different semi-meridians.

Some degree of asymmetry has been reported by all investigators, varying from the slight to the pronounced. In the horizontal meridian, differences between the temporal and nasal sides are associated with the tilt of the crystalline lens described by Tscherning. A detailed study of the effects of a tilted lens and cornea, and also of an off-axis translation of the cornea has been made by Barnes *et al.* (1987). The effects of corneal tilt and translation on the eye's entrance pupil were also considered. A corneal tilt was suggested as a reason for large amounts of asymmetry in peripheral astigmatism.

Retinoscopy has also been used as a means of estimating the ocular refraction at various degrees of obliquity, for example, by Hodd (1951) and Rempt *et al.* (1971). In this later study, both eyes of 442 subjects were examined. Further analysis of these results by Lotmar and Lotmar (1974) demonstrated a spread of astigmatism, most eyes showing between 1 and 5 D at 40° eccentricity, with no suggestion of a breakdown into types A and B. If angle alpha was taken as 4°, the nasal and temporal results were found to be symmetrical.

Figure 15.11 shows the importance of performing retinoscopy as close as possible to the patient's visual axis. If the axis of observation is to one side of it, the tangential meridian is horizontal and a minus cylinder axis vertical would be needed to correct the induced oblique astigmatism.

Aberrations of pseudophakic eyes

The spherical aberration of pseudophakic eyes will be reduced if the intra-ocular lens is designed to be almost convex-plano in form, with a shallow convex curve for the back surface. To minimize coma, a posterior chamber implant conversely requires a meniscus lens with an anterior concave surface. The retinal image size will be nearest that of the previously phakic eye with a posterior chamber implant of plano-convex form, so that its principal points lie close to those of the original crystalline lens. At present, intra-ocular lenses are manufactured with spherical surfaces, but aspherical surfaces could be employed to reduce aberrations. For further discussion, the reader is directed to papers by Smith and Lu (1988), Atchison (1989a,b) and González *et al.* (1996).

Aberrations of contact lens wearing eyes

Rigid lenses

When a rigid contact lens is worn on an eye, the tear lens neutralizes most of the refraction at the anterior corneal surface, and hence also its contribution to the reduction in ocular spherical aberration from its peripheral flattening. Thus a contact lens with a spherical front surface would be expected to increase the overall spherical aberration. Cox (1990) points out, however, that negatively powered lenses with their flatter front surfaces will induce less positive spherical aberration than plus powered lenses. Collins *et al.* (1992) fitted a group of low to moderate myopes with rigid lenses having spherical or flattening front surfaces. Nine subjects preferred the spherical lenses, three preferred lenses with a front surface of *p*-value 0.74, while all rejected lenses having a *p*-value of 0.49. A complication of rigid lens wear is that the lenses move relative to the visual axis. As Atchison (1995) points out, movement of lenses with aspherical front surfaces will induce coma, and thus may give a poorer image when poorly centred than a lens with spherical surfaces.

Rigid lenses with an aspherically flattening back surface are frequently fitted to provide a theoretically better mechanical fit on the cornea. The back surface has a reduced negative power towards the periphery, and although the effect on the eye is only about one-third of the effect in air, the overall action of the lens will be towards a relatively more positive power in the periphery compared to the centre.

Soft lenses

The back surface of soft lenses drapes closely to the cornea, and thus the front surface of low-powered lenses may adopt a similar asphericity to that of the cornea. Cox (1990) calculated that high-powered negative lenses became even more aspheric (lower *p*-value) while positively powered lenses transferred less of the corneal asphericity through to the front surface.

Because soft lenses centre much better to the cornea, aspherical surfaces may give more consistent changes to the overall ocular aberrations. Thus the peripheral back surface flattening of spun-cast lenses translates into peripheral steepening of the anterior lens surface. Similarly, there are lenses manufactured with peripheral steepening of the front surface (Patel, 1991) to counteract an assumed average spherical aberration of the eye. As has already been pointed out, there is considerable variation in ocular aberration, so that it seems unlikely that any single lens design could benefit all eyes.

Depth of field

Definitions

Largely because of the aberrations already described, there is a certain latitude in the eye's focusing. The terms 'depth of focus' and 'depth of field' tend to be used indiscriminately but their meanings are quite distinct.

Depth of focus

For a given object distance, the depth of focus is the distance through which the image-receiving surface can be moved without detriment to the quality of the image; or, given a fixed image-receiving surface, the greatest focusing error consistent with this requirement.

Depth of field

Applied to the eye in a given state of accommodation, the depth of field is the range of object distances (which may be expressed in dioptres) within which the visual acuity does not detectably deteriorate.

The depth of field in object space can be regarded as conjugate with the depth of focus in image space.

An eye seeing clearly an object at a dioptric distance L_o would obtain the same standard of vision for other objects lying between the distal end of the depth of field (dioptric distance L_d) and the proximal end (dioptric distance L_p). Expressed in dioptres, the depth of field is $(L_d - L_p)$. If L_d and L_p are equally spaced dioptrically about L_o, then

$$L_d = L_o + E$$

$$L_p = L_o - E$$

and depth of field $= \pm E$ (dioptres)   (15.12)

A low value of E denotes high sensitivity, inasmuch as the object position then becomes more critical and the depth of focus smaller.

Example (1)

$$L_o = -2.50 \,\text{D}; \quad E = \pm 0.25 \,\text{D}$$

$$L_d = -2.25 \,\text{D so that } \ell_d = -444 \,\text{mm}$$

$$L_p = -2.75 \,\text{D so that } \ell_p = -364 \,\text{mm}$$

(Linear) depth of field = 80 mm

However, if E has the larger value of $\pm 0.50 \,\text{D}$, these quantities become

$$L_d = -2.00 \,\text{D so that } \ell_d = -500 \,\text{mm}$$

$$L_p = -3.00 \,\text{D so that } \ell_p = -333 \,\text{mm}$$

(Linear) depth of field = 167 mm

The concept of 'hyperfocal distance', originating in photography, has also been applied to the eye. It denotes the value of L_o for which the distal end of the depth of field lies at infinity. In this case,

$$L_d = 0 \text{ and } L_o = -E \text{ so that}$$

$$L_p = L_o - E = -2E$$

Vision would thus remain at the same standard for all distances from infinity to the linear equivalent of $-2E$ dioptres.

Experimental determinations

The variables affecting the eye's depth of field have been studied by Campbell (1957). He found that the depth of field became smaller as illumination and luminance contrast were increased.

With increasing pupil diameters, the retinal blur circles become larger and so the retinal image goes more quickly out of focus, again reducing the depth of field. In exploring this relationship, Campbell kept the retinal illumination constant for all pupil diameters, taking into account the Stiles–Crawford effect. To a close

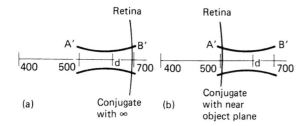

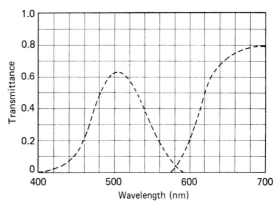

Figure 15.12. Depth of focus of the human eye. The bold arcs indicate the waist of the image focus over which acuity remains constant. The rear of the waist falls on the retina in distance vision (a), the front in near vision (b). Although spherical aberration contributes to the waist, the superimposed wavelength scale indicates the tendency for red or green focus in distance or near vision.

Figure 15.13. Transmittance curves of Courtoid Red 15 and Green 16 filter material, both 0.25 mm thick.

approximation his results are fitted by the empirical equation.

$$E = \pm\{(0.75/g) + 0.08\} \qquad (15.13)$$

in which the pupil diameter g is in millimetres.

Given optimum conditions of illumination and contrast, Campbell found the depth of field to be about $\pm 0.3\,D$ for a pupil size of 3 mm. This is somewhat larger than most previous determinations and estimates. However, as Ogle and Schwartz (1959) pointed out in their own study, experimental results are affected not only by the test method, but also by the criterion adopted for out-of-focus blurring. To the extent that comparison is possible, their own results are of the same order as Campbell's.

The manner in which the eye exploits its depth of focus merits attention. In distance vision (*Figure 15.12a*), it would clearly be advantageous to have the posterior end B′ of the depth of focus placed near the retina, with the anterior end A′ conjugate with infinity. Optimum vision would thus be obtained at all distances from infinity to the plane of B, conjugate with B′ in the depth of focus. In near vision at close range (*Figure 15.12b*) the situation is reversed because it would be advantageous for the depth of field to extend beyond the plane of regard. This change of retinal intercept with object distance minimizes the accommodative adjustment needed between distance and near vision and vice versa. It supports the resting-state theory of accommodation outlined in Chapter 7.

These theoretical assumptions have been confirmed experimentally by Ivanoff (1953). His method was to use the eye's chromatic aberration as a measuring scale and to determine which wavelength was focused on the retina in different states of accommodation. Ivanoff found that the relaxed eye focused a wavelength of approximately 680 nm on the retina. As accommodation was brought into play, the wavelength focused gradually moved towards the blue end of the spectrum, reaching about 500 nm with 2.50 D of accommodation in use. In terms of dioptres, this shift represents approximately 0.70 D or ± 0.35 D from a zero mean.

Results very similar to Ivanoff's were later obtained by Kellershohn *et al.* (1957), who also found that the eye's depth of focus is used in essentially the same way whatever the source of illumination used. Similar results were later reported by Millodot and Sivak (1973) who

made measurements over the extended range of accommodative stimuli from 0.65 to 8.3 D.

Bichromatic test filters

The clinical use of red–green bichromatic tests has been discussed on pages 96–97. For any such tests to operate efficiently, the coloured filters used must be chosen carefully.

The transmittance curves of two cellulose acetate materials meeting the requirements of the relevant British Standard* are reproduced in *Figure 15.13*. They are now called Courtoid Green 16 and Red 15 and both are 0.25 mm thick. Bichromatic tests are normally illuminated with tungsten-filament lamps. To assess the effect of the filters, the spectral luminous efficiency curve for the standard CIE observer weighted for Standard Illuminant A should be referred to (*see Figure 15.1b*). The numerical value at each wavelength must be multiplied by the transmittance of the filter, expressed as a fraction. *Figure 15.14* shows the result of this operation. For the green filter, the peak wavelength is at approximately 535 nm, while the peak for the red is at approximately 620 nm.

The scale above the graph shows the value of ΔK (chromatic difference of refraction) with its zero at 570 nm. It was constructed from the mean experimental values plotted in *Figure 15.5*, adjusted by the addition of +0.09 D to shift the zero point from wavelength 587.6 to 570 nm. For the green filter, the wavelength of peak luminous efficiency is at approximately 539 nm, corresponding to myopia of −0.21 D, while for the red filter the peak wavelength is at approximately 620 nm, corresponding to hypermetropia of +0.24 D. Thus, if the green half of the test is in focus, the addition of +0.50 DS would bring the red on to the retina.

It is important that the two filters should have approximately equal luminous transmittance (formerly known as integrated visible transmission). This quantity can be calculated from the data plotted in *Figure 15.14* and is proportional to the area enclosed by the curve

---

* BS 3668: *Red and green filters used in ophthalmic dichromatic and dissociation tests.*

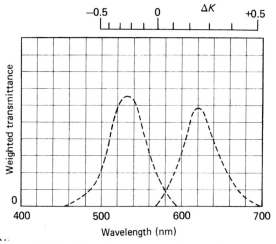

Figure 15.14. Transmittance curves of Courtoid Red 15 and Green 16 material of 0.25 mm thickness weighted for both the spectral luminous efficiency and Standard Illuminant A. Ordinate scale in arbitrary units from zero. The superimposed scale shows the chromatic difference of refraction.

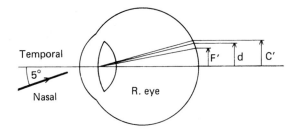

Figure 15.15. The transverse spectrum formed in the macular region when a positive angle alpha is associated with a centred pupil. View of right eye from above.

and the *x*-axis. It can be seen that the two materials in question are reasonably well matched in this respect. Their luminance transmittance is, in fact, about 18.6% for the green filter and 15.9% for the red.

For the protanope these figures are no longer valid and although the principle of the test is otherwise little affected, the marked reduction in the luminosity of the red panel must introduce a bias.

It was pointed out on page 289 that as accommodation is brought into play, the wavelength focused on the retina moves towards the blue end of the spectrum. If red–green equality is taken as the end-point in bichromatic near vision tests, the reading addition prescribed on that basis may be theoretically 0.25 D or even 0.50 D too strong. For this reason, Wilmut (1958) advocated the use of blue and yellow filters so as to shift the mid-point of the test by about 0.25 D in comparison with the normal green and red filters. In practice, the conventional red–green bichromatic test provides an excellent procedure for the presbyopic patient (*see* page 121). Nine out of 20 of Rosenfield *et al.*'s (1996) young subjects could not manage a blue–yellow test – the present writer suspects inadequate luminance to be the cause.

Chromatic stereopsis

Major factors

Surface areas in the same vertical plane but of different colours appear to some observers to be at different distances from the eyes. This phenomenon is called chromatic stereopsis. It is a true stereoscopic effect, disappearing when one eye is closed. According to a well-known saying among artists, red is an 'advancing' colour, whereas green and blue are 'retreating' colours. Though this may be a majority viewpoint, many people see the opposite effect.

Chromatic stereopsis appears most strongly when two colours from opposite ends of the spectrum are placed close together and viewed against a black ground. When viewed against a white ground a reversal of the effect is usually observed, though to a lesser extent.

Brucke (1868), one of the earliest investigators of the phenomenon, rightly concluded that it was caused by the eye's chromatic aberration, coupled with its optical asymmetry. He mentioned, in particular, the angle alpha. It was left to Einthoven (1885) to fill in the picture by drawing attention to the role of pupillary decentration. The illusion can be enhanced, neutralized or reversed by observing the scene through variably decentred pinhole apertures or horizontal prisms.

The effect of the angle alpha is explained by *Figure 15.15*. This represents an unaccommodated schematic emmetropic eye with the pupil centred on the optical axis but with a positive angle alpha of 5°. To be focused on the fovea, an incident pencil of parallel rays must be inclined at a horizontal angle of 5° to the optical axis, as shown. The distance *y* from this axis at which the ray passing through the centre of the pupil impinges on the retina can be calculated as outlined on pages 278–279. The results for three different wavelengths are as follows:

Wavelength (nm)	Distance *y* (mm)
F′ = 480.0 (blue)	1.442
d = 587.6 (yellow)	1.446
C′ = 643.8 (red)	1.448

In binocular vision, red would thus appear nearer than blue in the absence of other factors, if the angle alpha is positive. Though the dispersion of 0.006 mm shown by this table may seem extremely small, even modest levels of stereoscopic acuity depend on much smaller disparities than this (*see* pages 191–192). It should, however, be pointed out that the incident pencils of all out-of-focus wavelengths will form a series of overlapping blur circles (or ellipses) of varying size. The selected chief rays shown in *Figure 15.15* determine the geometrical centres of the respective retinal blurs. The effect of pupillary decentration is shown in *Figure 15.16*, which represents a horizontal section through the right eye viewed from above. In the schematic eye, the position of the exit pupil H′J′ varies very little with wavelength and in this context can be taken as fixed. The points B′ (blue) and R′ (red) refer to the foci for parallel incident pencils making an angle of 5° with the

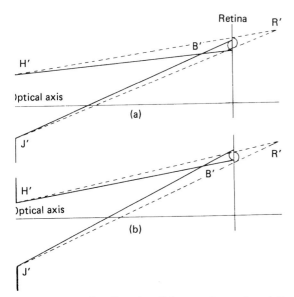

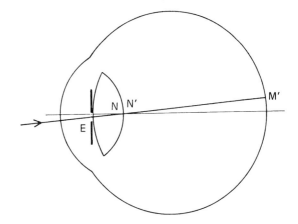

Figure 15.18. The chief rays of all wavelengths closely follow a common path to the fovea when the pupil is centred on the nodal axis.

Figure 15.16. The effect of pupil decentration on the relative positions of the red and green blur circles: (a) centred pupil, (b) pupil decentred nasally. Right eye viewed from above, with a positive angle alpha.

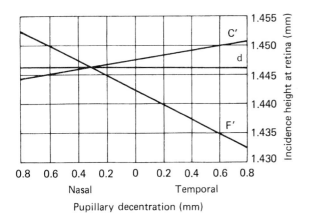

Figure 15.17. Incident height *y* on the retina of the chief ray through the pupil (from *Figure 15.15*) as a function of pupillary decentration. Plots of red (C′), yellow (d) and blue (F′) light.

optical axis, corresponding to a typical angle alpha. In *Figure 15.16(a)*, the pupil is centred with respect to the optical axis. If the retina is assumed to lie between the blue and red foci, overlapping blur circles will be formed on it, as indicated by the limiting ray paths. It is the red circle which, of the two, lies further from the optical axis. For clarity, their relative positions have been indicated by semi-circles drawn on opposite sides of the retina. If the pupil is sufficiently decentred inwards, the altered ray paths reverse the relative positions of the overlapping blur circles, as shown in *Figure 15.16(b)*.

Figure 15.15 shows the distance *y* from the optical axis at which the rays through the centre of the pupil impinge on the retina when the pupil is itself centred. If the pupil is decentred, a different ray of the incident pencil will pass through its centre and meet the retina at a different distance from the optical axis. *Figure 15.17* shows the variation in *y* with pupillary

decentration for three different colours, the d-line wavelength being assumed to be in focus on the retina. The calculations were based on the Gullstrand–Emsley unaccommodated schematic eye, with the angle alpha taken as 5°. It will be noted that the effect of such an angle would be neutralized by an inward pupillary decentration of about 0.3 mm.

It is most probably the relationship between these two major factors which determines individual awareness of chromatic stereopsis and especially whether red or green is seen in front in comparable conditions.

The conditions whereby rays of different wavelengths in the same incident pencil can re-unite at the fovea after following slightly different paths within the eye is illustrated in *Figure 15.18*. Like the eye's principal points, its nodal points are barely affected by changes of wavelength. Given a positive angle alpha, with the fovea on the temporal side of the optical axis, the principal ray path to the fovea via the nodal points is as shown in the figure. Consequently, if the pupil centre E is located on this ray path, the necessary condition is satisfied. Simple calculation shows that with a positive angle alpha of 5°, the required inward decentration of the pupil is approximately 0.3 mm. This agrees with the result given in *Figure 15.17*.

Chromatic stereopsis results from the binocular effects of transverse chromatic aberration. Rynders *et al.* (1995), using crosses of red or green light, or black on a red or green background, investigated the subjective TCA of 170 eyes. The mean value found was close to zero, suggesting that as a whole, the pupil is well centred to the nodal axis to the fovea both horizontally and vertically. If, however, the direction of the chromatic aberration is ignored, the mean TCA at the fovea was 0.83 minutes of arc, equivalent to a decentration of less than 0.4 mm of the pupil from the nodal axis.

A simple approximate equation relating the chromatic variation of magnification, CVM, and ΔK was derived for a simple reduced eye by Zhang *et al.* (1991):

$$CVM = EN\,\Delta K \qquad (15.14)$$

where EN is the distance between the entrance pupil and first nodal point, as in *Figure 15.18*. A more detailed formulation is given in Thibos *et al.* (1990), while Bradley *et al.* (1991) point out that an artificial pupil placed in front of the eye gives an exaggerated value for the chromatic variation of magnification because it increases the effective distance EN.

Reversal and other effects

Those who see red in front of blue on a black ground in good illumination may experience a reversal of the effect as the illumination is reduced. Although the precise reason for this is still uncertain, there is little doubt that it is the change of pupil diameter which is responsible. One theory is that pupillary dilation in such cases is eccentric. An alternative explanation by Vos (1960, 1963) is based on the directional sensitivity of the retina (Stiles–Crawford effect). Contrary to the eccentric dilation hypothesis, Sundet (1976) found that when the natural pupil is dilated and replaced by a series of carefully centred artificial pupils of different size, the reversal effect still occurred.

A partial explanation may be the eye's increasing spherical aberration as the pupil dilates. In *Figure 15.16*, the ray paths determining the outer extremities of the two blur circles are $H'R'$ (red) and $J'B'$ (blue). The effect of spherical aberration with a larger pupil would be to deviate both limiting ray paths further towards the axis, as a result of which they could well cross over before reaching the retina, even when the pupil is centred.

The reversal which normally occurs when the two coloured areas are viewed against a white ground was explained in principle by Einthoven (1885). It is due to the dispersion of light from the white areas at their lateral boundary with the coloured areas. The horizontal spectrum formed at the fovea by the effect of a positive angle alpha is similar to that produced by a base-in prism. If the object shown in *Figure 15.19(a)* is viewed through a horizontal prism with its base to the left, a blue fringe will appear along the right-hand side of the enclosed white area and a reddish fringe on the left-hand side. *Figure 15.19(b)* represents a red and a blue area, initially on a black ground. When viewed through a horizontal prism with its base to the left, the red area is displaced less than the blue, resulting in the appearance illustrated in *Figure 15.19(c)*. If, however, the background is white instead of black, the coloured areas are displaced as previously but modified by the fringes from the surrounding white area (*Figure 15.19d*). At their right-hand side (the left-hand side of the white surround) the red fringe extends the upper red area to the right while encroaching on the blue to give a whitish overlap. At the left-hand side, the blue fringe from the white surround extends the blue area to the left while encroaching on the red. The resulting effect can be neatly demonstrated by projecting a slide made from transparent coloured materials and holding a horizontal prism in front of the projector lens.

As commercial artists are aware, striking effects can be produced by black and white areas on a blue or red ground. *Figure 15.19(e)* represents a black and white

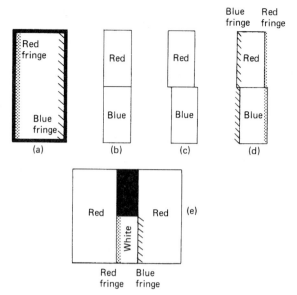

Figure 15.19. Modification of images by chromatic dispersion when the object is on a white or coloured background. (a) A black rectangular outline viewed through a prism with its base to the left, (b) an object, (c) its image seen through the prism and (d) its image with a spectrum fringe. (e) The similar effect produced when a black and white object on a red ground is viewed through a prism with its base to the left.

strip of equal width with their edges aligned, surrounded by a red area. Viewed by the right eye through a prism base in, the entire pattern would apparently be displaced to the right. Moreover, the left edge of the white strip would appear additionally displaced by the merging of the red fringe with the red surround. Similarly, the right-hand edge would seem additionally displaced to the right by the whitish overlap of the blue fringe and the red surround. Relatively to the black strip, the white strip is now seen temporalwards, suggesting that it is more distant than the black.

If black is seen nearer than white on a red ground, the reverse will appear on a blue ground. These are the effects normally observed by those who see red nearer than blue on a black ground. The corresponding opposite relationships also apply.

An interesting perceptual effect can be observed when two adjacent vertical strips, one black and one white, are mounted on a background divided horizontally into red and blue (or green) halves. Theory predicts that the two strips would appear broken, the top half of one seeming to be nearer than the bottom half, and vice versa for the other strip. Refusing to accept that the strips are not continuous, the mind adopts a compromise solution. To many observers the strips appear to remain continuous but tilted in opposite directions about a horizontal axis.

A similar effect is produced when two separated concentric rings, one red and the other blue, are mounted on a background divided vertically into black and white halves. In this case, the rings may appear to be tilted in opposite directions about a vertical axis. Steady fixation for several seconds or more may be needed to give both effects enough time to develop.

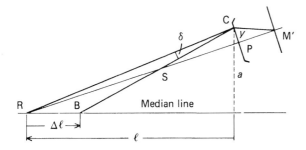

Figure 15.20. Narrow-beam stereoscopy: construction to determine the relationship between the various parameters.

Narrow-beam stereoscopy

Narrow-beam stereoscopy provides a means of increasing and measuring the effects of chromatic stereopsis. Results obtained in this way can then be compared with calculated figures. To isolate small areas of the pupil with variable horizontal decentration, adjustable pinhole or vertical stenopaeic apertures are placed before both eyes. Two adjacent vertical slits placed symmetrically about the median line (or one above the other) are illuminated by lights of different narrow wavebands of known peak values. One slit is fixed and the other movable along the median line. Both are seen against a black ground, with extraneous clues as to their location excluded as far as possible. With the pinhole or slit separations set for a range of different values in turn, the subject adjusts the position of the movable slit until it appears to be at the same distance as the other one.

The predicted result can be obtained from the geometry of *Figure 15.20*, in which R represents a fixed red object at a distance ℓ from the eyes and B a movable blue object. The visual axis is directed towards R and B has been moved a distance $\Delta\ell$ from R so that it appears in the same position as R. For simplicity, the pinhole aperture is assumed to be in contact with the eye. Its centre C is at a distance a from the median line and y from the visual axis, y being taken as positive when outwards (as in the diagram) and negative when inwards. The left eye, not shown in the diagram, is assumed to be in symmetrical relationship. Let S be the point on the visual axis where it is intersected by the ray BC. The eye's chromatic difference of refraction with respect to R is then given by

$$\Delta K = 1/PS - 1/PR$$

and the angle δ measured from the ray RC to BC by

$$\delta = y/PS - y/PR = y\Delta K \tag{15.15}$$

The angle δ can also be expressed as

$$\delta = \{a/(\ell + \Delta\ell)\} - a/\ell$$

Equating these last two expressions we get

$$\Delta\ell = \frac{-y\ell^2\Delta K}{a + y\ell\Delta K} \tag{15.15a}$$

in which all distances are in metres. Since the two peak wavelengths of the colour filters are known, the corresponding value of ΔK can be found from *Figure 15.5*.

Example (1)

Let the given wavelengths be 480 nm (blue) and 620 nm (red) and let $\ell = -1$ m, $y = +2$ mm, and $a = 32$ mm.

For the given wavelengths, ΔK is approximately -0.88 D. Equation (15.15a) then gives, with all distances in metres,

$$\Delta\ell = \frac{-0.002 \times (-0.88)}{0.032 + 0.00176} = +0.052 \text{ m (52 mm)}$$

For simplicity, the angle alpha has been ignored in this approach. When the viewing distance is 1 m, the necessary correction is of the order of $2\Delta K$ mm per degree of angle alpha, to be added algebraically to the value of $\Delta\ell$ for positive values of alpha and subtracted algebraically for negative values. In the above example, if angle alpha is $+5°$, the correction is $(2 \times -0.88) \times 5$ or -8.8 mm.

Confirmation of this principle is given by Ye *et al.* (1991). They measured the induced transverse chromatic aberration of five subjects as a function of the displacement y of small artificial pupils in front of the eye under monocular conditions. The position of the achromatic axis for each eye, i.e. where there was no transverse chromatic aberration, was also determined. Under binocular conditions, the artificial pupils were initially placed on each eye's achromatic axis. They were then moved symmetrically outwards or inwards, and the chromatic stereopsis measured. Excellent agreement was obtained between these experimental results and the predictions from the monocular transverse chromatic aberration. As expected, outwards decentration of the artificial pupils resulted in the red stimulus appearing in front of the blue, requiring it to be positioned further away from the observer to appear coincident.

An additional experiment showed that it was the distance between the two artificial pupils relative to the distance between the two achromatic axes which governed the chromatic stereopsis. Thus a decentration of only one pupil through 2 mm was equivalent to a decentration of both pupils through 1 mm in opposite directions.

Monocular diplopia and polyopia

Monocular diplopia may have pathological or neurological causes but the most common variety is optical in origin. Typically, a faint secondary image of a suitable test object is observed, nearly always displaced in an approximately vertical direction and usually upwards. This angular displacement is of the order of 3–6 minutes of arc, the mean being equivalent to about 0.12Δ. Either or both eyes may be affected, but usually only one. In a study of 70 eyes of subjects between the ages of 18 and 45, Fincham (1963) found no fewer than 40% with monocular diplopia.

Investigating possible optical causes, Fincham was led to exclude the cornea and the surfaces of the crystalline lens. Experiments with a rotatable luminous slit as test object and with stenopaeic and pinhole apertures moved across the pupil suggested that the origin was

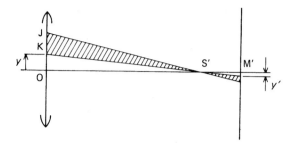

Figure 15.21. Monocular diplopia: region JK of the crystalline lens is more powerful, resulting in a ghost image indicated by the shaded ray bundle.

within the lens: specifically, in the upper part of the pupillary aperture. Within this area, a refractive index variation had the effect of a weak base-down prism. In many cases the faint secondary image was seldom noticed, even in visual tasks such as reading.

With the aid of his coincidence optometer (*see* previous editions of this text), Fincham was able to measure the ametropia in the upper and lower parts of the pupil separately. He found that although the horizontal refraction tended to remain unchanged, nearly every eye showed a difference in the vertical meridian. In all but 3 of the 70 eyes examined, the power of the eye was stronger in the upper part of the pupil, leading to relative myopia with respect to the lower half. The difference ranged from 0.50 to 1.75 D in 30 of the eyes. No monocular diplopia was detected in the remaining 37 eyes, having a difference less than 0.50 D. In nearly every case, the refraction in the lower half of the pupil agreed with the best correction found by subjective tests.

On the basis of Fincham's work it is possible to construct a hypothesis numerically consistent with his experimental findings. Monocular diplopia with the secondary image seen above the main image is evidently associated with relative myopia in an upper part of the pupillary area. This greater refractive power is accompanied by a base-down prismatic effect. It follows that the part of the crystalline lens associated with the secondary image must lie wholly above its optical centre and must also be relatively small, in keeping with the reduced brightness of this image.

In *Figure 15.21*, the actual crystalline lens is represented by a hypothetical thin lens placed at its optical centre O, about 2.4 mm behind its anterior vertex. The main image of an axial object point is formed on the fovea at M', while S' is the *optical* image formed in front of the retina by refraction through a relatively myopic upper area of the lens extending vertically from J to K. The secondary image *on the retina* is the blur bounded by rays through S' from J and K. If y is the height of K from the optical axis and y' the separation between the main and secondary images on the retina, then

$$y = -y'(OS'/S'M') \qquad (15.16)$$

Fincham's numerical results suggest that if the apparent angular separation of the diplopic images is 5 minutes of arc, this would correspond to relative myopia of about 1 D. If so, $S'M'$ would be approximately 0.4 mm while OS' would be about 17.5 mm in the Bennett–Rabbetts emmetropic eye. Also, to subtend 5 minutes at the nodal point, y' must be about −0.024 mm. With these values substituted in equation (15.16), we have

$$y = 0.024 \,(17.5/0.4) = 1.05 \,\text{mm}$$

which is a reasonable figure.

It is hard to visualize a local variation of refractive index capable of producing a relatively undistorted secondary image, unless it extends to the surfaces of the crystalline lens. We are therefore led to suppose an index variation such that a lens power of about +21 D is increased to + 22 D in a typical case. If the refractive indices of the humours and the lens are taken as 1.336 and 1.422 respectively, the necessary change Δn in the latter must be such that

$$22/21 = (1.422 + \Delta n - 1.336)/(1.422 - 1.336)$$

which gives

$$\Delta n \approx 0.004$$

This, too, is a not unreasonable figure. Partial occlusion of the pupil suggests that the affected area of the lens is narrow in width.

One of the authors (A.G.B.) had monocular polyopia in both eyes. Experiments in 1982 showed that the two perceived secondary images in the right eye were displayed obliquely downwards by about 6 minutes of arc from the main image at axes of approximately 60° and 120°. In the left eye, the similar patterns showed smaller displacements. At that time, each eye had about +2.50 D of absolute hypermetropia, with a VA better than 6/5 (20/15). Polyopia is sometimes attributed to incipient cataract, but no sign of this was then present. Polyopic images are most noticeable when the eye is out of focus for the object of regard. They may relate to the marked asymmetries of ocular wave-front aberrations of the type found by Walsh and Charman (1985) (*see* page 285).

In a comprehensive review and analysis by Amos (1982) of the previous literature, other possible optical causes (including corneal irregularities) are described. One is the presence of small extra-pupillary apertures in the iris, operating like the Scheiner disc to produce doubling of the retinal image when out of focus.

Irregular refraction

Irregular refraction may arise from a distortion or asymmetry of any ocular refracting surface or by index inhomogeneity of the crystalline lens. Corneal scars and early cataract are common causes. Keratoconus can produce very marked irregularity, though it is relatively uncommon, affecting only one in 10 000 or so.

Objective techniques will reveal irregularity but are seldom an adequate guide to the optimum correction.

Standard refractive procedures may be used in many cases and the best astigmatic correction found by the cross-cylinder technique. If the visual acuity is poor, the trial and error method described on page 105 may be adopted. The pinhole disc should be used to verify retinal integrity.

In cuneiform cataract, the crystalline lens is divided into areas which may differ in their refractive effect, with possibly more than one giving good acuity with the appropriate correction. In such cases, the lens power most similar to the previous prescription, or to that of the fellow eye, should be chosen. If monocular diplopia is experienced, its source may be located by gradually occluding the pupil from top to bottom or from side to side. A slight alteration to the correction may sufficiently reduce the intensity of the ghost image for the patient to ignore it.

The patient with irregular corneal curvature is best helped by a rigid contact lens because the tears layer between lens and cornea virtually neutralizes the latter's irregularities. Light scattered by anterior corneal scarring may be reduced for the same reason.

Scattered light

Sources of scatter

By reducing contrast, light scattered within the eye has an effect similar to aberrations, in that it degrades the retinal image. The crystalline lens and cornea are responsible for most of the scattered light but there are several other sources:

(1) diffuse reflection of obliquely incident light from peripheral parts of the retina and choroid, as at D in *Figure 15.22*;
(2) diffusion within the retina in the immediate vicinity of the image;
(3) multiple internal reflections, for example, light reflected back from the retina and returned by the crystalline lens or cornea;
(4) light penetrating the iris or sclera and choroid in the lightly pigmented eye, especially in albinos.

The angular distribution and wavelength dependence of the proportion of light scattered by an inhomogeneous substance depend upon the size of the scattering particle. Generalized equations for scattering by spherical particles were derived by Mie in 1908, and are described by Born and Wolf (1980). Particles a little larger than the wavelength of light mostly scatter in a forward direction. Work on corneal transparency (Farrell and McCally, 1976) showed that the wavelength dependency of scattering was proportional to λ^{-3}, but that in oedema, the scattered intensity became proportional to λ^{-2}. They considered that this was due to fibril-free 'lakes' about 230 nm in diameter. As the particle size decreases to significantly less than the wavelength of light, the scattered intensity becomes proportional to λ^{-4}, Rayleigh's law. Accordingly, blue light is scattered more than red. This is undoubtedly one reason for the yellowing of the crystalline lens with age, though the principal cause is pigmentation. Hemenger (1984) pointed out that Rayleigh scattering is in all directions, giving 'back-scattered' light. Hence the yellowing of the lens may be seen by the practitioner with a slit lamp. The entoptic phenomena of corneal and lenticular haloes are described in Chapter 22.

Because of the Stiles–Crawford effect, scattered light falling obliquely on the retina stimulates the retinal cones less than simple photometry would predict. The same undoubtedly applies to light diffusing within the retina. Nevertheless, the result is a veiling haze through which the true image has to be seen. A bright source of light near the object of regard is called a glare source. It can cause discomfort, or, indeed, disability glare. The sensitivity of the eye is then significantly depressed, as occurs when looking to one side of a low sun.

Experimental investigations

While 'back-scattered' light may be recorded objectively by, for example, slit lamp photography, investigations of 'forward-scattered' light which affects the subject's vision may be made by measuring:

(1) the effects of veiling glare on visual observation,
(2) scattered intensities in excised animal eyes,
(3) linespread function,
(4) contrast sensitivity function (discussed in the later section on Glare and contrast sensitivity).

Veiling glare techniques

A typical study is that by Fry and Alpern (1953). Two small rectangular fields of illumination, symmetrically placed above and below a fixation mark, are presented such that the upper field is seen only by the left eye and the lower one only by the right eye. A beam splitter before this eye introduces an overlying patch of veiling haze (H in *Figure 15.23a*) not seen by the left eye. With the luminance of the left field kept constant, the subject adjusts the luminance of the right field to match the left for various values of the veiling haze luminance. In a similar arrangement (*Figure 15.23b*), the right eye only is presented with two glare sources GG, the separation and intensity of which can be varied.

Both the veiling haze and the glare sources were found to reduce the apparent luminance of the affected (right eye's) test field. The luminance required for a match had to be increased with increasing haze or glare-source luminance and also with decreasing glare-source separations. Fry and Alpern concluded that the effect of a glare source was to produce, by scattering, a veiling haze which partially bleaches the retinal recep-

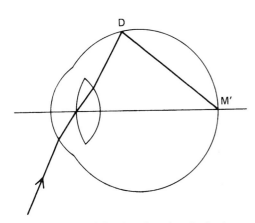

Figure 15.22.   Light diffusely reflected at the fundus at D veils the foveal image at M′.

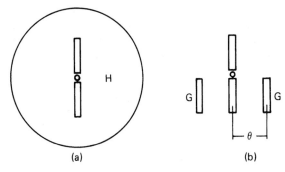

Figure 15.23. Veiling glare and scattered light. Upper rectangle is the left eye's field, lower is the right eye's. Arrangement (a) introduces a surrounding background haze H. Arrangement (b) uses two glare sources GG. Both H and GG are seen by the right eye only. (Redrawn from Fry and Alpern, 1953.)

tors. An increased luminance of the true image is then required to restore the same sensation. An alternative view which Fry and Alpern rejected is that the neighbouring glare sources produce lateral inhibition in the neural networks.

Le Grand (1956) also made a direct comparison of the luminance of the veiling haze with the illuminance of a glare source measured in the plane of the pupil. The graph of his results is shown in *Figure 15.24*. More recent experiments, for example those of Ijspeert *et al.* (1990), use a flickering annular glare source surrounding a central test area flickering alternately so that one is luminous when the other is off. The luminance of the test area is adjusted to give a minimum apparent flicker, thus matching that of the scattered light. These researchers found that the veiling glare depended on a function of the fourth power of the subject's age, doubling between ages 20 and 70. As expected, they also found that there was more veiling glare in Caucasian subjects with blue eyes compared with brown eyes, while dark-skinned non-Caucasian subjects showed even less.

Direct measurement

Using freshly excised bovine eyes from an abattoir, De Mott and Boynton (1958a) measured the illuminance of the scattered light from a glare source that emerged from a small hole cut at the posterior pole. The relative position of the source could be changed so as to vary the 'glare angle' – the angular separation between the retinal image of the source and the recording aperture. As the glare angle increased, a rapid fall was found in the illuminance of the scattered light relative to that of the glare source. At 1° glare angle the relative illuminance was about 0.5 but at 4° had fallen to 0.01. The results are shown in *Figure 15.24*, together with those for an elderly enucleated human eye and from psychophysical experiments of the type already described. As expected, all the curves are of similar form.

To try to identify the sources of scattered light in the eye, De Mott and Boynton (1958b) again used excised cattle eyes, but this time with the posterior third of the globe removed and replaced by a flat glass plate. A

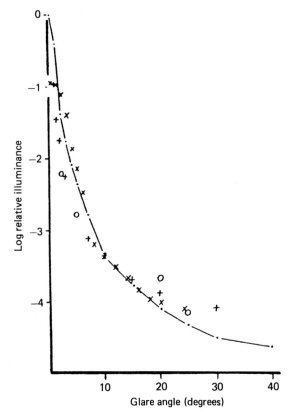

Figure 15.24. Comparison of the stray light distributions obtained by two methods. Direct measurement of illuminance: × Boynton ·—· De Mott and Boynton for the bovine eye. Veiling effect of glare sources on vision: + Le Grand, ○ Holladay. All curves arbitrarily equated at 10° glare angle. (Reproduced from De Mott and Boynton, 1958a, by kind permission of the publishers of *J. Opt. Soc. Am.*)

narrow beam of light was passed obliquely into the eye through the centre of the pupil and the scattered light recorded by photography through the glass plate. They concluded that about 70% of the scattered light comes from the cornea and the remainder from the lens, mainly from the subcapsular and nuclear portions. In order to study changes with oedema, Lovasik and Remole (1983) developed an instrument for investigating the light scattered by excised corneas. A horizontal arc up to 70° on either side could be measured.

Both Beckman *et al.* (1992) and Whitaker *et al.* (1994) give useful background theory and methods for measuring veiling glare, while Thaung *et al.* (1995) discuss modifications to the equation for the light-scattering function for the Pelli–Robson chart described in Chapter 3.

Linespread function

If a very narrow line is imaged by an optical system, a plot of the image luminance in a direction perpendicular to the line is called the linespread function (*see* page 49). Its shape, generally resembling a normal distribution curve, is conventionally indicated by its 'half-width', being the width of the curve at half the peak luminance. When the image is in best focus, the linespread function represents the combined effects of diffraction, light scatter and the eye's spherical and chromatic aberrations. Direct measurements were made by De Mott (1959) on excised cattle eyes, both for dark lines on a luminous ground and for a luminous slit. The latter gave a linespread with a half-width of 3 minutes of arc.

For human subjects, the linespread function is measured in a double-pass system similar to indirect ophthalmoscopy. Light reflected by the retina and returned through the eye's optical system forms an aerial image which can be monitored. Though the aerial image of the line has a much broader spread than that on the retina, the retinal linespread function can be calculated from the double-pass image. Thus, Westheimer and Campbell (1962) showed that the retinal linespread with the image in best focus could be indicated as follows:

Distance from centre of line image (minutes of arc)	Relative illuminance
0	1.0
1	0.5
3.2	0.1
6.5	0.01

These results show an angular half-width of 1 minute of arc compared with the 3 minutes found by Boynton for the bovine eye – doubtless due to a difference between species.

Charman and Jennings (1976b) suggested that the broad skirt at each side of the double-pass linespread function is caused by light scatter in the ocular media at short wavelengths and by penetration into the deeper layers of the retina and choroid at long wavelengths.

Westheimer and Liang (1994) investigated the closely related pointspread function to find an increase in light scatter with age. They suggested comparing the amount of light falling within a 14 minute of arc radius of the centre of the image with that in a surrounding annulus from $14'$ to $28'$. Their results suggest that more light falls into the peripheral annulus as age increases.

Practical importance of scattered light

Fry and Alpern (1953) showed that a glare source producing an illuminance E at the eye gave a veiling haze luminance proportional to $E/\theta^{2.5}$, where θ is the angle between the glare source and the visual axis (*Figure 15.23b*). This relationship was similar to previous results by Holladay, Stiles, and others.

The Building Research Station (cited by Durrant, 1977) found that discomfort glare due to artificial lighting was proportional to

$$\frac{B_s^{1.6}}{B_b} \times \frac{\omega^{0.8}}{p^{1.6}}$$

where B_s is the luminance of the source, B_b the luminance of the background, ω the solid angle subtended by the source and p a position index.

This formula might explain the relief obtained by some patients when wearing tinted lenses, despite the fact that B_s and B_b are reduced in the same proportion. If the luminous transmittance of the lenses is denoted by τ, B_s and B_b become τB_s and τB_b.

The value of $B_s^{1.6}/B_b$, which can be regarded as a glare index, is then reduced to the fraction $\tau^{0.6}$ of its previous value. Thus, lightly tinted lenses with a luminous transmittance of 0.85 would reduce the glare index to 0.91 of its previous value. With $\tau = 0.2$ (a typical value for sunglass lenses) the reduction would be 0.38 of the original glare index.

Glare and ageing changes

While scattered light may not have too detrimental an effect on vision in an eye with clear media, its effects can be marked in one with cloudy media or cataract. Such patients often complain of poor vision, especially when out of doors facing the sun or at night from vehicle headlamps. Hess, cited by Arden (1978) and Paulsson and Sjöstrand (1980), found that early changes in the crystalline lens can have a marked effect on contrast sensitivity, even when the visual acuity remains good. In a subsequent paper, Abrahamson and Sjöstrand (1986) showed that their 'glare score', a function involving the ratio of the contrast sensitivity with the glare to that without, was better related to patient symptoms and degree of lens opacification than it was to visual acuity. Measurement of contrast sensitivity with and without a glare source had been used by Griffiths et al. (1984, 1986) and Elliott et al. (1989) to investigate the increase in light scatter of the oedematous cornea and ageing crystalline lens. In these more recent studies, circular fluorescent lights concentric with the fixation axis to the contrast sensitivity television monitor have been used, both to provide more uniform glare and to reduce any tendency for fixation to wander to a localized glare source.

Hemenger (1984) points out that light scattered through angles of less than $1°$ is the most important in affecting contrast sensitivity. It is suggested by Sloane et al. (1988) that the light scatter function at first drops quite rapidly as a function of spatial frequency and then levels off at about 10 cycles/degree. Conversely, the contrast sensitivity function drops faster after this frequency.

Elliott et al. (1990), Beckman et al. (1992) and Regan et al. (1993) have studied the effects of glare and cataract on the visual acuity measured with low-contrast letter charts. Like contrast sensitivity measurements, all found that the drop in acuity with glare was more predictive of patient symptoms than a drop in normal high-contrast VA without glare. Moreover, Elliott and colleagues found that the binocular VA in the presence of cataract could be less than the best monocular VA. From a study of subjects with clear media, Birchão et al. (1995) suggested that at mesopic luminances, sudden transient glare in the peripheral field may be more disturbing than continuous glare. They felt this might particularly affect people with slight cataracts when driving at night.

Elliott (1993) gives a review of cataract and vision; *see also* pages 44–45

Exercises

15.1   (a) Taking the depth of field as ±0.3 D for a 3 mm pupil and a + 60 D emmetropic eye, calculate the size of the retinal blur circles corresponding to an object positioned at the extremity of the depth of field. (b) On the basis of blur circle geometry, what is the predicted linear depth of field of the same eye when accommodated by 2.50 D, the pupil size being 1 mm?

15.2   (a) A hypothetical avian eye of reduced form has an axial length of 6 mm, a pupil diameter of 0.75 mm and a cone-to-cone spacing of 0.015 mm. Taking this last value as the permissible blur-circle diameter, what is the dioptric depth of field? (b) If the eye has 6 D of accommodation, and when relaxed has its far point at the hyperfocal distance, what is the nearest point of clear vision?

15.3   In their experiments on the eye's depth of focus Tucker and Charman (1975) used a pinhole disc in front of the eye. In order to centre it (on the achromatic axis) the subject viewed a square, the top left and bottom right quarters of which were green, the opposite pair red. Show how and explain why the appearance of the square is altered by the transverse chromatic aberration of the eye when the pinhole disc is (a) above and (b) to the right of the axis.

15.4   By differentiating the expression $K = K' - F_e$ with respect to n, and then substituting $K' = F_e$ for approximate emmetropia, derive Zhang *et al.*'s (1991) equation for the chromatic difference in refraction of a reduced eye:

$$\Delta K = \frac{\Delta n'}{n'r}$$

where r is the corneal radius of curvature.

References

ABRAHAMSON, M. and SJÖSTRAND, J. (1986) Impairment of contrast sensitivity function (CSF) as a measure of disability glare. *Invest. Ophthalmol. Vis. Sci.*, **27**, 1131–1136

AMES, A. JR. and PROCTOR, C.A. (1921) Dioptrics of the eye. *J. Opt. Soc. Am.*, **5**, 22–84

AMOS, J.F. (1982) Diagnosis and management of monocular diplopia. *J. Am. Optom. Ass.*, **53**, 101–115

ARDEN, G.B. (1978) The importance of measuring contrast sensitivity in cases of visual disturbance. *Br. J. Ophthal.*, **62**, 198–209

ARTAL, P., IGLESIAS, I. and LÓPEZ-GILL, N. (1995) Double-pass measurements of the retinal-image quality with unequal entrance and exit pupil sizes and the reversability of the eye's optical system, *J. Opt. Soc. Am. A.*, **12**, 2358–2366

ATCHISON, D.A. (1989a) Third-order aberration of pseudophakic eyes. *Ophthal. Physiol. Opt.*, **9**, 205–212

ATCHISON, D.A. (1989b) Optical design of intraocular lenses. I, On-axis performance, II, Off-axis performance. *Optom. Vis. Sci.*, **66**, 492–506, 579–590

ATCHISON, D.A. (1995) Aberrations associated with rigid contact lenses. *J. Opt. Soc. Am. A.*, **12**, 2267–2273

ATCHISON, D.A., COLLINS, M.J., WILDSOET, C.F., CHRISTENSEN, J. and WATERWORTH, M.D. (1995) Measurement of monochromatic ocular aberrations of human eyes as a function of accommodation by the Howland aberroscope technique. *Vision Res.*, **35**, 313–323

BARNES, D.A., DUNNE, M.C.M. and CLEMENT, R.A. (1987) A schematic eye model for the effects of translation and rotation of ocular components on peripheral astigmatism. *Ophthal. Physiol. Opt.*, **7**, 153–158

BECKMAN, C., HÅRD, S., HÅRD, A. and SJÖSTRAND, J. (1992) Comparison of two glare measurement methods through light scattering modeling. *Optom. Vision Sci.*, **69**, 532–537

BEDFORD, R.E. and WYSZECKI, G. (1957) Axial chromatic aberration of the human eye (correspondence). *J. Opt. Soc. Am.*, **47**, 564–565

BENNETT, A.G. (1951) Oblique refraction of the schematic eye as in retinoscopy. *Optician*, **121**, 583–588

BIRCHÃO, I.C. YAGER, D. and MANG, J. (1995) Disability glare: effects of temporal characteristics of the glare source and of the visual-field location of the test stimulus. *J. Opt. Soc. Am. A.*, **12**, 2253–2258

BORN, M. and WOLF, E. (1980) *Principles of Optics*, 6th edn. Oxford: Pergamon Press

BRADLEY, A. (1992) Glenn A. Fry Award Lecture 1991: perceptual manifestation of imperfect optics in the human eye: attempts to correct for ocular chromatic aberration. *Optom. Vis. Sci.*, **69**, 515–521

BRADLEY, A., ZHANG, X. and THIBOS, L.N. (1991) Achromatizing the human eye. *Optom. Vis. Sci.*, **68**, 608–616

BRÜCKE, E. (1868) Uber asymetrische Strahlenbrechung im menschlichen Augen. *Sber. Akad. Wiss. Wien*, Abt. II, **58**, 321–328

CAMPBELL, F.W. (1957) The depth of field of the human eye. *Optica Acta*, **4**, 157–164

CAMPBELL, F.W. and GUBISCH, R.W. (1967) The effect of chromatic aberration on visual acuity. *J. Physiol.*, **192**, 345–358

CAMPBELL, M.C., HARRISON, E.M. and SIMONET, P. (1990) Psychophysical measurement of the blur on the retina due to optical aberration of the eye. *Vision Res.*, **30**, 1587–1602

CHARMAN, W.N. (1991) Wavefront aberration of the eye: a review. *Optom. Vis. Sci.*, **68**, 574–583

CHARMAN, W.N. and JENNINGS, J.A.M. (1976a) Objective measurements of the longitudinal chromatic aberration of the human eye. *Vision Res.*, **16**, 999–1005

CHARMAN, W.N. and JENNINGS, J.A.M. (1976b) The optical quality of the monochromatic image as a function of focus. *Br. J. Physiol. Optics*, **31**, 119–134

CHARMAN, W.N. and TUCKER, J. (1978) Accommodation and color. *J. Opt. Soc. Am.*, **68**, 459–471

COLLINS, M.J., BROWN, B., ATCHISON, D.A. and NEWMAN, S.D. (1992) Tolerance to spherical aberration induced by rigid contact lenses. *Ophthal. Physiol. Opt.*, **12**, 24–28

COOPER, D.P. and PEASE, P.L. (1988) Longitudinal chromatic aberration of the human eye and wavelength in focus. *Am. J. Optom.*, **65**, 99–107

CORNSWEET, T.N. and CRANE, H.D. (1970) Servo-controlled infrared optometer. *J. Opt. Soc. Am.*, **60**, 548–553

COX, I. (1990) Theoretical calculation of the longitudinal spherical aberration of rigid and soft contact lenses. *Optom. Vis. Sci.*, **67**, 277–282

COX, M.J. and MERINO, N. (1996) The reliability of a computerised crossed-cylinder aberroscope for measuring the optical aberrations of the human eye. *Ophthal. Physiol. Opt.*, **16**, 253

DE MOTT, D.W. (1959) Direct measures of the retinal image. *J. Opt. Soc. Am.*, **49**, 571–579

DE MOTT, D.W. and BOYNTON, R. (1958a) Retinal distribution of entoptic stray light. *J. Opt. Soc. Am.*, **48**, 13–22

DE MOTT, D.W. and BOYNTON, R. (1958b) Sources of entoptic stray light. *J. Opt. Soc. Am.*, **48**, 120–125

DESCARTES, R. (1637) *Discours de le méthode, plus la dioptrique, les météores et la géometrie*. Leyden: Jan Maire

DUNNE, M.C.M., BARNES, D.A. and CLEMENT, R.A. (1987) A model for retinal shape changes in ametropia. *Ophthal. Physiol. Opt.*, **7**, 159–160

DURRANT D.W. (ed.) (1977) *Interior Lighting Design*, 5th edn, p.29. London: The Electricity Council and The Lighting Industry Federation

EINTHOVEN, W. (1885) Stereoscopie durch Farbendifferenz. *Albrecht v. Graefes Arch. Ophthal.*, **31**, Abt. III, 211–238

ELLIOTT, D.B. (1993) New clinical techniques to evaluate cataract. In *Cataract, Detection, Measurement and Management in Optometric Practice*, pp. 32–45 (Douthwaite, W.A. and Hurst, M. A., eds). Oxford: Butterworth-Heinemann

ELLIOTT, D.B., GILCHRIST, J. and WHITAKER, D. (1989) Contrast sensitivity and glare sensitivity changes with three types of cataract morphology: are these techniques necessary in a clinical evaluation of cataract? *Ophthal. Physiol. Opt.*, **9**, 25–30

ELLIOTT, D.B., HURST, M.A. and WEATHERILL, J. (1990) Comparing clinical tests of visual function in cataract with the patient's perceived visual disability. *Eye*, **4**, 712–717

FARRELL, R.A. and McCALLY, R.L. (1976) On corneal transparency and its loss with swelling. *J. Opt. Soc. Am.*, **66**, 342–345

FERREE, C.E. and RAND, G. (1932) The refractive conditions for the peripheral field of vision. In *Report of a Joint Discussion on Vision*. London: Physical Society

FINCHAM, E.F. (1963) Monocular diplopia. *Br. J. Ophthal.*, **47**, 705–712

FRY, G. and ALPERN, M. (1953) The effect of a peripheral glare source upon the apparent brightness of an object. *J. Opt. Soc. Am.*, **43**, 189–195

GLIDDON, G.H. (1929) An optical replica of the human eye for the study of the retinal image. *Archs Ophthal. N.Y.*, **2**, 138–163

GONZÁLEZ, C., PASCUAL, I., BACETE, A. and FIMIA, A. (1996) Elimination and minimization of the spherical aberration of intraocular lenses in high myopia. *Ophthal. Physiol. Opt.*, **16**, 19–30

GRIFFITHS, S.N., DRASDO, N. and BARNES, D.A. (1984) A method of measuring the light scattering properties of the cornea and crystalline lens using the contrast sensitivity function. *The Frontiers of Optometry: First International Congress 1984*, Vol. 2, pp. 173–180. London: British College of Ophthalmic Opticians

GRIFFITHS, S.N., DRASDO, N., BARNES, D.A. and SABELL, A.G. (1986) Effect of epithelial and stromal oedema on the light scattering properties of the cornea. *Am. J. Optom.*, **63**, 888–894

HELMHOLTZ, H. VON (1962) *A Treatise on Physiological Optics*, Vol. 1, translated by Southall, J.P.C. from the German 1909 ed., reprinted Dover, New York, pp. 172–188

HEMENGER, R.P. (1984) Intra-ocular light scatter in normal vision loss with age. *Appl. Opt.*, **23**, 1972–1974

HEMENGER, R.P., TOMLINSON, A. and OLIVER, K. (1996) Optical consequences of asymmetries in normal corneas. *Ophthal. Physiol. Opt.*, **16**, 124–129

HODD, F.A.B. (1951) The measurement of spherical refraction by retinoscopy. *International Optical Congress 1951*, pp. 191–231. London: British Optical Association

HOWARTH, P.A. and BRADLEY, A. (1986) The longitudinal chromatic aberration of the human eye and its correction. *Vision Res.*, **26**, 361–366

HOWARTH, P.A., ZHANG, X.X., BRADLEY, A., STILL, D.L. and THIBOS, L.N. (1988) Does the chromatic aberration of the eye vary with age? *J. Opt. Soc. Am. A.*, **5**, 2087–2092

HOWLAND, H.C. and HOWLAND, B. (1977) A subjective method for the measurement of monochromatic aberrations of the eye. *J. Opt. Soc. Am.*, **67**, 1508–1518

IJSPEERT, J.K., DE WARD, P.W.T., VAN DEN BERG, T.J.T.P. and DE JONG, P.T.V.M. (1990) The intraocular straylight function in 129 healthy volunteers; dependence on angle, age and pigmentation. *Vision Res.*, **30**, 699–707

IVANOFF, A. (1953) *Les Aberrations de l'Oeil*. Paris: Editions de la Revue d'Optique

IVANOFF, A. (1956) About the spherical aberration of the eye. *J. Opt. Soc. Am.*, **46**, 901–903

JACKSON, E. (1888) Symmetrical aberration of the eye. *Trans. Am. Ophthal. Soc.*, **5**, 141–150

JENKINS, T.C.A. (1963) Aberrations of the eye and their effects on vision: Part II. *Br. J. Physiol. Optics*, **20**, 59–91, 161–201

KELLERSHOHN, C., CHATELAIN, P. and ROUBAULT, H. (1957) Répartition spectrale d'une source lumineuse et l'accommodation de l'oeil. *C.r. Séanc. Soc. Biol.*, **151**, 985–987

KOCZOROWSKI, P. (1990) Axial chromatic aberration: linear or power function of wavenumber? *Ophthal. Physiol. Opt.*, **10**, 405–408

KOOMEN, M., SCOLNIK, R. and TOUSEY, R. (1956) Spherical aberration of the eye and the choice of axis. *J. Opt. Soc. Am.*, **46**, 903–904

KOOMEN, M., TOUSEY, R. and SCOLNIK, R. (1949) Spherical aberration of the eye. *J. Opt. Soc. Am.*, **39**, 370–376

KRUGER, P.B., MATHEWS, S., AGGARWALA, K.R. and SANCHEZ, N. (1993) Chromatic aberration and ocular focus: Fincham revisited. *Vision Res.*, **33**, 1397–1411

LE GRAND, Y. (1956) *Optique Physiologique*, Vol. 3: *l'espace visuel*. Paris: Editions de la Revue D'Optique. English translation by Millodot, M. and Heath, G.G. (1967) *Form and Space Vision*, pp. 31–36. Bloomington: Indiana University Press

LEWIS, A.L., KATZ, M. and OEHRLEIN, C. (1982) A modified achromatizing lens. *Am. J. Optom.*, **59**, 909–911

LIANG, J., GRIMM, B., GOELZ, S. and BILLE, J.F. (1994) Objective measurement of wave aberrations of the human eye with the use of a Hartmann–Shack wave-front sensor. *J. Opt. Soc. Am. A.*, **11**, 1949–1957

LOTMAR, W. and LOTMAR, T. (1974) Peripheral astigmatism in the human eye: experimental data and theoretical model predictions. *J. Opt. Soc. Am.*, **64**, 510–513

LOVASIK, J.V. and REMOLE, A. (1983) An instrument for mapping corneal light-scattering characteristics. *Ophthal. Physiol. Opt.*, **3**, 247–254

MANDELBAUM, T. and SIVAK, J.G. (1983) Longitudinal chromatic aberration of the vertebrate eye. *Vision Res.*, **23**, 1555–1559

MILLODOT, M. (1976) The influence of age on the chromatic aberration of the eye. *A. Graefes Arch. Klin. Exp. Ophthalmol.*, **198**, 235–243, cited in Howarth *et al.* (1988)

MILLODOT, M. (1981) Effect of ametropia on peripheral refraction. *Am. J. Optom.*, **58**, 691–695

MILLODOT, M. and SIVAK, J.G. (1973) Influence of accommodation on the chromatic aberration of the eye. *Br. J. Physiol. Optics*, **28**, 169–174

MILLODOT, M. and SIVAK, J.G. (1974) Measurement of the spherical aberration of the crystalline lens *in vivo*, a preliminary report. *Atti Fond. Giorgio Ronchi*, **29**, 903–908

MORRELL, A., WHITEFOOT, H.D. and CHARMAN, W.N. (1991) Ocular chromatic aberration and age. *Ophthal. Physiol. Opt.*, **11**, 385–390

NAVARRO, R., SANTAMARÍA, J. and BESCÓS, J. (1985) Accommodation-dependent model of the human eye with aspherics. *J. Opt. Soc. Am. A.*, **2**, 1273–1281

OGLE, K.N. and SCHWARTZ, J.T. (1959) Depth of focus of the human eye. *J. Opt. Soc. Am.*, **49**, 275–280

PATEL, S. (1991) The influence of hydrogel contact lens shape on the spherical aberration of the eye. *J. Br. Contact Lens Assoc.*, **14**, 189–191

PAULSSON, L.E. and SJÖSTRAND, J. (1980) Contrast sensitivity in the presence of a glare light. *Invest. Ophthal.*, **19**, 401–406

PEASE, P.L. and BARBEITO, R. (1989) Axial chromatic aberration of the human eye: frequency or wavelength? *Ophthal. Physiol. Opt.*, **9**, 215–217

POWEL, I. (1981) Lenses for correcting chromatic aberration of the eye. *Appl. Optics*, **20**, 4152–4155

REGAN, D., GIASCHI, D.E. and FRESCO, B.B. (1993) Measurement of glare sensitivity in cataract patients using low-contrast letter charts. *Ophthal. Physiol. Opt.*, **13**, 115–123

REMPT, F., HOOGERHEIDE, J. and HOOGENBOOM, W.P.H. (1971) Peripheral retinoscopy and the skiagram. *Ophthalmologica*, **162**, 1–10

ROSENFIELD, M., PORTELLO, J.K., BLUSTEIN, G.H. and JANG, C. (1996) Comparison of clinical techniques to assess the near accommodative response. *Optom. Vis. Sci.*, **73**, 382–388

RYNDERS, M., LIDKEA, B., CHISHOLM, W. and THIBOS, L.N. (1995) Statistical distribution of foveal transverse chromatic aberration, pupil centration, and angle ψ in a population of young adult eyes. *J. Opt. Soc. Am. A.*, **12**, 2348–2357

SANTAMARIA, J., ARTAL, P. and BESCÓS, J. (1987) Determination of the point-spread function of human eyes using a hybrid optical-digital method. *J. Opt. Soc. Am. A.*, **4**, 1109–1114

SIMONET, P. and CAMPBELL, M.C.W. (1990) The optical transverse chromatic aberration on the fovea of the human eye. *Vision Res.*, **30**, 187–206

SIVAK, J.G. and MANDELBAUM, T. (1982) Chromatic dispersion of the ocular media. *Vision Res.*, **22**, 997–1003

SIVAK, J.G. and MILLODOT, M. (1974) Axial chromatic aberration of the eye with achromatizing lens. *J. Opt. Soc. Am.*, **64**, 1724–1725

SLOANE, M.E., OWSLEY, C. and ALVAREZ, S.L. (1988) Ageing, senile miosis and spatial contrast sensitivity at low luminance. *Vision Res.*, **28**, 1235–1246

SMITH, G. and LU, C. (1988) The spherical aberration of intra-ocular lenses. *Ophthal. Physiol. Opt.*, **8**, 287–294

SMITH, G., APPLEGATE, R.A. and HOWLAND, H.C. (1996) The crossed-cylinder aberroscope: an alternative method of calculation of the aberrations. *Ophthal. Physiol. Opt.*, **16**, 222–229

SUNDET, J.M. (1976) Two theories of colour stereoscopy. *Vision Res.*, **16**, 469–472

THUANG, J., BECKMAN, C., ABRAHAMSSON, M. and SJÖSTRAND, J. (1995) Importance of stimulus geometry, contrast definition and adaptation. *Invest. Ophthalmol. Vis. Sci.*, **36**, 2313–2317

THIBOS, L.N., BRADLEY, A., STILL, D.L., ZHANG, X. and HOWARTH, P.A. (1990) Theory and measurement of ocular chromatic aberration. *Vision Res.*, **30**, 33–49

THIBOS, L.N., BRADLEY, A. and ZHANG, X. (1991) Effect of ocular chromatic aberration on monocular visual performance *Optom. Vision. Sci.*, **68**, 599–607

THOMSON, L.C. and WRIGHT, W.D. (1947) The colour sensitivity of the retina within the central fovea of man. *J. Physiol.*, **105**, 316–331

TSCHERNING, M. (1924) *Physiologic Optics*, 4th edn (trans. Weiland, C.). Philadelphia: Keystone Publishing Co.

TUCKER, J. and CHARMAN, W.N. (1975) The depth of focus of the human eye for Snellen letters. *Am. J. Optom.*, **52**, 3–21

VOS, J.J. (1960) Some new aspects of colour stereoscopy. *J. Opt. Soc. Am.*, **50**, 785–790

VOS, J.J. (1963) An antagonistic effect in colour stereoscopy. *Ophthalmologica*, **145**, 442–445

WALD, G. and GRIFFIN, D.R. (1947) The change in refractive power of the human eye in dim and bright light. *J. Opt. Soc. Am.*, **37**, 321–336

WALSH, G. and CHARMAN, W.N. (1985) Measurement of the wavefront aberration of the human eye. *Ophthal. Physiol. Opt.*, **5**, 23–31

WALSH, G. and CHARMAN, W.N. (1988) The effect of pupil centration and diameter on ocular performance. *Vision Res.*, **28**, 659–665

WALSH, G. and COX, M.J. (1995) A new computerised video-aberroscope for the determination of the aberration of the human eye. *Ophthal. Physiol. Opt.*, **15**, 403–408

WESTHEIMER, G. and CAMPBELL, F.W. (1962) Light distribution in the image formed by the living human eye. *J. Opt. Soc. Am.*, **52**, 1040–1045

WESTHEIMER, G. and LIANG, J. (1994) Evaluating diffusion of light in the eye by objective means. *Investig. Ophthalmol. Vis. Sci.*, **35**, 2652–2657

WHITAKER, D., ELLIOTT, D.B. and STEEN, R. (1994) Confirmation of the validity of the psychophysical light scattering factor. *Invest. Ophthalmol. Vis. Sci.*, **35**, 317–321

WILMUT, E.B. (1958) Chromatic selectivity of the eye in near vision. *Optician*, **135**, 185–187

YE, M., BRADLEY, A., THIBOS, L.N. and ZHANG, X. (1991) Inter-ocular differences in transverse chromatic aberration determine chromostereopsis for small pupils. *Vision Res.*, **31**, 1787–1796

YOUNG, T. (1801) On the mechanism of the eye. *Phil. Trans. R. Soc. 1800*, **92**, 23–88 + plates

ZHANG, X., BRADLEY, A. and THIBOS, L.N. (1991) Achromatizing the human eye: the problem of chromatic parallax. *J. Opt. Soc. Am. A.*, **8**, 686–691

ZHANG, X., THIBOS, L.N. and BRADLEY, A. (1991) Relation between the chromatic difference of refraction and the chromatic difference of magnification for the reduced eye. *Optom. Vision Sci.*, **6**, 456–458

16

Visual examination of the eye and ophthalmoscopy

Introduction: focal illumination

Like the ophthalmologist, the optometrist must examine the eye to make sure that there is no abnormality or pathology present, and if there is, to try to identify the condition. Examination is conveniently divided into two areas:

(1) the anterior segment comprising the bulbar conjunctiva, anterior sclera, cornea, aqueous humour, iris and anterior part of the crystalline lens;
(2) the posterior segment, which for this purpose can be taken as the remainder of the eye including the crystalline lens, vitreous humour and the fundus (the view through the pupil of the retina, choroid, sclera and optic nerve head).

The anterior segment, together with the eyelids, should first be examined in good general diffuse illumination. The cornea, aqueous, and anterior crystalline lens may then be examined under localized illumination. While the instrument of choice is the slit lamp, to be described below, historically the method of focal illumination was employed. An electric lamp bulb was imaged on the eye by means of a condensing lens of power approximately +13.0 DS and aperture 50 mm. The anterior segment was then examined either with the unaided eye or with a hand or binocular headband magnifier.

The hand slit lamp provides a more convenient method of focal illumination (*Figure 16.1*). In the majority of such instruments a low-voltage bulb has a filament of uncoiled wire shaped like a goal post, an image of which is projected on to the cornea by a high-powered condenser. The better instruments have a compound condensing system so as to reduce aberrations and give sharper definition to the filament image. To increase the depth of focus, the condenser aperture may be stopped down with a rectangular diaphragm parallel to the bulb filament. A useful technique is to position the instrument so that the beam is initially out of focus. Corneal opacities are best revealed by a beam about 1 mm wide. The distance of the instrument from the eye can then be adjusted to focus the filament image on the cornea, thereby obtaining a more detailed picture of

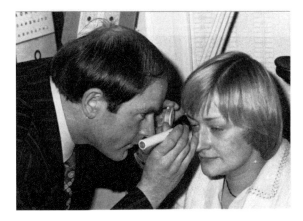

Figure 16.1. Focal illumination using a hand slit lamp and loupe.

the cross-section. An 8× or 5× magnifier held in the other hand or a binocular headband magnifier aids the examination. Corneal opacities may also be detected by the method of scleral scatter, in which the beam is aimed at the sclera just to the side of the limbus: light enters the cornea through its edge, and is totally internally reflected at both surfaces. As a result, the cornea appears dark but any opacity will scatter light and show up as a lighter area.

These methods are useful for general routine examination, but for more precise inspection the major slit lamp is essential because of its luminance, binocular viewing and magnification.

The slit lamp

The term 'slit lamp' is now usually reserved for the major stand instrument or biomicroscope. There are two main parts, the illuminating system and the observation system, mounted on a movable trolley. Both parts are rotatable about the same vertical axis, which also coincides with their respective foci. By this means, the slit image illuminating the eye and the observing microscope remain simultaneously in focus on the same part of the eye.

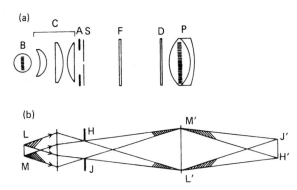

Figure 16.2. Illuminating system of the major slit lamp. (a) B lamp bulb, C condenser, A aperture controlling slit length, S slit, F colour filter, D diffuser, P projection lens. (b) Basic principles of illumination system. LM extremities of lamp filament, HJ extremities of slit, M′L′ inverted image of lamp filament, J′H′ inverted image of slit.

A well-designed illuminating system will have the following features:

(1) The slit image projected on to the eye will be adequately and uniformly illuminated over its entire area. For example, graduations of corneal opacity which could be masked by uneven illumination are then more easily discerned.
(2) The width of the slit image will be reducible to 0.02 mm or less to illuminate a very narrow 'optical section' of the cornea or lens.
(3) The slit image should present a good luminance contrast, with its edges well defined.
(4) There should be adequate depth of focus so that a reasonably thin section can be obtained throughout, say, the thickness of the crystalline lens.

The optical system now used and shown diagrammatically in *Figure 16.2*, is that of the slide projector and was first used in the instrument by Vogt. To illustrate the principle more clearly, the system has been reduced to its simplest form in *Figure 16.2(b)*. The lamp filament LM is imaged by the condenser lens at L′M′ in the plane of the projection lens. This, in turn, forms an image of the slit aperture HJ at H′J′. As shown in the diagram, a part of the full pencil of rays from L passes through the slit and is focused at L′ on the projector lens. After refraction, the rays cross over and become divergent, at the same time being deviated towards the optical axis by the prismatic effect of the lens and thereby passing through the image H′J′. Since the whole of the slit was evenly illuminated by the pencil from L, it follows that the slit image is evenly illuminated. In a similar manner, pencils from every point on the filament are capable of passing through both the slit and the projection lens, thus contributing to the illumination of the image.

Most instruments allow a continuous variation of slit width, while the length may be altered by means of aperture stops or an iris diaphragm near the condenser. The depth of focus of the slit image is mainly dependent on the width of the lamp filament image in the plane of the projection lens. As a means of controlling this,

some slit lamps incorporate an aperture stop of variable width placed near the lens.

In some instruments, the slit can be rotated from its customary vertical orientation. Coloured filters can often be inserted: for example, a green 'red-free' filter for viewing blood vessels, and a blue filter to accentuate fluorescein-stained areas of damaged epithelium. The contrast of fluorescein-stained areas may be further enhanced by placing a yellow barrier filter in front of the microscope, thus absorbing the blue light but transmitting the yellow–green fluorescence. Suitable filters are Lee 101 yellow[*] and Kodak Wratten 15. Neutral-density filters can be used as an alternative to voltage control of illumination, while a diffuser may be fitted over the projection lens to give a larger field of illumination.

Figure 16.3 illustrates a modern instrument. In these, the illuminating system is essentially vertical, a mirror or prism reflecting light on to the patient's eye. This vertical layout (either above or below the microscope) was originated by H. C. Binstead, and allows the lamp on its shorter arm to be moved easily from one side of the microscope to the other, or even directly in front of it.

The eye is observed through a binocular stereoscopic microscope, often called a Greenhough microscope, although it was Czapski who first used it on the slit lamp. Like the illuminating system, the microscope can be freely swung around their common axis of rotation. The principle of keeping the microscope and slit lamp simultaneously focused on their centre of rotation had been introduced in 1923 by E. F. Fincham, who achieved the effect by mounting the two systems on a circular arc.

The microscope provides magnification from about 5× to 40× or occasionally higher, but the constant tiny movements of the eye and the very small depth of field at high magnifications set an upper limit to the useful range. Various means are used to alter the magnification:

(1) Changing the objectives, which usually give initial magnifications between 1× and 2×,
(2) Changing the eyepieces (often 10×, 12.5×, 15× 20×),
(3) The use of a zoom system,
(4) The incorporation of a revolving turret of small Galilean telescopes, a device due to Mueller. As shown in *Figure 16.4*, this is placed between a large objective which collimates the light from the object, and two small objectives which form the aerial images magnified by the eyepieces. If the convex component of the telescope is placed nearer the microscope objective, the magnification is increased, but if the telescope is reversed the magnification is decreased.

A low magnification (about 7× or 8×) with its correspondingly wide field of view is ideal for such things as observing the relative movements of a soft contact lens on the eye, and removing ingrowing eyelashes. These

[*] Lee Filters, Central Way, Walworth Industrial Estate, Andover, Hants SP10 5AN.

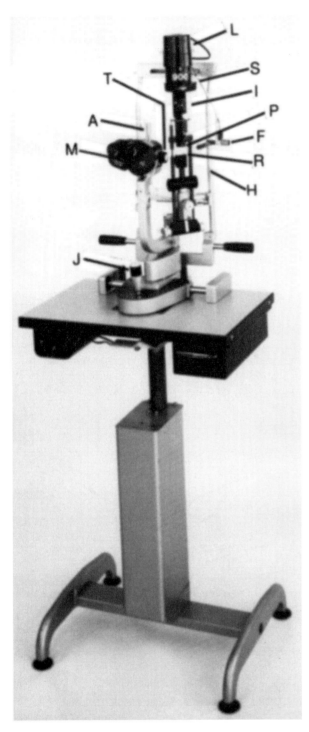

Figure 16.3. The Haag–Streit 900BQ slit lamp. An attachment fitting for tonometer, pachometer, etc, F fixation lamp, H headrest, I illuminating system, J joystick control, L lamp house, M microscope, P projection lens, R mirror, S slit assembly, T turret magnification changer. Photograph reproduced by kind permission of Clement Clarke International Ltd.

The axes of the twin eyepieces may be parallel or convergent. While parallel axes are theoretically more restful as the accommodation and convergence are relaxed, the proximal convergence and accommodation frequently exerted by younger observers may lead them to prefer instruments with a convergent system. Eyepiece adjustment for ametropia is usually incorporated. Alternatively, and especially if the observer is markedly astigmatic, eyepieces with extra-long eye relief allowing spectacles to be worn may be of service.

The performance of the instrument as a whole depends on several factors:

(1) the intensity of illumination of the slit beam, especially when the slit is at its narrowest;
(2) the width and definition of the beam;
(3) the quality of the microscope;
(4) the accuracy with which the focus of the slit projection system is positioned above the common axis of rotation – otherwise, the beam may be in focus when incident from the left but not from the right;
(5) the accuracy with which the foci of the slit projection system and of the microscope coincide.

One method of judging the performance of the instrument is to look for the relatively dark line formed by the epithelium in a cross-section of the cornea, using a very narrow beam coming first from one side of the instrument, then from the other. The angular separation between slit lamp and microscope should be about 50° and the magnification about 20×. Another test is whether the instrument provides a good view of the corneal endothelium, using the method of specular reflection. (Particular aspects of the basic optical design of the instrument are brought out in the Exercises at the end of the chapter.)

The use of the slit lamp in clinical practice is described by Sheridan (1989) and Morris and Stone (1992), the latter giving a useful bibliography of texts on pathology.

In addition to providing a view of the anterior segment, the slit lamp may also be used for viewing the angle of the anterior chamber (gonioscopy), examining the fundus, measuring corneal and anterior chamber depths, tonometry and photography.

Gonioscopy

Gonioscopy is the technique for viewing the angle of the anterior chamber where the cornea meets the root of the iris. It enables the skilled observer to assess the width or narrowness of the angle. A narrow angle predisposes to a disease known as angle-closure glaucoma where the pressure of the fluid in the eye rises rapidly, causing pain and damage. Even when the angle is relatively wide, the pressure may rise if the drainage through the trabecular meshwork is deficient. A distinction is necessary in determining the medical treatment.

Because of refraction at the strongly curved anterior corneal surface, it is not possible to view the angle of the anterior chamber without special aid (*Figure 16.5a*). The principle of the gonioscopy contact lens is that the corneal surface is approximately neutralized by

tasks are helped if a diffuser can be attached between the prism or mirror of the illumination system and the patient's eye to provide a large field of illumination. Magnifications of 30× or more are needed for observing the corneal endothelium.

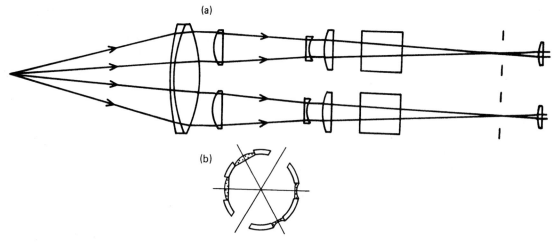

Figure 16.4. (a) Plan view of the binocular microscope of the Carl Zeiss slit lamp. (b) Side view of rotating Galilean magnification changer. (Redrawn from illustrations kindly supplied by Carl Zeiss Ltd.)

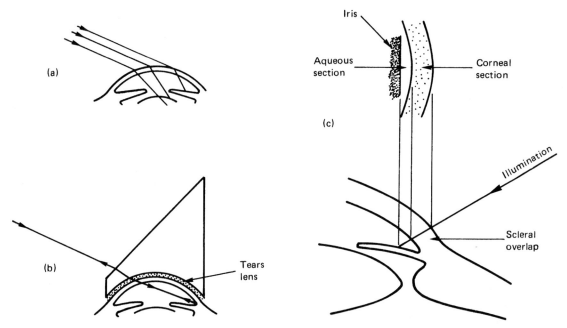

Figure 16.5. Gonioscopy: (a) ray paths showing that the angle of the anterior chamber is not visible without aid, (b) a prism type of gonioscopy contact lens, (c) the Van Herick technique for estimating anterior chamber depth.

the rear surface of the contact lens and the tears lens formed between this surface and the cornea. Light from the slit lamp can thus pass into the angle and return to the microscope. *Figure 16.5(b)* shows a simple gonioscopy lens, the slit lamp and microscope being directed approximately normal to the inclined surface of the lens.

There are many different types of gonioscopy lens: illustrations are given by Sabell (1970) and Stone (1989). Prokopich and Flanagan (1996; 1997) give an introduction to the technique, while an extensive treatment is given by Fisch (1993).

The gonioscopy lens is an awkward diagnostic tool for a quick analysis of the angle of the anterior chamber. An indirect but simple technique for assessing the width of the angle with the major slit lamp was introduced by Van Herick *et al.* (1969). A very narrow illuminating beam is aimed at the temporal side of the cornea

as near as possible to the limbus (*Figure 16.5c*). The patient looks at the microscope which should be set at 60° to the slit lamp, so that the illumination strikes the cornea approximately at right angles. With low magnification to obtain sufficient depth of field, the observer relates the apparent thickness of the dark space between the posterior surface of the cornea and the illuminated patch on the iris – the aqueous section – to the apparent thickness of the corneal section.

Polse (1975) suggested that the depth at the nasal limbus should also be evaluated: the microscope will need to be set somewhat temporally so that the illumination will pass the patient's nose. Van Herick showed that the slit lamp appearance may be related to gonioscopy grades as follows:

Grade 4 Aqueous section equal to or greater than corneal section.

Grade 3 Aqueous section between $\frac{1}{2}$ and $\frac{1}{4}$ of corneal section.

Grade 2 Aqueous section approximately $\frac{1}{4}$ of corneal section.

Grade 1 Aqueous section less than $\frac{1}{4}$ of corneal section.

An eye with a grade 2 chamber has a relatively narrow angle which could give rise to angle-closure glaucoma.

A grade 1 chamber is dangerously narrow. Sympathomimetic or parasympatholytic drugs should be avoided both topically and orally. Thus, mydriasis to allow better inspection of the fundus would be unwise, while referral for gonioscopy or provocative tests for potential angle-closure glaucoma may be worthwhile.

Slit-lamp examination of the fundus

Contact-lens devices

The slit lamp and microscope are designed to illuminate and observe objects at a finite distance, about 100 mm from the microscope lenses. It is therefore unable to provide a view of the ocular fundus, the image of which (in the eye's far point plane) may be at any distance up to infinity.

Koeppe (1918) introduced a glass flat-fronted contact lens which approximately neutralizes the whole refractive power of the eye. The fundus is then brought directly into the focusing range of the instrument.

A modified plastics form of the Koeppe lens[*] due to Goldmann (1938) has a slightly convex anterior surface of radius 70 mm and a concave rear surface giving adequate corneal clearance (*Figure 16.6*). A surrounding black hood allows the observer to manipulate the lens while preventing the patient's eyelids from sweeping across it. The space between the rear surface and cornea is filled with viscous artificial tears, forming a liquid lens that is generally of low positive power. When this is taken into account, the total power added by the Koeppe lens is in the neighbourhood of -55 to -60 D. Consequently, if the eye is emmetropic, the fundus M' is imaged at M'' in the focal plane of the Koeppe lens, about 18 mm behind its front surface. Since the Koeppe lens and the eye are usually of similar but opposite power, the fundus image is not inverted and its magnification is negligible.

With all fundus-viewing lenses, whether of the contact-lens type or not, the slit lamp and microscope are initially placed as close together as possible. Most modern instruments allow the slit lamp to be placed immediately in front of the microscope, between the objectives, though often at a slightly lower level. The patient's pupil needs to be dilated. When the fundus image is in focus, the slit lamp may be displaced sideways through about $10°$ to give slightly oblique illumination of the fundus, enhancing the stereoscopic view through the microscope.

[*] Produced by Haag–Streit, Berne.

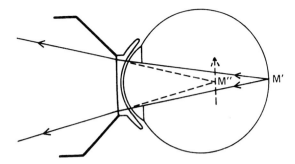

Figure 16.6. The Koeppe fundus contact lens.

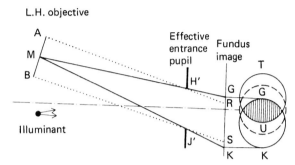

Figure 16.7. Simplified diagram of fields of view of the slit lamp and Koeppe lens: TU, GK are the monocular fields, GU the binocular field.

Though a rigorous study of the field of view obtained with this arrangement involves many complications, a sufficiently accurate picture can still be obtained if the problem is reduced to its barest essentials. In *Figure 16.7* the left-hand microscope objective is directed towards the centre of the fundus image, which has to be viewed through a centrally placed diaphragm H'J', an image of the pupil. Straight lines through AH' and BJ' meet the fundus image at R and S. Every point within these limits – bounding the field of full illumination – is clearly capable of sending a pencil filling the microscope objective. Outside this area is a zone bounded by the points G and K lying respectively on MH' and MJ' produced. Pencils from these limiting points can still cover half the width of the objective and the circle through G and K is taken to be the useful field of view. The symmetrically placed circle TU marks the field provided by the right-hand objective, the shaded area of overlap GU representing the binocular field of view.

To illuminate the fundus, the lamp is placed approximately mid-way between the two objectives. Since the source is relatively small, the illuminated area is of similar diameter to the monocular fields GK and TU. This area of illumination is indicated in the diagram by the dotted outline and can be seen to cover a good part of both monocular fields. The remainder will be relatively dark, being illuminated only by light reflected or scattered within the eye.

The area of fundus observed may be altered by asking the patient to turn his eye sideways or up or down. Despite this, it is not possible to view the whole fundus with such a simple lens. Other designs incorporating a prism or mirrors, somewhat similar to gonioscopy lenses, are described in the references previously

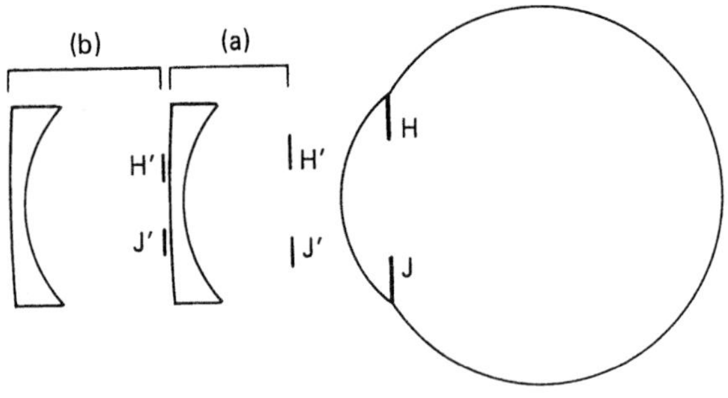

Figure 16.8. The Hruby lens: image H′J′ of the actual entrance pupil HJ formed by the lens in two positions (a) and (b), the longer vertex distance reducing the field of view.

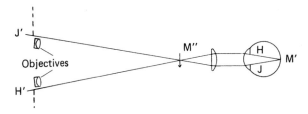

Figure 16.9. The El Bayadi lens.

quoted. These allow a view of the peripheral fundus even up to the ora serrata.

The Hruby lens

Contact lenses for fundus viewing have the disadvantage that the patient's cornea needs anaesthetizing. This can be overcome by a lens of similar negative power placed before but not in contact with the eye. Introduced by Lemoine and Valois (1923), a lens of this kind was popularized by Hruby (1941, 1942).

The lens power is usually about −55 D, the concave surface being placed as close to the cornea as possible. Reflections from the surfaces are reduced though not eliminated both by coating the lens and tilting it slightly. In addition, the front surface of the lens is sometimes made slightly convex to reduce the size of the reflections from it.

The slit-lamp beam and microscope axis should initially be placed as close together as possible. If the lens is spring-mounted on the microscope to bear against a bar on the headrest, the whole instrument should be slowly moved forward until the fundus image comes into focus. If the lens is mounted on the instrument's headrest, the slit lamp should first be focused on the lens and then moved towards the patient.

Though the field of view through the Hruby lens is proportional to the size of the patient's pupil, the distance of the lens from the eye is also of importance. The entrance pupil of the lens–eye system is the virtual image H′J′ of the eye's own entrance pupil HJ formed by the Hruby lens. This image not only becomes smaller

but also moves forward as the lens is moved away from the eye (*Figure 16.8*). As a result, the field of view is reduced by more than one-quarter when the distance of the lens from the eye is increased from 10 to 20 mm. For the same reason, the Koeppe lens fitted in contact with the eye gives a larger field of view than the Hruby lens.

The El Bayadi and Volk lenses

Unlike the Hruby lens which approximately neutralizes the dioptric power of the eye, these positive lenses form a real and inverted image of the fundus as shown in *Figure 16.9*. In effect, the slit lamp is converted into a stereoscopic indirect ophthalmoscope (*see* pages 318–323).

The original El Bayadi lens (1953) was of power +55–60 D and, if of plano-convex form, was placed with its convex face towards the patient's eye. Kajiura (1978, cited by Rumney, 1988) suggested using aspherical surfaces to improve the field of view of the El Bayadi lens. A recent development is the introduction by Volk of a range of anti-reflection coated lenses in bi-convex form with both surfaces aspherical, with powers between 60 and 150 D (*Table 16.1*), and smaller ranges from Nikon and Ocular Instruments.

To optimize viewing conditions, the distance of the lens from the patient's eye must be such that an enlarged image H′J′ of the eye's entrance pupil HJ is formed in the plane of the microscope objectives, completely surrounding them. The 90 D and SuperField NC (non-contact) lenses should be held about 6.5–7 mm from the cornea. Assuming that the microscope's objectives are 27 mm from outer edge to outer edge, the patient's pupil must be at least 3 mm in diameter. This, however, allows no latitude in positioning the lens nor

Table 16.1 Details of the Volk fundus biomicroscopy lenses

Lens type	Lens aperture (mm)	Field of view (°)	Working distance from cornea (mm)	Fundus magnification	Pupil magnification
60 D	31	67	11	−1	−1/6
78 D	31	73	7	−0.77	−1/7.8
90 D	21.5	69	6.5	−0.67	−1/9
SuperField NC (90 D)	26	120	6.5	−0.67	−1/9
SuperPupil NC (150 D)	16	120	2 to 4	−0.4	−1/15

The fundus magnification is based on a power of +60 D for the patient's eye, while the pupil magnification is the ratio q/q' in *Figure 16.23*, i.e. the magnification with which the slit lamp objectives are imaged into the patient's pupil. The microscope is assumed to have a working distance of 100 mm to the fundus image.

Table 16.2 Slit-lamp examination of the fundus: comparison of useful fields of view with different supplementary lenses

Ocular refraction (K)	Koeppe lens −66 D		Hruby lens −55 D		El Bayadi lens +55 D		Aspherical +90 D (at 9 mm aperture)	
	Monocular (mm)	Binocular (mm)	Monocular (mm)	Binocular (mm)	Monocular (mm)	Binocular (mm)	Monocular (mm)	Binocular (mm)
−10.00	7.3	2.7 (5.7)	3.7	0.5 (2.6)	7.4	4.3 (6.4)	14.6	11.0 (13.4)
Emmetropia	7.1	3.5 (6.0)	4.1	1.7 (3.3)	6.2	3.0 (5.0)	12.1	8.6 (10.9)
+5.00	7.0	3.8 (5.9)	4.3	2.1 (3.5)	5.7	2.5 (4.6)	11.1	7.8 (10.0)

for the movement of the objective's image within the pupil as the instrument is scanned across the fundus image, so a larger pupil is preferable. If the eye is emmetropic, the fundus image M'' lies in the focal plane of the lens. The magnification is then $-F_e/F$, where F_e is the equivalent power of the eye and F that of the lens. This is, however, augmented by the magnification of the slit lamp's microscope, though the use of higher magnifications is often limited by the quality of the patient's media.

In use, the slit lamp is usually positioned symmetrically between the two microscope objectives, and, if possible, the beam tilted up to reduce reflections from the aspheric lens. A neutral filter to reduce brightness will aid patient comfort, while a yellow filter or a yellow-coated lens will minimize any hazard from excess blue light. The slit lamp is first focused on the patient's cornea. While viewing from the side, the lens is positioned in front of the eye, and then viewing through the eyepieces the instrument is next withdrawn some 25 mm from the eye until the inverted fundus image is seen in focus.

As the maximum beam width of many slit lamps is 9 mm, this value has been adopted for the diameter of the lens when calculating the fields of view given in *Table 16.2*. In practice, the width of the illuminating beam is reduced to 2–3 mm for patient comfort and to reduce reflections, and hence a narrower field of view is given at any one instant. The aperture of the lens is utilized by traversing either the illuminating beam (by dissociating the illuminating and observation systems) or the whole instrument across the lens. If the image in one eyepiece becomes relatively dimmer than the other, equality is often restored by slightly moving the lens sideways towards the dimmer image. While dilated pupils are greatly advantageous, the Volk Instruction Manuals for the 90 D and SuperField NC lenses suggest that, with practice, a view of about 3 mm of the fundus (2–3 disc diameters) can be obtained through an undilated pupil of 2.5–3 mm diameter. Pupil miosis as a reflex to the light may restrict the pupil diameter to less than this and lens position becomes critical. The Super-Pupil lens has a much greater power so that the microscope objectives are imaged closer together into the patient's pupil, thus allowing a better view without dilation.

The lower power lenses in *Table 16.1* give larger fundus images, allowing detail to be more readily observed, and can be held further from the patient's eye so that they are less likely to be soiled by the lashes. The lateral position will possibly be more critical. The

SuperField lens seems the most practical, especially as there are a range of auxiliary lenses both to increase the lens power and hence field of view or to decrease it to give a similar magnification to the 78 D lens. Two contact lens adaptors are also available to convert it to a Koeppe-type lens.

Apart from the manufacturer's handbooks, Austen (1993), Cavallerano *et al.* (1994) and Flanagan and Prokopich (1995) give advice. Field and Barnard (1993) point out that for habitual users of the direct ophthalmoscope (described later in this chapter), observation of the inverted image requires thought: drawing is simplified by turning the record sheet upside down, while viewing adjacent areas is best achieved by imagining that the fundus is on the outside of a convex surface, so that one moves in the opposite direction to that normally used.

The Panfunduscope

This instrument, originally suggested by Goldmann in 1965 and developed by Schlegel, is a high-powered optical system forming an inverted image of the fundus in close proximity to the eye. Like the El Bayadi lens, the Panfunduscope acts as the condensing system of an indirect ophthalmoscope, the inverted image being viewed through and magnified by the slit-lamp microscope. The name given to the instrument reflects the claim by the manufacturers* that the whole posterior hemisphere can be viewed without movement of either lens or eye. The field of view is, in fact, limited by that of the microscope itself.

The optical system of the instrument is shown in *Figure 16.10(a)*, drawn approximately to scale. A pencil from the macula M' is converged by a high-powered contact lens and then refracted by a complete sphere which forms an inverted but virtual image of the fundus at M''. The system also forms an enlarged image $H'J'$ of the eye's entrance pupil HJ, approximately in the plane of the microscope objectives. In round figures, the magnification of the fundus image at M'' is -0.7, while the magnification of the entrance pupil is -7.5.

To show the path of the rays through the sphere in more detail, a separate drawing has been inserted (*Figure 16.10b*) with the angles exaggerated. The axial pencil from M' is converged by the contact lens towards the point B_1, which becomes a virtual object for the first surface of the sphere. After refraction, this pencil is

---

* Produced by Rodenstock, Munich.

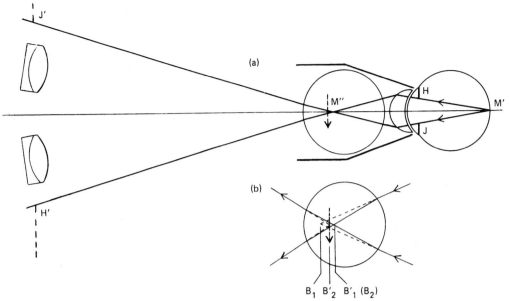

Figure 16.10. Optics of the Panfunduscope. (Redrawn from material kindly supplied by G. Rodenstock Instrumente GmbH.)

converged to the image point B'_1, which becomes the object point B_2 for the second surface of the sphere. The emergent pencil diverges from the virtual image point B'_2, which fixes the position of the fundus image M'' presented to the microscope.

Comparison of fields

Table 16.2 gives an indication of the fields of view of the fundus given by the four types of supplementary lens. The figures refer to the useful fields of view represented by GK (monocular) and GU (binocular) in *Figure 16.7*.

In all cases, the diameter of the eye's entrance pupil was taken to be 7 mm and the objective aperture 5 mm at a working distance of 100 mm to the fundus image. The centres of the objectives were taken to be separated by 23 mm, corresponding to the 13° angular separation subtended at the object that has been adopted by Haag-Streit. The effective aperture of the El Bayadi lens (placed at its optimum distance of approximately 18.5 mm from the corneal vertex) was taken as 8 mm. The Hruby lens was assumed to be 10 mm from the cornea. These dimensions should be understood to be no more than broadly representative.

Of all the lenses, the aspherical is seen to perform best of all, thus vindicating its popularity. Of the three older types of lens, the El Bayadi lens is seen to perform best in myopia, while the Koeppe lens is the best in emmetropia and hypermetropia. The Hruby lens has the smallest field throughout the range investigated. A further comparison may be made with the fields obtained in direct and indirect ophthalmoscopy (techniques which are discussed on pages 312–324). The direct method gives about 2 mm with a 4 mm pupil, while the indirect method gives about 7 mm or more.

The calculations show that the binocular field is very much less than the monocular. To improve on this, the Haag-Streit 900 BQ slit lamp introduced in 1986 can be fitted with a Stereo-Variator, which reduces the effec-

tive separation of the objectives to 4.5°, or about 8 mm. This greatly increases the field of view, as indicated by the figures in brackets in *Table 16.2*, though with some reduction in stereoscopic effect. Although the introduction of the Volk aspheric lenses has reduced the need for this device, it still remains useful with fundus contact lenses. The Stereo-Variator also provides a binocular view of the corneal endothelium and the posterior pole of the crystalline lens when using the method of specular reflection, thus giving better resolution.

Ocular measurements with the slit lamp

The slit lamp provides a convenient means of measuring the corneal thickness and the depth of the anterior chamber. In *Figure 16.11*, a ray from the back vertex A_2 of the cornea emerges as though from the image of the back surface formed at A'_2 by refraction at the front surface.

By focusing the microscope first on the front vertex A_1 and then measuring* the travel required to focus on the image point A'_2, the apparent thickness d' can be determined. The true thickness d can then be calculated from the conjugate foci relationship. Let r_1 denote the radius of curvature, F_1 the power of the anterior corneal surface and n the refractive index of the corneal substance, normally taken as 1.376. Then, in outline,

---

* Some early instruments allowed the microscope to be moved forwards against a linear scale, independently of the instrument as a whole. A different arrangement on modern instruments is to measure the travel of the whole instrument. Perkins (1988) determined the anterior chamber depth and lens thickness by adding a pointer arm to the slit lamp's trolley axle. If the diameter of the trolley wheels is known, the angle of rotation can be measured against a protractor scale and converted into a linear distance.

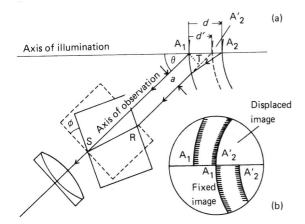

Figure 16.11. (a) Measurement of the apparent thickness of the cornea by the pachometer method of Jaeger. (b) Appearance of doubled image in correct setting. (Diagram not to scale.)

$\ell = -d$ (d is taken as +ve)

$L = n/\ell$

$L' = L + F_1$

$\ell' = 1/L' = -d'$ (d' also +ve)

which gives

$$d = \frac{n}{1/d' + F_1} \tag{16.1}$$

$$= \frac{n}{1/d' + (n-1)/r_1} \tag{16.1a}$$

Measurement of the anterior chamber depth involves the complication that refraction takes place at both surfaces of the cornea. For many purposes, however, it is sufficient to assume a single-surface cornea and to regard the depth of the anterior chamber as including the corneal thickness. If so, equation (16.1) can still be used, provided that n now denotes the refractive index of the aqueous humour.

The pachometer

One drawback of the successive focusing method is that an involuntary movement of the subject's head may take place between the two settings. This difficulty is overcome by a device designed by Jaeger (1952) and generally known as a pachometer, which fits over one of the slit-lamp microscope objectives. The mode of action of the Haag–Streit model is shown schematically in *Figure 16.11*. A vertical section of the anterior segment is illuminated by directing a very narrow beam through an aperture stop projecting from one side of the pachometer. The intended angle (40°, for example) is thus obtained between the axes of observation and illumination, the patient looking at the light. Variable doubling of the observed optical section is produced by two glass plates positioned in front of the microscope objective so as to bisect its aperture horizontally. The fixed lower plate is normal to the optical axis, but the upper plate can be tilted about a vertical axis. As a result, rays passing into the objective through this plate undergo a lateral displacement a which varies with the angle of tilt ϕ. A duplicate image is thus formed.

The diagram shows the tilt adjusted such that the ray

$A_2'R$ refracted by the upper plate emerges along the same path as the ray A_1S through the fixed plate. In this setting, the appearance is as suggested by *Figure 16.11(b)*. The arrangement described would, in fact, produce a complete doubling of the image, but a special eyepiece incorporating a bi-prism and slit aperture in the exit pupil plane is used to remove the unwanted half of each image. This makes coincidence setting easier.

The lateral displacement a produced by a plate of thickness t can be found from

$$a = \frac{t \sin(\phi - \phi')}{\cos \phi'} \tag{16.2}$$

where ϕ is the angle of incidence of the given ray and ϕ' the corresponding angle of refraction. In this case, ϕ is also the angle through which the plate has been tilted from its zero setting. A tilt of about 25° is needed for a cornea of typical thickness.

From the triangle $A_1A_2'T$ it will be seen that

$$d' = A_1T \operatorname{cosec} \theta = a \operatorname{cosec} \theta \tag{16.3}$$

These two expressions enable the angle of tilt to be plotted against the apparent corneal thickness d'. Hence, by assuming particular values for r_1 and n in equation (16.1), the pachometer can be calibrated to give a direct reading of the corneal thickness or depth of anterior chamber. To measure the latter, a separate model with thicker plates (about 5.5 mm instead of 1.25 mm) is made in order to give the larger displacement required.

An idea of the apparent thickness a is obtained by regarding the cornea as a flat parallel plate of thickness 0.5 mm and index 1.375. For an observation angle θ of 40°, the thickness d' is about 0.26 mm, giving an apparent thickness a of about 0.20 mm. Exact ray tracing is necessary to take into account both the obliquity of the ray from A_2 and the curvature of the cornea. Equations are given by Patel (1981) and in the Appendix of Brennan *et al.* (1989). Alternatively, experimental calibration on contact lenses could be used.

Correction tables are provided for use when the actual corneal radius differs from the standard value assumed. If this difference is denoted by Δr_1, it can be deduced from equation (16.1a) that the resulting error E is given by the reasonable approximation

$$E = \frac{-(n-1)d^2\Delta r_1}{nr_1^2} \tag{16.4}$$

Taking, as average values, 7.8 mm for r_1, 0.5 mm for the corneal thickness and 3.6 mm for the depth of anterior chamber, we should have

$$E = -0.0011\,\Delta r_1 \text{ for the cornea}$$

and

$$E = -0.053\,\Delta r_1 \text{ for the anterior chamber}$$

The effect of refractive index changes in the media should also be considered. If the true value is $(n + \Delta n)$ instead of the assumed value n, the value of d obtained from equation (16.1) will be $n/(n + \Delta n)$ times the correct figure. For average ocular values, the resulting error in corneal thickness will be approximately

0.0004 mm for every 0.001 variation in the corneal refractive index and the error in the depth of anterior chamber will be approximately 0.003 mm for every 0.001 variation in the refractive index of the aqueous.

In monitoring thickness changes, accuracy depends on measuring exactly the same part of the cornea or anterior chamber on each occasion. One method is to direct the patient to look into the beam. The lateral position of the instrument is then adjusted so that the beam reflected from the cornea forms a narrow patch of light symmetrically distributed about the pachometer's aperture stop (Clark and Lowe, 1973; Stone, 1974). Another method (Mandell and Polse, 1969) is to fit small lamps above and below the microscope objective and to adjust the instrument so that the reflections of these lights are immediately above and below the corneal section when viewed through the microscope. It is now the observation, not the illuminating beam, that is normal to the cornea. In the Holden–Payor technique, the illuminating beam is 40° to the side of fixation, observation 25° from the other, while the angle of tilt of the pachometer plates is monitored by a computer so that many instrument settings may be recorded very quickly.

A micropachometer

The thickness of the corneal epithelium is less than 100 μm (microns). To measure it *in vivo* and without touching the eye, apparatus called a micropachometer has been devised by Wilson *et al.* (1980). A projection system incorporating variable doubling plates was used to form two bright slit images, each of about 0.007 mm in width, very close to the corneal apex. Observation was made through a Zeiss (Jena) slit lamp with a magnification up to 100×. For the three subjects examined, the mean results from 40 measurements on each were 55.3, 65.4 and 65.5 μm.

Depth of anterior chamber

A clinically orientated technique for measuring the depth of anterior chamber with a slit lamp alone has been described by Smith (1979). The instrument used was a Haag-Streit 900 which has a scale recording the length of the slit. With the slit horizontal and of moderate thickness, the beam is focused on the subject's cornea from the temporal side at an angle of 60° from the visual axis. Observation is made along the visual axis. The length of the slit is adjusted so that the intersection of its leading edge with the crystalline lens appears in alignment with the intersection of the opposite edge with the posterior surface of the cornea. The depth of anterior chamber is found by multiplying the required slit length by 1.117 and adding 0.5079 mm; or, more simply, multiplying by 1.1 and adding 0.5 mm. The derivation of this formula is described in detail.

Douthwaite and Spence (1986) modified Smith's technique by using a horizontal slit of fixed 2 mm length (governed by what is normally the height control), and varying the obliquity of observation, the patient fixating the slit. A conversion table was provided to give the anterior chamber depth. A change of 0.1 mm in depth

is equivalent to a 1° change in angle between slit lamp and microscope.

Another method of measuring the depth of anterior chamber is to photograph a slit-lamp section of the anterior chamber, the method used by Sorsby *et al.* (1961). Clark and Lowe (1973, 1974) have discussed the mathematical treatment of the measurements from the resulting photographs.

Other methods of measuring corneal thickness and depth of anterior chamber, less suitable for routine clinical use, are described in Chapter 20.

The applanation tonometer

The Goldmann applanation tonometer is a reliable device for measuring the intra-ocular pressure. A plane surface is pressed against the anaesthetized cornea with a variable force until a circular area of 7.35 mm² (diameter 3.06 mm) is flattened. The force then applied can be shown to equal the pressure within the globe. One of the factors determining the above choice of diameter was that 1 g weight of force is then equal to the pressure of 10 mmHg.

In the original Goldmann design, the truncated cone used to apply the force incorporates a prismatic doubling device to ensure that the applanated area is of the correct diameter. In *Figure 16.12(a)*, illustrating a

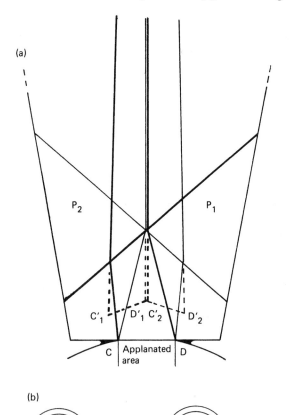

Figure 16.12. (a) Cross-section of the Goldmann applanation cone for measuring intra-ocular pressure: $C'_1D'_1$ is the image of CD formed by prism P_1; $C'_2D'_2$ the image formed by prism P_2. (b) Appearance of the split ring at the correct setting.

cross-section of the Goldmann cone, prism P_1 should be visualized as lying above the plane of the diagram and prism P_2 below it, the two adjacent plane edges being in contact. The points C and D mark the horizontal diameter of the area to be flattened. The upper half of this circle is deviated to the left by prism P_1, which images CD at C_1D_1. The lower half is imaged by prism P_2 at C_2D_2. The dimensions and angles of the prisms are so arranged that D_1 and C_2 are just in contact when CD has its predetermined value of 3.06 mm.

Fluorescein stain is used so that the prismatic ring of tears liquid surrounding the applanated area becomes luminous under blue light. Since it is the internal periphery of this ring which defines the applanated area, the correct setting is that shown on the left in *Figure 16.12(b)*. The setting shown on the right is incorrect and would give too low a reading.

This tonometer is conveniently used in conjunction with a slit lamp, on which it is mounted in front of the patient's headrest. As well as giving the necessary support, adequate magnification and illumination with blue light are also provided.

It is important to adjust the level of the cone so that the circle appears symmetrically split into two equal halves. Just before the cone touches the eye, the reflection of its tip in the cornea may be seen through the microscope and this, together with the pupil, will aid initial alignment. Only a small final adjustment will then be necessary after contact with the cornea has been made. The prism dividing line is usually set at horizontal, but when the cornea is markedly astigmatic should be set at $43°$ to the minus cylinder axis to allow for the elliptical area of contact.

The Goldmann cone is also used in the Perkins hand-held applanation tonometer,[*] which gives a comparable standard of accuracy.

Photography of the anterior segment

External eye photography

A satisfactory view of the face can be obtained with an ordinary camera, using natural lighting, flood lighting or electronic flash. For close-up photography (macrophotography) with object image reductions of 2:1 or even 1:1, a single-lens reflex camera can be used, preferably with a special macro-lens. The appropriate close-up lens and extension tube or bellows must be fitted. A headrest is required to keep the patient's head steady, while the camera is best mounted on a sliding base similar to that of the slit lamp. Informative papers written for ophthalmic practitioners have been published by Wagstaff (1970), Bishop (1976) and Zantos and Pye (1980). Larger works on this topic by Hansell (1957), Justice (1982) and Long (1984) may also be consulted.

Slit-lamp photography

Photography through the slit lamp with a relatively broad beam of illumination may be undertaken by attaching a camera to the eyepiece (Holden and Zantos, 1979; Thaller, 1983). Khaw and Elkington (1988) recommended the use of a single-lens reflex camera with an exposure meter recording from a small area in the centre of the viewfinder.

Photography of a narrow section of the cornea requires special apparatus. First, the illumination must be increased. One method is to boost the voltage supply to the ordinary tungsten-filament bulb at the moment of photographic exposure. Even so, relatively long exposures of perhaps 1/30 second may be needed, increasing the risk of an eye movement during this time. A much superior method using electronic flash requires a modification or addition to the slit-lamp system. One arrangement is to mount the flash tube in the position previously occupied by the tungsten-filament lamp. The latter is moved further away from the projection lens and imaged on the flash tube by an extra condensing system. Since the flash tube is transparent, it does not interfere with the illumination provided by the ordinary lamp for routine use of the slit lamp and focusing for photography. When fired, the flash tube has a light output many times greater than that of the lamp, but for a duration of only about 1/1000 second.

The camera of the conventional photo slit lamp may either have its own objective giving a magnification in the range −0.5 to −2.0, or may view through one of the microscope objectives. In this case the magnification is usually that of the microscope objective, possibly multiplied by the zoom or Galilean magnification changer incorporated in the instrument. Depending on the particular model, it is in the range −0.65 to −6.5. Both still and continuous video displays using the normal tungsten lamp and a CCD camera are also coming into use.

Tilted image plane

At magnifications in the neighbourhood of unity, the depth of field is very limited, even if the apertures of both the camera lens and slit projector are reduced. As a result, only a portion of the slit-lamp section can be accurately in focus. This problem was overcome by Brown (1972) and Brown *et al.* (1987) in a research instrument designed to record anterior chamber geometry and the relative amounts of light scattered by the media. By using Scheimpflug's principle of tilting the plane of the film with respect to the optical axis of the camera lens, a focused image of the complete slit-lamp section of the anterior segment can be obtained.

Photography of corneal endothelium

To obtain the higher magnification needed to record details of the corneal endothelium, a conventional single-lens reflex camera can be mounted behind one of the microscope eyepieces. The latter then contributes to the final magnification (Holden and Zantos, 1979; Bellisario-Reyes *et al.*, 1980). Alternatively, Long and

---

[*] Supplied by Clement Clarke International Ltd, Edinburgh Way, Harlow, Essex CM20 2TT.

Murphy (1987) suggested doubling the magnification of a conventional slit-lamp camera by adding a teleconverter immediately in front of the camera body. They also recommended the use of fine-grain black and white film such as Kodak Technical Pan 2415.

The endothelium is best observed by the method of specular reflection, in which an obliquely incident narrow illuminating beam is reflected by the cornea into the observation system. The Eisner lens (1985), a hand-held contact lens giving a 2.2× magnification, has been developed for visual observation. A number of specular photo-microscopes have been designed for this method. For example, the Nikon instrument uses a conventional photo slit-lamp illuminating system and a× or 10× camera objective to form an image directly on the film.* The Leitz design follows earlier research instruments in using a plano-convex lens to applanate an area of the cornea, thus increasing the area that can be photographed in one exposure.

Automated non-contact specular microscopes are now available. Viewing a video monitor, the observer places the instrument in approximately the correct position in relation to the patient's eye. When the image of the endothelium is in focus, the computerized system triggers the flash. The image is stored digitally, displayed on the monitor and can be printed out on a video printer at about 120× magnification. The cell density may also be calculated and displayed.

Photographic recording of a cataract

The conventional photo-slit lamp may be used to photograph lens changes, either in slit section or by retro-illumination, the slit beam passing through the dilated pupil and preferably being reflected from the optic disc. For research purposes, a more precise recording of areas and densities of the opacities is needed. In addition to the tilted image plane camera described above, Brown *et al.* (1987) and Brown (1987) describe a retro-illumination system specifically designed for this. The illuminator and camera are positioned at right-angles, the illuminating beam being directed into the eye by a semi-reflecting mirror. The Purkinje images are almost eliminated by using a polarized hollow conical illuminating beam, with a crossed analyser in the viewing pathway. Devices of the types described on page 44 for assessing what is termed the retinal visual acuity are mounted on slit lamps.

Lasers in eye treatment

Lasers can be incorporated in specialized slit lamps for various therapeutic or surgical procedures. An account has been given by Brown (1986). As these intense sources of light can be aimed and focused very precisely, the energy can be used to heat localized areas of tissue

in order to photo-coagulate it. Alternatively, if sufficient energy is concentrated in an exposure of only a few nanoseconds, the atoms of the tissue are ionized to form a gaseous plasma, thus obliterating it. For this purpose, the laser radiation must be of a wavelength which the tissue absorbs strongly.

The cornea transmits radiation of wavelengths between 300 and 1500 nm and can therefore be reshaped by the ultra-violet energy of shorter wavelength from an excimer laser. The word 'excimer' is derived from 'excited dimers', a term denoting a highly unstable combination of an inert gas with a halogen, for example, argon fluoride. As these molecules decay, ultra-violet light is emitted in extremely short pulses. For argon fluoride, the wavelength is 193 nm. A more detailed account of this technique has been given by Marshall (1988). The infra-red energy emitted continuously from a carbon dioxide laser at 10 600 nm or from the holmium laser may also have application here.

The neodymium–YAG (neodymium ions within a yttrium-aluminium-garnet crystal) pulsed laser emits in the near infra-red at 1063 nm. Radiation of this wavelength passes through the cornea and can be used for cutting the posterior capsule if it should become cloudy after an extra-capsular cataract implant operation. Punching a small hole in the iris of patients with potential angle-closure glaucoma is another of its uses.

The diode laser's near infra-red radiation (810 nm) and the krypton laser's red light (647 nm) are absorbed by melanin, and may be used for treatment of retinal conditions. As the krypton laser's wavelength is transmitted by the yellow pigment of the macula, it may have applications where coagulation is required close to the fovea. The diode laser may be employed in conjunction with indocyanine green dye, since this absorbs at this wavelength, re-emitting also in the near infra-red. The dye may be used to photograph choroidal vessels, or for photocoagulation since it will accumulate in zones of leakage.

The argon laser emits both blue (488 nm) and green light (514 nm), which are absorbed by both melanin and haemoglobin. This laser is used to seal leaking blood vessels, and, with the addition of a green filter to absorb the blue light, may also be used near the macula. Both this and the krypton lasers give continuous emission of light as distinct from pulses. A low-intensity beam is produced for aiming, a high-power flash being triggered when required. Instruments having ultra-violet, infra-red or pulsed lasers need to incorporate low-powered lasers as well to give a continuous emission of visible light for aiming purposes.

The direct ophthalmoscope

Basic principle

The ophthalmoscope is the standard instrument for examining the posterior segment of the eye and fundus, as well as allowing a view of the anterior segment in general diffuse illumination. In normal conditions, the pupil of the eye appears dark to an observer. *Figure 16.13* represents a myopic eye, with H and J the edges

---

* A 10× objective lens had previously been used in a similar way by Brown (1970).

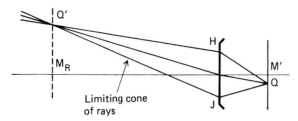

Figure 16.13. Observation of the fundus point Q. Both the light source and the observer's eye must lie within the cone Q'HJ.

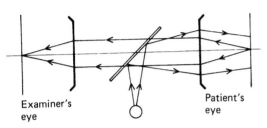

Figure 16.14. The simplest form of direct ophthalmoscope.

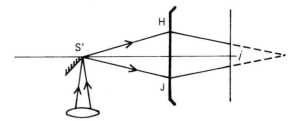

Figure 16.15. Illumination of the fundus by the ophthalmoscope.

Table 16.3 Diameter in millimetres of illuminated retinal patch in direct ophthalmoscopy

g (mm)	$w = -25$ mm			$w = -35$ mm		
		K			K	
	-10 D	0	$+10$ D	-10 D	0	$+10$ D
2	1.0	1.3	1.7	0.6	0.9	1.3
4	2.0	2.7	3.3	1.2	1.9	2.6
6	3.0	4.0	5.0	1.9	2.9	3.9

of the pupil, Q a point on the retina and Q' its image in the eye's far-point plane. The point Q would be illuminated by a source of light placed anywhere within the cone Q'HJ. For Q to be visible to an observer, the observer's eye must also be placed within this same cone. Normally, the observer's head prevents illumination entering the eye from within the cone. The ophthalmoscope is a device incorporating some form of beam splitter to allow a beam of light to enter the eye, undergo diffuse reflection at the fundus and return to the examiner's eye by the same or a neighbouring path. At its simplest, the beam splitter is an inclined glass plate (*Figure 16.14*) reflecting light into the eye and allowing direct observation of the patient's fundus. This method of ophthalmoscopy is accordingly called direct to distinguish it from the 'indirect' method described on pages 318–324.

The detailed design of the direct instrument is considered later in this section. In outline, a modern system usually consists of a small low-voltage bulb whose filament is imaged on an inclined mirror or reflecting prism. This image acts as the immediate source of light. Just above the reflector is a sight hole through which the patient's eye is viewed. One of a series of lenses can be placed behind the sight hole to allow any part of the media of fundus of an emmetropic or ametropic eye to be brought into focus. These lenses could simultaneously correct the spherical component of the examiner's own ametropia.

Illumination of the fundus

The cone of rays leaving the filament image or immediate source will, in general, more than fill the patient's pupil. The instrument is held close to the patient's eye, but at its closest the immediate source will be at a negative distance w, some 25 mm from the patient's cornea and usually nearer 35 mm. This is well beyond the anterior focal point of the eye so that, after refraction, the rays of light converge to a focus behind the retina, illuminating an area of diameter j smaller than that of the pupil (*Figure 16.15*).

If the size of the source is ignored, the illuminated area of the fundus can be regarded as a blur circle. Its diameter j can thus be obtained from equation (4.16a) by substituting $W(= 1/w)$ for L. Thus

$$j = g\frac{(K - W)}{K'} \tag{16.5}$$

Table 16.3 gives specimen values for j over a range of values of g, K and w, the dioptric length of the eye, K', being taken as $+60$ D.

Two points should be noted. The field of illumination in an emmetrope with a 4 mm pupil is about the same size as the optic disc, which is approximately 2 mm vertically by 1.5 mm horizontally. Secondly, irrespective of refractive error, the field of illumination reduces rapidly with increasing distance between instrument and eye.

In reality, the source has a finite size, say about 1 mm. This would increase the diameter of the illuminated area by about 0.5 mm.

The angular divergence of the cone of illumination, angle HS'J in *Figure 16.15*, need be no greater than would fill a fully dilated pupil of about 7 mm at a working distance of 35 mm, an angle of about 11.5°. A wider angle than this would not increase the area of fundus illuminated.

With a normal, smaller sized pupil, the cone of illumination overlaps its margins, allowing some inexactness in the position of the instrument relative to the patient's eye. Controlling the area of fundus illuminated is important and is discussed below.

Observation system

The optical system of the unaccommodated emmetropic eye of power about $+60$ D forms an erect image of the fundus at infinity. For an unaccommodated emmetropic

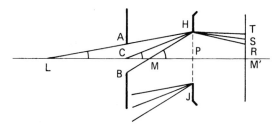

Figure 16.16. Fields of view of the direct ophthalmoscope. Limiting ray paths: THB (maximum field); SHC (field of half illumination); RHA (field of full illumination).

or corrected observer, it thus acts like a magnifier of power 15×. The same observer would also obtain a clear view of the fundus of an ametropic eye by placing the appropriate lens before the sighthole, thereby correcting the spherical element of the subject's ametropia. Although the ophthalmoscope can provide an approximate estimate of the mean refractive error, a number of factors lead to inaccuracies (Emsley, 1952).

Small amounts of astigmatism do not impair the view but higher amounts have marked effects. Because of the different magnifications in the two principal meridians, some scissors distortion may be evident and the optic disc may appear to be unusually oval. Retinal blood vessels running in directions approximately parallel to one of the principal meridians may appear blurred in comparison with others perpendicular to it, needing a different sighthole lens to bring them into focus.

A much clearer view of the fundus of a highly astigmatic eye is usually obtained by observation through the patient's spectacles. (For reasons discussed later, this is also true of the highly myopic eye.) The highly astigmatic examiner should wear his correction or mount a lens or lenses of the appropriate power in a supplementary cell or disc behind the sighthole.

Fields of view

The fields of view are governed by the subject's pupil diameter g, the sighthole aperture a, and their separation w. Given an eye with only moderate ametropia, the pencil of rays emerging from any point on the retina will be approximately parallel. In *Figure 16.16*, the various semi-fields of view are determined by rays emerging from the upper extremity H of the pupil and passing respectively through the upper extremity A, the centre C and lower extremity B of the sighthole.

Maximum field of view

The limiting ray is HB which originates from the point T on the retina and just enters the sighthole after intersecting the axis at M. The field of view is twice the angle HMP. For the typical values of $g = 4\,\text{mm}$, $a = 2\,\text{mm}$ and $w = 35\,\text{mm}$ (neglecting its minus sign), the maximum field of view is 9.8°.

Field of half illumination

Because of vignetting, the illumination falls to zero at the extreme edge of the maximum field of view. A more realistic value is that given by the 'field of half illumination'. The meaning of this term is that the illumination at the edge does not fall below 50% of its value at the centre. This reduction is relatively unimportant because physiologically and psychologically the observer adapts to the difference, and can also turn the instrument to bring the object of regard into the centre of the field of view. The limiting ray is HC, originating from the point S on the retina. It can be visualized from *Figure 16.16* that the full pencil of refracted rays from S covers the lower half of the sighthole. For the same values of g and w as previously, the field of half illumination would be 6.5°.

Field of full illumination

This is the field within which *every* incident pencil fills the sighthole. The limiting ray is HA, originating from the retinal point R and meeting the axis at L. The field is twice the angle HLP. On the same basis as before, its value would be only 3.3°, but this figure is of little importance in practice.

Linear extent of fields

The diameter of the observation field of half illumination (also known as the 'useful field of view') may be obtained by regarding C, the centre of the sighthole, as an object for the patient's eye and calculating the blur-circle diameter on the patient's retina. Equation (16.5) and *Table 16.3* can thus be regarded as giving the useful linear field of view as well as the field of illumination. In practice, the sighthole is often 2–5 mm behind the filament image, thus making the useful field of observation slightly smaller than the field of illumination. There is also a slight displacement, approximately $1\frac{1}{2}°$, between these two fields because the bulb filament is imaged just below the sighthole.

The other linear fields can be obtained in the same way, taking L and M as object points. For the reduced emmetropic eye and other values as before, the results would be 2.86 mm (maximum) and 0.95 mm (full illumination).

Magnification

Although it is easy to determine the ratio of image size on the observer's retina to an object size on the patient's fundus, a more informative approach is to compare the apparent subtense of a fundus element with the angle that the same element would subtend if placed at the assumed reference seeing distance, i.e. $-250\,\text{mm}$ or $-4\,\text{D}$. This is analogous to the method used to determine the conventional magnification of the ordinary magnifying glass (*see page 248*) and similarly neglects any difference between observers due to their own refractive errors.

Figure 16.17(a) illustrates the relationship for an emmetropic eye. The fundus element M′Q of height h subtends an angle u at the eye's principal point P. The image, being formed at infinity, subtends the same

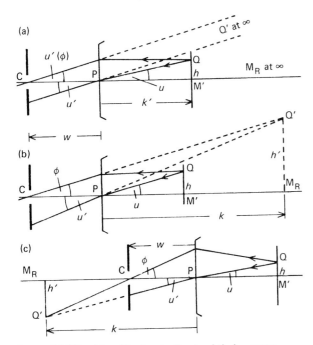

Figure 16.17. Magnification in direct ophthalmoscopy. Patient's eye: (a) emmetropic, (b) hypermetropic, (c) myopic.

angle u' at the centre of the sighthole C as at P. In radians, these angles are given by

$$u = h/k'$$

and

$$u' = n'u = n'h/k' = hK'$$

Viewed directly from a distance of 250 mm or 0.25 m, this same fundus element would subtend an angle u_o equal to $h/0.25$. The magnification M under which it is seen through the ophthalmoscope is therefore

$$M = u'/u_o = 0.25K' = K'/4 \qquad (16.6)$$

Thus, for the standard reduced eye, $M = 15$.

A hypermetropic eye is illustrated in *Figure 16.17(b)*. The fundus is imaged behind the eye at M_RQ' where it subtends a smaller angle at C than at P. The reverse applies to the myopic eye, as shown in *Figure 16.17(c)*. In both cases, the image height h' is given by

$$h' = hK'/K \qquad (16.7)$$

and the angle ϕ which it subtends at the sighthole by

$$\phi = \frac{M_RQ'}{CM_R} = \frac{h'}{CP + PM_R}$$

$$= \frac{h'}{-w + k} = \frac{h'K}{1 - wK}$$

Using equation (16.7) we can replace $h'K$ in this last expression by hK', giving

$$\phi = \frac{hK'}{1 - wK} \qquad (16.8)$$

As previously, for the unaided eye we have

$$u_o = h/0.25 = 4h$$

The magnification M can therefore be put in the form

$$M = \phi/u_o = \frac{K'}{4} \times \frac{1}{1 - wK} \qquad (16.9)$$

Since w is a negative quantity, the term $(1 - wK)$ is greater than unity in hypermetropia and less than unity in myopia. Consequently, for a given value of K' the magnification is greater for the myopic than for the hypermetropic eye. For example, if K' is taken as $+60$ D and w as -35 mm, the magnification is 18.2 when $K = -5.00$ D but only 12.8 when $K = +5.00$ D. On the other hand, as shown by *Table 16.3*, the field of view is greater in hypermetropia than in myopia. It has already been pointed out that this table and equation (16.5) apply also to the useful linear field of view. If equations (16.5) and (16.9) are multiplied together, the result can be reduced to

$$M = -gW/4j \qquad (16.10)$$

showing that for given values of g and w the magnification is inversely proportional to the useful linear field of view j.

In medium and high myopia, it is often advantageous to examine the central fundus through the patient's own spectacles. The field of view is enlarged, while the fundus does not go out of focus so rapidly should the examiner move away from the patient.

In with-the-rule astigmatism, the disc will appear more oval than usual because of the higher magnification in the eye's stronger (vertical) principal meridian. However, if the patient is made emmetropic by means of a contact lens, the working distance w no longer affects the magnification, which now becomes $K'/4$. Consequently, the disc may not appear quite so oval, though in high astigmatism its actual shape is possibly abnormal. In myopia, the disc may indeed be larger than normal, as well as the increased magnification making it appear so.

Design requirements

Several criteria must be satisfied for the instrument to provide a clear view of the fundus. These are:

(1) Adequate illumination of the fundus. Halogen lamps of higher intensity are tending to replace the conventional tungsten-filament types but should not be used any brighter than is necessary.
(2) Control over the intensity of illumination. This is often provided by a variable resistance, either in the instrument handle or in the transformer circuit.
(3) Control over the area of fundus illuminated (the reason for this is described on pages 317–318 on clinical use of the direct ophthalmoscope).
(4) Freedom from harmful radiation: the low-voltage, low-wattage lamps normally used emit negligible ultra-violet radiation and the amount of infra-red is too small to cause trouble. Strong illumination by blue light, which can easily penetrate the ocular media, especially that of an aphakic, may also be a possible cause of trouble (*see* 1980 Symposium on Intense Light Hazards and Ophthalmic Diagnosis and Treatment, particularly the paper by Calkins *et al.*, 1980). In general, examination of any one area of the retina with the direct ophthalmoscope is

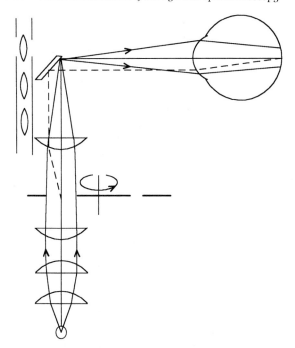

Figure 16.18. Optical system of the Keeler Vista Specialist ophthalmoscope. (Redrawn from material kindly supplied by Keeler Instruments Ltd.)

unlikely to be prolonged enough to cause trouble, but the indirect instrument and fundus cameras to be described below need careful design and use. To reduce both the blue light hazard and glare to the patient, the use of yellow-coated indirect ophthalmoscopy lenses is recommended.

(5) Freedom from stray light reflected from the edges of the sighthole and lens mounts, known as sighthole flare.

(6) Minimization of the corneal reflex.

The corneal reflex

The cornea acts as a convex mirror and forms an image of the immediate source about 3.6 mm behind its vertex. When the sighthole lenses are adjusted to view this region of the eye, the corneal reflex forms a tiny bright spot in the field of view. When the lenses are changed to bring the fundus into focus, a much larger though dimmer blur patch is formed on the observer's retina, veiling the view of the central fundus. The size of this blur patch may be reduced by decreasing the diameter of the sighthole to between 2 and 3 mm, but this also reduces the apparent brightness of the fundus.

Early ophthalmoscopes often consisted of a silvered mirror which reflected light from an external lamp into the eye, while the fundus was observed through a pierced hole in the mirror. This gave rise both to sighthole flare and to a corneal reflex positioned in the centre of the field of view. The corneal reflex may be decentred by reflecting the light from just below the sighthole. In many instruments, the immediate source is an image of the lamp filament which is formed on and reflected by an inclined stainless steel mirror which extends only as far as the bottom of the sighthole (*Figure*

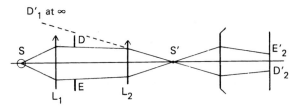

Figure 16.19. Imagery of the field stop DE in the direct ophthalmoscope (mirror omitted for clarity). The source S is imaged at S' on the mirror by the condensing lenses L_1 and L_2, and the stop at infinity by lens L_2. A second image ($D_2'E_2'$) of the stop is thus formed on the retina of the emmetropic eye.

16.18). Sighthole flare is eliminated at the same time. The lamp filament must be compact and special pre-centred bulbs allow accurate positioning of the filament image on the mirror without requiring centring adjustments on the instrument itself.

The corneal reflex and specular reflexes from the retinal blood vessels and internal limiting membrane may be eliminated by placing a piece of Polaroid material in the illumination system below the mirror, and a crossed analyser behind the sighthole. Since the diffusely reflected light from the fundus does not remain polarized, it is not extinguished by the analyser. The bulb output has to be increased by about four times because the polarizer absorbs approximately 50% of the light, while a further 50% of the scattered light from the fundus is absorbed by the analyser.

Typical designs

Figure 16.18 illustrates a modern ophthalmoscope. Light from the bulb is collected by the multi-element condensing system and is imaged to form the immediate source on the inclined stainless steel mirror just below the sighthole. A series of diaphragms of different sizes are mounted in the first focal plane of the last element of the condensing system. They are therefore imaged in sharp focus on the fundus of an emmetropic eye. Round stops give illuminated field diameters subtending approximately 6, 12 and 30Δ at the eye's nodal point. *Figure 16.19* shows these diaphragms to be aperture stops with regard to the filament image, but field stops for the instrument and eye together. Other shaped stops, graticules and filters may also be provided. The sighthole lenses are mounted in individual metal cells which are driven round a channel in the instrument by means of a cog wheel. This type of lens arrangement, dating from 1883, was introduced by Morton as an improvement on Couper's original system.

Figure 16.20 illustrates a somewhat different type of instrument. The condensing system consists of two lenses and the convex lower face of a prism, which also reflects the light into the patient's eye. This is a modification of the instrument introduced in 1914 by May. The sighthole lenses are mounted around the circumference of a disc – a development of the Rekoss disc of about 1852. This type of arrangement is also often called a May head. The May disc has fewer lenses than the Morton race, but both instruments are often provided with an auxiliary lens disc with further strong

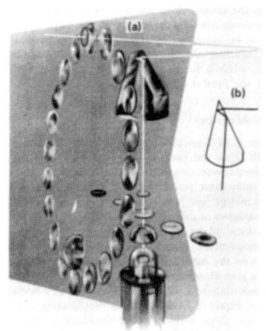

Figure 16.20. (a) Optical system of the AO Fulvue ophthalmoscope, using a modified May prism, also shown in (b). (Reproduced by kind permission of American Optical Corporation.)

positive and negative lenses in order to extend the range.

Although the aperture stops and graticule are imaged sharply only on the fundi of emmetropes, a sharp image will still be formed in marked ametropia if the patient wears his refractive correction. In the Keeler Acuity Scope, a graticule incorporating gratings of decreasing size is projected onto the fundus to evaluate the clarity of the ocular media. In some other instruments the graticule is mounted on an axial slide between the elements of the condensing system, so that compensation for the patient's refractive error can be made within the instrument. The slide is calibrated in dioptres to give a rough indication of the ametropia.

Clinical use of the direct ophthalmoscope

It is essential to follow a routine in ophthalmoscopy so that the eyes are examined thoroughly. With the widest field stop in place, the instrument provides a uniform illumination for inspecting the lids and tarsal and bulbar conjunctiva with the naked eye. With the instrument now held against the observer's brow and a positive lens of power +10.00 DS to +15.00 DS in the sighthole, a magnified view of these structures can be obtained. The homogeneity of the cornea and crystalline lens may also be checked, irregularities in structure often showing up as shadows against the fundus glow – light reflected back from the fundus. This glow usually becomes whiter and brighter if the ophthalmoscope is aimed at the optic disc, but peripheral lens opacities will not then be visible.

Still looking through the sighthole, the eye may be approached to a distance of about 35 mm or less, while the lens power is reduced to focus progressively backwards in the eye to the fundus. The instrument should be kept continuously in motion, angling it up and down and from side to side to view neighbouring regions of media and fundus. The patient is also requested to look up, down, left, right or in oblique positions of gaze so that the entire periphery of the fundus may be seen.

If the patient has small pupils, the largest field stop on the ophthalmoscope will illuminate the iris. Light reflected by a light-coloured iris can make observation of the fundus very much more difficult. Selection of a medium-sized aperture will reduce the angle of the cone of light and area of iris illuminated, making conditions easier.

If the fovea is illuminated with the large field stop in position, reflex miosis of the pupil is often very great: pupil reaction is more pronounced when the central rather than the peripheral retina is stimulated. This effect could be reduced by dimming the illumination, but it is then more difficult to see fine detail. The colour of the illumination will also become more red, upsetting the observer's judgement of colour. A small field stop – the macular stop of about 6Δ size – reduces the pupil constriction because a smaller area of the retina is illuminated, even though the full intensity of light is maintained. This macular stop is, however, too small to allow easy observation of peripheral regions of the retina.

Because of the small field of view with the macular stop, the macula may be difficult to find, though the optic disc can usually be found easily. From the disc, the ophthalmoscope beam is moved temporally through about three disc diameters, when the relatively vessel-free, darker red macula should be seen. The fovea is easily found if the patient is asked to look directly at the light, but it is then dangerously easy to miss a paramacular lesion, and pupil miosis seems to be even greater with active than with passive fixation. This 'lazy' method is, however, useful at times and can help in detecting eccentric fixation. Care should be taken to look at the region one to two disc diameters on the temporal side of the fovea. This seems to be particularly prone to diabetic retinopathy.

The observer's right eye should be used to view the patient's right eye, and left eye for left. For the right eye, the ophthalmoscope should be held in the right hand, while the left hand rests either on the back of the patient's chair, or on the patient's forehead to make observation steady. This second position is preferable when the pupil is small since it enables the practitioner to come as close as is safely possible to the patient's eye, thereby increasing the field of view (*see Table 16.3*). When the patient is looking down, the thumb of the left hand can gently raise the upper lid, holding it about 10 mm above the margin. This allows the patient to make a partial blink and is more comfortable than when the lid is held immediately above the lashes.

Irregularities in the contour of the fundus, such as cupping or elevation of the disc, may be detected in three ways. First, a change in the power of the sighthole

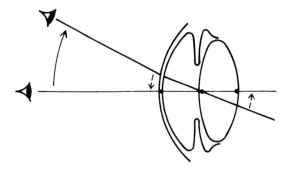

Figure 16.21. Location of opacities in the media by parallactic motion.

lens may be needed to focus on the structure at different levels. This difference can be expressed in dioptres or converted approximately to millimetres by the rule $1 D = \frac{3}{8}$ mm (*see* page 64). (Clinically, the area of cupping of the disc is often more important than the depth. Probably because there is less scattered light within the patient's eye, the colour, contrast and demarcation of the cup are frequently enhanced if viewed with the macular stop.) Secondly, if a streak of light is projected on to the fundus, irregularities of contour may be observable as deviations in the edge of the streak. Some ophthalmoscopes have a slit aperture stop which can be used for this purpose. Alternatively, the edge of the largest field stop might serve as a substitute for a light streak. In this use of the instrument, however, the very small angle between the axes of illumination and observation becomes a disadvantage. For this reason, observation with a slit lamp in conjunction with a Volk or similar lens as described earlier is much more satisfactory. Parallactic motion is the third clue to a difference in level. It may be observed, for example, with respect to blood vessels at the margin of a cupped disc or shallow retinal separation as the axis of observation is moved across the pupil.

Parallax may also be used to locate opacities in the media relative to the pupil margin (*Figure 16.21*). Opacities anterior to the pupillary plane appear to move 'against' the movement of the instrument, those in the crystalline lens 'with' the ophthalmoscope. The corneal reflex, although positioned near the middle of the crystalline lens, cannot be used to judge parallax since it also moves 'with' the motion of the ophthalmoscope.

The presence of extensive lenticular opacities always hinders fundus observation. A medium or small stop in the instrument is helpful and the ophthalmoscope should be held as close as is safely possible to the patient's eye so that any clear region of the media will subtend the maximum angle at the observer's eye. Dilation of the pupil with a mydriatic often helps, but care must be taken not to dilate the pupil of an eye with a very narrow anterior chamber angle.

It is sometimes said that since a lens opacity or irregularity at the posterior pole of the crystalline lens is near the nodal point of the eye, it will cause a greater deterioration in vision than a similar opacity placed anteriorly. In fact, an anterior cataract will spoil the definition of both central and peripheral images on the retina, while the posterior defect may not affect periph-

eral vision at all. This can be seen from *Figure 15.10*. Because of convergence, the area of an axial pencil at the rear of the crystalline lens is about 75% of its area at the pupil (*see Figure 22.7* on page 425). An opacity on the axis of the lens will therefore obstruct a greater proportion of light directed towards the fovea if positioned near the rear rather than the front of the lens. A posterior cataract is perhaps more difficult to see than an anterior one, especially by focal illumination or the slit lamp and thus may need to become more severe before being discovered. The impairment of vision on eventual diagnosis will thus be greater.

Occasionally, disturbances in the deeper layers of the fundus are better observed by illuminating a region neighbouring the suspected area, which is then illuminated by light scattered within the retina.

The fundus appears red because of blood and pigment in the retina and choroid. If the fundus is illuminated by red-free light (usually obtained by placing a green filter in the illumination system and increasing the voltage supplied to the bulb), the retinal blood vessels appear black against a greenish ground. The contrast of small haemorrhages or aneurysms is therefore increased. An even more dramatic enhancement of contrast of the vascular system is obtained by the technique of fluorescein angiography, in which fluorescent dye is injected into a vein and the fundus photographed in blue light. Fundus cameras are described on pages 324–327.

Because the sighthole is usually placed above the immediate source, the conventional ophthalmoscope gives poorer illumination of the fundus at the handle end of the field of view. The effect is worst when the instrument is held vertically and angled to view the inferior fundus, mainly because of the foreshortening of the pupil due to the obliquity of observation. A contributory factor is that more light is lost by surface reflections when the angle of incidence is very large, as in this case at the anterior surface of the crystalline lens. If the instrument is held horizontally and rotated about the axis of its handle, the inferior fundus may often be seen more brightly.

The indirect ophthalmoscope

Basic principle

The method of indirect ophthalmoscopy differs from the direct in that a positive lens is used to form a real inverted image of the patient's fundus. This intermediate aerial image is viewed by the observer, who may need a sighthole lens to bring it into focus.

The principle of the method is shown in *Figure 16.22*. The immediate source (usually an image of the actual source) is placed in close proximity to the observer's pupil (or sighthole) and both are imaged by a condensing lens into the plane of the subject's entrance pupil. Since the condenser also forms the aerial image of the fundus, its diameter controls the size of the field of observation as well as of illumination. The retinal fields of illumination and observation are of the same size and very nearly coincident, a small discrepancy arising

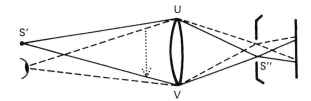

Figure 16.22. Basic principle of indirect ophthalmoscopy: the observer's and patient's pupillary planes are made conjugate by the condensing lens UV. The immediate source S' is thus imaged at S''. The dashed rays show the limits of the possible field of view and the dotted arrow the visible extent of the illuminated aerial image.

from the separation of immediate source and sighthole. In practice, it is the *effective* aperture of the lens which limits the fields – the diameter within which its image aberrations remain unobtrusive.

The traditional power of the condenser is +13 D, though a power of +20 or 25 D may be easier to use. To steady the condenser, the outstretched little finger of the hand holding it should be able to rest on the patient's forehead. This limits the distance between patient and examiner. On the other hand, for comfortable viewing, the examiner should not be too close to the aerial image. If a +13 D lens is held at about 91 mm from the patient's entrance pupil, the correct distance for the examiner is about 500 mm from the condenser. The illuminated patch on the retina would then have a diameter of about 7 mm, assuming the condenser to have an effective aperture of 40 mm. This is in the neighbourhood of three times its diameter in the direct method at normal working distances.

By using aspherical surfaces to minimize aberrations, it has been possible to increase both the actual and effective diameters of the traditional condenser, and also to produce a range of considerably higher powers. For example, the current Nikon range[*] comprises the following nominal powers with the effective apertures shown in parentheses: +14 D (52 mm), +20 D (48.6 mm) and +28 D (38.8 mm). Their centre thicknesses range from 12 to 14.5 mm; these lenses cannot be treated as thin. In the following discussion the power F of the condensing lens is therefore to be taken as its equivalent power. Also, the distances q and q' in *Figure 16.23* are measured from the respective principal points of the lens, which are internal, uncrossed, and separated by about one-third of the centre thickness. As a result, the vertex distance from the lens to the eye will be somewhat shorter than q, while the overall distance from the patient's eye to the observer's is increased by a trifling amount.

The purpose of the higher powered lenses is to increase the field of view by holding the lens closer to the eye without increasing the overall working distance. For example, the +14 D aspherical lens held at 84 mm from the eye would give an illuminated retinal patch of about 10 mm diameter while slightly *decreasing* the overall distance. The +20 D lens, designed to be held at 58 mm from the eye, gives an even larger illuminated

patch and substantially decreases the overall distance. On the other hand, compared with the traditional +13 D lens, the magnification is reduced – the price usually paid for an enlarged field of view, and vice versa.

As pointed out by Calkins *et al.* (1980), lenses of power +20 D and higher give a lower retinal illuminance than a +14 D lens because the illuminating beam is spread over a larger area. They also have the advantage of needing a smaller pupil and so a less powerful mydriatic can be used.

Magnification

Figure 16.23 shows the limiting ray paths from an illuminated point R on the retina of a hypermetropic eye and the formation of the aerial image. The distances k and k' are still regarded as positive, but for the return beam the direction of the light is reversed, so that q is negative and q' positive. For calculation, $Q(= 1/q)$ is conveniently regarded as -11.25 D and $Q'(= 1/q')$ as $+2.75$ D, the power F of the condenser being +14 D. The linear distances q and q' are then -88.9 and $+363.6$ mm respectively. By virtue of the returning light, an image H'J' of the subject's pupil HJ is formed in the plane of the sighthole by the condenser. Given $Q = -11.25$ D and $Q' = +2.75$ D, the image H'J' is 4.1 times the size of HJ. Every full pencil emerging from the subject's pupil and able to pass through the condenser must fill the exit pupil H'J'. Consequently, the full field of view will be obtained provided that the sighthole is positioned anywhere within H'J'. Without such latitude, indirect ophthalmoscopy in this simple form would be impracticable.

The subject's eye forms an image of R at R_1' in its far-point plane. The emergent pencil of rays from R therefore appears to diverge from R_1' and is bounded by the rays HA and JB. After refraction by the condenser, the ray HA is bound to pass through H' because H' and H are conjugate points. Similarly, the ray JB is bound to pass through J'. The point at which these two refracted rays intersect, R_2', is therefore the aerial image of R_1', their virtual origin. In addition, the central ray path R_1' PGC also passes through R_2'. *Figure 16.24* shows the corresponding construction for a myopic eye.

When the sighthole is at the correct distance q' from the condenser, it is unnecessary to determine h_2' in order to calculate the magnification. The angle u subtended by h_1 at P and its conjugate angle u' (OPG) are expressed by

$$u = h_1/k'$$

and, because of the reverse ray trace

$$u' = n'u = n'h_1/k' = h_1K' \qquad (16.11)$$

The aerial image subtends the angle ϕ at the sighthole. From the triangles OCG, OPG it can be seen that

$$\phi/u' = OP/OC = q/q' = Q'/Q$$

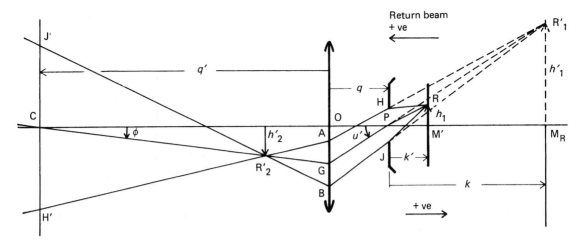

Figure 16.23.   Formation of the fundus images R'_1 and R'_2 in indirect ophthalmoscopy with a hypermetropic patient. Positive distances are measured towards the right in the incident beam (labelled below the optical axis) but towards the left in the return beam (labelled above the axis).

so that, from equation (16.11)

$$\phi = u'(Q'/Q) = h_1 K'(Q'/Q) \qquad (16.12)$$

Viewed directly from the reference seeing distance of 250 mm, on which the determination of conventional magnification is based, the fundus element of height h_1 would subtend an angle u_o equal to $h_1/0.25$ or $4h_1$. Consequently, the magnification M can be found from the expression

$$M = \phi/u_o = (K'/4)(Q'/Q) \qquad (16.13)$$

Thus, given the conjugates Q and Q', the magnification is directly proportional to the dioptric length of the eye and inversely proportional to its axial length. If $K' = +60$ D, $Q = -11.25$ D and $Q' = +2.75$ D, Q'/Q is -0.244 and the magnification is -3.66, the minus sign denoting inversion of the image. This is much lower than in the direct method.

If the $+14$ D lens is used with the conjugates $Q = -10.50$ D   ($q \approx -95$ mm)   and $Q' = +3.50$ D ($q' = +285.7$ mm), Q'/Q becomes -0.333. The magnification when $K' = +60$ D is then increased to -5.0.

The ratio Q'/Q depends on the power of the condensing lens and the distance chosen to separate the patient's and observer's eyes. When these quantities are fixed, the necessary value of q can be found from conjugate foci relationships, leading to Q and Q'. When aspheric condensers of increasing power are used, the working distance is progressively reduced and with it the ratio Q'/Q. It varies from about -0.25 for a $+14$ D lens to about -0.12 for a $+28$ D lens. For the $+90$ D BIO lens (page 306) it is about -0.1.

The position of the aerial image varies considerably with the subject's ametropia. In emmetropia it is formed in the anterior focal plane of the condenser. In hypermetropia, the pencils leaving the eye are divergent, causing the image to be formed at a greater distance from the condenser. The reverse applies in myopia.

A rough idea of the subject's ametropia can be obtained by moving the condenser closer to the examiner's eye. Calculation based on the conventional values of

Table 16.4   Calculation of aerial image size and magnification

Given data	$K = +6$ D, $K' = +64$ D
	$h = 3$ mm, $q = -90$ mm
	$F = +13$ D, $d = +480$ mm

Calculating scheme	Worked example
Refraction by eye	
$h'_1 = hK'/K$	$+32$ mm
$k = 1000/K$	$+166.67$ mm
Refraction by condenser	
$\ell = q - k$	-256.67 mm
$L = 1000/\ell$	-3.90 D
$L' = L + F$	$+9.10$ D
$\ell' = 1000/L'$	$+109.89$ mm
$h'_2 = h'_1 L/L'$	-13.71 mm
Angular subtense at eye	
$d - \ell'$	$+370.11$ mm
$\phi = h'_2/(d - \ell')$	-0.0370
Magnification	
$u_o = h/250$	0.012
$M = \phi/u_o$	-3.08

Q, Q' and F shows that if the magnification decreases, it indicates hypermetropia in excess of about $+3$ D. Other refractive states give rise to an increase in magnification.

A general 'step along' method of determining the position and size of the aerial images, together with the magnification obtained, is set out in *Table 16.4*, which should be used in conjunction with *Figure 16.25*. It is applicable to cases in which the sighthole is not necessarily at the correct distance q' from the condenser but at some specified distance d from it.

Reflex-free observation

In direct ophthalmoscopy, the corneal reflex of the source can be displaced from the centre of the field of view and reduced in size by appropriate design of the

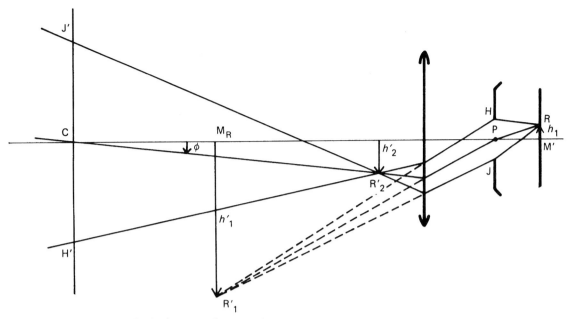

Figure 16.24. Formation of the fundus image for a myopic eye.

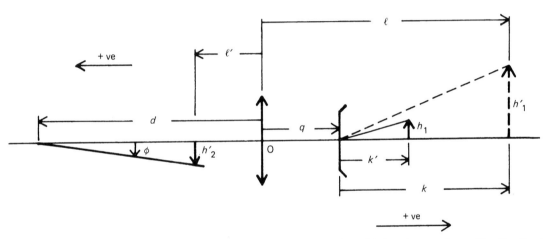

Figure 16.25. Magnification in indirect ophthalmoscopy. For dimensions indicated below the axis, the positive direction is to the right. For dimensions above the axis, it is to the left.

geometrical optics of the instrument. Similarly, in the indirect method, the corneal reflex and light reflected back or scattered by the crystalline lens can be rendered harmless, provided that certain conditions are met. Both the immediate source and the entrance pupil of the observer's eye are imaged in the plane of the patient's pupil at a magnification of Q'/Q, say about 0.2. These images are thus quite small. The image of the observer's pupil acts as the exit pupil for the return beam. Only those rays emerging from within this area can enter the observer's pupil. Being small, the two images in the patient's pupil can be completely separated. Given enough separation, any overlap between the entering beam and the return beam through the exit pupil can be avoided in the region of the cornea and crystalline lens. Specular reflections from the entering beam at the various surfaces are then unable to affect the return beam. This condition, due to Gullstrand, is illustrated in *Figure 16.26(a)*.

If the separation is insufficient, the corneal reflex may possibly be eliminated but the beams will overlap within the crystalline lens as in *Figure 16.26(c)*. Light scattered by lenticular opacities may then cause flare visible in the return beam.

In most systems of indirect ophthalmoscopy, further reflections could arise from the surfaces of the condenser lens. They can be reduced by anti-reflection coating the lens and displaced by tilting it slightly.

In general, a fairly large or even a pupil dilated by mydriasis is required for the indirect method.

Types of indirect ophthalmoscopes

Instruments for indirect ophthalmoscopy can be divided into two main categories: those which use the same condenser for both illumination and observation and those which do not. The principle of the first category is illustrated in *Figure 16.22*.

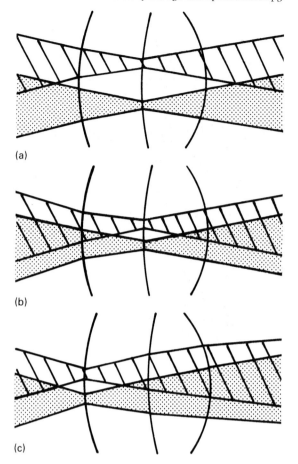

(a)

(b)

(c)

Figure 16.26. Paths of the entrance and exit bundles through the anterior segment of the eye in indirect ophthalmoscopy: (a) complete separation of the beams giving reflex-free conditions, (b) inadequate separation giving both corneal reflex and lens flare, (c) focus readjusted to eliminate corneal reflex at the expense of increased lens flare, the beams having the same separation as in (b).

Single-condenser instruments

To observe the patient's right fundus, the light source is held in the right hand and the condenser between the thumb and forefinger of the left hand, the little finger resting on the patient's forehead or zygomatic bone.

The lens is held close to the patient's eye, and moved to centralize the fundus glow within the condenser. The lens is then withdrawn from the patient's eye until the expanding fundus glow fills the condenser. At this separation, the patient's pupil is imaged in the plane of the observer's. The observer will have to accommodate for a distance closer than the condenser, possibly by wearing a near correction.

An ordinary direct ophthalmoscope could be used, but this is not very satisfactory as the internal condensing system produces a beam with too wide an angle. A modified condensing system is needed to provide a narrower spread of light, so that the aperture of the hand-held condenser is only just covered. If the examiner views the fundus image through the normal sighthole, the image will appear even duller. Since the sighthole usually has a diameter between 2 and 3 mm and is imaged into the patient's eye with a magnification of -0.2 or less, the exit pupil for the return beam is very small. Moreover, the separation of the illuminating and observation systems is too small to allow reflex-free observation. Some direct ophthalmoscopes can be converted for indirect use by increasing the separation between the immediate source and sighthole and by using larger than normal sighthole lenses. Alternatively, the top of the instrument is removed, allowing the observer to look above the ophthalmoscope. His own pupil then forms the aperture stop for the system.

An early stand instrument of this type was the large simplified Gullstrand ophthalmoscope. The photometry of the indirect method is discussed further by Martin (1951).

Binocular indirect ophthalmoscopy (BIO)

This method of indirect ophthalmoscopy has been elaborated into a binocular system. An example is shown in *Figure 16.27*. A lamphouse, mounted above and between the examiner's eyes on a headband or spectacle frame, illuminates the condenser which images the source at the bottom of the patient's pupil. Paired mirrors before the observer's eyes reduce the inter-pupillary distance so that the effective entrance pupils are imaged side by side near the top of the patient's pupil.

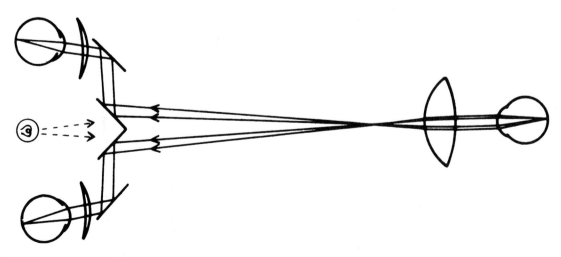

Figure 16.27. Layout of the headband or spectacle binocular indirect ophthalmoscope.

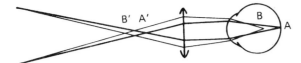

Figure 16.28. Stereopsis in binocular indirect ophthalmoscopy. The view of the image of B by the left eye is to the right of the image of A, exactly as when viewing B and A directly.

On some modern instruments, the distance between these paired mirrors and also between them and the lamphouse are adjustable. The narrowest separation is employed if the patient has small pupils, while the wider separation gives better stereopsis and less media flare. This type of device was originally introduced by the French ophthalmologist Giraud-Teulon and independently by Schepens (1947, 1951). The right eye is imaged at the left of the patient's pupil and vice versa for the left eye. This inversion of the exit pupils does not give pseudoscopic vision because the aerial image is also inverted. *Figure 16.28* shows two objects, A on the fundus and B in front of the fundus. The image B′ of B is nearer the observer than the image A′. To his left eye it appears on the right on A′, and to his right eye on the left of A′. This crossed projection is exactly the same as if A′ and B′ were real objects instead of inverted images. The stereoscopic view produced by this instrument is extremely useful clinically, while the head-mounted illuminator allows one hand to remain free to manipulate the patient's eyelids, draw the fundus and so on. Potter *et al.* (1988) and the Volk Optical Instruction Manuals (*see* References) are useful sources describing the clinical techniques needed for this type of ophthalmoscopy.

A binocular stand instrument was introduced by Bausch and Lomb in the 1930s. In the Zeiss Jena Binocular Ophthalmoscope 110, the aerial image of the fundus is further magnified by an additional system in front of the eyepiece, giving final magnifications of 15×, 20× and 40×; the corresponding fields of view are 40°, 29° and 14.5°.

The El Bayadi and aspherical lenses discussed on pages 306–307 convert the slit-lamp biomicroscope to a binocular indirect ophthalmoscope.

Instruments with separate condensers

In this second category of indirect ophthalmoscopes, separate condensers are used for illumination and observation. One of the earliest stand instruments – the Gullstrand reflex-free ophthalmoscope – uses this system, which is now incorporated in the modern hand instrument illustrated in *Figure 16.29*. The lamp filament is imaged by a multi-lens condenser system and semi-reflecting mirror into the bottom of the subject's pupil. Instead of a series of stops, an iris diaphragm is used to vary the field of view. Observation is made by means of a second multi-lens condenser, the aerial image being re-inverted by an erecting system before being viewed through the eyepiece. The instrument thus shows the fundus in the same orientation as the direct ophthalmoscope. The eyepiece is adjustable to

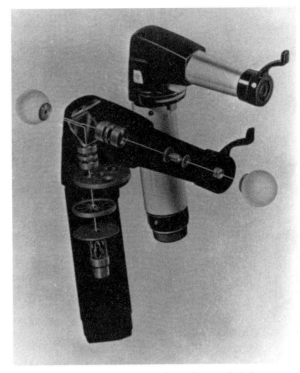

Figure 16.29. The AO monocular indirect ophthalmoscope. (Photograph reproduced by kind permission of the American Optical Corporation Inc.)

focus on the erect aerial image, the position of which varies with the subject's refractive error. With a typical eye, the magnification is about 5×, while the angular field of view can be extended to 20°. This instrument could be particularly useful for practitioners who have only one eye with good acuity.

Comparison of methods

The advantages of indirect ophthalmoscopy over the direct method are that:

(1) a much larger field is obtained, giving a general view of the fundus and of changes over a large area (especially useful in myopia);
(2) flare caused by poor media can be reduced, a reasonable view of the fundus often being obtained where no useful view can be achieved with the direct instrument;
(3) the fundus periphery is seen more clearly, perhaps because the small exit pupil and lower magnification reduce the effects of oblique image aberrations;
(4) a stereoscopic view can be obtained.

The disadvantages are:

(1) The much lower magnification, 2–4× as opposed to about 15×, though specially designed instruments incorporating a telescope can narrow or restore this discrepancy. Important but tiny foveal lesions can easily be missed.
(2) The technique is rather more difficult to use, especially with a patient who cannot keep his eye still.

It is very easy to lose the image completely when the patient's eye is turned so that the fundus periphery may be viewed.

(3) The indirect system normally gives an inverted image, which is confusing to practitioners who rarely use the method since the instrument has to be moved in the opposite direction to that in the direct method.

(4) Unfortunately, the larger field of illumination tends to produce greater pupillary contraction than the direct method so that a mydriatic is usually needed to dilate the pupil.

On balance, the direct method is more useful generally to optometrists, the indirect method being used when appropriate.

Development of the ophthalmoscope

Three stages can be discerned in the development of the ophthalmoscope, the first being the illumination of the fundus in such a way that the pupil appears luminous to an observer. Everyone is familiar with the bright reflex in the pupils of cats and dogs caught in the beams of vehicle headlights. This reflex is easily seen because of the large proportion of incident light reflected at the retinal tapetum and the wide pupillary aperture. In 1823, Purkinje described how the pupils of dogs, and then humans, were made luminous by light reflected into their eyes from a concave front surface of the spectacle lenses worn to correct his myopia. William Cumming, while at the Royal London Ophthalmic Hospital, took the investigation of the reflex a stage further in his attempt to relate its colour and luminosity to various pathological conditions. In 1846, he described optimum conditions for clinical observation of the pupillary reflex and noted that the axes of illumination and observation should be as close together as possible.

To obtain a useful view of the illuminated fundus was the next stage. The first true ophthalmoscope, in the sense of an instrument providing such a view, was made in about 1847 by the English mathematician Charles Babbage, best known for his pioneer work on computing engines. His simple device consisted of a plane mirror with perforations in the silvering. Because Babbage's idea was never developed into a clinical instrument, Hermann von Helmholtz is usually regarded as the inventor of the ophthalmoscope. His first model, announced in 1850, used three microscope cover-glasses, bound together and mounted at an angle to the sighthole, to reflect light into the subject's eye from an oil lamp placed beside his head. Provision was made for incorporating lenses for the correction of ametropia, but a later model in 1852 used the more convenient rotating disc of lenses suggested by Rekoss. A large number of different instruments using light reflected from an external source were produced during the years up to the early part of the twentieth century.

The final major development into the now familiar type of hand ophthalmoscope arose from the invention of the electric lamp. In 1885, the American ophthalmologist Dennett produced the first ophthalmoscope in which it was used. At that time, however, the very short life of the electric bulb and the bulk of the battery were serious drawbacks. It was the development of miniature low-voltage bulbs and torch batteries which could be housed in the instrument handle that led to the variety of instruments available today. In recent years, halogen bulbs have been introduced because of their higher luminance, colour temperature and longer life.

Although Helmholtz had realized that indirect ophthalmoscopy was possible, he thought it would have little advantage over the direct method. Ruete, in 1852, was the first to use the indirect method.

Descriptions of the development of the ophthalmoscope are available in the excellent text by Rucker (1971) and details of some of the early instruments are also to be found in Helmholtz's treatise (English edition 1924) and of a number of later designs in the work by Emsley (1952).

As Rucker points out, the term ophthalmoscope – derived from the Greek *ophthalmos* (eye) and *skopos* (target) – was not used by Helmholtz but soon came into use in America. Helmholtz called the instrument an Augenspiegel (eye mirror), the term still in use in German-speaking countries.

The fundus camera

The fundus camera is based upon the reflex-free indirect ophthalmoscope. Reflections from lenses within the instrument must also be eliminated by careful design of lens-surface curvatures and the positioning of internal aperture stops.

The illuminating system consists of a tungsten bulb to set up and focus the instrument, with an electronic flash or strobe (a xenon arc discharge tube) for the photographic exposure. As in some photo slit lamps, the tungsten bulb can be focused on to the flash tube by means of a relay condenser. When the flash is fired, its intensity is many times greater than that of the tungsten lamp, the effective exposure being about 1/500 second or less. Alternatively, the light from the tungsten bulb can be reflected towards the eye by means of an inclined glass plate, light from the flash passing straight through it.

In the system shown in *Figure 16.30*, the illuminating beam enters the eye through the lower part of the pupil, observation and photography being through the upper part. In the different arrangement shown in *Figure 16.31*, illumination from the flash enters the eye through an annular area, observation being made through the centre of the pupil. During photography, the mirror (3) reflecting light from the flash into the system swings up and another mirror (15) folds down to allow exposure of the film. The head (18) may be interchanged to allow stereoscopic fundus photography, while the alternative lenses (13) provide a 50° field at 1.5× or a 30° field at 2.5× on the film.

A blue filter can be inserted in the illumination beam and a yellow filter in the observation path in order to photograph the passage of fluorescein dye through the

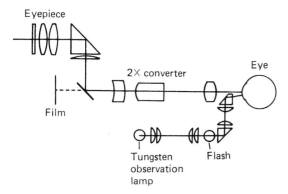

Figure 16.30. Simplified diagram of the optical system of the Kowa RC2 fundus camera. (Redrawn from information kindly given by Keeler Instruments Ltd.)

retinal vessels, a process called fluorescein angiography. The power supply for the flash has to be capable of allowing exposures every few seconds. Black and white monochrome film is normally used in this technique. For normal work, a high-contrast colour film with good colour discrimination at the red end of the spectrum is needed.

Details in the photographs may be enhanced for specific purposes by dark-room methods (*see*, for example, Shakespeare, 1987), or computer processing (Gilchrist, 1987a,b; Cox and Wood, 1991a,b).

The patient's pupil must first be dilated with a cycloplegic or strong mydriatic. With the patient seated comfortably with the head on the rest, the camera is moved so that the image of the aperture stop of the illuminating beam is in focus on the patient's iris. A slight movement of the camera will then allow the light to pass into the eye with the camera's illumination and observation pupils correctly positioned for reflex-free observation and maximum field of view. Rotation of the eye to photograph another part of the fundus will almost always require repositioning of the camera.

Modern fundus cameras can provide fields up to 45° and over. Aspheric condensing lenses are often used and some cameras now have an additional lens placed in contact with the cornea. By this means, fields up to 100° can be obtained.

Non-mydriatic fundus cameras

Non-mydriatic fundus cameras incorporate an infra-red video camera to allow alignment with the patient's eye and focusing on the fundus. Working in a darkened room enables the pupil to remain naturally dilated, whereas the focusing beam of the usual fundus camera would constrict the pupil. Provided that it dilates to about 4–4.5 mm, satisfactory photographs can be obtained because the electronic flash is quicker than the pupillary reflex. Some patients find the resulting brightness and after-image more disturbing but are spared the time needed for a mydriatic both to work and wear off. Polaroid film is often employed for convenience, though 35 mm film records finer detail. Still video or computer recording with the image captured by a CCD camera needs less light than conventional photography. Pupil dilation is probably still required in the presence of media opacities.

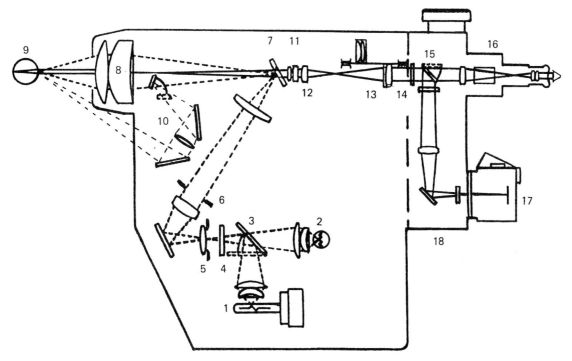

Figure 16.31. Optical system of the Zeiss Oberkochen stereo fundus camera FK 50. Key: 1 flash tube, 2 tungsten lamp, 3 swing-in mirror, 4 filter, 5 illumination aperture stop, 6 illumination field stop, 7 annular mirror, 8 aspheric objective, 9 patient's eye, 10 internal viewing system (for camera alignment, ray path incomplete for clarity), 11 astigmatism compensator, 12 internal focusing, 13 50°/30° field-selection system, 14 filter, 15 swing-in mirror, 16 stereo-binocular tube with eyepieces, 17 film plane, 18 interchangeable ocular head (the secondary photographic or observation system within head 18 has been omitted for clarity).

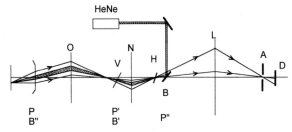

Figure 16.32. Optical system of the Scanning Laser Ophthalmoscope. Key: HeNe helium–neon laser, B beam diverter, H, V horizontal and vertical scanning mirrors, N, O concave mirrors, L lens, P pupil, A confocal aperture, D detector. For simplicity, the deviation produced by all the mirrors except B has been ignored. The input beam is shown shaded.

Measurement of fundus details

The image height on a fundus photograph of a structure such as the optic disc may depend upon several variables, for example the axial length of the patient's eye, the amount of ametropia, the design of the camera and the photographic format such as 35 mm or Polaroid.

Littman (1982, 1992), cited by Rudnicka *et al.* (1992), developed a Zeiss fundus camera with its objective based on telecentric principles. Like the Badal optometer illustrated in *Figure 4.25*, the angle u is given by the relation:

$$u = n'h/k'$$

where h is the height of the fundus detail. These workers showed that h can be expressed as a function of the image size h' by an expression of form:

$$h = pk'h'/57.296n' = pk'h'/76.539 \qquad (16.14)$$

where p is a value depending on the camera and n' is assumed to be 1.336. The value for k' for any particular patient can only be surmised. The combination of corneal power and refractive error K would give a clue, while the addition of ultrasonography would refine the estimate further. For the original Zeiss camera, p took the value 1.37, but this could be ascertained experimentally for any camera by photographing an object of known size on the 'retina' of a model eye for various degrees of ametropia. A camera of telecentric design should give a constant value for p irrespective of the ametropia while Rudnicka and colleagues showed that p was linearly proportional to the ametropia for a camera that was not telecentric.

Scanning laser ophthalmoscopes

Scanning laser ophthalmoscopes are video fundus cameras, in which a laser is used to illuminate a very small area of the fundus at any one instant. A red helium–neon laser at 633 nm is generally employed, giving a spot about 25–30 μm in diameter. The full picture is obtained by sweeping the illuminating beam across the fundus while the electron beam of the video-display moves in harmony. Even though the spot is relatively bright, very much less radiation is entering the patient's eye than with a conventional indirect ophthalmoscope

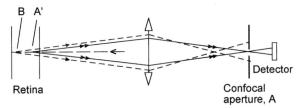

Figure 16.33. The confocal principle. The confocal aperture A is imaged at A′, so light returning from A′ strikes the detector. Most of the light returning from deeper in the retina at B is occluded by the aperture surround.

so that the scanning instrument may be used in a non-mydriatic mode.

Webb *et al.* (1987) give a detailed description of both the optical and electronic arrangement of the instrument. They point out that because the observation beam is only about 10^{-5} the intensity of the illuminating beam, if lenses were incorporated in the instrument, reflections would grossly reduce the clarity of the image. Hence imaging in the part traversed jointly by the illuminating and observation beams is performed by mirrors.

In *Figure 16.32*, which gives a simplified schematic of the laser ophthalmoscope, the illuminating beam is directed by a small mirror B towards the patient's eye. This is scanned horizontally across the fundus by means of a rotating polygonal mirror H. Since this is placed in the image plane P″ of the pupil formed by mirrors O and N, the beam passes through a stationary zone 1 or 2 mm in diameter in the middle of the patient's pupil, even though the beam is moving across the fundus. Similarly, the vertical scanner V is placed in the first image plane P′ produced by mirror O, which is equivalent to the normal ophthalmoscopy lens.

The observation beam is formed by light leaving the eye through the annular zone between the pupil margin and the image B″ of the beam diverter. The third aerial image of the fundus is positioned at A. These instruments have been further developed to provide confocal imaging. In this, not only is a small region illuminated, but the image is recorded from light scattered back from only a small volume surrounding the illuminated point. The instrument is made confocal by placing a small aperture here, as shown in *Figure 16.33*. A narrow illuminating beam is shown passing perpendicularly into the retina. Light returning from around point A′ will pass through the confocal aperture A, whereas light from deeper in the retina, say at B, is mostly occluded. The ophthalmoscope records information from a depth of about 300 μm around the illuminated point. This greatly reduces loss of definition by light scattered from the media, or from deeper or more superficial layers of the fundus. Thus contrast of structures such as the lamina cribosa of the optic disc are much clearer than in a conventional fundus photograph, though conversely, thick scattering layers such as exudate show up less well. Alternatively, a small occluder at A will eliminate light returned from the volume around this point, but records light scattered from deeper or shallower layers, in a manner reminiscent of dark-field microscopy. The instrument may also be used with no aperture here, in which case it performs more like a normal fundus camera.

The ability to image defined depths in the eye enables the instrument to provide sections of the eye in a plane perpendicular to the axis of illumination. Thus the Heidelberg retina tomograph can, for example, record 32 confocal sections of the nerve head, from which it can plot out a cross-section showing the depth and width of the cup.

An argon laser providing blue light allows fluorescein angiography to be undertaken, while a diode laser operating in the near infra-red at 805 nm allows indocyanine green angiography. If the output from the laser is modulated, test stimuli can be projected on to the retina and simultaneously viewed by the examiner. The retinal region employed for reading by patients suffering from macular damage can then be observed (e.g. Culham, 1991). Reviews of the instrument are given by Woon *et al.* (1992), Culham (1991) and Bhandari and Fitzke (1994).

Exercises

16.1 A slit-lamp microscope has an objective diameter of 8 mm and a working distance of 80 mm. Calculate the limit of resolution. What is the necessary magnification for this limit to subtend 2 minutes of arc at the observer's eye?

16.2 A slit lamp has a projector aperture (horizontal) of 8 mm and working distance of 80 mm. Calculate the depth of focus for the beam such that its width does not exceed: (a) 0.02 mm, (b) 0.05 mm, the slit width itself being assumed to be infinitesimal. (Compare these results with the thickness of the cornea.)

16.3 In pachometry, a narrow beam of nearly parallel light is incident on the cornea, its width at the cornea being 0.05 mm. Calculate the width of the reflected beam at the pachometer stop 100 mm away, assuming the radius of curvature of the cornea to be 8 mm.

16.4 In measuring anterior chamber depth, the patient looks at the slit lamp while observation is made from $45°$ to the side. On the basis of paraxial theory, what is the transverse linear doubling required to obtain coincidence of the anterior corneal and lens surfaces? Assume a single-surface cornea of radius 8.0 mm and values of 3.6 mm and 1.336 respectively for the anterior chamber depth and refractive index of the aqueous.

16.5 Calculate the sighthole lens power needed by an unaccommodated emmetrope to view the fundus of: (a) a hypermetrope of $+10.00$ D, (b) a myope of -10.00 D spectacle refraction, both at 15 mm vertex distance. Assume a 35 mm separation between the subject's cornea and the ophthalmoscope lens. (Note the difference in these results.)

16.6 In direct ophthalmoscopy the subject is an unaccommodated uncorrected myope of -10.00 D spectacle refraction and the observer an uncorrected myope of -5.00 D spectacle refraction. The spectacle plane is 15 mm from the eye in each case. If the observer obtains a clear view of the fundus with a -20.00 D lens in the sighthole, how much (spectacle) accommodation is he exerting? Assume the eyes to be separated by 50 mm with the sighthole 20 mm from the observer's eye.

16.7 Calculate the magnification in direct ophthalmoscopy, assuming the subject's eye to be 25 mm from the sighthole, when the subject has: (a) -4.00 D of axial myopia, (b) -4.00 D of refractive myopia. Also determine in each case the linear extent of fundus visible, assuming the subject's pupil to have a diameter of 4 mm.

16.8 A myope of ocular refraction -10.00 DS is corrected by spectacles at a vertex distance of 12 mm. His fundus is examined by direct ophthalmoscopy both with and without his spectacles. Assuming the power of the (reduced) eye to be $+57$ D,

the pupil diameter to be 4 mm and the ophthalmoscope sighthole and immediate source to be at 37 mm from the cornea, calculate the field of illumination on the fundus and magnification for both cases.

16.9 In direct ophthalmoscopy, what are the apparent magnifications of the fundus in the principal meridians of an astigmatic eye of ocular refraction $+4.00/-6.00 \times 180$, the ophthalmoscope being 40 mm from the eye's principal point. Assume K' to be $+62$ D.

16.10 In direct ophthalmoscopy, what proportion of the fundus may be seen without moving the instrument? Assume an emmetropic reduced eye with pupil diameter 5 mm, $F_e +60$ D, working distance 40 mm and a maximum possible field with instrument movement of only the posterior hemisphere, the radius of which may be taken as 12 mm.

16.11 The image of the bulb filament formed on the mirror of a direct ophthalmoscope is 2 mm in height. Calculate the position and size of the Purkinje I image when the mirror is: (a) 40 mm, (b) 25 mm from the patient's cornea, the radius of which is 8 mm.

16.12 Indirect ophthalmoscopy is carried out on a hypermetrope of $+4.00$ D (axial error) with the aid of a $+16.00$ D condenser held 75 mm from the subject's eye. Determine: (a) the correct position of the observer's eye for optimum viewing conditions, (b) the position and size of the aerial image of the optic disc (1.5 mm diameter) and (c) the magnification under which the fundus would be seen by an accurately placed observer.

16.13 The fundus of an emmetropic eye of normal length is viewed in indirect ophthalmoscopy by means of a $+16.00$ D condenser held 500 mm from the observer's eye. How far should the condenser be placed from the subject's eye and what would be the linear extent of fundus visible if the condenser had a useful aperture of 36 mm?

16.14 (a) In indirect ophthalmoscopy, an eye of power $+60$ D is observed with a $+20$ D condenser lens placed with its second principal focus coincident with the eye's first. The observer's eye is placed in the plane of the aerial image of the patient's eye. Calculate the diameter of that area of the patient's pupil utilized by the return beam filling the observer's entrance pupil of 4 mm diameter. (b) Calculate the magnification of the fundus for: (i) an emmetrope, (ii) an axial myope of -5.00 D.

16.15 In indirect ophthalmoscopy, an eye is observed with a $+20$ D lens held 55 mm from the apparent pupillary plane of the patient's eye, while the observer's eye is 250 mm from the condenser. What diameter of the condenser is filled with light, assuming the observer's pupil diameter to be 4 mm?

16.16 What are the requirements, in both direct and indirect ophthalmoscopy, for maximizing the field of view? Are there any disadvantages if these conditions are obtained?

16.17 A range of aspheric indirect ophthalmoscopy lenses has the following particulars:

	Equivalent power (D)	q (mm)	Diameter (mm)
(a)	$+14$	-89.7	52
(b)	$+20$	-60.0	48
(c)	$+28$	-40.8	39

Calculate for each: (i) the magnification that will be given for a patient's eye of standard dioptric length $+60$ D, the observer's eye being placed in the optimum position; (ii) the angular field of view as given by the subtense of the lens aperture at the patient's eye. (The distance q as given is measured from the principal point of the lens nearer to the patient's eye, but for the purpose of this question all the lenses may be regarded as thin.)

References

AUSTEN, D.P. (1993) Binocular indirect ophthalmoscopy. *Optom. Today*, 22 March, 13–19

BELLISARIO-REYES, J.P., KEMPSTER, A.J. and SABELL, A.C. (1980) A method of observing and photographing human corneal endothelial cells *in vivo. Ophthal. Optn*, **20**, 661–662

BHANDARI, A. and FITZKE, F. (1994) Scanning laser ophthalmoscopy – an update. *Optician*, **207**(5444), 15–17

BISHOP, C. (1976) Basic aspects of ophthalmic photography. *Ophthal. Optn*, **16**, 719–731, 762–769, 817–820, 845–853

BRENNAN, N.A., SMITH, G., MACDONALD, J.A. and BRUCE, A.S. (1989) Theoretical principles of optical pachometry. *Ophthal. Physiol. Opt.*, **9**, 247–254

BROWN, N. (1970) Macrophotography of the anterior segment of the eye. *Br. J. Ophthal.*, **54**, 697–701

BROWN, N. (1972) An advanced slit image camera. *Br. J. Ophthal.*, **56**, 624–631

BROWN, N.A.P., BRON, A.J., AYLIFFE, W., SPARROW, J. and HILL, A.R. (1987) The objective assessment of cataract. *Eye*, **1**, 234–246

BROWN, N.P. (1986) Lasers in eye treatment. *Optician*, **192** (5063), 15–19; (5068), 22–27

BROWN, N.P. (1987) Cataract recording cameras. *Optician*, **194** (5108), 23–29

CALKINS, J.L., HOCHHEIMER, B.F. and d'AUNA, S.A. (1980) Potential hazards from specific ophthalmic devices. *Vision Res.*, **20**, 1039–1053 (See also the whole of issue 12.)

CAVALLERANO, A.A., GUTNER, R.K. and SEMES, L.P. (1994) Enhanced non-contact examination of the vitreous and retina. *J. Am. Optom. Assoc.*, **65**, 231–234

CLARK, B.A.J. and LOWE, R.F. (1973) Alignment of eye and slit-lamp beam. *Ophthalmologica, Basel*, **166**, 194–198

CLARK, B.A.J. and LOWE, R.F. (1974) Slitlamp measurement of anterior chamber geometry. *Ophthalomologia, Basel*, **168**, 58–74

COX, M.J. and WOOD, I.J.C. (1991a) Computer-assisted optic nerve head assessment. *Ophthal. Physiol. Opt.*, **11**, 27–35

COX, M.J. and WOOD, I.J.C. (1991b) Image variability in computer-assisted optic nerve head assessment. *Ophthal. Physiol. Opt.*, **11**, 36–43

CULHAM, L. (1991) Scanning laser ophthalmoscopy, a review. *Optician*, **202**(5326), 20–23

DOUTHWAITE, W.A. and SPENCE, D. (1986) Slit-lamp measurement of the anterior chamber depth. *Br. J. Ophthal.*, **70**, 205–208

EISNER, G. (1985) Endothélioscopie à large champ simplifiée. *Bull. Mém. Soc. fr. Ophtal.*, **96**, 129–134

EL BAYADI, C. (1953) New method of slit-lamp micro-ophthalmoscopy. *Br. J. Ophthal.*, **37**, 625–628

EMSLEY, H.H. (1952) *Visual Optics*, 5th edn, Vol. 1, pp. 230–231, 246–254. London: Hatton Press

FIELD, A. and BARNARD, S. (1993) Imaginary convex eye (ICE). An aid to indirect ophthalmoscopy. *Optom. Today*, 31 May, 22

FISCH, B.M. (1993) *Gonioscopy and the Glaucomas*. London: Butterworth-Heinemann

FLANAGAN, J.G. and PROKOPICH, C.L. (1995) Indirect fundus biomicroscopy. *Ophthal. Physiol. Opt.*, **15**, suppl. 2, s38–s41

GILCHRIST, J. (1987a) Computer processing of ocular photographs – a review. *Ophthal. Physiol. Opt.*, **7**, 379–386

GILCHRIST, J. (1987b) Analysis of early diabetic retinopathy by computer processing of fundus images – a preliminary study. *Ophthal. Physiol. Opt.*, **7**, 393–399

GOLDMANN, H. (1938) Zur technik der spaltlampenmikroscopie. *Ophthalmologica, Basel*, **96**, 90–97

GULLSTRAND, A. (1924) Appendix VI. Ophthalmoscopy. In Helmholtz, H. von, *Physiological Optics*, Vol. 1, pp. 443–482. English translation ed. J.P.C. Southall. New York: Optical Society of America. (Reprinted 1962 by Dover Publications, New York)

HANSELL, P. (1957) *A System of Ophthalmic Illustration*. Springfield, Ill.: Thomas

HOLDEN, B.A. and ZANTOS, S.C. (1979) The ocular response to continuous wear lenses. *Optician*, **177**(4581), 50–57

HRUBY, K. (1941) Ueber eine wesentliche Vereinfachung der Untersuchungstechnik des hinteren Augenabschnittes im Lichtbüschel der Spaltlampe. *Albrecht v. Graefes Arch. Ophthal.*, **143**, 224–228

HRUBY, K. (1942) Spaltlampmikroscopie des hinteren Augenabschnittes ohne Kontaktglas. *Klin. Mbl. Augenhcilk.*, **108**, 195–200

JAEGER, W. (1952) Tiefenmessung der menschlichen Vorderkammer mit planparallen Platten (Zusatzgerät zur Spaltlampe). *Albrecht v. Graefes Arch. Ophthal.*, **153**, 120–131

JUSTICE, J. JR. (1982) *Ophthalmic Photography*. Boston: Little, Brown & Co.

KAJIURA, M. (1978) Slit-lamp photography of the fundus by use of aspherical convex preset lens. *Jpn J. Ophthalmol.*, **22**, 214–228

KHHAW, P.T. and ELKINGTON, A.R. (1988) Slit-lamp photography made easy by a spot metering system. *Br. J. Ophthal.*, **72**, 473–474

KOEPPE, L. (1918) Die Mikroscopie des lebendes Augenhintergrundes mit starken Vergrösserungen im fokalen Lichte der Gullstrandschen Nernstspaltlampe. *Albrecht v. Graefes Arch. Ophthal.*, **95**, 282–306

LEMOINE and VALOIS (1923) Ophtalmoscopie microscopique du rond d'oeil vivant. *Bull. Mem. Soc. fr. Ophtal.*, **36**, 366–373

LITTMANN, H. (1982) Zur Bestimmung der wahren Grösse eines Objektes auf dem Abductsdes lebenden Auges. *Klin. Mbl. Augenjeilk.*, **180**, 286–289 (Trans. T.D. Williams (1992) Determination of the true size of an object in the fundus of the living eye. *Optom. Vis. Sci.*, **69**, 717–720.)

LONG, W.F. (1984) *Ocular Photography*. Chicago: Professional Press

LONG, W.F. and MURPHY, M. (1987) Alternative technique for photographing the corneal endothelium with a conventional photo slit-lamp. *Am. J. Optom.*, **64**, 217–220

MANDELL, R.B. and POLSE, K.A. (1969) Keratoconus: spatial variation of corneal thickness as a diagnostic test. *Archs Ophthal., N.Y.*, **82**, 182–188

MARSHALL, J. (1988) Potential of lasers in ophthalmology. *Trans. Br. Contact Lens Assoc. Int. Contact Lens Centenary Congr.*, **5**, 43–46

MARTIN, L.C. (1951) The optics of the ophthalmoscope. In *International Optical Congress 1951*, pp. 1–10. London: British Optical Association

MORRIS, J.A. and STONE, J. (1992) The slit lamp biomicroscope in optometric practice. *Optom. Today*, 7 Sept, 26–28; 5 Oct, 16–19; 2 Nov, 28–30 and reprint from *Optom. Today*

PATEL, D. (1981) Some theoretical factors governing the accuracy of corneal-thickness measurement. *Ophthal. Physiol. Opt.*, **1**, 193–203

PERKINS, E.S. (1988) Depth measurement with the slit-lamp microscope. *Br. J. Ophthal.*, **72**, 344–347

POLSE, K.A. (1975) Technique for estimating the angle of the anterior chamber with the slit lamp. *Optom. Wkly*, **66**, 524–527

POTTER, J.W., SEMENS, L.P., CAVALLERANO, A.A. and CARSTON, M.J. (1988) *Binocular Indirect Ophthalmoscopy*. Boston: Butterworths

PROKOPICH, C.L. and FLANAGAN, J.G. (1996) Gonioscopy: evaluation of the anterior chamber angle. *Ophthal. Physiol. Opt.*, **16**, Suppl. 2, S39–S42

PROKOPICH, C.L. and FLANAGAN, J.G. (1997) Gonioscopy: evaluation of the anterior chamber angle. *Opthal. Physiol. Opt.*, **17**, Suppl. 1, 59–513

RUCKER, C.W. (1971) *A History of the Ophthalmoscope*. Rochester, Minn.: Whiting

RUDNICKA, A.R., EDGAR, D.F. and BENNETT, A.G. (1992) Construction of a model eye and its applications. *Ophthal. Physiol. Opt.*, **12**, 485–490

RUMNEY, N.J. (1988) Slit-lamp examination of the fundus. *Optician*, **196**(5174), 32–38

SABELL, A.C. (1970) Some notes on diagnostic contact lenses. *Ophthal. Optn*, **10**, 1160–1162, 1173–1178

SCHEPENS, C.L. (1947) A new ophthalmoscope demonstration. *Trans. Am. Acad. Ophthal. Oto-lar.*, **51**, 298–301

SCHEPENS, C.L. (1951) Progress in detachment surgery. *Trans. Am. Acad. Ophthal. Oto-lar.*, **55**, 607–615

SHAKESPEARE, A.R. (1987) Dark-room methods of enhancing details in diabetic fundus photographs: a preliminary study. *Ophthal. Physiol. Opt.*, **7**, 387–392

SHERIDAN, M. (1989) Keratometry and slit lamp biomicroscopy. In *Contact Lenses*, 3rd edn (Phillips, A.J. and Stone, J., eds), pp. 243–259. London: Butterworths

SMITH, R.J.H. (1979) A new method of estimating the depth of the anterior chamber. *Br. J. Ophthal.*, **63**, 215–220

SORSBY, A., BENJAMIN, B. and SHERIDAN, M. (1961) Refraction and its components during the growth of the eye from the age of three. *Spec. Rep. Ser. med. Res. Coun.*, No. 301, Appendices C and D. London: HMSO

STONE, J. (1974) The measurement of corneal thickness. *Contact Lens*, **5**(2), 15–19

STONE, J. (1989) Special types of contact lenses and their uses. In *Contact Lenses*, 3rd edn (Phillips, A.J. and Stone, J., eds), pp. 870–901. London: Butterworths

THALLER, V.T. (1983) An inexpensive method of slit-lamp photography. *Br. J. Ophthal.*, **67**, 63–66

VAN HERICK, W., SHAFFER, R.N. and SCHWARTZ, A. (1969) Estimation of width of anterior chamber. Incidence and significance of the width of the narrow angle. *Am. J. Ophthal.*, **68**, 626–629

VOLK OPTICAL (no date) Instruction Manuals. For example, for the Volk double aspheric 90 D BIO lens. Mentor, Ohio: Volk Optical

WAGSTAFF, D.F. (1970) External eye photography in ophthalmic practice. *Ophthal. Optn.*, **10**, 17–20, 25–28

WEBB, R.H., HUGHES, G.W. and DELORI, F.C. (1987) Confocal scanning laser ophthalmoscope. *Appl. Optics*, **26**, 1492–1499

WILSON, C., O'LEARY, D.J. and HENSON, D. (1980) Micropachometry: a technique for measuring the thickness of the corneal epithelium. *Invest. Ophthalmol. Vis. Sci.*, **19**, 414–417

WOON, W.H., FITZKE, F.W., BIRD, A.C. and MARSHALL, J. (1992) Confocal imaging of the fundus using a scanning laser ophthalmoscope. *Br. J. Ophthalmol.*, **76**, 470–474

ZANTOS, S.G. and PYE, D.C. (1979) Clinical photography in ophthalmic practice. *Aust. J. Optom.*, **62**, 279–285 (Reprinted in *Optician*, 1980, **179**(10), 13–15, 19)

Retinoscopy (skiascopy)

Objective refraction

Subjective refraction as described in Chapter 6, though an accurate method for determining any optical correction required, does depend upon the patient's ability to discern changes in the clarity of the test object as the trial lenses are changed. In objective refraction, it is the practitioner who decides with the aid of auxiliary apparatus which lens combination gives the best optical correction for the ametropia. The examiner's opinion replaces the patient's preference. Some apparatus replaces even the human examiner with an electronic system. The findings of objective refraction should, if possible, be checked subjectively, and even these results may need modification to increase the comfort of the lenses prescribed.

Objective refraction is not only useful but often essential, for example, when examining young children and patients with poor communication due to mental or language difficulties. Moreover, a refraction will be much easier and quicker if it is based on an objective estimate instead of only a knowledge of the unaided vision.

There are many different techniques of objective refraction, but they fall into three basic classes:

(1) retinoscopy,
(2) objective optometers (refractionometers),
(3) automated optometers.

This chapter deals only with retinoscopy. Other objective methods and apparatus are described in Chapter 18.

Retinoscopy

Retinoscopy is an offshoot of ophthalmoscopy. In ophthalmoscopy, the principal aim is to inspect the fundus. In retinoscopy, the fundus acts as a fixed screen over which a spot of light is moved. The practitioner watches the shape and movement of the patch of reflected light within the pupil (the 'reflex') and, by placing trial lenses in front of the patient's eye, modifies the speed of movement of the reflex to arrive at a particular condition called 'reversal'.

The technique of retinoscopy was introduced in 1873 by the French ophthalmologist Cuignet (d.1889) and was brought to Paris by his pupil Mengin in 1878. At

Table 17.1 Comparison between neutralization and retinoscopy

Neutralization	Retinoscopy
Stationary test object	Test object moves across retina
Lens under test is moved	Eye examined is stationary
Lens power indicated by direction and speed of image movements	Refractive error indicated by by direction and speed of reflex movement (fundus glow in pupil)
Trial lenses of known power added to neutralize movement	Trial lenses added to obtain 'reversal'
End-point: no movement	End-point: extremely rapid movement and disappearance of reflex

the same clinic (1880–81), Parent introduced the term 'retinoscopie', since he believed that the source of the reflex was the retinal pigment layer. This method of refraction was popularized in the USA by Jackson. The terminology is rather confused. Especially with poor illumination, the movement of shadows in the pupil is easier to follow than that of the light reflex. Hence, names such as umbrascopy, skiascopy and skiametry were introduced, the last two being widely used in the USA. The term retinoscopy – although a misnomer – is generally accepted in Great Britain and some other countries.

Retinoscopy is a process having similarities with neutralization (the method of determining the power of a lens by adding another lens or lenses of approximately equal and opposite power to produce an afocal combination). *Table 17.1* sets outs a comparison.

The sighthole of the instrument acts in a similar way to the knife edge in the Foucault test for aberrations. The retina is made conjugate to the sighthole, so that if the eye were aberration free, there would be an instantaneous cut-off of the return beam entering the examiner's eye as the light patch moves over the patient's retina.

The self-luminous retinoscope

It was seen (pages 312–313) that the direct ophthalmoscope needed the source of light and observer's eye to be placed very close together in order that light entered the patient's eye and returned to the observer. The simplest way to do this is to reflect the light from a bulb off an inclined semi-silvered mirror and view by transmission through the mirror, i.e. to use a beam splitter. An alternative method is to use a fully silvered mirror and to view the pupil through a perforation in the silvering.

Self-luminous retinoscopes often have a bulb with a tiny coiled filament about 1–2 mm in size. This is imaged by a lens of about 20 mm focal length to give a divergent beam of light. In some instruments, the lens may be moved along its axis to give a vergence of light after refraction from −0.50 D to −7.00 D. The virtual image of the source, called the immediate source, is then positioned between 2 m and 140 mm behind the instrument. *Figure 17.1* shows two instruments (not to scale) with perforated and semi-reflecting mirrors. Note that a sighthole is still required in the latter instrument to give definition to the appearance of the reflex. A diameter of about 1.5 mm is satisfactory, although a larger diameter giving a brighter reflex may be useful in the early stages of learning retinoscopy.

A slightly different type of instrument – the streak retinoscope – uses a bulb with an uncoiled linear filament and also provides a greater range of vergences. It can even give a real image of the filament in front of the instrument (*see* pages 347–349).

In the past, instruments were designed which could be modified from an ophthalmoscope to a retinoscope. In principle, the only modification needed is an extra condensing lens so that the immediate source may be positioned on the mirror for ophthalmoscopy; removal gives a divergent beam for retinoscopy. In practice, separate instruments left in permanent adjustment perform better, though economies can still be made in the form of an interchangeable handle.

Principles of retinoscopy

In retinoscopy, the instrument is moved so that the beam travels across the patient's pupil. Simultaneously, the immediate source (the image of the real source formed by the retinoscope lens and mirror) moves transversely to the axis of the patient's eye so that a patch of light moves across the fundus. In *Figure 17.2*, which refers to a self-luminous retinoscope, the instrument has been rotated through an angle θ. Since the bulb is fixed in relation to the mirror, the immediate source also rotates through angle θ, moving from S' to S''. The incident ray path S''P makes an angle u with the eye's optical axis, and the conjugate refracted ray PQ the angle u'.

When the immediate source is behind the retinoscope, θ, u and u' all have the same sign. Thus the illuminated fundus patch moves across the retina in the same direction as the mirror rotation.

In general, the immediate source does not lie in the eye's far-point plane. So the image formed by the eye is blurred and the illumination falls away at the edges. Near reversal, when the retina is conjugate with the

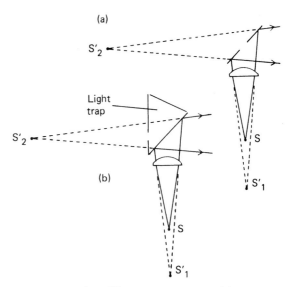

Figure 17.1. The self-luminous retinoscope: (a) an instrument with perforated mirror, (b) one with a semi-silvered reflector. The immediate source is the bulb image S'_2.

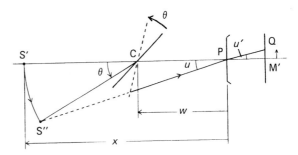

Figure 17.2. Rotation of the retinoscope through angle θ gives a source movement through angle u with respect to P.

mirror, the blur-circle diameter and the basic image height are both small, about 0.02 and 0.05 mm respectively. For simplicity, the illuminated fundus area is considered to be a point.

Figure 17.3 illustrates a myopic eye (or an eye rendered myopic by trial lenses). Light reflected back from the fundus at M' must pass through the far-point M_R. At the mirror, the emergent beam diameter is larger than the sighthole AB. Only light in the dotted part of the beam will enter the observer's eye, so that the pupil will appear dark with a bright glow in the centre. This glow, irrespective of size or position, is the reflex.

When the trial lenses are changed so that the (artificial) far-point closely approaches the sighthole, all the light leaving the patient's eye reaches the observer's

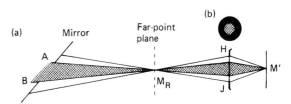

Figure 17.3. (a) Formation of the reflex in a myopic eye. (b) Appearance in the pupil.

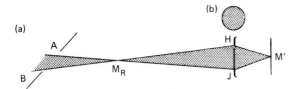

Figure 17.4. (a) Formation of the reflex in a myopic eye, the far-point approaching the sighthole. (b) Appearance in the pupil.

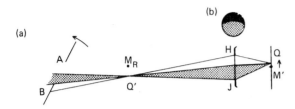

Figure 17.5. (a) Effect of retinoscope tilt on the formation of the reflex: against movement. (b) Appearance in the pupil.

(*Figure 17.4*). The whole pupil then appears to be luminous.

Effect of rotation

Suppose the retinoscope is angled slightly so that the patch of light passes upwards over the patient's eye. The illuminated patch on the fundus will move upwards from M′ to Q, while its image in the far-point plane moves downwards to Q′. *Figure 17.5* shows that only light leaving through the lower part of the pupil passes through the sighthole. The remainder of the light is occluded by the mirror to give a crescent-shaped shadow at the top of the pupil. The reflex has moved downwards in the opposite direction to the instrument rotation. This is therefore called an against movement.

Condition for reversal

When the retina is made conjugate with the plane of the sighthole (*Figure 17.6*), the emergent pencil of light is either wholly admitted or totally occluded. The reflex would then appear and disappear instantaneously when the retinoscope is moved. In reality, this does not happen quite instantaneously because of the finite size of the illuminated retinal patch and sighthole, and the effect of ocular aberrations. It is this part of the process that resembles the Foucault knife-edge test.

Analysis of the reflex: introduction

It is useful to precede the algebraic analysis of the reflex

by a diagrammatic demonstration of the stages in its formation. In all these diagrams, the patient's eye will face left and there is therefore no change in the sign of k and K. The incident light (illuminating beam) travels as usual to the right.

Six elements are involved in the analysis of the reflex:

(1) illumination of an area of the fundus,
(2) formation of an image of this fundus patch (the fundus image),
(3) the potential reflex,
(4) formation of the actual reflex,
(5) direction of motion of the reflex,
(6) the end-point or reversal.

As shown in *Figure 17.2*, all relevant distances will be measured from the patient's eye, the point P being considered both as principal point and pupil centre. The retinoscope is at a distance w (which is always negative), called the working distance. It is normally two-thirds of a metre, so that the practitioner can easily reach the trial frame or refractor head with his free hand to change lenses.

The immediate source S′ is at a linear distance x (dioptric distance X), depending on the instrument and technique used.

Formation of the fundus image

The fundus image is important for the following reasons:

(1) A reflex will be visible if light can pass from the patient's pupil into the observer's pupil via the fundus image.
(2) The fundus image indicates the behaviour of the reflex. When viewed from the sighthole, the reflex invariably moves in the same direction as the fundus image.

Myopia: $|K| > |X|$

In myopia in which the far-point plane is between the eye and immediate source (*Figure 17.7*), the image of S″ formed by the eye must lie in front of the retina, say at S‴, on the refracted ray PQ. Drawing the pencil of rays from the centre of the immediate source S″ to the pupil margins H and J, we can construct the refracted rays HU and JV through S‴ to define the illuminated circle on the retina.

Since the far-point plane is conjugate with the retina and ray paths are reversible, Q′, the image of Q, is the intersection of S″P with the far-point plane. Similarly, U′ and V′ are the images of U and V.

Therefore the circle in the far-point plane bounded by

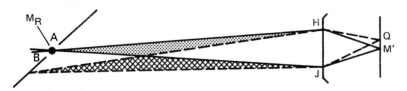

Figure 17.6. Complete transmission or occlusion of the reflex at reversal.

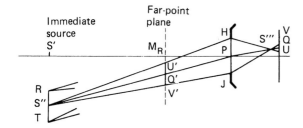

Figure 17.7. Formation of the blurred retinal image UV of the immediate source and the resulting fundus image U'V' in the far-point plane in a myopic eye.

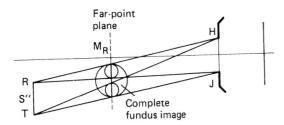

Figure 17.8. The fundus image of an extended source RT.

U' and V' is the image of the illuminated fundus patch due to the pencil from S''. This general theorem makes it unnecessary to consider the detailed course of the rays within the eye in the other cases.

In reality, the immediate source has a finite size, say RT. A fundus image circle may be drawn in the far-point plane to correspond to each point of the source. The complete fundus image is the envelope of all such circles (*Figure 17.8*).

Hypermetropia

In all degrees of hypermetropia (*Figure 17.9*), the fundus image will be formed in a far-point plane behind the patient's eye and is constructed by producing the rays S''H and S''J. The source image, S''', will also lie behind the eye.

Myopia: $|K| < |X|$

A third similar construction could be drawn for myopia

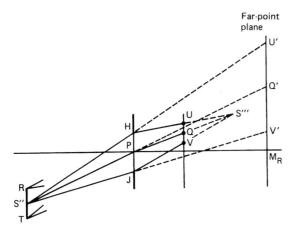

Figure 17.9. The fundus image in hypermetropia.

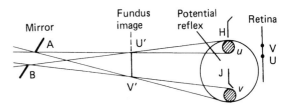

Figure 17.10. Projection from the sighthole AB through the fundus image U'V' to give the potential reflex in a myopic eye.

of low degree such that the far point lies beyond the plane of the immediate source.

Formation of the reflex

The fundus image, governed by the position of the immediate source and pupil margins, is bounded by U' and V', as shown in *Figure 17.10* which follows on from *Figure 17.7*.

Projection from the sighthole margins A and B through U' locates circle *u* in the pupillary plane. If the pupil were of unlimited size, a pencil from U on the retina could emerge through circle *u* to enter the sighthole via U'. The area *u* of the pupil would therefore appear luminous. Similarly the circle *v* is defined by projection from A and B through V'.

The envelope of all such circles constitutes what may be called the potential reflex.

The visible reflex is bounded by the overlap of the potential reflex upon the actual pupil. If the retinoscope is tilted to move the potential reflex upwards, the actual reflex will be seen to move upwards across the pupil. In *Figure 17.10* it nearly fills the pupil, leaving a crescent-shaped 'shadow' at the top. It will then proceed to fill the pupil, making the whole of it glow and then its lower edge will travel upwards, leaving a shadow in its wake.

Figure 17.11, following on from *Figure 17.9*, illustrates the formation of the reflex in hypermetropia. In this diagram, the potential reflex overlaps the upper part of the pupil. This is therefore the illuminated area, the lower part remaining dark.

Direction of the reflex movement

Only a single point of the immediate source and fundus

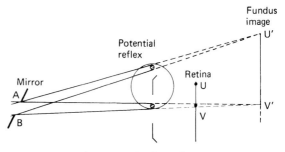

Figure 17.11. The potential reflex in hypermetropia. Direction of the reflex movement.

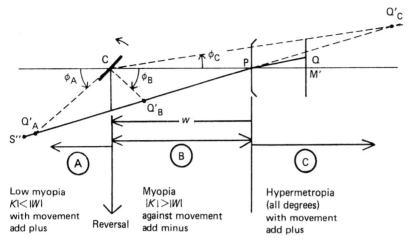

Figure 17.12. The direction of reflex movement in the three main categories of ametropia.

image need be considered. In *Figure 17.12*, as the mirror with its sighthole at C is rotated through angle θ from its central position, the immediate source moves from S′ to S″. The ray S″P to the centre of the pupil is refracted to Q.

The fundus image Q′ must lie on the ray S″P, produced if necessary in either direction, according to the position of the far-point plane. The reflex is seen in the direction CQ′, making an angle φ with the axis.

The relative speed of reflex movement is the ratio φ/θ. A plus sign denotes a with movement, in that the reflex moves upwards when the path of light from the retinoscope beam on the patient's face also moves upwards. A minus sign denotes an against movement.

The direction of the reflex movement depends upon the position of the far-point. There are three distinct ranges, as shown in the diagram. In range B, where the myopia is such that the far-point plane lies between the patient and sighthole, a negative lens is indicated by the against movement, exactly as in neutralization. Negative lenses of increasing power are added until reversal is obtained, a condition described more precisely below.

In the two regions A and C, the with movement indicates the need for a plus lens in the spectacle plane to obtain reversal. In hypermetropia (region C), a gradual addition of plus power will move the resulting artificial far point to infinity on the right of the diagram. It will then approach the sighthole from infinity in region A.

Reversal

The end-point for retinoscopy, called reversal, occurs when the far-point plane coincides with the plane of the sighthole (*Figure 17.13*). If the working distance w is two-thirds of a metre, giving $W = -1.50$ D, reversal would be obtained with an uncorrected myope of ocular refraction $K = -1.50$ D. In general, lenses are placed in the subject's spectacle plane to give an artificial far-point positioned in the plane of the sighthole. If the patient were actually a -2.00 D myope, there would be an initial against movement with no trial lenses in place. If a -1.00 DS lens were inserted, the artificial far point would now be behind the mirror, resulting in a with movement. The end-point is the lens power from which a change of 0.25 DS or less converts an against movement to a with movement, or with to against.

The lens giving reversal can be considered as the sum of two components:

(1) a lens of power F_{sp} representing the distance spectacle correction,
(2) a positive lens of power $-W$ to make the patient artificially myopic for the plane of the sighthole.

Thus, *Figure 17.14* shows a pencil from M′ converging towards the true far-point M_R on emerging from the eye. A lens of power F_{sp} renders it parallel and a pos-

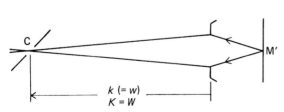

Figure 17.13. Condition for reversal: the fundus image is formed in the plane of the sighthole, the residual error K then being equal to the dioptric working distance W.

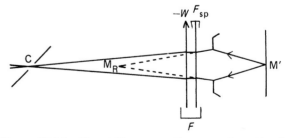

Figure 17.14. The trial lens power F at reversal considered as a combination of the spectacle correction F_{sp} and a plus lens of power $-W$ to compensate for the working distance.

itive lens of power $-W$ converges the pencil to the plane of the sighthole. In clinical work, F_{sp} is more important than the ocular refraction K, though for simplicity in the next section, K will be used.

Let F be the power of the single reversing lens. Then

$$F = F_{sp} + (-W)$$

which gives

$$F_{sp} = F + W \qquad (17.1)$$

For example, if $F = -6.00\,D$ and $W = -1.50\,D$

$$F_{sp} = -6.00 - 1.50$$
$$= -7.50\,D$$

For $F = +4.00\,D$, with W as before, then

$$F_{sp} = +4.00 - 1.50$$
$$= +2.50\,D$$

It is easier to remember that one always algebraically subtracts $+1.50$ DS (or $+1.00$ DS if working at 1 m, $+2.00$ DS if at 0.5 m) than to add negative power.

This alteration to be made to the lens power at reversal is called the 'allowance for working distance'. One possible routine is to keep a pair of lenses of power $+1.50$ DS in the trial frame while retinoscopy is performed. Their subsequent removal then leaves the distance correction of power F_{sp} in the trial frame. Drawbacks are the additional weight and reflections. Some manufacturers of refractor heads apply anti-reflection coatings to all the lenses in their instruments.

Relative speed of the reflex movement

The simple equation derived below is the key to the critical use of the instrument.

In *Figure 17.15*, the mirror is assumed to have rotated anticlockwise through an angle θ so that the immediate source has moved through an identical angle from the optical axis of the patient's eye. The resulting position of the fundus image must be found and hence the angle ϕ, subtended at the sighthole by its displacement.

From the triangles $PM_R Q'$, $CM_R Q'$ in the diagram we have

$$\frac{\phi\,(-ve)}{u\,(+ve)} = \frac{PM_R\,(-ve)}{CM_R\,(+ve)} = \frac{PM_R}{CP + PM_R}$$

$$= \frac{k}{-w + k} = \frac{k}{k - w}$$

Multiplying throughout by $K\,(= 1/k)$ and $W\,(= 1/w)$ gives

$$\frac{\phi}{u} = \frac{W}{W - K} \qquad (17.2)$$

The main variable in this factor is the ametropia. Also,

$$\frac{u\,(+ve)}{\theta\,(+ve)} = \frac{CS'\,(-ve)}{PS'\,(-ve)} = \frac{CP + PS'}{PS'}$$

$$= \frac{-w + x}{x} = \frac{x - w}{x}$$

Multiplying throughout by X and W gives

$$\frac{u}{\theta} = \frac{W - X}{W} \qquad (17.3)$$

This factor is dependent on the optical arrangement of the retinoscope. Finally, multiplying equations (17.2) and (17.3) we obtain

$$\frac{\phi}{\theta} = \frac{\text{angular movement of reflex}}{\text{mirror rotation}} = \frac{W - X}{W - K} \qquad (17.4)$$

Factors affecting the speed of the reflex movement

Amount of ametropia

The relative speed ratio given by equation (17.4) can be considered as the product of two factors, one varying with the ametropia and the other with the retinoscopy arrangement. If W and X are held constant, the effect of K on the speed of reflex depends solely on equation (17.2), the ametropia factor. By way of illustration, suppose that the dioptric working distance W is $-1.50\,D$. The ametropia factor then becomes

$$\frac{-1.50}{-1.50 - K}$$

This plots as a hyperbola (*Figure 17.16*) which is asymptotic to the vertical at $K = W = -11.50\,D$ but approaches zero as the ametropia increases in either direction.

If it is also supposed that the immediate source is at a

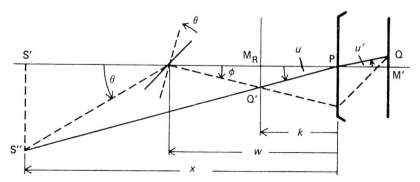

Figure 17.15. Derivation of relative speed of reflex.

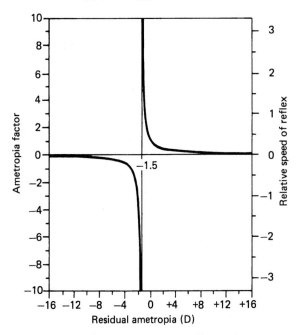

Figure 17.16. The ametropia factor $W/(W - K)$ plotted as a function of residual ametropia. Dioptric working distance -1.50 D. The right-hand ordinate is scaled for relative speed of reflex when $X = -1.00$ D.

dioptric distance of -3.00 D from the retinoscope mirror, then it is also at a linear distance x of -1 m from the eye, so that $X = -1.00$ D. The retinoscope factor, equation (17.3), then assumes the value $(-1.50 + 1.00)/-1.50$ or $1/3$. The right-hand ordinate scale in *Figure 17.16* represents the total relative speed ratio, which in this case is one-third of the ametropia factor.

If K is considered, not as the subject's ametropia but as the residual ametropia at any stage when trial lenses are placed before the eye, *Figure 17.16* shows the relative speed of the reflex to increase more and more rapidly as reversal is approached. Theoretically, the speed then becomes infinitely great.

Distance of the immediate source

The distance x of the immediate source from the eye is not a completely independent variable since it is affected by the adjustment of the retinoscope and the working distance w. It may, however, be regarded as a variable if w is kept constant.

The relationship expressed by equation (17.3) could be called the retinoscope factor because u/θ, equal to $(W - X)/W$, is the ratio of the angular movement of the immediate source (with respect to the patient's eye) to the rotation of the mirror. In *Figure 17.17(a)* the retinoscope factor is plotted as a function of the distance x when W is fixed at -1.50 D. It takes a positive value when the immediate source S' is on the far side of the patient's eye (region C). Should the source be imaged between the patient's eye and the mirror (region B), the retinoscope factor takes a negative value; the direction of the reflex for a particular residual ametropia is reversed. A moderately myopic eye will then show a with movement instead of the customary against movement. Regions A, B and C correspond exactly to those of *Figure 17.12*.

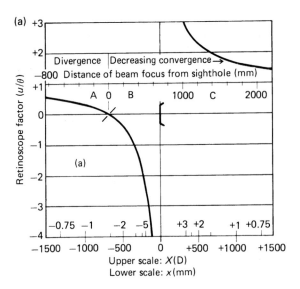

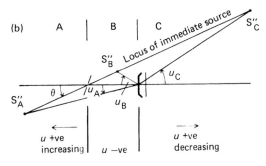

Figure 17.17. (a) The retinoscope factor $(W - X)/W$ plotted as a function of the distance x for $W = -1.50$ D. (b) The sign and relative size of angle u when the immediate source is in each of the regions A, B and C.

When x is zero, X is infinite and thus so is the speed of the reflex movement. An apparent reversal has been reached, but it is independent of the residual ametropia. This condition is called false reversal and occurs if the immediate source lies in the pupillary plane. As shown by *Figure 17.18*, a slight angling of the mirror from the central position will displace S' to S'', where the light is totally occluded by the iris. The reflex therefore suddenly disappears. Although the self-luminous spot retinoscope cannot usually be adjusted to image the filament on the patient's eye, this can occur with the streak retinoscope. Care must therefore be taken not to generate this condition during use.

Figure 17.17(a) shows that altering the adjustment of the instrument varies the speed of the reflex movement for a particular ametropia. When the ametropia is high, the ametropia factor is low, giving a slow reflex movement. It is therefore an advantage to make the retinoscope factor as large as possible so that there is a perceptible movement in the reflex. This can be done by

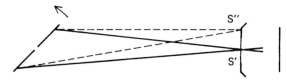

Figure 17.18. False reversal: the immediate source lies in the patient's pupil plane.

making the beam diverge as little as possible. If the immediate source is moved from 200 mm to 500 mm behind the mirror, X falls from −1.15 to −0.86 D and the retinoscope factor almost doubles from 0.23 to 0.43.

Near reversal, the higher value for the retinoscope factor means that the reflex movement is faster than it need be. The trial lens consequently appears closer than it really is to the power needed for true reversal. If preferred, the reflex movement can now be slowed down by making the beam as divergent as possible. This is illustrated in the following example.

Example (1)

Residual error	Beam divergence	Retinoscope factor	Relative speed of reflex
0.50 D			0.69
	Maximum	0.23	
0.25 D			1.38
0.50 D			1.29
	Minimum	0.43	
0.25 D			2.58

Approximately the same final reflex speed is obtained with the less divergent retinoscope beam at 0.50 D from reversal, as occurs with the more divergent beam at only 0.25 D from reversal.

Figure 17.17(b), drawn in register with *Figure 17.17(a)*, shows the sign and relative size of the angle *u* when the immediate source, after a mirror rotation θ, is in each of the three regions A, B and C.

If no adjustment of the vergence is possible, an instrument with a fixed divergence between −3 and −5 D is preferable to one with a nearly parallel beam.

Non-luminous retinoscopes: a retrospect

Retinoscopy was originally performed with an external light source such as an oil lamp. Later, an opal or pearl glass electric lamp bulb masked to give a range of apertures (known as a Lister lamp) was placed to the side of the patient's head. The retinoscope often consisted of a small plane mirror with a perforated sighthole. Since relatively little light reached the patient's eye, the reflex was dim.

To overcome this drawback, a 'long-focus' concave mirror could be used, giving an immediate source positioned behind the patient's head.

Such a mirror might have a radius of curvature of 1 to 1.5 m, concentrating light towards the patient's eye. The disadvantage was that the resulting reflex movement was very much quicker for the same angular movement of the mirror. It must be noted that whenever the source is external to the instrument, as in all non-luminous instruments, the immediate source moves through double the angle that the mirror is turned. The right-hand side of equation (17.3) and (17.4) must therefore be doubled.

A 'short-focus' concave mirror having a radius of curvature about $\frac{1}{3}$ m was also used. This, too, gives a brighter reflex than the plane mirror, but reverses the direction of the reflex movement because the immediate source falls within range B of *Figure 17.17*.

For streak retinoscopy, toroidal mirrors were used.

Working distance

Reversal is obtained when the far-point plane coincides with the mirror. In moderate and high ametropia, the far-point is much closer to the eye than the normal working distance. The reflex moves very slowly and its direction may be difficult to determine. If so, the reflex speed may be increased by approaching much closer to the eye. This can readily be deduced from equation (17.4) giving the relative speed of the reflex.

Table 17.2 shows the relative speed for a range of different values of the ametropia *K* and dioptric working distance *W*. The immediate source was assumed to remain at 250 mm behind the mirror, whatever the working distance. It can be seen that in all refractive conditions the speed increases with a shorter working distance, but more so in high myopia than in high hypermetropia.

Brightness of the reflex and ametropia

In *Figure 17.19*, the fundus image with the far-point

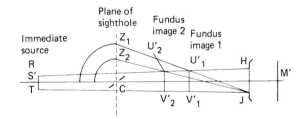

Figure 17.19. The influence of the relative positions of far-point and sighthole on reflex brightness.

Table 17.2 Effect of working distance on relative speed of reflex

W	W − X	Ametropia (D)						
(D)	(D)	−10.00	−5.00	−2.50	−1.50	0	+5.00	+10.00
−1.00	−0.20	−0.022	−0.050	−0.133	−0.400	0.200	0.033	0.018
−1.50	−0.41	−0.048	−0.117	−0.409	∞	0.272	0.063	0.036
−2.00	−0.67	−0.083	−0.222	−1.333	1.333	0.333	0.095	0.056
−2.50	−0.96	−0.128	−0.385	∞	0.962	0.385	0.128	0.077
−3.00	−1.29	−0.184	−0.643	2.572	0.857	0.428	0.161	0.099

plane in position 1 is formed by the intersection of the limiting rays RH and TJ with this plane. The image is thus bounded by $U_1' V_1'$.

The cross-section of the return beam from the eye is found by projecting from H and J through U_1' and V_1'. Thus, in the plane of the mirror, the cross-section is bounded by Z_1 on JU_1' produced, and forms circle 1 of radius CZ_1.

In the less-myopic eye with the far-point plane in position 2, the fundus image is bounded by U_2' and V_2', and the cross-section of the beam in the plane of the mirror by Z_2' determining circle 2 of radius CZ_2.

Although light distribution in the beam is not uniform because of vignetting, intensity per unit area is obviously higher in position 2 because the same quantity of light is spread over a smaller area.

Hence the brightness of the reflex increases as neutralization is approached and the fundus image moves nearer to the mirror.

Sighthole shadow

If the mirror is pierced, or the silvering removed, no light is reflected from the sighthole. With respect to the immediate source, the mirror acts like a clear window with an opaque central spot. There is thus a narrow occluded cone within the pencil from each point on the immediate source (*Figure 17.20*).

The area bounded by DAEB is common to all the occluded cones and is therefore a blind area in the illuminating beam.

The fundus image is the intersection of the illuminating beam with the far-point plane. Hence, if the far-point plane lies between D and E, the fundus image will have a dark central spot, giving rise to a 'sighthole shadow' in the centre of the reflex. This occurs only when close to reversal.

If the fundus image lies exactly in the plane of the mirror, its dark area coincides with the sighthole. Consequently, no reflex should be visible. This prediction has been demonstrated with a well-corrected artificial eye by Bentall and Diprose (1932).

In reality, the aberrations of the eye and light scatter within it give rise to some residual illumination. The shadow tends to be more obvious the smaller the immediate source. Since, however, it is the edge of the reflex rather than the centre which is important, sighthole shadow is not necessarily a disadvantage. The shadow may be eliminated by using a semi-reflecting mirror in conjunction with a separate small aperture (*Figure 17.21b*).

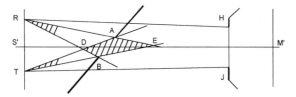

Figure 17.20. Formation of sighthole shadow. RT the immediate source, AB the sighthole.

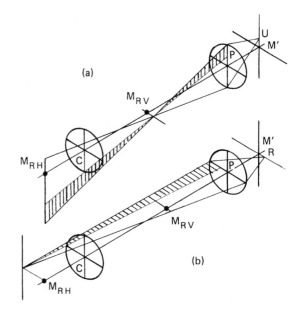

Figure 17.21. Retinoscopy in astigmatism with the rule. P represents the patient's pupil centre, C the sighthole centre. (a) The vertical section of the return beam, the retinoscope beam having been tilted upwards, (b) the horizontal section of the return beam, the retinoscope beam having been tilted to the right. In both diagrams, the hatched area shows that portion of the beam cut off by the edge of the sighthole.

Retinoscopy in astigmatism

Retinoscopy is of very great value in estimating the astigmatic error, particularly if large. In order to simplify the initial discussion, the behaviour of the reflex will be considered in a myopic eye for which the far-points in the two principal meridians are on opposite sides of the sighthole (*Figure 17.21*). The astigmatism is with the rule. Consequently, in the axial position the return beam will form a horizontal focal line at M_{RV} the far-point for the vertical meridian, and a vertical line at M_{RH} the far-point for the horizontal meridian.

If the mirror is now tilted so as to move the illuminated retinal patch upwards to U (*Figure 17.21a*), the return beam with its focal lines will move downwards. Rays emerging from the top of the pupil are the first to be occluded as the beam crosses the sighthole boundary. The reflex is therefore seen to move downwards, showing an against movement. *Figure 17.21(b)* shows the situation in the horizontal meridian after the mirror has been tilted anticlockwise about a vertical axis so that the illuminated fundus patch moves rightwards to R from the examiner's point of view. The first occluded rays are those emerging from the left-hand side of the pupil, thus showing a with movement of the reflex. Thus each principal meridian behaves like an eye with spherical ametropia of the identical amount. If the direction of either one of them were known in advance, retinoscopy of the astigmatic eye would present no special problem.

There are two different clues to the axis direction of the correcting cylinder. First, in *Figure 17.21*, suppose that the horizontal focal line is just in front of the sighthole, a position close to reversal for the vertical meridian. (This apparent paradox arises from the fact that every point on the horizontal focal line is the focus of a pencil of rays in a particular vertical section of the pupil.) As a result, the cross-section of the beam in the plane of the sighthole is elongated horizontally, causing the reflex to be drawn out vertically and to have approximately straight edges. Similarly, if the vertical line were brought close to the sighthole, the reflex would show a horizontal elongation. In general, the shape and edges of the reflex near reversal in either meridian give an approximate indication of the astigmatic axis. The higher the astigmatism, the more obvious and accurate this indication will be.

The usual procedure is to obtain reversal with spherical lenses in the meridian of greater hypermetropia or lower myopia first, leaving the far-point in the other meridian in front of the sighthole. Suppose retinoscopy to be performed on an eye with a refractive error of

$+4.75/-2.25 \times 140$

the working distance being (minus) two-thirds of a metre ($W = -1.50$ D). When the beam is driven along the $140°$ meridian, reversal will be nearly attained with $+6.00$ DS before the eye. The reflex would appear elongated in this meridian, showing a border at the top and bottom roughly aligned with it. After completion of reversal, the speed of reflex movement when the beam is driven along the $50°$ meridian will give some indication of the cylinder power needed. Minus cylinders are now placed before the eye at axis $140°$ until reversal is obtained in the $50°$ meridian also. To allow for the working distance, 1.50 D would have to be subtracted (from the spherical power only) of the final retinoscopic findings.

With low astigmatic errors, the elongation of the reflex may be insufficient to give an accurate indication of cylinder axis. The second clue is particularly useful in such cases. If the retinoscope beam is driven across an astigmatic eye in a direction oblique to the principal meridians, the reflex will move in a different direction. This may be inferred from the different speeds of the reflex movements in the principal meridians.

In the following examples, W is assumed to be -1.50 D and X to be -1.00 D.

Example (1)

$K = -2.25/-0.50 \times 120$

In *Figure 17.22(a)*, O represents the centre of the pupil and the retinoscope beam is driven rightwards from O to B along the horizontal meridian. Perpendiculars BM, BN are dropped from B to the principal meridians. The arbitrary length OB can be considered as the resultant of a travel OM along the $30°$ meridian and ON along $120°$. From equation (17.4), the relative speed of the reflex μ when resolved along these meridians is found to be:

	Along 30°	Along 120°
K	-2.75 D	-2.25 D
μ	-0.4	-0.67

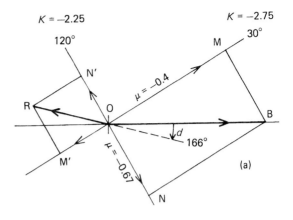

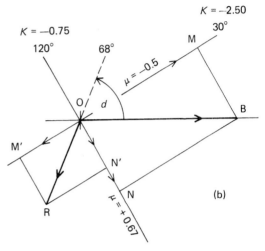

Figure 17.22. The relative speed and direction of reflex movement in astigmatism. The beam is driven from O to B. OM and ON represent the eye's principal meridians, OM′ and ON′ the components of reflex movements along these meridians, and OR the resultant movement. (a) $K = -2.25/-0.50 \times 120$, (b) $K = -0.75/-1.75 \times 120$.

Since both movements are against, we construct the point M′ on the $30°$ meridian on the side of O opposite from M such that $OM′ = -0.4$ OM. Similarly, N′ is located on the $120°$ meridian on the side of O remote from N such that $ON′ = -0.67$ ON. The diagonal OR of the completed rectangle OM′N′R indicates both the relative speed (compared to OB) and direction of the reflex movement. It is seen to be an against movement along the $166°$ meridian, thus making an angle d of $14°$ with the direction along which the beam was driven.

Example (2)

$K = -0.75/-1.75 \times 120$

We now obtain

	Along 30°	Along 120°
K	-2.50 D	-0.75 D
μ	-0.5	$+0.67$

The construction (*Figure 17.22b*) proceeds as before except that, since there is now a with movement along

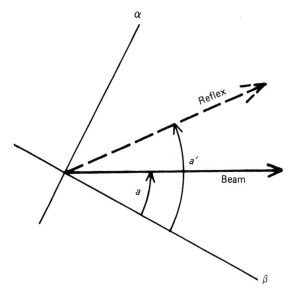

Figure 17.23. Angular separation of beam and reflex movements in retinoscopy along an oblique meridian of the astigmatic eye. The eye's principal meridians are designated alpha and beta, the latter corresponding to the axis of the minus correcting cylinder.

the 120° meridian, N′ lies on the same side of O as N. The construction shows an against reflex movement along 68°, a considerable angle from the direction of the beam. Such angles do not occur when there is a with or an against movement in both principal meridians, as in Example (1).

In principle, this graphical method is identical with Figure *13.7* on page 235 illustrating the analysis of astigmatic line rotation and the resulting 'scissors effect'. It leads to the general relationship shown in Figure *17.23*, in which α refers to the eye's principal meridian of greater power and β to the meridian of lower power. The beta meridian is therefore the axis of the minus correcting cylinder. The refractive errors in these two meridians are denoted by K_α and K_β respectively. If the retinoscope beam is driven at an angle a from the beta meridian, the reflex movement makes an angle a' from the beta meridian such that

$$\tan a' = \frac{W - K_\beta}{W - K_\alpha} \tan a \qquad (17.5)$$

Angles a and a' are subject to the usual sign convention.

Scissors reflex movements in retinoscopy are also very apparent when trial cylinders are placed before the eye at an incorrect axis. Suppose the refractive error to be

$$+6.00/-1.50 \times 20$$

and retinoscopy performed at $W = -1.50\,\text{D}$ and with $X = -1.00\,\text{D}$. With $+7.50$ DS before the eye, reversal is obtained in the 20° meridian. Now suppose a -1.00 DC trial cylinder is added at axis 10°. Calculation (*see* pages 87–89) shows the residual refractive error to be

$$+0.08/-0.66 \times 36$$

The residual astigmatic axis is 26° oblique to the trial cylinder axis (*Figure 17.24a*). From the construction of *Figure 17.22* it can also be determined that if the retinoscope beam is passed along the 10° meridian, the move-

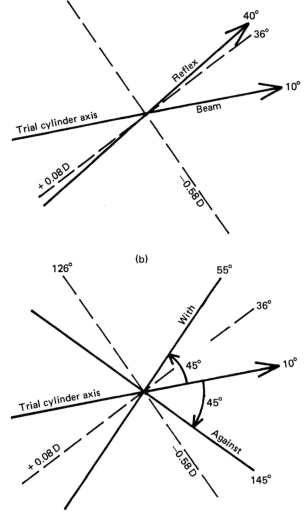

Figure 17.24. (a) The trial cylinder is placed at the incorrect axis 10° instead of the correct position of 20°. The resulting reflex direction (40°) is close to the axis (36°) of the residual error. (b) The principle of Lindner's method for verifying the astigmatic axis.

ment of the reflex will be along the 40° meridian. This is anticlockwise from the trial cylinder axis, indicating that the latter should be moved in this direction. If necessary, the procedure is then repeated.

If the trial cylinder is of the correct power C but is set at ϕ degrees from the true direction, the residual refractive error can be found from equation (6.1). The resultant principal meridians are at 45° on each side of the mean direction of the true and incorrect cylinder axes, while the refractive errors in these meridians are numerically equal to $C \sin \phi$ but are opposite in sign. Though affected numerically, these relationships are not changed fundamentally if the trial cylinder power is inaccurate but close to that required and ϕ is small.

The above is the basis of Lindner's method of refining the cylinder axis, cited by Pascal (1930) and Freeman and Hodd (1955). Reversal is first obtained in the more hypermetropic meridian. Then, with the minus trial cylinder in position at the estimated axis, the retinoscope beam is driven along the two meridians at about 45° to the cylinder axis, which are close to the principal meridians of the residual refractive error (*Figure 17.24b*). This diagram refers to the same example as *Figure 17.24(a)*. A with movement will be seen when the retinoscope is driven along the 55° meridian and an against movement when driven along 145°. Since a with movement is required, the cylinder axes should be rotated towards the 55° meridian. When the cylinder is at the correct axis, the movement in the two meridians at 45° to it should be the same, both with or both against, depending on whether the astigmatism is under- or over-corrected.

When the true cylinder axis has been determined, by whatever method, the cylinder power should be adjusted to obtain reversal in the second meridian. The practitioner should then lean forward about 50 mm and check that a with movement is obtained in both meridians. Leaning backwards by the same amount should produce an against movement in all meridians, confirming that sphere and cylinder are both correct. If the patient's accommodative state has changed between the two reversals, both sphere and cylinder will be wrong.

Positive cylinders may be used in retinoscopy, in which case the more myopic or less hypermetropic meridian should be corrected first, leaving a with movement in the second meridian. When the trial plus cylinder is inserted, the retinoscope beam should be passed along its axis, the practitioner leaning forward slightly to obtain a with movement. If the reflex movement deviates anticlockwise from the trial axis, the latter should be rotated slightly in the opposite direction. If Lindner's method of driving the beam at 45° on each side of the trial axis is used, the cylinder axis should be rotated towards the meridian showing the against movement.

A disadvantage of plus cylinders may occur when the patient is young and has active accommodation. When reversal is obtained in the less hypermetropic meridian, the astigmatic image plane for the second meridian lies behind the retina if the astigmatism is more than 1.50 D (or greater than $|W|$). This may act as a stimulus to accommodation because the eye is fogged in both meridians only when the plus cylinder has been put in place. The same problem arises in a subjective examination if plus cylinders are changed without temporary occlusion. Another possible disadvantage of plus cylinders is that difficulties may arise during the subjective examination if the fan and block technique is used.

Plus cylinders of power less than +1.50 D (or $|W|$) do have the advantage of giving a less diffuse reflex. When reversal has been obtained in the less hypermetropic meridian, the eye's artificial far point for the other meridian is closer to the immediate source. For the same reason, the reflex is improved when minus cylinders are used by setting the retinoscope beam at maximum divergence.

One interesting paradox concerning retinoscopy of the astigmatic eye has already been mentioned. A second one arises with marked astigmatism and concerns the apparent path of the reflex. In *Figure 17.25*, a horizontal band reflex is shown in three positions as the beam is directed downwards along the 110° meridian. It first appears at the top of the pupil, then extends

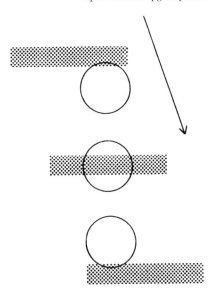

Figure 17.25. A possible illusion affecting the apparent movement of an elongated reflex when the retinoscope beam is driven along an off-axis meridian. The direction of the reflex movement appears to be perpendicular to the edge of the reflex (shown stippled).

horizontally across it and finally disappears at the bottom. Exactly the same appearance would be caused if the band reflex were moved vertically downwards. This is the interpretation placed on it by the observer.

Spot retinoscopy in practice

Static retinoscopy

The trial frame or refractor head is correctly adjusted and centred before the patient's eyes. Working distance lenses may be inserted or not according to preference or practical convenience. The consulting room should be darkened; the patient's pupil will dilate a little and the low ambient illumination will make the reflex much easier to see.

Accommodation should be relaxed by asking the patient to look at a distant fixation object. The spot light of the test cabinet is often used, but the green of the bichromatic panel, being a larger stimulus, is less likely to provoke spasm of accommodation in the young patient. To examine the right eye, the practitioner should sit so that the patient can just see the fixation object to the right of the practitioner's head. The latter's right eye will then be very close to the patient's right visual axis. A quick look with the retinoscope is made at the patient's left eye to check that there is an against movement. If not, as is usually the case, sufficient positive spherical power must be placed before the left eye to produce an against movement. The left eye is then fogged, so helping to ensure that accommodation is relaxed.

Retinoscopy is now performed accurately on the right eye. The movement of the reflex is observed as the retinoscope is tilted slightly to drive the patch of light slowly in the horizontal, vertical and mid-way oblique meridians. If the reflex movements in these meridians are a mixture of with and against, indicating at least a moderate amount of astigmatism, an approximate cylinder axis may be discernible. The same applies if the reflex tends to follow a fixed direction irrespective of the beam direction. Usually, however, the reflex shows the same variety of movement in all meridians. There may then be no useful clue to an axis direction until reversal is approached with plus or minus spheres. With experience, the lens power needed for reversal in the more hypermetropic or less myopic principal meridian can be found with only a few trials. An against movement remains in the meridian at right-angles. If the retinoscope is now moved in this meridian, the orientation of the edge of the reflex will often give a good indication of the astigmatic axis. One of the procedures described on pages 338–341 should then be used to refine the axis and check the cylinder power. It is often an advantage to lean forward slightly when driving the retinoscope beam along the cylinder axis to check its orientation. Reversal then changes to a moderate with movement and any discrepancy between the directions of reflex and beam is then easier to see.

If a spot retinoscope with focusing adjustment is used, a less divergent beam will give a brighter reflex than a more divergent one: this is helpful when examining patients with high ametropia or small pupils. On approaching reversal, a more divergent beam should be used, both to slow down the relative speed of reflex movement and to provide a crisper reflex for identifying the astigmatic axis and for neutralizing the relatively myopic second meridian.

While examining the right eye of a markedly hypermetropic patient, an occasional quick look should be made at the left eye to ensure that an against movement remains. Accommodation may have relaxed as positive power is increased before the right eye, leaving the left eye unfogged. This can be best demonstrated by an example. Suppose the patient is a +4.00 DS bilateral hypermetrope accommodating about 3.00 D. Initially, there is no lens before the right eye and +2.50 DS is found to be needed before the left to produce an against movement. Retinoscopy now shows that a +4.50 DS lens gives reversal for the right eye, apparently indicating that this eye is only +3.0 DS hypermetropic. The patient's accommodation may now have relaxed from 3.00 to about 1.00 D enabling him to see clearly with the supposedly fogged left eye. If maintained, this 1.00 D of accommodation will upset the measurement for the right eye. A further look at the left reflex at this stage would indicate the need for additional plus power to keep the eye fogged. Reversal for the right eye will now be given by +5.50 DS, indicating the true manifest error of +4.00 DS. This procedure is set out in *Table 17.3*.

The practitioner should now move his stool so that he sits to the left of the patient, who can just seen the fixation object past the practitioner's left ear. The retinoscope is held in the left hand in front of the left eye, so that retinoscopy is again as near as possible to the visual axis.

At the end of the procedure, the trial frame or refractor head should be removed to give the patient a brief rest while the results are noted, and the allowance for

Table 17.3   Procedure for static retinoscopy in hypermetropia

	Right eye	*Left eye*
Error	+4.00	+4.00
Start of retinoscopy		
Trial lens	0	+2.50 ⎱ against
Accommodation	+3.00	+3.00 ⎰
Total	+3.00	+5.50 → fogged
During retinoscopy		
Trial lens	+4.50 ⎱ reversal	+2.50 ⎱ with
Accommodation	+1.00 ⎰	+1.00 ⎰
Total	+5.50 → fogged	+3.50 → clear
Add more plus to L eye		
Trial lens	+5.50 ⎱ reversal	+6.00 ⎱ against
Accommodation	0 ⎰	0 ⎰
Total	+5.50 → $(F_{sp} - W)$	+6.00 → fogged

the working distance made. It might, however, be inadvisable to remove the correction if the patient is a young hypermetrope.

If more convenient, a working distance other than the usual two-thirds of a metre can be adopted, in which case the allowance must be altered correspondingly.

When the patient has a strabismus of more than a few prism dioptres, the safest procedure to ensure refraction near the visual axis of the normally deviating eye is to occlude the eye not under examination. Distance fixation can be made as before. The patient will usually say if the refractionist's head obscures the fixation object. Observation of the corneal reflection of the retinoscope light relative to the pupil centre will show if the retinoscope axis is too oblique to the patient's axis.

A suggested routine for static retinoscopy on the astigmatic eye is as follows:

(1) Add spherical lenses to approach reversal.
(2) (a) If reflex elongated and approximate axis direction apparent, proceed to obtain reversal in the more hypermetropic or less myopic principal meridian. Note orientation of reflex margins at reversal.
    (b) If axis direction uncertain, drive the retinoscope along the 180°, 90°, 45° and 135° meridians, noting direction and speed of reflex movements. From these observations it should become apparent if there is any astigmatism present. If so, its approximate axis direction should also be suggested.
(3) Add a minus trial cylinder of the estimated power at the axis found in procedure (2).
(4) Drive retinoscope beam along trial cylinder axis.
(5) If reflex moves anticlockwise to trial cylinder axis, rotate trial cylinder anticlockwise (or if it moves clockwise, rotate trial cylinder clockwise).
(6) When reflex moves along trial cylinder axis, the axis is correct.
(7) Check that reversal is still maintained in cylinder axis meridian.
(8) Determine cylinder power required for reversal in second meridian.

Stafford and Morris (1993) give a useful guide to retinoscopy in practice.

The Barrett method

This technique of retinoscopy was advocated for routine use by Barrett (1945) with the object of bringing the patient's fixation line close to the retinoscope. For various reasons, some practitioners are unable to do accurate retinoscopy with both eyes, in which case the Barrett method may provide a good alternative. The retinoscope should have a bright luminous fixation object on the body of the instrument, near the mirror. The patient looks with both eyes at this fixation object, which is devoid of fine detail that might stimulate the accommodation. Retinoscopy at the normal working distance is then undertaken on both eyes in turn, the observer's better eye being used. As with normal retinoscopy, the patient's left eye must be fogged before the right eye is examined. In general, since the convergence to the fixation object will stimulate some accommodation, an allowance for this is made as follows. When reversal has been obtained for both eyes, the patient's attention is redirected towards a distant fixation object such as the green bichromatic panel. If the practitioner's left eye is the better, he re-examines the patient's left eye with the patient looking past his left ear. A small increase in the positive (or decrease in the negative) sphere power will often be required, though the astigmatic element should not change appreciably. The resulting spherical adjustment is made for both eyes, since accommodation is presumed to be stimulated equally in each of them.

This adjustment is fairly reliable in all except young school children, who may have exerted an excessive amount of proximal accommodation. When fixation returns to the distant object, the accommodation may not relax sufficiently to give an accurate result.

The convergence required may induce a small amount of miosis, which makes retinoscopy more difficult. Another disadvantage of the Barrett method is that the patient's heterophoria may sometimes be broken down into a heterotropia. The retinal illumination from the immediate source is often many times greater than from the fixation object and therefore dazzles the patient. This tends to dissociate the eyes, resulting in a manifest deviation.

The Barrett method may also be useful in the domiciliary situation where a convenient distance fixation object may not be available. For elderly patients, the allowance for accommodation will be unnecessary, though to ensure that the eye being examined is the one fixating, it may be advantageous to occlude the other.

Mohindra near retinoscopy

This technique was developed by Mohindra (1975) to allow the refraction of infants without the use of cycloplegics. Retinoscopy is undertaken in a completely dark room, the patient fixating the immediate source, i.e. the retinoscope filament image. The child's attention should be held by interesting audible effects. While trial case lenses or the refractor head may be used for older patients, the use of retinoscopy racks is advocated for infant patients. The racks should be painted matt black to avoid distracting the patient, and, unlike the paired racks used for dynamic retinoscopy (*see* pages 345–347), are for one eye only. The suggested lenses are +0.50 to +3.50 DS in 0.50 D steps in one rack, and +4.00 to +8.00 D in 1.00 D steps together with +10.00 and +13.00 D lenses in another. A similar range of minus lenses is provided by another two racks. The racks enable different meridians of the eye to be examined in quick succession, thus avoiding the use of cylindrical lenses.

The recommended working distance is 0.5 m, but an allowance of only 1.25 D should be deducted from the retinoscope findings. This suggests that, on average, infant patients accommodate by approximately 0.75 D during the examination. Owens *et al.* (1980) have concluded, however, that this amount of accommodation is not induced by an active effort to focus the source image but is a form of inadequate stimulus myopia (*see* pages 132–138), caused by the absence of any visual detail in the darkened room and the lack of any structure in the source itself.

Older patients could be expected to react similarly. The present writer (RER) has compared conventional static and Mohindra near retinoscopy, though not with infants. Some young children appear to go into accommodative spasm, while others do not: this could perhaps be a reflection of the varying amounts of inadequate stimulus myopia found in the general population. The technique was useful with those patients whose fundi appear to be tilted in relation to the visual axis and with those unable to maintain the fixation required in the static method. It has also been advocated for the measurement of the eye's resting state of accommodation, provided that the eye not being refracted is occluded to eliminate any control of accommodation by the convergence pathway.

Errors and accuracy of retinoscopy

Although the principles of retinoscopy can be described in simple optical terms, there are several possible sources of error. Despite these difficulties, experience makes the retinoscopy findings an extremely useful estimate of the refraction. An accuracy better than 0.50 D on the ametropia in either principal meridian and within 15° on the astigmatic axis of 1.00 DC should easily be obtained, given a medium-sized pupil and no irregular refraction.

The typical eye with relaxed accommodation has positive spherical aberration in which the refractive power increases from the paraxial region outwards (*see* pages 281–284). Spherical aberration becomes apparent in retinoscopy when the pupil is large, especially when dilated with mydriatics or cycloplegics. As a result, the reflex may simultaneously show a with movement in the centre of the pupil and an against movement in the periphery. It is important in retinoscopy to watch the reflex in the centre of the pupil, ignoring the remainder.

The split (or scissors) reflex

Particularly in the vertical meridian, the reflex may occasionally appear to be split, moving simultaneously in opposite directions from the centre of the pupil. There is no easy rule to decide what should constitute reversal in such an eye. Usually the refraction may be 'bracketed', an overall with movement being obtained when, for example, a −0.50 DS is added, and an overall against movement when +0.50 DS is added. Roorda and Bobier (1996) have demonstrated that coma is the probable cause of the split reflex. Large-scale irregularities in the media due to corneal scarring or lens changes will considerably reduce the accuracy of all objective methods of refraction.

Off-axis errors

As mentioned on pages 286–287, oblique astigmatism of the beam leaving the eye can cause significant errors if retinoscopy is performed more than 5° from the visual axis. *Figure 15.11* for the schematic eye shows that an induced astigmatic error of about −0.50 DC × 90 would arise at 10° horizontal obliquity of observation.

Ocular abnormalities and asymmetries

As the result of a localized bulge (perhaps due to a tumour) or a depression (for example, posterior staphyloma as in high myopia), that part of the fundus forming the source for the returning light may be situated nearer or further from the principal planes of the eye than the fovea. The accuracy of the estimated spherical component of refraction would be affected by this (Hodd, 1951). It is also possible that the errors arising from obliquity of observation could be increased by various ocular asymmetries. Spherical aberration, in particular, is seldom symmetrical. Because of the Stiles–Crawford effect, a tilted fovea might also have optical ramifications as yet unexplored in this context.

Accommodative tonus

The spherical element of the refraction may not be confirmed subjectively if the fogging of the working distance lenses forces a young hypermetrope to relax his accommodative tonus. A higher positive error is often found by retinoscopy than is manifested subjectively, especially if the patient has been previously uncorrected or does not need to wear the full refractive findings constantly. The typical subject is a young +3.00 D hypermetrope, wearing the correction only for critical vision indoors and with no problems of oculo-motor imbalance.

Position of the reflecting surface

The reflex in the human eye is distinctly red, suggesting that the reflection occurs at the pigment epithelium layer since the retina itself is transparent. If so, the axial length of the eye for retinoscopy would be longer than the true length to the retinal receptor layer, resulting in a slightly myopic estimate of the refraction. On the other hand, because chromatic aberration gives the eye a slightly lower power for red than for white light, this factor would result in a slightly hypermetropic estimate. Charman (1975), taking into account the spectral variations of the source emittance, the retinal reflectivity and the eye's refractive power, concluded that retinoscopy findings would be about 0.1 D more hypermetropic than the subjective refraction. Further experiments by Charman involving retinal photography and electronic objective optometry with light of various colours suggested that the longer wavelengths are reflected from deep within the retina.

Glickstein and Millodot (1970) and Millodot (1974) have reintroduced the contrary idea that the reflection takes place in front of the retinal receptors. Their argument is as follows. In animals with eyes very much smaller than those in man but of equal retinal thickness, reflection at an anterior layer such as the internal limiting membrane would give a result several dioptres more hypermetropic than reflection at the retinal receptor level. Their experiments with the electroretinogram (ERG), in man with visually evoked cortical response (VECR) and several other animal studies, confirmed that the refraction thus measured was significantly less hypermetropic than the retinoscopy findings, especially in small animal eyes. Indeed, there would be no advantage to an animal in being excessively hypermetropic. This discrepancy between retinoscopy and physiological findings is sometimes termed the 'artefact of retinoscopy'. Since chromatic aberration alone is insufficient to account for the discrepancy, its cause must be that reflection takes place at or near the vitreous–retinal boundary – *see* Exercise 17.15.

Millodot and O'Leary (1978a) rationalized this as follows: using 1078 records from three practitioners, they investigated the mean difference between retinoscopy and subjective findings in various age groups, to find a nearly linear drop from +0.35 D on the 5–15 age group to almost −0.1 D in the over-65 group. In the young patient, they postulated that the reflex originates predominantly from the internal limiting membrane, but with sufficient reflection from the deeper layers to give the red coloration. To confirm this, they (1978b) undertook retinoscopy on 305 eyes of various ages with a retinoscope providing a polarized beam. The sighthole was fitted with an analyser, which when aligned with the polarizer, tended to select light reflected at the internal limiting membrane, while with a crossed analyser, the reflex is produced predominantly by light diffusely reflected from the retina. The latter results gave a similarly myopic bias to retinoscopy at all ages, while the results with the aligned analyser gave results similar to those of the first study. This can be explained, since, with increasing age, the refractive index difference at, and hence reflectance from, the internal limiting membrane decreases. Also, changes in the plane of polarization of light passing through the eye (e.g. van Blokland, 1985; and Gorrand, 1986), mean that even with aligned polarizers, some of the light will be reflected at surfaces other than the internal limiting membrane.

Error in the working distance

The spherical component will obviously be in error if the working distance is incorrect. This can easily occur if refracting a young child or a patient with small pupils, when one tends to get closer than usual without realizing it. The sphere balance will obviously be upset if the refraction for the two eyes is done at different distances. An error of about 100 mm is required at two-thirds of a metre to give an error of 0.25 D in the refraction.

Subjective checks

Despite these possible errors, retinoscopy gives a good estimate of the refraction of most patients, and has to be relied on in certain circumstances. Since the patient's vision in everyday life is, however, a subjective response, a subjective check of the retinoscopy findings should always be made or attempted, except in the youngest of patients. If the response to the subjective test is poor, but the vision with the retinoscopy findings is good, then, and only then, may the subjective tests be abandoned. The final sections of Chapter 6 describe a routine to follow retinoscopy.

Dynamic retinoscopy

Basic principle

In the techniques described so far, a common factor is the aim of inhibiting or minimizing the patient's accommodation. Although the Barrett method requires fixation at the normal working distance, there is little stimulus to accommodation because the fixation object is relatively large and luminous. Some proximal and convergence-induced accommodation may occur. Both of these techniques, together with Mohindra's, are forms of static retinoscopy inasmuch as active accommodation is not required.

In dynamic retinoscopy, introduced by Cross in 1902 (*see* Cross, 1911), the aim is to investigate the accommodative state of the eye in near vision. There are two distinctly different techniques:

(1) The patient observes a separate fixation object while the retinoscope is held behind it. The distance between the object and retinoscope at reversal indicates the accuracy of accommodation.
(2) The fixation object is on the retinoscope, the level of accommodation being measured by trial lenses placed before the eyes.

In both techniques the patient wears the distance correction, usually as found by the subjective tests. The fixation object must be well illuminated and finely detailed so as to provide a good stimulus for accommodation. An Anglepoise type of light, positioned about 30–40 cm above the patient's head and aimed downwards, will give adequate illumination of the stimulus while keeping both the patient's and retinoscopist's faces in the shade. Alternatively, an internally illuminated fixation stimulus could be used, either separately or as an illuminated aperture on the retinoscope. The retinoscope beam, however, should be as dim as possible to reduce any tendency to dissociate the eyes. The beam is moved in a continuous path to investigate the horizontal meridians of the two eyes in rapid succession.

Separate fixation method

The fixation object, which should be well illuminated, is held in the median plane at the patient's customary reading or working distance. The practitioner holds the retinoscope just behind and above the fixation object and passes the beam across the pupils. A with movement indicates that the retinoscope should be moved further away from the eyes, the fixation object remaining stationary.

In general, the with movement will change to an against movement for both eyes at the same distance of the retinoscope from the fixation object. Provided that the patient's astigmatism is properly corrected, this indicates that the spherical component of the refraction is balanced in near vision.

Should reversal in the two eyes be obtained at different distances, low positive or negative lenses are added before one eye until simultaneous reversal in both is obtained in a single sweep of the retinoscope. This is easily checked by leaning forward slightly with the retinoscope, when a with movement should occur in both eyes, or leaning back when an against movement should be seen.

Any change required in the spherical balance may indicate that the distance findings are incorrect. Dynamic retinoscopy can thus be a useful method of checking the subjective balance when confirmation is desired. A genuine change in the spherical balance when vision switches from distance to near could, of course, arise from unequal accommodation or from eye to spectacle plane effectivity in marked anisometropia.

A change in the astigmatic component of the refraction is indicated if the reflex moves obliquely instead of exactly along the horizontal meridian of the eye. This may be due to astigmatic changes in the crystalline lens in its accommodated state.

Dynamic lag of accommodation

In dynamic retinoscopy, the patient must try to maintain accurate fixation and accommodation for the fixation object. This should have small letters, for example, a reduced Snellen chart or a series of small dots to be counted. Despite this stimulus, the reversal position of the retinoscope usually lies about 120 mm behind the fixation object. The difference in the dioptric distances of fixation object and retinoscope sighthole from the patient's eyes is known as the dynamic lag of accommodation. As explained later, a more specific term for it is the 'low neutral' dynamic lag.

Woodhouse *et al.* (1993) mounted an internally illuminated fixation stimulus on an accommodation rule, thus enabling the accommodative demand and the position of the retinoscope to be measured accurately.

The researches summarized on pages 288-289 show

that in white light the wavelength focused on the retina is in the green region in near vision but approaches the red region in distance vision. Subjectively, this can easily be shown with the bichromatic apparatus. If the test patterns on the two colours are made equally clear in distance, the subject will nearly always report that the green is clearer in near vision. A lag of accommodation in dynamic retinoscopy could therefore be expected. Rosenfield *et al.* (1996), comparing this technique of retinoscopy with the near bichromatic test and the near cross cylinder test, found that retinoscopy gave the best agreement for the accommodative response as measured with an infra-red aurorefractor (*see* Chapter 18).

The possible errors of static retinoscopy apply equally to the dynamic method, except those arising from obliquity of observation. There is, however, the added risk that normal binocular vision might be disturbed by the glare source of the retinoscope lamp. The accommodation could also be affected even if binocular vision is properly maintained. Good illumination of the fixation stimulus is therefore essential.

Variation in dynamic lag

If the lag is very high, the accommodation must be insufficient. This could suggest that:

(1) The amplitude of accommodation is low and extra positive power is needed for near vision. Sometimes the dynamic lag is initially normal, but rapidly increases, showing the accommodative effort to be ill-sustained. Extra help is again indicated. Near additions in presbyopia may be estimated by adding positive spheres until a normal lag is obtained.
(2) The distance refractive error has been wrongly determined, for example, hypermetropia either under-corrected or with a large latent component, or myopia over-corrected. A refraction under cycloplegia is probably indicated.
(3) The patient is a low myope, infrequently wearing the distance correction for near vision. The accommodative mechanism is therefore sluggish.
(4) An esophoria in near vision. Inhibition of convergence to prevent a breakdown into a manifest deviation may also inhibit accommodation.

Reversal may be obtained near or in the plane of the fixation object or there may even be an against movement with the retinoscope in that position. The small dynamic lag thus shown may indicate:

(1) Spasm of accommodation in near vision. This could occur normally when a previously under-corrected young hypermetrope is given a marked increase in correction. The patient is habitually used to accommodating both for the refractive error and for the distance of regard and now has to accommodate only for the latter element. This effect does not always occur but may sometimes be seen when the refractive correction for a young patient is increased by about +2.00 DS.
(2) Spasm of accommodation in near vision unrelated to distance refraction.

(3) Exophoria in near vision, accommodation being stimulated through the mechanism of convergence-induced accommodation.

The amplitude of accommodation in a juvenile patient may be checked objectively by bringing the fixation object closer and closer to the patient, the retinoscope following behind. An against movement will initially be seen, changing to a with movement near the face. At this point, the dioptric distance of the sighthole from the spectacle plane is a measure of the amplitude.

The quick and useful techniques described above follow approximately those of Nott (1925) and Freeman and Hodd (1955).

Method using trial lenses

An alternative technique is for the patient to observe a detailed fixation stimulus attached to the retinoscope, which is held at the near working distance. The patient again wears the distance subjective or static retinoscopy findings. A with movement will usually be seen in both eyes as the retinoscope is passed quickly across their horizontal meridians. Equal positive power is added before each eye until reversal is obtained. This process can be simplified by using dynamic retinoscopy racks, holding a paired series of lenses of increasing plus power, and with a cut-out slot for the patient's nose. The lowest lens power giving reversal is the dynamic low neutral, which corresponds to the finding of the previous technique. In the normal pre-presbyopic patient, this will be about 0.50 or 0.75 DS.

If the plus lens power is increased, the neutral reflex appearance will remain over a significant change, up to about + 1.50 DS. Beyond this point an against movement will occur. The strongest reversing lens is known as the 'high neutral': the difference between the high and low neutrals is assumed to correspond to negative relative accommodation – the amount by which accommodation can be relaxed while accurate and constant convergence is maintained (*see* pages 164–165).

This method of retinoscopy using additional trial lenses and its various techniques have been described by many authors including Swann (1944) and Borish (1970).

Whitefoot and Charman's (1992) study into this technique of dynamic retinoscopy found that the mean results of the low and high neutrals for pre-presbyopic patients were 1.10 ± 0.58 D and 1.52 ± 0.36 D respectively. The size of the standard deviations, however, indicated a wide spread of values in the normal population, indicating that a deviation from the mean did not mean an abnormal result. As expected from the effects of convergence-induced accommodation (*see* pages 163–164) with binocular fixation, there was a tendency for both neutrals to be higher in esophoria and lower in exophores. They concluded that dynamic retinoscopy might have a role in binocular balancing in near vision, and in the investigation of patients with specific near-vision symptoms.

MEM retinoscopy

In the method of dynamic retinoscopy described above, the stimulus to accommodation is altered by the presence of the trial lenses. In the monocular estimate method, described by Greenspan (1974), Rouse *et al.* (1982) and Eskridge (1989), the patient again binocularly fixates a stimulus mounted on the retinoscope. Instead of the binocular rack, a single lens is briefly held in front of one eye and the beam passed across. With practice, it may be possible to refract the eye faster than it can react to the change in stimulus (about 0.3 sec – *see* page 130). The method is applied to one eye at a time, though both should be checked if it is wished to use the technique to verify the near binocular balance or accommodative response. The lens giving reversal gives the value of the low neutral.

Streak retinoscopy

The idea underlying streak retinoscopy is to elongate the illuminated fundus patch and hence the potential reflex while simultaneously narrowing its width. The presence of low astigmatism then becomes more apparent and its axis direction more easily determined. To this end, the coiled-filament lamp of the spot retinoscope is replaced by a goalpost filament lamp mounted to give a very narrow linear source perpendicular to the axis of the condensing lens. The lamp can be rotated so that its rectangular beam can be set at any orientation. At all times, the beam is passed across the pupil at right-angles to its length.

In streak retinoscopy, the *orientation* of the streak reflex or its borders is of great importance. It cannot be exactly parallel to the illuminating streak unless this is itself parallel to one of the eye's principal meridians or unless no astigmatism is present. Another important fact is that because of the illusion illustrated in *Figure 17.25*, the direction of travel of the streak reflex always *appears* to be perpendicular to its length, provided that it extends over the entire width of the pupil.

Streak retinoscopy is performed somewhat similarly to spot retinoscopy. With a divergent beam the patient's right eye is examined first, the left eye having been fogged. Then, with the beam always kept perpendicular to the meridian explored, the direction of the reflex movement is noted in the horizontal, vertical, 45° and 135° meridians. Unless the astigmatism is high, the reflex will be nearly parallel to the beam and will show the same kind of movement, with or against, in each meridian. Spherical lenses as appropriate are then added to approach reversal.

Figure 17.26 illustrates the stages in the subsequent procedure, the refractive error being taken as +5.00/−1.00 × 110. With +6.00 DS before the eye, there will be a with movement in the vertical meridian and an against movement in the horizontal, the same as in spot retinoscopy. When the beam is horizontal, that is to say, at 20° from the orientation required, the reflex will appear tilted as shown in *Figure 17.26(a)*. As the beam is rotated anticlockwise about the pupil centre, the reflex will gradually come into line with the ends of

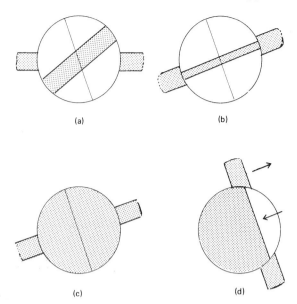

Figure 17.26. Streak retinoscopy in astigmatism: minus cylinder axis 110°, indicated by the line. (a) Streak horizontal, scanning vertical, the reflex is oblique; (b) streak rotated until reflex appears parallel and both are now parallel to the required axis; (c) reversal in 110° meridian, reflex filling the pupil; (d) beam rotated to 110° meridian to examine the 20° meridian, initial against movement.

the beam that spill over on to the lens surrounds, as in *Figure 17.26(b)*. The beam is then at right-angles to the cylinder axis, which can be read by temporarily focusing the beam on to the cylinder axis scale.

With the beam made divergent again, it is swept along the 110° meridian and the sphere power adjusted to obtain reversal. As shown in *Figure 17.26(c)*, the reflex then fills the pupil (unless there is pronounced spherical aberration). An against movement will now be seen when the beam is swept along the 20° meridian. The reflex still covers the width of the pupil (*Figure 17.26d*) and reversal is obtained with a minus cylinder at axis 110°.

An alternative procedure can be followed by the experienced practitioner after reversal has been obtained in the more hypermetropic meridian. The beam vergence is then adjusted to position the immediate source between the retinoscope and the patient's eye. The reflex now shrinks to a well-defined band in the pupil. A relatively rapid *with* movement is produced, neutralized as before with a minus cylinder.

Francis (1973) has devised the following alternative method of determining the presence of astigmatism and its axis direction:

(1) Reversal with spherical lenses is obtained in the more hypermetropic or less myopic meridian, in the normal manner.
(2) The retinoscope beam is set for maximum divergence, so that the immediate source then lies about 1 m from the patient's eye, with a working distance of two-thirds of a metre.
(3) The lens power for reversal is reduced by +0.50 DS so that the immediate source becomes focused on the retina in the meridian neutralized. As a result,

the reflex shrinks to a narrow line instead of filling the pupil.

(4) The beam is now rotated through 90°. If the reflex remains narrow, no astigmatism is present, but even the smallest amount will cause the reflex to fill the pupil as the beam completes its rotation. Its orientation when the reflex is at its narrowest is perpendicular to the axis of the required minus cylinder.

(5) The +0.50 DS deducted is restored and reversal obtained in the second meridian in the usual manner.

Width of the potential reflex

The length of the potential reflex, corresponding to the length of the immediate source, is of no particular interest because it is nearly always greater than the pupil diameter. Its width, however, is important in streak retinoscopy. For simplicity, the cross-sectional diameter of the filament can be neglected and the immediate source regarded as an axial point at a dioptric distance X from the patient's eye. The refractive error, or residual refractive error when a lens is placed before it during retinoscopy, is denoted by K, the dioptric length of the eye by K' and the pupil diameter by g. In *Figure 17.27*, h is the half-width of the blurred retinal image of the point source and h' half the size of its image in the eye's far-point plane. From equation (4.16a), replacing L by X and j by $2h$, we then have

$$2h = g \times \frac{K - X}{K'} \qquad (17.6)$$

while the conjugate foci relationship gives

$$h' = hK'/K \qquad (17.7)$$

Viewed from the centre C of the sighthole, its diameter being ignored, the total width q of the potential reflex is equal to $2y$. From the similar triangles in the diagram we get

$$q = 2y = 2h' \times \frac{w}{w - k}$$
$$= 2h' \times \frac{K}{K - W} \qquad (17.8)$$

Finally, multiplying together equations (17.6)–(17.8) produces

$$q = g \times \frac{K - X}{K - W} \qquad (17.9)$$

which can also be put in the form

$$q/g = (K - X)/(K - W) \qquad (17.10)$$

This gives the width of the potential reflex in terms of its

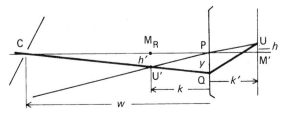

Figure 17.27. The potential reflex in streak retinoscopy. Q is the edge of the potential reflex, not the edge of the pupil.

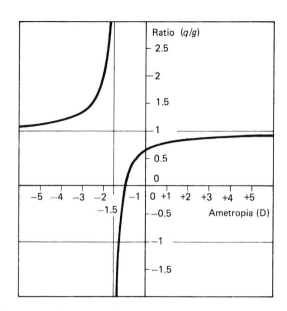

Figure 17.28. Graph showing the ratio of the width of the potential reflex to the pupil diameter, plotted against ametropia. Dioptric working distance −1.50 D. (After Francis, 1973.)

ratio to the pupil diameter. The width of the *observed* reflex cannot, of course, exceed the pupil diameter.

In *Figure 17.28*, the ratio q/g is plotted as a function of the ametropia K when $W = -1.50$ D and $X = -1.00$ D. The graph is a hyperbola, asymptomatic to the vertical at $K = W$ (reversal). It will be seen that as a hypermetropic (but not a myopic) meridian is gradually brought to reversal, the width of the reflex decreases, becoming theoretically zero (an Euclidean line) when $K = X$.

The hypothetical point source is then in focus on the retina and the actual reflex observed is at its narrowest. It then expands rapidly to fill the pupil when reversal is obtained. A more detailed discussion is given by Francis (1973), on whose graphs *Figure 17.28* is based.

Orientation of the reflex

In *Figure 17.29*, the refractive error of the eye represented is

$$-1.75/-0.25 \times 50$$

so that $K_\alpha = -2.00$ D and $K_\beta = -1.75$ D. If $W = -1.50$ D and $X = -1.00$ D, the relative speed of reflex movement μ in the two meridians is found to be, $\mu_\alpha = -1$ and $\mu_\beta = -2$. The illuminating streak IS is horizontal and has been moved vertically downwards from the pupil centre O. To find the corresponding position of the streak reflex SR, it is merely necessary to consider the points C and D at which the illuminating streak intersects the principal meridians. In the 140° (alpha) meridian where $\mu_\alpha = -1$, C′ is located on the side of O remote from C such that OC′ = −OC. Similarly, in the 50° (beta) meridian where $\mu_\beta = -2$, D′ is located on the side of O remote from D such that OD′ = −2 OD. The streak reflex therefore lies along the line C′D′.

Let ϕ denote the angle from the beta meridian to the illuminating streak and ϕ' the angle to the streak reflex. Then, from the geometry of the diagram,

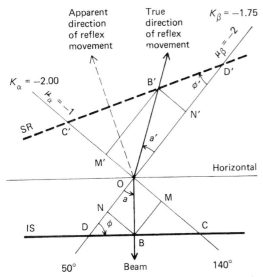

Figure 17.29. Derivation of orientation and true and apparent directions of movement of the reflex in streak retinoscopy.

$$\frac{\tan \phi'}{\tan \phi} = \frac{OC'/OD'}{OC/OD} = \frac{\mu_\alpha}{\mu_\beta} \tag{17.11}$$

Using equation (17.4), this relationship can also be written as

$$\tan \phi' = \frac{W - K_\beta}{W - K_\alpha} \tan \phi \tag{17.12}$$

In the example shown in *Figure 17.29* we should have

$$\tan \phi' = \frac{-1.50 + 1.75}{-1.50 + 2.00} \tan (-50°)$$

$$= 0.5 \tan (-50°)$$

giving $\phi' = -30.8°$. If ϕ and ϕ' are measured from the alpha meridian, the coefficient of $\tan \phi$ in equation (17.12) need merely be inverted. In the same example, ϕ would become $40°$ and we should have

$$\tan \phi' = 2 \tan 40°$$

giving

$$\phi' = 59.2°$$

Some interesting deductions can be made from equation (17.12). For example, when reversal occurs in the beta meridian, the term $(W - K_\beta)$ becomes zero. Consequently, ϕ' remains zero irrespective of the value of ϕ. That is to say, the reflex remains aligned with the beta meridian whatever the orientation of the streak. Similarly, when reversal occurs in the alpha meridian, ϕ' becomes $90°$ for all values of ϕ, the reflex thus remaining aligned with the alpha meridian.

Direction of the reflex movement

In *Figure 17.29*, the angle a' gives the direction of the reflex movement when the illuminating streak moves at an angle a, both angles measured from the beta meridian. The relationship between them, stated without proof as equation (17.5), can be derived very simply.

To locate B', the point on the reflex corresponding to B on the illuminating streak, the procedure illustrated in

Figure 17.22 can be used. Perpendiculars BM and BN are dropped from B to the principal meridians. Then, M' and N' are located from $OM' = \mu_\alpha OM = -OM$ and $ON' = \mu_\beta ON = -2(ON)$. The point B' is the fourth corner of the completed rectangle OM'N'B'. The construction is confirmed by finding B' to lie on C'D'. Thus, the centre of the streak reflex has moved in a direction OB' which is not only oblique to that of the illuminating streak but also to its own apparent movement, which, as shown in *Figure 17.25*, is perpendicular to its length. From the geometry of *Figure 17.29* we have

$$\frac{\tan a'}{\tan a} = \frac{N'B'/ON'}{NB/ON} = \frac{OM'/ON'}{OM/ON} = \frac{\mu_\alpha}{\mu_\beta}$$

Since this expression is identical in form to equation (17.11), it can similarly be written as in equation (17.12), with a' and a substituted for ϕ' and ϕ.

A new method

An interesting variation of streak retinoscopy was introduced by Parker (1966). The retinoscope is fixed in alignment with the patient's pupil and the vergence control adjusted to give minimum reflex width. Lenses are added to increase this width by reducing the ametropia. Neutralization occurs when the reflex fills the pupil.

Exercises

17.1 Retinoscopy is performed at a working distance of two-thirds of a metre with a self-luminous retinoscope. The bulb filament is 1 mm across and is imaged to the immediate source by a lens of power +20.00 D. Neglecting the distance between this lens and the mirror, find the overall size of the illuminated patch on the retina when the vergence of the retinoscope beam, measured at the mirror, is (a) −1.00 D, (b) −5.00 D, (c) +3.00 D. Assume the patient's pupil to be 5 mm in diameter, the ocular refraction −3.75 D and the axial length of the eye 24 mm.

17.2 Retinoscopy is carried out at a working distance of half a metre, the immediate source being 25 mm in diameter and 750 mm behind the mirror. Find the size of the image of the illuminated fundus patch, given that the subject has a 4 mm pupil and is (a) myopic −0.50 D, (b) myopic−5.00 D, (c) hypermetropic +1.00 D.

17.3 A myopic eye of $26\frac{2}{3}$ mm axial length has an ocular refraction of −12.50 D and a 6 mm pupil. Light is reflected from an illuminated point on the retina 0.3 mm directly below the optical axis. On a diagram with the actual size along the axis and five times the actual size vertically, show the emergent pencil of rays and shade that part of it which would enter the 4 mm pupil of an observer's eye placed 120 mm from the reduced surface of the subject's eye. On a separate drawing five times actual size, show what part of the subject's pupil would appear to be illuminated.

17.4 (a) An astigmatic eye has ocular refraction of

−1.00 DS/−3.00 DC axis 180

Assuming light to be reflected from a single point on the retina, draw a scale diagram showing a section through the emergent pencil in each principal meridian. Hence construct a separate diagram showing the appearance of the reflex as seen by an observer at 1 m. Assume both pupils to have a diameter of 4 mm. (b) How would the reflex appear to move if the luminous point were to move across the retina (i) horizontally, (ii) vertically, (iii) in the 45° meridian?

17.5 (a) Retinoscopy is performed at two-thirds of a metre. The immediate source, assumed to be a point, is placed −800 mm from the subject's eye. Calculate the diameter of the potential reflex when the ametropia is: -0.50, -1.00, -2.00, $-2.50\,\text{DS}$. Assume $K' = +60\,\text{D}$ and pupil diameter $4\,\text{mm}$. (b) Suppose the bulb filament image or immediate source is now made $2\,\text{mm}$ in diameter. Calculate the new potential reflex dimensions. Since the actual reflex diameter cannot exceed the pupil diameter, discuss the practical difference between these results. (c) The point-source retinoscope is adjusted so that the immediate source is $-400\,\text{mm}$ from the subject's eye. Calculate the new potential reflex dimensions. Comment in relation to streak and spot retinoscopy.

17.6 A streak retinoscope is used at a working distance of two-thirds of a metre. From first principles find the angular movement of the reflex when the mirror rotates $0.1\,\text{rad}$, in each of the following cases: (a) patient's eye myopic $-1.00\,\text{D}$, beam vergence at the mirror $+4.00\,\text{D}$; (b) patient's eye hypermetropic $+5.00\,\text{D}$, beam vergence at the mirror $+1.00\,\text{D}$.

17.7 Retinoscopy is performed at $-0.5\,\text{m}$ on a patient with refractive error $-1.75\,\text{D}$. Find the angular speed of the reflex relative to the retinoscope movement when the immediate source is positioned $-0.5\,\text{m}$, $-0.17\,\text{m}$ and $+0.17\,\text{m}$ from the retinoscope.

17.8 (a) Retinoscopy is performed with a luminous instrument on a myopic eye of $-12.50\,\text{D}$ ocular refraction, the immediate source being $500\,\text{mm}$ behind the mirror. By what factor is the speed of the reflex movement increased when the working distance is reduced from two-thirds to one-tenth of a metre? (b) Repeat (a) for an aphakic eye of $+12.50\,\text{D}$ ocular refraction.

17.9 (a) Retinoscopy is performed at a working distance of $-\frac{2}{3}\,\text{m}$ on a patient with a $5\,\text{mm}$ diameter pupil. The instrument uses a point source and a $+30\,\text{D}$ lens which can be positioned to give a beam divergent (i) $-2\,\text{D}$, (ii) $-5\,\text{D}$ on leaving the retinoscope lens. For both adjustments, calculate the diameter of that area of the retinoscope lens through which light can pass into the patient's pupil, and also the solid angle subtended by this area at the actual source. For which adjustment is the reflex brighter? (b) Repeat for a different instrument with a lens of power $+10\,\text{D}$ but giving the same beam vergences.

17.10 In static retinoscopy, the patient's right eye looks just past the refractionist's right ear, so that the retinoscope is $25\,\text{mm}$ to the side of the right visual axis. Calculate the obliquity of the axis of retinoscopy to the visual axis for the right eye, and also for the patient's left eye, the examiner not moving. Assume the patient's PD to be $68\,\text{mm}$, the working distance $\frac{2}{3}\,\text{m}$, and no vertical discrepancy.

17.11 In static retinoscopy, working $4°$ temporally to the visual axis, the refractive error is found to be $1\,\text{D}$ more myopic than the subjective finding. Assuming this to be caused by a slope in the retina (of a reduced eye of power $+60\,\text{D}$), calculate the angle between the visual axis and the plane of the retina.

17.12 (a) Reversal having been obtained at a working distance w, the retinoscope is tilted so that the ray from the centre of the patient's pupil just grazes the upper edge of the sighthole, which has an effective vertical diameter a. At the same time, a ray from the upper extremity of the pupil just grazes the lower edge of the sighthole. Derive an expression for K, the relative refractive error at the pupil margin, equal in amount but opposite in sign to the zonal spherical aberration. (b) Tabulate the values of K for sighthole diameters 1, 2 and 3 mm and pupil diameters 2, 4 and 6 mm, the working distance being $\frac{2}{3}\,\text{m}$.

17.13 In dynamic retinoscopy, the fixation object is $350\,\text{mm}$ from the mid-point between the patient's eyes. If the retinoscope is held (a) 80, (b) 100, (c) 120 mm behind the test object at reversal, what is the dioptric value of the dynamic lag (with respect to the mid-point between the eyes)? Calculate also the horizontal angle between the visual and retinoscopic axis, assuming both the fixation object and retinoscope to be held in the median plane, and a PD of $64\,\text{mm}$.

17.14 On comparing retinoscopy with the method of parallax used on an optical bench to locate the position of an image, what similarities and differences could be listed?

17.15 Calculate the artefact of retinoscopy produced for eyes of axial length (a) 5, (b) 7.5, (c) 10, (d) 15, (e) 20 and (f) 25 mm if, (i) the reflection takes place $0.1\,\text{mm}$ in front of the plane of the receptors and if (ii) the discrepancy is caused by chromatic aberration. Assume the eyes to be of simple reduced

form, emmetropic for the d-line with index $n = 1.336$ and index $n = 1.334$ for red light.

References

BARRETT, C.D. (1945) Sources of error and working methods in retinoscopy. *Br. J. Physiol. Optics*, **5**, 35–40

BENTALL, W.K. and DIPROSE, D.R. (1932) A practical examination of certain theoretical aspects and anomalies connected with static retinoscopy. *Trans. Inst. Ophthal. Optns*, Nov. 1932

VAN BLOKLAND, G.J. (1985) Ellipsometry of the human retina *in vivo*: preservation of polarization. *J. Opt. Soc. Am. A.*, **2**, 72–75

BORISH, I.M. (1970) *Clinical Refraction*, 3rd edn. Chicago: Professional Press

CHARMAN, W. (1975) Some sources of discrepancy between static retinoscopy and subjective refraction. *Br. J. Physiol. Optics*, **30**, 108–118

CROSS, A.J. (1911) *Dynamic Skiametry in Theory and Practice*. New York: A. Jay Cross Optical Co.

ESKRIDGE, J.B. (1989) Clinical objective assessment of the accommodative response. *J. Am. Optom. Assoc.*, **60**, 272–275

FRANCIS, J.L. (1973) The axis of astigmatism with special reference to streak retinoscopy. *Br. J. Physiol. Optics*, **28**, 11–22

FREEMAN, H. and HODD, F.A.B. (1955) Comparative analysis of retinoscopic and subjective refraction. *Br. J. Physiol. Optics*, **12**, 8–36

GLICKSTEIN, M. and MILLODOT, M. (1970) Retinoscopy and eye size. *Science*, **168**, 605–606

GORRAND, J.M. (1986) Separation of the reflection by the inner limiting membrane. *Ophthal. Physiol. Opt.*, **6**, 187–196

GREENSPAN, S.B. (1974) M.E.M. retinoscopy. *Bausch & Lomb Today*, **18**, cited in Eskridge (1987)

HODD, F.A.E. (1951) The measurement of spherical refraction by retinoscopy. In *International Optical Congress 1951*, pp. 191–231. London: British Optical Association

MILLODOT, M. (1974) Some aspects of experimental optometry. *Ophthal. Optn*, **14**, 99–104

MILLODOT, M. and O'LEARY, D. (1978a) The discrepancy between retinoscopic and subjective measurements: effect of age. *Am. J. Optom.*, **55**, 309–316

MILLODOT, M. and O'LEARY, D. (1978b) The discrepancy between retinoscopic and subjective measurements: effect of light polarization. *Am. J. Optom.*, **55**, 553–556

MOHINDRA, I. (1975) A technique for infant vision examination. *Am. J. Optom.*, **52**, 867–870

NOTT, I.S. (1925) Dynamic skiametry, accommodation and convergence. *Am. J. Physiol. Opt.*, **6**, 490–503

OWENS, D.A., MOHINDRA, I. and HELD, R. (1980) The effectiveness of a retinoscope beam as an accommodative stimulus. *Invest. Ophthalmol. Vis. Sci.*, **19**, 942–949

PARKER, J.A. (1966) Stationary streak retinoscopy. *Can. J. Ophthal.*, **1**, 228–239

PASCAL, J.I. (1930) *Modern Retinoscopy*. London: Hatton Press

ROORDA, A. and BOBIER, W.R. (1996) Geometrical technique to determine the influence of monochromatic aberration on retinoscopy. *J. Opt. Soc. Am. A.*, **13**, 3–11

ROSENFIELD, M., PORTELLO, J.M., BLUSTEIN, G.H. and JONES, C. (1996) Comparison of clinical techniques to assess the near accommodative response. *Optom. Vis. Sci.*, **73**, 382–388

ROUSE, M.W., LONDON, R. and ALLEN, D.C. (1982) An evaluation of the monocular estimate method of dynamic retinoscopy. *Am. J. Optom.*, **59**, 234–239

STAFFORD, M. and MORRIS, J. (1993) Retinoscopy in the eye examination. *Optom. Today*, 8 Feb, 17–25, and reprint from *Optom. Today*

SWANN, L.A. (1944) *Dynamic Retinoscopy*. London: Raphaels Ltd

WHITEFOOT, H. and CHARMAN, W.N. (1992) Dynamic retinoscopy and accommodation. *Ophthal. Physiol. Opt.*, **12**, 8–17

WOODHOUSE, J.M., MEADES, J. S., LEAT, S.J. and SAUNDERS, K.J. (1993) Reduced accommodation in children with Down's syndrome. *Invest. Ophthalmol. Vis. Sci.*, **34**, 2382–2387

18

Objective optometers

Introduction

While retinoscopy is an excellent method of objective refraction, it is a procedure that not every practitioner manages to accomplish accurately. Moreover, in some countries it is illegal for opticians to perform retinoscopy, and they must therefore rely on some other objective method.

Instruments called optometers or refractionometers offer an alternative means for evaluating the optical correction of the eye.

Automated electronic optometers, often termed autorefractors, offer the advantage of greater speed. Also, they can be operated by trained auxiliaries, thereby saving the practitioner's time.

Developments in autorefractors have rendered the visual optometers and some of the early electronic instruments obsolete. In the first edition of this work we gave detailed accounts of the different optical principles on which the three pioneering autorefractors were based. Their manufacturers were more ready to publish details of the optical design than is now generally the case. Since many of the currently available models appear to embody no new optical principles, as opposed to electronic refinements, we have continued to describe the older instruments as well as some of the newer designs. The older visual instruments were described in previous editions of this book. Other treatments of the subject are to be found in the work by Henson (1996) and the contribution by Wood (1988) to another work.

Visual instruments

We have seen (see pages 314 and 317) that the direct ophthalmoscope can give an approximate idea of the spherical ametropia but lacks accuracy. Accommodation by either patient or observer affects the result and the sighthole lens is about 20 mm from the spectacle plane. Some improvement can be made by incorporating an axially sliding graticule in the illumination system that can be focused on the retina, the position of the graticule indicating the amount of ametropia. Even so, the accuracy is not greatly improved, and estimation of astigmatism and axis detection are particularly difficult by this means.

Most objective optometers, whether designed for clinical or research purposes, are based on the method of indirect ophthalmoscopy. A simple system could be designed as in *Figure 18.1*, using two objectives or condensing lenses and a beam splitter. As in normal indirect ophthalmoscopy, the immediate source is imaged near the edge of the pupil, shown inferiorly for convenience in the diagram. A test object T can be moved along the axis of the projection system; when in the anterior focal plane of the projection lens L_1, its image T' will be at infinity and will therefore be sharply focused on the retina of an emmetropic eye. If the patient is myopic, the test object will have to be moved towards L_1 in order to be imaged on the fundus. The reverse applies in hypermetropia. If the second focal plane of L_1 coincides with the average position of the spectacle plane, the illumination system also becomes a Badal optometer (see page 75) and the scale indicating the position of T relative to the anterior focal plane of L_1 can be calibrated linearly in terms of spectacle refraction.

When attempting to measure the refraction of the eye with such an instrument, the first adjustment would be to focus the source image on the patient's iris by moving the whole instrument towards or away from the eye. This will simultaneously position L_1 at the correct distance from the eye required by the optometer graduation. With the instrument then moved sideways slightly so that the fundus is illuminated, the observation telescope would be focused to give a reasonable view of it. Finally, the test object's position would be adjusted to give a clear image. In astigmatism, there are two positions where the two mutually perpendicular meridians of the test object become clear in turn. Hence, for the detection and measurement of astigmatism, a test object with a ring of dots, a pattern of radial lines or a rotating cross is required.

The accuracy and speed of operation will be increased if movement of the test object is simultaneously coupled with focusing of the observation system. To the observer, the test object will then appear to go in and out of focus at twice the rate that occurs when only the test object is moved.

A combination of Scheiner disc and coincident alignment at the correct focus can also be used in subjective optometers, for example, as described by Fry (1937) and Allen (1949).

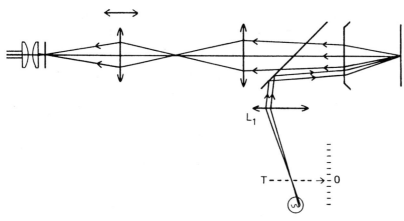

L_1

T - - - - - → O

Figure 18.1. Indirect ophthalmoscope modified to act as an optometer.

Moses (1971) and Jaschinski-Kruza (1988) developed an elegantly simple hand optometer. The eye is centred behind a 4 mm artificial pupil covered by two abutting pieces of Polaroid filter with their polarizing axes at right-angles. On the opposite side of the +5.0 D Badal optometer lens is a narrow bar of light-emitting diodes (LEDs) orientated parallel to the dividing line between the Polaroid filters. These LEDs are also covered by two pieces of Polaroid, so that each half of the bar is viewed through only half the pupil, thus providing a simple subjective Scheiner-disc vernier-alignment optometer. The LEDs are flashed on for only 200 ms so as not to stimulate the accommodation.

Some general considerations

With all objective optometers, the patient can see the test graticule and may be required to fixate it. As a result, accommodation may be stimulated and lead to an incorrect low hypermetropic or high myopic reading. Because the patient is looking into an instrument positioned very close to his face, proximal accommodation may well be induced. For these reasons the graticule should be moved to a position of hypermetropia before measurements are taken. The graticule will then appear fogged to the patient, helping to relax accommodation.

Some instruments provide a second graticule for the patient to observe through an auxiliary optical system, so that it appears adjacent to the measuring graticule. The fixation stimulus is moved with the measuring graticule, but is arranged to be fogged in relation to the measuring beam. This will also aid in relaxation of accommodation, especially when measuring the less hypermetropic or more myopic meridian, when the patient could accommodate to keep the first meridian's image in focus if the normal measuring graticule served as fixation. Alternatively, a fixation stimulus could be mounted on the carrier of the measuring graticule, but positioned a little further away from the objective or intermediate lens than this test graticule.

Several instruments incorporated an orange filter in the illuminating system. This reduced the amount of light entering the patient's eye and hence moderated

the glare. Since the light reflected by the fundus was orange–red in colour, very little light was lost to the observer.

Electronic optometers

The objective optometers formerly used relied on the examiner's decision on when the image is clearest or in coincidence setting; they were objective only in the sense that the patient's subjective choice has been replaced by the choice of an experienced examiner.

Electronic optometers fall into two classes:

(1) Instruments designed to measure automatically the refraction of the eye and capable of being operated by auxiliary staff; these may be called objective optometers in the fullest sense.
(2) Instruments designed for research on accommodation, when a fast and continuous response is required.

In most cases, all these instruments use infra-red radiation instead of visible light to ascertain the focus of the eye. Research instruments can thus measure accommodation without distracting the subject or stimulating accommodation. Similarly, the clinical instruments should be able to refract the relaxed eye: a visible fixation stimulus has to be provided, however, and this may stimulate the accommodation unless the eye is fogged.

Autorefractors

As explained in detail by Bennett and Rabbetts (1978), some electronic optometers operate in various forms on the principle of meridional refraction. There is a persistent fallacy that a sphero-cylindrical lens has a focal 'power' equal to $(S + C \sin^2 \theta)$ in the meridian at $\theta°$ from the cylinder axis. In fact, those rays passing through any oblique meridian of an astigmatic lens undergo skew convergence or divergence and fail to reunite at any focus. The expression quoted does, however, correctly express the prismatic power of the lens along a specified meridian, ignoring the prismatic component at right-angles to it.

It had previously been shown by Bennett (1960) that if Scheiner disc refraction is performed with spherical lenses, it is the prismatic power of the eye in the meridian parallel to the Scheiner disc apertures that is measured. From three determinations of $(S + C \sin^2 \theta)$ in different meridians, it is possible to calculate the separate values of the three quantities S, C and θ which define the optical correction needed. The prediction was made that this was a possible basis for automated refraction.

Electronic optometers fall into six main classes depending on the operational method used:

Analysis of image quality
(Dioptron, early Canon Autorefractors, Hoya Autorefractor)
Retinoscopic scanning
(Ophthalmetron, Nikon 5000 and 7000)
Scheiner disc refraction
(6600 Autorefractor, Nidek autorefractors)
Knife edge refraction
(Humphrey Auto Refractor)
Analysis of image dimensions
(Topcon Autorefractors)
Vergence measurement
(Canon autorefractors)

The first electronic optometer to appear was the Collins Electronic Refractionometer, designed and patented by the English optometrist Collins (1937). It has been appraised in the light of subsequent developments by Charman (1976) and Bennett (1978). Its basic features were incorporated in the Dioptron instrument to be described, but it was less sophisticated in that the optical system was adjusted manually to determine the endpoint.

To simplify the descriptions, the aligning and patient's fixation optical systems have been ignored in most of the following explanations. Most instruments employ an infra-red camera and video display to enable the operator to place the instrument approximately in the correct position in front of the eye; the instrument will then automatically centre itself to the pupil at the correct working distance. A visible fixation stimulus is incorporated on the optical axis – this is generally positioned to appear fogged to the patient, the vergence being adjusted according to the measured refractive error.

The author is indebted to Dr C. Campbell of Humphrey Instruments (Carl Zeiss Inc.) for details of some of the newer instruments.

The Dioptron

The Dioptron (manufactured by Coherent Radiation but now obsolete) consists of a measuring head, digital computer and printer. The measuring head is illustrated schematically in *Figure 18.2*. Infra-red radiation illuminates the test graticule T, formed by a series of slits in the cylindrical surface of a drum rotating about the optical axis. The beam splitter P_2 and lens L_1 collimate the beam from T, while the movable lens L_2 forms an aerial image T'_1 of the graticule. This image forms an object for the Badal optometer lens L_3 and is moved by L_2 along the axis of the instrument until it is conjugate with the patient's fundus. It then lies in the artificial far-point plane of the eye as formed by lens L_3.

The returning beam, after refraction by lens L_3, forms an image T'_3 of the fundus in the same plane as T'_1. It is then collimated by lens L_2 and imaged by lens L_1 as T'_4 in the plane of a mask M in front of the photoelectric detector system D. If the mask is made as a positive replica of an aperture in the revolving drum, the radiation forming the aerial image T'_4, when this is in focus on

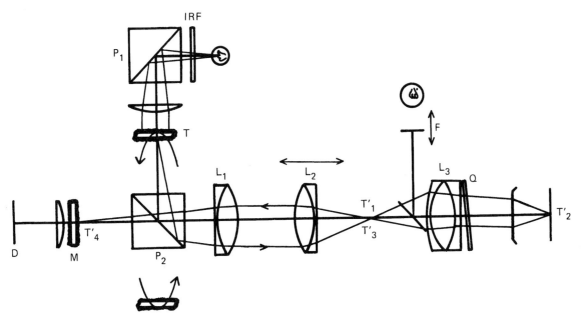

Figure 18.2. Simplified optical layout of the Coherent Radiation Dioptron. IRF infra-red transmitting filter, F auxiliary fixation system. (Redrawn from an illustration kindly supplied by Coherent Radiation Inc.)

the mask, will pass through it to the detector with little loss except from aberrations. When it is well out of focus, a much greater proportion of the energy will be intercepted by the mask, thus giving a low input to the detector. As the drum revolves, successive images T_4' of its slits pass laterally across the mask. When these images are in focus, they are alternately passed and occluded by the mask to give a high-amplitude output from the detector. When the images are slightly out of focus, the alternating amplitude is lower, while when greatly out of focus a steady output results. An AC electronic amplifier tuned to maximum response at the 'chopping' frequency feeds the computer, which positions the lens L_2 to maximize output.

An aperture stop placed between L_1 and L_2 is imaged near the patient's pupil. This stop has a round aperture extended by four slits in the form of a cross. Their purpose is to add a contribution of radiation passing through the pupil periphery to the more important central zone. To reduce the effects of stray light, the first reflecting prism P_1 polarizes the light. The beam splitter P_2 reflects light of this orientation towards the patient's eye, while the double passage through the quarter-wave plate Q rotates the plane of polarization through $90°$ so that the returning beam is now transmitted through P_2 to the detector.

The operator aligns the instrument with the patient's eye by means of an auxiliary observation system. The illuminating system, the beam splitter P_2, mask and quarter-wave plate all rotate simultaneously to investigate various meridians of the eye. A peak response due to either of the eye's two principal astigmatic meridians is first sought, after which the instrument measures the refraction in six different meridians. If only the minimum of three readings are taken, a small error in any one or more of them can lead to a disproportionately large error in the calculated refraction. The six readings are analysed by a computer to obtain the best-fitting refraction, while the degree of consistency between them is used to express a 'confidence factor'. The mathematical procedures involved in this analysis have been detailed by Long (1974, 1981).

Further descriptions of the instrument have been given by its inventor (Munnerlyn, 1978) and by Wood and French (1981). A review of its accuracy was given by French and Wood (1982).

The early Canon autorefractors

These were based on a similar operating system to the Dioptron. The now obsolete AutoRef R-1 had the unique feature of utilizing an imaged refraction system, an example of which is illustrated in *Figure 19.3* (page 371). The patient was thus allowed a binocular view of a real object through the inclined semi-reflecting mirror which reflected the measuring infra-red radiation from and to the autorefractor positioned below the line of sight. Thus, myopic patients could view a real object across the room, helping to relax accommodation. This instrument is now proving useful in research into accommodation, allowing an objective measurement of the ocular response to stimuli at known distances from

the eye. Like all clinical instruments, it was designed to provide a single measurement of refractive error in each operating cycle. Modifications described by Pugh and Winn (1988), Davis *et al.* (1993) and Wetzel *et al.* (1996) make possible the continuous measurement of accommodation, including its micro-fluctuations. Descriptions of the AutoRef R-l are given in the papers by Pugh and Winn (1988) and McBrien and Millodot (1985). Clinical evaluations are given both in this latter paper and by Berman *et al.* (1984).

The Ophthalmetron and Nikon autorefractors

The Bausch and Lomb Safir Ophthalmetron, no longer in production, described by Knoll and Mohrman (1972), was the first instrument to be based on the principle of streak retinoscopy. A somewhat similar system, to be described, is used by Nikon. An infra-red LED and condensing lens L_1 are surrounded by a chopper drum (*Figure 18.3*) which sweeps the beam across the pupil, and hence fundus, in a manner analogous to retinoscopy. The returning beam passes through a beam splitter to be received by a positive lens L_2 which forms an image of the patient's pupil on a four-element detector. The upper and lower infra-red detectors, being basically parallel to the chopper's slit apertures, record whether the resulting reflex has a with or an against movement, depending on which cell of the pair is stimulated first. If the scanning direction is not aligned with the eye's principal astigmatic meridians, the returning reflex will be twisted, and hence will strike the two lateral receptors at different times.

The amount of meridional ametropia is calculated from the time interval between the returning beam striking the upper and lower detectors. The sighthole of conventional retinoscopy is replaced by a slit aperture S parallel to the scanning apertures. S is positioned in the second focal plane of the lens L_2, so that the retinoscopy working distance is infinite. Alternatively, S may be regarded as being imaged at S' in the focal plane within the patient's eye. The returning beam from the illuminated fundus patch has to pass through S', and then through H' or J', the images of the photodetectors in the pupil. For the myopic eye illustrated in the inset, the upwards moving fundus patch will leave the eye

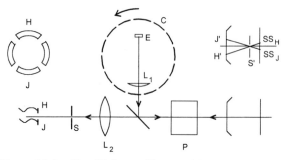

Figure 18.3. Simplified optical layout of the Nikon Autorefractometer. C chopper drum, E LED, H and J detector system, L_1 and L_2 positive lenses, P Pechan prism for astigmatic scanning, S slit aperture.

first though J′ and then H′. The nearer the eye is to emmetropia, the closer the two secondary sources SS$_J$ and SS$_H$ on the fundus, and hence the shorter the time interval between the responses of the detectors.

A Pechan prism is used in some of the instruments to rotate the direction of scan of the beam around the instrument's axis, thus allowing the measurement of the refractive error. The annular shape of the detector allows the instrument to centre itself to the pupil, but inevitably means that the peripheral rays are being measured. A more sophisticated design discards the Pechan prism by employing oblique slits in the chopper drum, a circular sighthole and more complex computer processing of the time data from the four-element detector.

A description of these instruments has also been given by Wood (1988).

The 6600 Auto-Refractor

Another objective optometer, the 6600 Auto-Refractor, was based on the Scheiner principle, being a development of a research instrument (Cornsweet and Crane, 1970). It was introduced in that year but is no longer available. Four LEDs of wavelength 935 nm are positioned in the anterior focal plane of the collimating lens L$_1$ (*Figure 18.4*). The lens L$_2$ images these sources in the plane of the pupil and acts as a Badal optometer lens with a circular aperture (target) as the test object. Opposite pairs of LEDs are powered alternately and cause the aperture to be imaged on or near the retina through two separate but neighbouring regions of the patient's pupil. When the aperture T is out of focus, the illuminated fundus patch oscillates, with or against the source alternation depending on whether the focus is in front of or behind the retina. When in focus, there is no movement of the illuminated patch.

Lens L$_3$ is of the same power and positioned at the same optical distance from the eye as the illuminating optometer lens L$_2$. A fundus image T$_2'$ is formed by L$_3$ in the plane of lens L$_4$ which acts as a field lens. Lenses L$_5$ and L$_6$ form an image T$_3'$ of the fundus on the four photodetectors. The positions of the aperture T and lenses L$_4$ and L$_5$ are adjusted automatically to give a

nil-difference signal from the corresponding pair of photodetectors. This position gives the refractive error in spherical ametropia.

A second pair of LEDs and photodetectors are provided, both arranged orthogonally to the first. These LEDs are powered at a different frequency from the first and effectively allow the detection of astigmatic scissors rotation of the oscillating light patch on the fundus. The sources and detectors are automatically rotated to align with the astigmatic meridians of the patient's eye, while the axially moving system moves to measure the two refractive powers.

Auxiliary systems are incorporated to allow accurate alignment of the instrument including the vertex distance setting and to provide a diffuse green fixation source (McDevitt, 1977).

The Nidek Autorefractors

These are similar to the 6600 Auto-Refractor, being based on the Scheiner disc principle. These use a pair of LEDs, initially, say, along the 180° meridian. A four-element detector again records whether the fundus patch is oscillating obliquely or if the system is aligned with the eye's principal meridians. The LEDs and detector assembly are rotated simultaneously, and allow the test aperture T to be positioned conjugate to the fundus and the refractive error determined.

Descriptions have also been given by Wood *et al.* (1984), and Wood (1988). The Nidek ARK-2000 also combines the function of an automatic keratometer.

The Humphrey Auto Refractors

The Humphrey Auto Refractor was the first instrument which, as well as providing an automatic refraction, also allowed the practitioner to measure the resulting visual acuity and to obtain a subjective confirmation of the spherical component of the refraction. The simplest of their three present instruments no longer provides the spherical confirmation facility, but its optical system is the same as in the more comprehensive models.

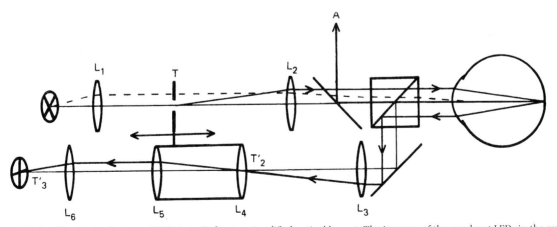

Figure 18.4. The Acuity Systems 6600 Auto-Refractor: simplified optical layout. The imagery of the quadrant LEDs in the pupil is indicated by the dashed line, a theoretical raypath that would not pass through the aperture T. The path to the fixation and alignment systems is indicated by A. (Redrawn from McDevitt, 1977.)

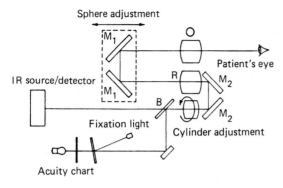

Figure 18.5. Simplified optical layout of the Humphrey Auto Refractor. (Reproduced by kind permission of Humphrey Instruments Inc.)

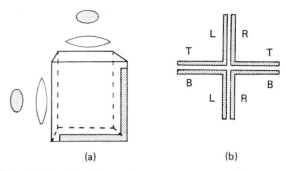

Figure 18.6. The infra-red source arrangement of the Humphrey Auto Refractor: (a) one of the four prism components together with its associated LEDs (shaded ellipses), condenser lenses and L-shaped aperture, (b) the complete source assembly, forming an illuminated hollow cross. L and R denote left and right pairs, T and B top and bottom pairs of parallel source elements.

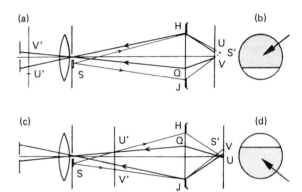

Figure 18.7. A schematic construction for the formation of the pupil reflex in the Humphrey Auto Refractor in (a) relative hypermetropia, (c) relative myopia. The arrowed areas in (b) and (d) show that part of the pupil which appears luminous to the detector for radiation originating below the optical axis of the instrument.

Tracing the ray path shown in *Figure 18.5* backwards from the patient's eye, O is a Badal optometer lens whose posterior focal plane is positioned in the eye's pupil. The mirrors M_1 fold the optical path within the instrument to reduce space and also provide the variable spherical element by altering the distance between the optometer lens O and the intermediate aerial image formed by the relay lens R. A second pair of mirrors M_2 again fold the light path. The cylindrical assembly is positioned in the anterior focal plane of the relay lens and so is imaged in the pupil plane irrespective of the spherical adjustment. The assembly is formed by two sets of Stokes lenses, which are arranged to correct astigmatism in the 90°/180° and 45°/135° meridians, the two corrections being compounded to give a single correcting cylinder.

The beam splitter B is designed to reflect visual light from the acuity chart, while transmitting infra-red light to and from the source and detector. The whole pupil area is used for both incident and emergent beams. To investigate the returning light, the instrument performs a Foucault knife-edge test in horizontal and vertical meridians simultaneously. As in retinoscopy, the reflex is interpreted to arrive at the optical power adjustments needed for reversal. The system then provides a complete ocular correction through which the test charts can be viewed, whereas many automated refractors use only spherical optometer systems from which spherocylindrical refractions are calculated.

The infra-red source comprises eight LEDs arranged around the edge of an assembly of four prisms to provide an illuminated hollow cross (*Figure 18.6*). The aligning pairs, for example, the lower horizontal right and left sources, may be regarded as a single source, while the horizontal aperture between the upper and lower pairs constitutes the knife-edge or sighthole for these pairs. A positive lens behind the aperture forms an image of the pupil on a photosensitive detector. *Figure 18.7(a)* shows schematically the construction of the pupil reflex for that part of the source below the optical axis of the eye.

If the instrument's sphere adjustment provides too little positive power, the source S is imaged behind the retina at S', giving a blur patch UV on the retina, as indicated by the broken lines. This blur forms the source for the returning beam, limited by the image U'V' formed in the artificial far-point plane, which is behind

the source plane because there is relative hypermetropia. The Foucault slit further restricts the beam falling on the detectors, so that only the lower part is illuminated as indicated by the solid lines from H and Q.

The stippled upper part of the pupil in *Figure 18.7(b)* appears luminous to the photodetector. Conversely, in relative myopia (*Figure 18.7c*) the lower region of the pupil appears luminous (*Figure 18.7d*).

The area of illumination falling on the detector depends on the relative ametropia. The detector is divided vertically and horizontally into four separately registering quadrants. Each pair of LEDs has a power supply of different frequency, while each quadrant of the detector is linked to four amplifiers, one tuned to each LED frequency. In this way, the illumination on each quadrant of the detector from each source pair can be determined.

Figure 18.8(a) represents the four quadrants numbered for reference. The nature of the reflex, whether crossed or uncrossed, arising from sources B and T is determined electronically by comparing their contribution to quadrants (1 + 4) with that to (2 + 3). The information thus obtained is used to adjust the position of mirrors M_1 and hence alter the spherical correction.

The presence of an astigmatic error with exactly hori-

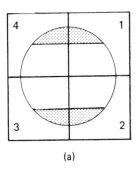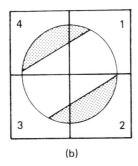

(a)   (b)

Figure 18.8. The quadrant photodetector of the Humphrey Auto Refractor. The circle denotes the pupil margin, which is imaged on the detector and centred automatically. The stippled areas denote radiation reaching the detector from sources T and B in: (a) spherical ametropia, (b) uncorrected astigmatism at an oblique axis.

zontal and vertical meridians is ascertained from the difference in response to the horizontal and vertical sources. An astigmatic correction can therefore be introduced by the 90°/180° cross cylinder in order to give a spherical response. In oblique astigmatism, the returning pupil reflex is rotated, exactly as in streak retinoscopy (*see* pages 347–349). Thus, in *Figure 18.8(b)*, the illumination due to sources B on quadrant 4 is increased relative to that on quadrant 1. Similarly sources T give rise to a larger area of illumination on quadrant 2 than on 3. The same effect, but in the opposite direction because of scissors movement, will occur for the vertical bars. This information is used to alter the 45°/135° Stokes lens.

The instrument is initially positioned by the operator, who aligns the corneal reflection of a red LED between two yellow ones, the first LED turning green on alignment. The instrument subsequently maintains alignment automatically by summation signals from the quad-detector. Acuity charts are presented initially to obtain unaided vision if this is wanted. On pressing the 'measure' button, the chart is switched off and the infrared source/detector system operates. The sphere adjustment is first driven through its range to find an approximate reversal, after which the two astigmatic systems come into operation. Since the summation signals for each system are independent, all three correction systems drive simultaneously towards reversal.

The instrument then makes an infra-red to visual wavelength compensation of 0.75 DS towards myopia, thus generating a 'spherical error signal', and switches on the acuity chart which the patient attempts to read. Line sizes of 20/15 (6/4.5) to 20/400 (6/120) are available. Positive spherical power is then slowly added (automatically) to fog the eye, while the error signal is simultaneously monitored. If it remains constant as power is increased, accommodation is relaxing. When accommodation will relax no further, the error signal begins to increase. The computer notes this value, then adds an extra 0.50 D to check that no further relaxation occurs. If no more hypermetropia is revealed, the instrument returns to the noted position. The acuity is then checked.

The two more sophisticated models then allow the operator to fog the eye by pressing the '+Sph' button, say to the 20/60 (6/18) level, and then to reduce the power in 0.12 or 0.25 D steps until the smallest line can just be read. In addition, they allow binocular fixation and provide many extra subjective tests: for example, a bichromatic target, and cylinder and axis refinement with both a cross-cylinder target and the Humphrey fan target described in the footnote on page 373. Near-vision testing and low-contrast charts are incorporated, while the most sopisticated model also allows glare testing.

Both the objective and subjective corrections and resulting acuities can be printed out, together with a note of the vertex distance and a reflex number. This effectively denotes the amount of useful light returning to the detector, small pupils or hazy media giving a low signal. Eyes with a pupil diameter down to just under 3 mm can be examined. Although it is the ocular refraction that is measured, it can be converted if required to the corresponding spectacle refraction at any vertex distance within the range 10.5–16.5 mm.

The Topcon Autorefractor

This uses a modified Badal optometer system to generate an annulus of infra-red radiation on the fundus, the dimensions of which are determined by the patient's refractive error. Radiation from a small LED, E (*Figure 18.9*), is collimated by lens L_1, and forms an image E' after passing through the illuminating system's optometer lens L_2. The beam between these two lenses is intercepted by an annular aperture T, which is eventually imaged on the fundus. Because the beam has to pass through the small zone at E', this forms an optometer arrangement, and therefore the angle between the beam and optical axis at E' is a constant, irrespective of the position of T. The hollow beam is then passed through a second annular aperture A, which is imaged in the plane of the pupil by relay lens L_3, which also images the LED at E'' in front of the pupil. The eye is therefore illuminated by a hollow beam of infra-red radiation.

The test aperture T (and E and L_1) can all be moved along the optical axis, in order to focus T on the fundus. For an emmetropic patient, T is positioned further from L_2 than its focal length, so that it is imaged at T' in the anterior focal plane of L_3. Hence the zero position of T is not in the usual position for a Badal optometer.

The detector beam is restricted to the central zone of the pupil since the relay lens L_3 and beam splitter BS image the stop C into the pupil. An element of the fundus, B, is imaged at B', which, in turn, is imaged by the detector optometer lens L_4 at B''. The camera lens L_5 in turn images B'' on the CCD detector D. The camera lens and detector assembly are linked to the test object T, so that when T is imaged on the fundus, the fundus is also in focus on the detector, thus enabling more accurate measurement to be made of the image dimensions.

The ray paths entering the eye are similar to those

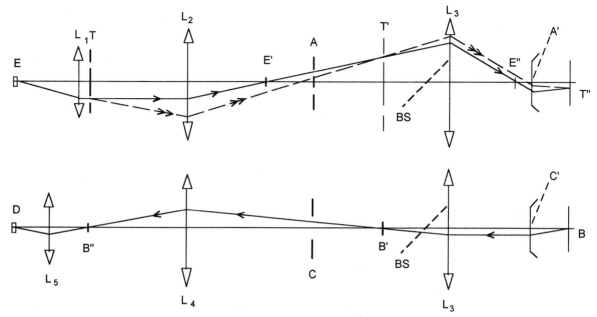

Figure 18.9. The Topcon Autorefractor. For clarity, the illuminating and detecting pathways have been shown under each other rather than joined by the beam splitter. E, LED, L_1 collimating lens, L_2 illuminating optometer lens, L_3 relay lens, L_4 detector optometer lens, L_5 camera lens, A annular aperture, C central aperture, BS beam splitter, D detector, T target annulus.

forming the extreme rays of a blur patch on the retina, and are the same whether or not T is in focus on the fundus. Hence, if the diameter of the annulus image A' is taken as g, the basic size of the corresponding fundus dimension j is given by:

$$j = g\frac{(K - L)}{K'} \qquad (4.16a)$$

It is thus larger in hypermetropia, smaller in emmetropia and elliptical in astigmatism.

The size j' of the first aerial image of the fundus dimension j is given by:

$$j' = \frac{\text{Object vergence}}{\text{Image vergence}} = \frac{K'}{K} \cdot j = g\frac{(K - L)}{K}$$

so the unknown, the dioptric length of the eye K', is eliminated from the expression. This would suggest that the refractive error could than be calculated. When T is in focus on the fundus, however, the image on the detector bears a constant ratio to the size of the test annulus, irrespective of the amount of ametropia. The instrument presumably calculates the refractive error from the basic image height when the test annulus and optometer lenses are set for various known amounts of ametropia.

The Topcon RM-700 needs a 2.5 mm pupil diameter.

The Canon Autorefractors

These measure the vergence of light leaving the eye by combining a Scheiner disc to select two beams, one on each side of the pupil, and prisms to give a double image of the secondary source on the fundus. Thus, in *Figure 18.10*, an infra-red-emitting LED, E, is placed at the anterior principal focus of a collimator lens C, while a relay lens L_1 forms an image E_1' in the central aperture of the beam splitter. A second relay lens forms an

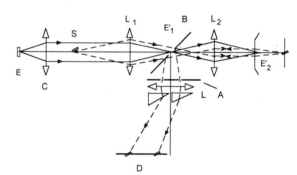

Figure 18.10. The Canon Autorefractor. A annular aperture, B beam splitter, C collimating lens, D linear detector, E, LED, L_1, L_2 and L_3 relay lenses, S slit aperture.

image E_2' at the centre of the patient's pupil. A horizontal slit, S, between the collimator and first relay lens is imaged at infinity, and so is in focus on the fundus if the eye is emmetropic. By using a small LED and a small aperture, the pinhole effect ensures that the illuminated patch on the fundus is not grossly out of focus even in high ametropia. The returning beam from the eye is reflected by the beam splitter and passes through an annular aperture A so that only radiation leaving the eye in a zone between 2.0 and 2.9 mm diameter is recorded. This radiation is then focused on a linear position detector D by lens L_3. The two ray bundles would combine in emmetropia to form a single image on D, while they would give crossed or uncrossed 'images' in myopia or hypermetropia. This ambiguity is resolved by covering the two halves of lens L_3 with unequal prisms, so that even in emmetropia, a double image is formed on D. The spacing between the two 'images' now varies continuously with ametropia.

In order to calculate refractive error, measurement is provided in three meridians simultaneously. The illuminating slit aperture is three bladed, with apertures at 120° to each other, L_3 is covered with an array of three pairs of prism sectors, with three radiating detectors positioned to receive their respective aperture 'images'.

Research instruments

The accommodative response of the eye to changes in object vergence may be determined indirectly by photography of the Purkinje III image, described in more detail on page 398. During accommodation, the anterior surface of the crystalline lens becomes steeper, thereby reducing the size of an image formed by reflection at its anterior surface. From calibration photographs, the difference between the image sizes can be interpreted in terms of accommodative response (*see*, for example, Allen, 1949).

The anterior surface of the crystalline lens has a cellular structure and gives rise to a diffuse reflection, often termed 'shagreen' or 'orange peel'. Measurements of such images are therefore imprecise. Furthermore, relatively little light is reflected by the surface since the change in refractive index is low: cine photography is therefore more difficult than static photography with electronic flash. More precise and direct results have been obtained by studying the retinal image. In general, infra-red illumination is used to prevent interference by the measuring system with the subject's vision.

Several research instruments have been based on the Scheiner disc principle. The earliest of them and probably the next electronic instrument after Collins (1937) was produced by Campbell and Robson (1959). It needs no description because the instrument of Cornsweet and Crane described above is in many ways similar to it. Heron *et al.* (1989) developed a binocular system, also based on the Scheiner disc principle, to investigate the symmetry of accommodation responses in the two eyes.

The recording infra-red coincidence optometer designed by Roth (1962) used a system in which Scheiner disc doubling was combined with a prism to displace one image below the other on the fundus. The horizontal separation of the two images, which varied with the accommodation, was monitored photomechanically.

In a continuously recording optometer by Lovasik (1983), infra-red radiation filtered from a tungsten lamp is focused near the anterior focal plane of the eye after passing through a Scheiner disc. It thus enters the eye through two peripheral zones of the pupil to form two streaks on the retina. These are imaged, via the whole pupil area by a beam splitter and a lens on to two photovoltaic cells, one on each side of the axis. One beam thus falls on each cell. As the accommodation of the subject's eye alters, it changes the separation of the streaks on the retina and also of their images on the photocells. This effect is monitored by masking the cells to a wedge shape, one with the base towards the optical axis, the other away from it. If the streaks move closer together towards the axis, a longer strip of one photocell and a shorter strip of the other are illuminated. As a result, the respective signals are increased and decreased proportionately. The two outputs are fed to a differential amplifier.

The Scheiner principle was again employed by Fitzke *et al.* (1985) to investigate the refraction of pigeon eyes. The illuminating system is the same as that of the Cornsweet and Crane instrument, but the focus is determined electrophysiologically by measuring the electroretinogram (ERG, *see* page 39), the peak response occurring when the test grating is conjugate to the retina.

A different approach was made by Allen and Carter (1960). Their optometer (*Figure 18.11*) is effectively based upon the reflex-free indirect ophthalmoscope using two separate objectives. The lamp S is imaged by lens L_1 on to the upper part of the patient's pupil. The measuring graticule T, a narrow rectangular aperture, is placed in the anterior focal plane of the same lens. If the subject is emmetropic, a clearly focused image T_1' is formed on the axis of the subject's eye.

An aperture stop A_o immediately in front of the photomultiplier tube is imaged by lens L_2 in the lower

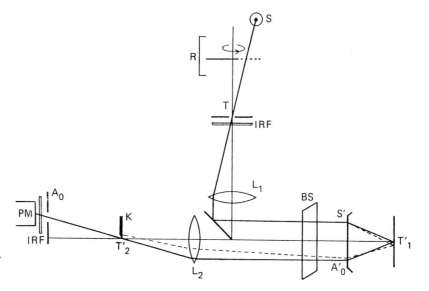

Figure 18.11. Simplified optical layout of the recording infra-red optometer of Allen and Carter (1960). BS gold-coated beam splitter permitting a view of the test stimulus, K knife-edge, PM photomultiplier, R rotating sector disc.

part of the patient's pupil at A_o. Thus, radiation from T'_1 will leave the patient's eye through A_o to form an aerial image T'_2. Part of this image is occluded by the knife edge K.

When the subject accommodates, the image T'_1 on the retina will move downwards. The aerial fundus image T'_2 will move upwards (and axially towards the lens L_2), so that a greater proportion of the energy will be occluded by the knife edge. A lower response by the photomultiplier tube will therefore result. Infra-red-transmitting filters IRF are placed near the measuring aperture T and also in front of the photomultiplier tube to absorb ambient illumination. The rotating chopper disc gives a pulsating radiation level and hence a pulsating output from the photomultiplier, which in turn may be fed into a tuned electronic amplifier. Ambient infra-red radiation gives a constant photomultiplier output. This DC component will be rejected by the amplifier, so that the final AC signal may be fed to a pen recorder which is calibrated in terms of the subject's accommodation.

Kruger (1979) developed an infra-red recording retinoscope for monitoring accommodative response. Its optical system is very similar to the Nikon instrument shown in *Figure 18.3*, but does not incorporate the Pechan prism since it monitors only the vertical meridian of the eye. The time interval between the reflex passing over each of the two photoreceptors, and its direction of movement, were evaluated by the electronic recording system to give a linear response over the range +6 to −6 D of refractive error or change in accommodation.

Design and calibration of infra-red optometers

Since the eye is not achromatic, an allowance has to be made for the difference in ocular refraction between visible light and whatever wavelength of infra-red radiation is used. This is usually about 880 nm, for which the eye is 0.75–1.00 DS hypermetropic relative to 550 nm (Cornsweet and Crane, 1970). Provided that the lenses of the optometer itself are achromatic, their refractive power should not differ too greatly between visible and near-infra-red radiation, while any mirrors used are naturally free from chromatic aberration.

As with retinoscopy, uncertainty over the position of the plane of reflection within the eye of visible and infra-red radiation may invalidate theoretical calibration of an instrument. Although Kruger (1979) found his optometer read 0.8 D hypermetropic, Cornsweet and Crane's optometer gave a reading about 1.50 DS more hypermetropic than the subjective visual focus obtained simultaneously. Thus there may be about 0.50–0.75 D allowance to be made in addition to the effects of chromatic aberration. This suggests that the infra-red radiation is either being reflected from the capillary bed of the retina, about 0.3 mm in front of receptors, or that it is reflected from several layers, the mean effect being equivalent to reflection from a single plane in front of

the receptors. Within the visible spectrum, however, Charman and Jennings (1976) found that while blue light was reflected from a plane anterior to the receptors, yellow and red light appeared to be reflected from a plane very close to the receptors. Moreover, observation of the fundus with infra-red radiation, as occurs with some fundus cameras, shows that the choroidal features can be seen through the partially transparent retina. Hence, reflection must be regarded as arising throughout a depth rather than from a surface within the fundus, though Dr C. Campbell (pers. comm., 1995) suggests that the mean position is near the retina–pigment epithelium interface.

Charman (1980) points out that the reflectance of the fundus increases towards the red end of the spectrum, from about 0.003 at 400 nm to almost 0.1 at 700 nm, while Campbell gives a figure of 0.35 for 880 nm. As this reflectance is diffuse, there are multiple reflections of scattered radiation within the eye, which, acting as an integrating sphere, degrade the image. Thus, Cornsweet and Crane found a linespread function (*see* page 49) of at least 1° as compared with a few minutes of arc in the visible part of the spectrum. It is therefore not possible to measure the eye's refractive error accurately by means of a simple best-focus optometer.

Another result of the diffuse retinal reflectance is the need for bright sources. Only a small proportion of the incident radiation is reflected back out through the pupil. A 2 mm diameter pupil, for example, subtends only about 1/100 of a steradian at the retina, so depending on the instrument design, only about 1/100 to 1/500 of the incident radiation is returned to the instrument for measurement purposes. Fortunately at the required levels, the infra-red radiation is not harmful to the eye, but care has to be taken in the instrument design to avoid reflections from relay lenses or mirrors in the common illuminating and observation paths.

The simplest method of calibrating a clinical instrument would be to determine a zero error by examining a few eyes under cycloplegia and comparing with the subjective results. With all instruments, the patient or subject must be positioned at the correct distance from the instrument or else the calibration will be upset by effectivity factors.

Charman and Heron (1975) discuss the linearity of several of the research optometers from a mathematical viewpoint. Several of these instruments are seriously affected by changes in pupil size while accommodation is being investigated. For example, the instrument designed by Allen and Carter depends upon the amount of radiation that is not occluded by a knife edge positioned near the fundus image. If the pupil size decreases, the energy reaching the photocell will be reduced in the absence of a change in accommodation. Campbell and Robson's (1959) instrument is also affected. Artefacts due to changes in pupil size may be greatly reduced by dilating the pupil with a mydriatic that has either little affect on accommodation or whose cycloplegic effect occurs considerably later than the mydriatic effect. Campbell and Robson also suggested that a small artificial pupil placed before the eye gives a fixed pupil area as far as the instrument is concerned and does not require medication. The small pupil area does reduce the precision of the instrument.

Several of the research instruments use beam splitters to allow the subject to view a test stimulus while accommodation is being monitored. These beam splitters may be formed by interference techniques or by coating the surface with a thin layer of a metal such as gold, which has a high reflectance for infra-red radiation. Both these techniques result in non-uniform transmission in the visible spectrum, the gold film appearing green. A filter of a similar colour may be required before the other eye if satisfactory investigation under binocular conditions is required (Allen and Carter, 1960).

Clinical results with electronic autorefractors

Objective optometers are subject to many of the uncertainties of retinoscopy with regard to accuracy of measurement. The plane of reflection of the radiation may or may not be at the percipient layer of the retina. Proximal accommodation may be much more troublesome with the optometer, though most designs incorporate a fogging system for the fixation object, which is often a pictorial representation of a distant scene in order to minimize this effect. The fixation point is aligned with the measuring system, so that measurement is made very close to the fovea.

Especially when the ametropia is high, the distance between the instrument and eye must be capable of being set very accurately or else effectivity errors arise. Corrections to the results for different vertex distances can usually be calculated automatically.

A minimum pupil diameter of around 2.5–3.0 mm is needed, depending upon the instrument design.

Several reports have been published comparing the results obtained by clinical objective optometers with subjective examination: Knoll *et al.* (1970), Safir *et al.* (1970), Sloan and Polse (1974), Polse and Kerr (1975), Wood (1982), French and Wood (1982). All have suggested that these objective instruments give fairly accurate results similar to those achieved by retinoscopy. Large differences between objective and subjective findings occurred occasionally. In general, proximal myopia did not appear to cause difficulties in the age groups surveyed.

Proximal myopia would be expected, however, to affect the refractions of younger patients. In a study of patients under 40 years of age, Ghose *et al.* (1986) analysed the distribution of the differences between autorefractor and subjective results. For emmetropes, low hypermetropes and low myopes, the results were skewed towards more minus or less plus with the autorefractor. The mean difference in the equivalent spherical refraction (or mean refractive error) was -0.58 D ± 0.79 D. In a similar study but using cycloplegia, the same team (Nayak *et al.*, 1987) found much better agreement between the instrument and clinical results. The percentage showing the difference to be within $+0.25$ D increased from 32% without cycloplegia to 86% with it. The respective figures for $+0.50$ D were

Table 18.1 comparability of infra-red optometers and final subjective refraction (percentage of results given where differences in power or axis are less than or equal to the stated amount). Mean results for 790 patients

Lens power	±0.25 D	±0.50 D	±1.00 D
Cylinder axis	±5°	±10°	±20°
Sphere	78.5	91.0	96.5
Cylinder	81.2	95.1	98.5
Axis	40.9	62.4	82.7

Figures abstracted from McCaghrey and Matthews (1993).

44% and 96%, while for $+1.00$ D they were 68% and 100%. This would effectively confirm the accuracy of the manufacturers' calibration.

In a survey conducted in optometric practice, Griffiths (1988) found a similar bias. In 75% of the cases where the difference in the mean refractive error exceeded $+0.26$ D, it was the autorefractor which gave the more minus or less plus result. Agreement within this amount was found for about 45% of the patients, with rather more consistent results for the myopes than for the hypermetropes.

Conversely, a study of eight different autorefractors by McCaghrey and Matthews (1993) showed little evidence of consistent bias towards myopia (or hypermetropia). In this investigation, each of the instruments in turn was used to examine 90–100 consecutive patients, and then the instrument reading compared with the final subjective results. The mean comparability for the 790 patients over all the instruments is given in *Table 18.1*.

They also evaluated the residual refractive error between the autorefractor and subjective findings. Between 21 and 45% (mean 35%) of results were within a residual error of $+0.50$ to -0.25 DS combined with a residual astigmatic error not greater than 0.25 DC. If the residual error allowed was increased to $+0.75$ to -0.50 DS with a cylinder not more than 0.50 DC, the percentage of acceptable results increased to 64% (52–75% depending upon the instrument).

They also evaluated the test–retest repeatability[*] of the instrument that appeared best in their comparability study. For example, one of their subjects had a subjective refraction of $+2.25$ DS/-0.50 DC $\times 140$. The mean and standard deviation of 50 autorefractor results was: $+2.07 \pm 0.31/-0.35 \pm 0.20 \times 148 \pm 26°$. A second individual with a slightly more astigmatic eye ($-9.00/-1.25 \times 175$) gave results of $-9.27 \pm 0.20/-1.80 \pm 0.21 \times 3 \pm 2.4°$. As expected, the standard deviation of the axis findings decreases with increased astigmatism, even though in this case the result is not particularly valid.

The techniques of astigmatic analysis on pages 88–89 may be used to analyse differences between autorefractor and subjective findings.

An extensive evaluation of autorefractors was undertaken at Glagow Caledonian University for the British

---

[*] The terms 'accuracy', 'precision' and others having specialized meanings in this context, are explained at the end of Chapter 1.

Department of Health's Medical Devices Agency (1996 – evaluation report number MDA/96/36). In the first part of the study, test model eyes were constructed from polymethyl methacrylate, with axial lengths varying to provide refractive errors over a range of nominally ±20 D. A myopic adjustment was made to the paraxial error to allow for the effects of spherical aberration. Many, but not all, of the six different manufacturer's instruments tested gave good agreement between their results and the adjusted refractive error. One design, however, underestimated hypermetropia of more than +8 D by about 2 D, while another showed a negative shift of 1.5 D or more for eyes with errors arithmetically greater than 10 D. Even when a reading was obtained, pupil diameters of less than 3 mm tended to give erroneously hypermetropic results.

Two hundred and sixty-one patients in the University Eye Clinic were examined on all six instruments, by retinoscopy and by subject refraction (student refractions verified by experienced staff). To gauge the validity of the results, the research team adopted a 95% confidence level of ±0.82 D for the mean sphere, being twice the standard deviation of Adams *et al.*'s (1995) investigations. Almost 14% of retinoscopy results were outside this limit, as were the measurements by three of the autorefractors. Two autorefractors were only slightly poorer, while the sixth showed just over 21% of its findings to be outside the limit. The 95% confidence limits for the mean sphere as found by the autorefractors was about ±1.5 D, while by retinoscopy it was ±1.3 D. Despite measuring closer to the visual axis than retinoscopy, the results for the astigmatic component appear only a little more precise (by 0.02 D in their standard deviation). The researchers found slight evidence for more consistent results in myopic patients than in hypermetropes, but no obvious variation with age.

They also compared the intolerance rate for spectacles prescribed directly from the autorefractor with those made up to the subjective findings (without modification on the basis of the previous spectacle prescription). Out of their 47 patients, '19.1% of the subjects were unable to adapt to wearing the autorefractor result. This compares with 12.8% of the subjects wearing the subjective prescription. A higher percentage (42.6% compared to 29.8%) of subjects also reported experiencing some kind of headaches or eye strain over the two week period when wearing the autorefractor prescription in comparison to the subjective result'.

The team found that the instruments coped well in measuring eyes wearing both rigid and soft contact lenses, but in the hospital environment they performed badly on patients with cataract (as did retinoscopy), and performed worse than retinoscopy for patients with intra-ocular lenses or keratoconus, and were virtually incapable of measuring patients with nystagmus (*see* page 184). Four of the instruments were poorer than retinoscopy for patients with amblyopia (*see* pages 41–43), while age-related macular degeneration proved a problem only for the instrument based on analysis of image quality, being upset by fundus changes causing poor reflection. Short reviews of this study are given by Ehrlich (1996) and Strang *et al.* (1997).

Conclusion

Although the subjective refraction is frequently taken as being correct, there will be small variations in this, particularly if performed by different refractionists who may take different end-points or use slightly different techniques. Thus small differences between autorefractor and subjective results are to be expected, and should not be taken to imply that the instruments are poor. These studies suggest, however, that it would be inadvisable to rely on any instrument findings alone for prescribing. Thus the ability of a patient to read 6/6 or even 6/5 through an objective refraction (retinoscopic or autorefractor) does not necessarily mean that the correction gives the sharpest vision or that it will be the most comfortable. At present, all the instruments refract monocularly. If lenses are to be prescribed, autorefractors, like retinoscopy, have the important role of providing an initial result for refinement by subjective refraction and binocular balancing.

If operated by a technician, automatic optometers save the practitioner's time by replacing retinoscopy. This does not necessarily save the patient's time because setting up takes longer than for retinoscopy even though measuring time is less. Moreover, the uniformity or irregularity of a retinoscopic reflex may provide the examiner with more information about the ocular media than an instrument's 'confidence factor', if one is provided. Some autorefractors show the regularity of the media on the monitor screen when aligning the instrument with the eye, although this may not be as sensitive as distortions in the retinoscopy reflex which, for example, demonstrate keratoconic corneae, pronounced spherical aberration of the crystalline lens and very early spoke cataracts clearly. The small pupil zones effectively sampled by some autorefractors may cause errors if they are partly occluded by opacities, whereas visual retinoscopy may allow the practitioner to evaluate the whole pupil area. In general, autorefractors cannot be used in the domiciliary situation, for very young children or for assessing near-vision performance.

Photorefraction

This technique, introduced by Howland and Howland (1974), uses a photographic method to deduce the refractive or accommodative state of the patient's eyes. Because the photographs can be taken immediately the patient appears to be looking at the camera, this method can be used with young infants whose span of attention is too short for retinoscopy. In such cases, an automated objective optometer is equally unsuitable because the eye has to be positioned accurately in relation to the instrument. Atkinson and Braddick (1982) recommend photorefraction as a screening test for significant refractive errors in young infants.

The photorefractor consists essentially of a small source of light (S in *Figure 18.12*) mounted in front of a suitable camera. The source is formed by an electronic flash illuminating one end of a fibreoptic lightguide, the other end being mounted centrally in front of the

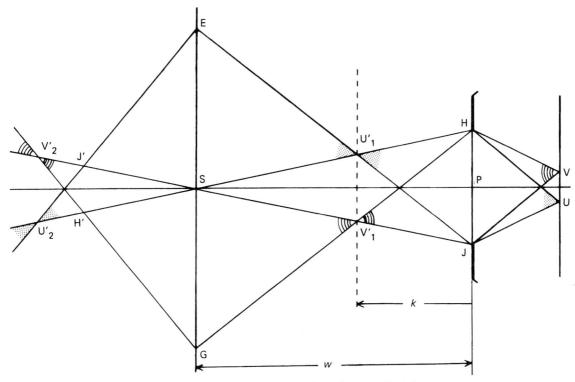

Figure 18.12. The optical principles of photorefraction, the patient's eye being on the right.

camera lens. It illuminates the patient's face and is imaged on the fundus of both eyes. The retinal image may be regarded as a secondary source giving rise to a fundus image in the plane conjugate with the retina.

If the eye is in focus for the source, the light leaving the eye returns to the source and is thus occluded from the camera lens. As a result, the pupil appears dark in the photograph. When the eye is out of focus, a blur circle or ellipse is formed on the fundus, producing in turn an illuminated zone around the source. The size of this zone varies with the ocular focusing error relative to the source.

Figure 18.12 shows the principle of the technique applied to a myopic eye at a distance w from the camera lens (assumed to be thin and in contact with the source). As in *Figure 17.7*, the rays from S filling the pupil form the retinal blur UV, imaged as $U_1'V_1'$ in the plane conjugate with the retina. If the eye is unaccommodated, this will be the far-point plane at a distance k from the eye's principal point P. The reflected ray SHU retraces its original path, while the ray UJU_1' through the opposite extremity of the pupil reaches the camera lens plane at E. In the case of the myopic eye illustrated, it is this latter ray which defines the size of the blur in the lens plane.

If SE and HJ (g) are taken as positive, the triangles $U_1'JH$, $U_1'ES$ give

$$\frac{SE}{g} = \frac{w - k}{k}$$

The blur diameter b, equal to 2 SE, is then given by

$$b = 2g(K - W)/W \qquad (18.1)$$

The term $(K - W)$ is the residual ametropia relative to

the camera. If the eye is accommodating by A dioptres, K should be replaced by $(K - A)$.

As shown in *Figure 18.12*, if the camera is in focus for the pupil, its sharp image $H'J'$ on the film is unaffected by the blur in the camera lens plane. To determine the ametropia, the camera must be defocused from the pupillary plane by a known amount.

Orthogonal photorefraction

This system of photorefraction was the original technique introduced and is now known as orthogonal photorefraction. To record the ametropia in two mutually perpendicular meridians simultaneously, an auxiliary lens composed of four quadrants is placed in front of the camera lens. Two opposite quadrants form part of a convex plano cylinder of power about +1.50 DC, with the cylinder axis across the centre of the camera lens. The other pair of opposite quadrants also form part of a +1.50 DC plano cylinder with its axis perpendicular to that of the first pair. In this way the photographic image is drawn out into a cruciform shape, the overall length in each of the two meridians being proportional to the corresponding blur dimension 2 SE in the camera lens plane. Photographs are taken with the composite lens axes horizontal and vertical and also at 45° and 135°, the camera lens itself being focused on the patient's pupil. The pupil size is determined by an additional photograph without the composite lens. (For a detailed explanation and analysis of this technique, *see* Howland and Howland, 1974; Howland *et al.*, 1983).

Isotropic photorefraction

Because orthogonal photorefraction does not determine the astigmatic meridians of the eye directly, Howland *et al.* (1979) developed the isotropic method. In this technique the cylindrical lens assembly is not used. Photographs are taken with the camera focused first for an object distance nearer than the pupil, then on the pupil to record its diameter and finally for an object distance beyond the pupil. The blur dimensions on the film in the out-of-focus settings depend both on the ametropia and on the degree to which the camera is defocused. The reason for two out-of-focus exposures is to resolve an ambiguity. Because a blur circle can be either erect or inverted, the quantity b in equation (18.1) could have either a plus or a minus sign. Thus, for given values of g and W, the same numerical value of b could result from two different values of K. For example, with $g = 4\,\mathrm{mm}$ and $W = -1.50\,\mathrm{D}$, the same blur diameter of $24\,\mathrm{mm}$ would be given both by $K = +3.00\,\mathrm{D}$ and by $K = -6.00\,\mathrm{D}$. Similarly, the cross-sectional diameter of the refracted beam in any given position of the film plane is consistent with two different values of K, but only one of these is consistent with the dimension recorded in another position of the film. In general, the blur is smaller in the setting where the camera is focused nearer to the plane conjugate with the subject's retina.

Atkinson and Braddick (1982) suggest a working distance w of $-0.75\,\mathrm{m}$ ($W = -1\frac{1}{3}\,\mathrm{D}$) with the camera defocused by an equal dioptric amount E on either side of the pupil setting. The value suggested for E is $\pm\frac{2}{3}\,\mathrm{D}$. The shorter focusing distance would thus be $-0.5\,\mathrm{m}$ ($-2.00\,\mathrm{D}$) and the longer distance $-1.5\,\mathrm{m}$ ($-\frac{2}{3}\,\mathrm{D}$).

Figure 18.12 illustrates a simple method of constructing the beam in camera image space. In principle, it can be applied to similar diagrams representing other refractive states. First, the pupil image formed by the camera lens (of power F) is at a known dioptric distance $(W + F)$ from the lens. Its extremities H' and J' must lie in this image plane on the undeviated rays from H and J through S, which also represents the optical centre of the camera lens. Then, since the ray $JU_1'E$ must pass through J' after refraction, the intersection of the refracted ray with $HU_1'H'$ gives the second fundus image point U_2'. The image point V_2' is located in a similar manner.

It can be seen that the refracted beam has three distinct sections, in any of which the film plane may lie. A single expression for the blur diameter would thus be cumbersome. By deriving equations to the rays $EJ'U_2'$, $GH'V_2'$ and $SJ'V_2'$, it can be shown that the diameter j of the blur in the film plane is given by the larger arithmetic value of the two expressions

$$j = \frac{-gW}{F + W + E} \tag{18.2}$$

and

$$j = 2g\left(\frac{-W/2 - E + KE/W}{F + W + E}\right) \tag{18.3}$$

In these last expressions, as in equation (18.1), W is regarded as negative in sign.

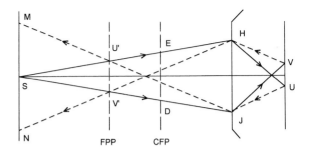

Figure 18.13. The myopic 'dead space' in isotropic photorefraction. FPP the eye's far-point plane, CFP camera focusing plane, S source and camera lens.

A number of simplifications were made in the above analysis. As Howland and colleagues point out, the size of the camera blur is affected by the finite size of the source, its vignetting or occluding effects on the returning light and the distance of the source from the principal planes of the camera lens. For these reasons they recommend an experimental calibration.

Bobier *et al.* (1992a,b), in extensive discussions of photorefraction, point out that there is a 'dead space' in which the blur is independent of the refractive error. Thus *Figure 18.13* shows a myopic eye where the far point plane FPP lies between the camera's focusing plane CFP and the source. The rays defining the size of the blur patch, DE, in the focusing plane are those from the source to the extremities HJ of the pupil, and are therefore independent of the precise amount of myopia. Thus, when the camera is defocused to its closer setting, myopia between $-1\frac{2}{3}\,\mathrm{D}$ and $-4\,\mathrm{D}$ gives a constant blur, while in the further setting, refractive errors between low myopia of $-1\frac{2}{3}\,\mathrm{D}$ to low hypermetropia of $+1\frac{2}{3}\,\mathrm{D}$ are indistinguishable. With the pair of photographs from each camera setting, these errors may be evaluated.

In the isotropic method, astigmatism produces an elliptical blur, its axes identifying the principal ocular meridians. The use of colour film provides a separate clue to the sign of the refractive error, since the chromatic aberration of the eye gives rise to a blue fringe in a myopic meridian and an orange–red fringe in a hypermetropic meridian.

Eccentric photorefraction

For typical values of the working distance and camera aperture, the lens plane blur fills the lens at about 4 D of ametropia, equations for these values being given by Bobier and colleagues. Higher refractive errors are therefore beyond the scope of both the orthogonal and isometric methods. A further technique described by Kaakinen (1979) and discussed by Howland (1980) may then be used. It is called eccentric photorefraction or static photographic skiascopy. In this method, the light-guide is decentred to the edge of the camera lens or beyond so that, as in retinoscopy, a crescent of light appears in the pupil.

In *Figure 18.14*, the source S produces an out-of-focus

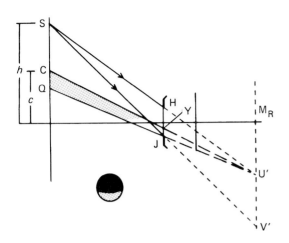

Figure 18.14. The optical principles of eccentric photorefraction; the inset shows the appearance of the pupil, the stippled zone being luminous.

blur on the retina which in turn is imaged at U′V′ in the far-point plane of the unaccommodated eye. If C is the upper edge of the camera's aperture, only the pencil of rays bounded by U′YC and U′JQ will enter the camera lens. For the hypermetropic eye illustrated, the width JY of the illuminated pupillary crescent is given by the equation

$$\text{Crescent width} = g + \left\{ \frac{(h-c)W}{K-W} \right\} \qquad (18.4)$$

where h is the distance of the light source from the camera axis and c the linear semi-aperture of the camera lens. In hypermetropia relative to the plane of the flash, the luminous crescent is on the side of the pupil opposite to the flash.

In myopia relative to this plane, the luminous crescent is on the same side as the flash. Equation (18.4) for the crescent width remains valid if the plus sign between the two terms is changed to minus.

An alternative method is to vary the distance h until a crescent is just seen within the pupil. An analysis of refractive error and theoretical and experimental crescent width is given by Bobier and Braddick (1985). They point out that the sensitivity of the film also affects the apparent size of the blur since it governs the threshold of light intensity that can be recorded. The crescent is therefore slightly larger than the photographs would suggest. The eye's aberrations also cause errors, so for these reasons the technique requires experimental calibration. Analyses of the technique are also given by Howland (1985), Crewther *et al.* (1987) and Bobier *et al.* (1992b). An interesting variation on the method, introduced by Abramov *et al.* (1990) is to leave the flash at a fixed small eccentricity, and photograph the eyes at various working distances. The type of refractive error can be deduced from the changes in crescent size. An alternative technique, originally introduced for animal research (Schaeffel *et al.*, 1987) employs a series of LEDs arranged along a radius of the camera aperture – these are triggered in succession, with a separate photograph for each, thus reproducing the moving

reflex of normal retinoscopy. This was subsequently adapted for continuous recording of accommodation response (Schaeffel et al., 1993).

The Cambridge and other paediatric videorefractors

Video recording and a constant light source instead of flash photography may be used with any of the methods described.

In the UK, the main centre of experimental research in photorefraction and its practical application in routine screening of infants has been the Visual Development Unit[*] of Cambridge University, headed by Dr Janette Atkinson and Dr Oliver Braddick. A broad picture of both these aspects of the unit's work is given in the paper by Braddick and Atkinson (1984). An important development was the appearance of the Cambridge Paediatric Videorefractor VPR-1 which was based on the isotropic method. The three photographs, having been recorded by the computer, are displayed in turn on the monitor screen, simultaneously with a cursor for measurement of the pupil or blur dimensions. The computer then calculates the refractive error. Rapid screening of large numbers of infants is made possible by this system.

Hodi and Wood (1994) compared the performance of the Cambridge videorefractor with the findings of cycloplegic spot retinoscopy. For the highest hypermetropic or least myopic meridian, non-cycloplegic videorefraction gave mean results 2 D less hypermetropic, but with a wide scatter. As would be expected, comparing both findings when made under cycloplegia gave much better agreement, though still with a wide scatter. The results for astigmatism were poorer, and they cite Ehrlich *et al.* (1994) who found marked changes in some infants' refraction with change of fixation. In their experiments, the infant looked at a toy held above the camera lens, while retinoscopy was performed with the child looking at the light (immediate source). Hence, oblique astigmatism may be the likely explanation. The occluding affect of the fibreoptic flash lead to the videorefractor may also affect results.

Searle *et al.* (1990) and Hodi (1994) evaluated the refractor for screening purposes. Provided the refraction was done under cycloplegia, the instrument was found to give acceptable results for identifying those infants needing further investigation. (Hodi's results for hypermetropia of ≥ 4.00 D gave a sensitivity 83.3%, specificity 90.6%, while for any degree of myopia the sensitivity was 92.3% with specificity of 98.7% – these terms are defined at the end of Chapter 1.)

Ehrlich *et al.* (1995) compared infants showing a hypermetropic error of ≥ 1.50 D when they should have been accommodating for a fixation toy at -0.75 m, i.e. they were showing an accommodative lag of ≥ 2.8 D, with those who showed more accurate accommodation. Inspection of their result confirms that non-cycloplegic

---

[*] The Visual Development Unit is situated at 22 Trumpington Street, Cambridge.

videorefraction fails to identify a small proportion of those infants who are more than 4.0 D hypermetropic, while a larger proportion of poor accommodators were false positives, i.e. were less than 4.0 D hypermetropic.

The Topcon PR-2000 is a more recent infra-red paediatric refractor.

Exercises

18.1 Compare and contrast the effects of residual ametropia in photorefraction, retinoscopy and the Foucault test as used in both the Humphrey Automatic Refractor and in the Dioptron.

18.2 (a) What is the blur dimension at the camera lens in photorefraction, given a working distance of -1 m, $K = -4.00$ D and pupil diameter 6 mm? (b) In orthogonal refraction with a camera lens of focal length 50 mm and a $+4.00$ D composite cylinder, with all other details as in (a), what is the overall length of the image on the film?

References

ABRAMOV, I., HAINLINE, L. and DUCKMAN, R.H. (1990) Screening infant vision with paraxial photorefraction. *Optom. Vis. Sci.*, **67**, 538–545

ADAMS, C.W., BULLIMORE, M.A., FUSARO, R.E., COTTERAL, R.M., SARVER, J. and GRAHAM, A.D. (1995) The reliability of automated and clinical refraction. *Invest. Ophthal. Visual Sci.*, **36**(4), S947

ALLEN, M.J. (1949) An objective high speed photographic technique for simultaneously recording changes in accommodation and convergence. *Am. J. Optom.*, **26**, 279–289

ALLEN, M.J. and CARTER, D.B. (1960) An infrared optometer to study the accommodative mechanism. *Am. J. Optom.*, **37**, 403–408

ATKINSON, J. and BRADDICK, O. (1982) The use of isotropic photorefraction for vision screening in infants. *Acta Ophthal.*, suppl. 157, 36–45

BENNETT, A.G. (1960) Refraction by automation? New applications of the Scheiner disc. *Optician*, **139**, 5–9

BENNETT, A.G. (1978) Methods of automated objective refraction. *Ophthal. Optn*, **18**, 8–13, 19

BENNETT, A.G. and RABBETTS, R.B. (1978) Refraction in oblique meridians of the astigmatic eye. *Br. J. Physiol. Optics*, **32**, 59–77

BERMAN, M., NELSON, P. and CADEN, B. (1984) Objective refraction: comparison of retinoscopy and automated techniques. *Am. J. Optom.*, **61**, 204–209

BOBIER, W.R. and BRADDICK, O.J. (1985) Eccentric photorefraction: optical analysis and empirical measures. *Am. J. Optom.*, **62**, 614–620

BOBIER, W.R., CAMPBELL, M.C.W., McCREARY, C.R., POWER, A.M. and YANG, K.C. (1992a) Co-axial photorefractive methods: an optical analysis. *Appl. Opt.*, **31**, 3601–3615

BOBIER, W.R., CAMPBELL, M.C.W., McCREARY, C.R., POWER, A.M. and YANG, K.C. (1992b) Geometrical optical analysis of photorefractive methods. *Ophthal. Physiol. Opt.*, **12**, 147–152

BRADDICK, O. and ATKINSON, J. (1984) Photorefractive techniques: applications in testing infants and young children. *The Frontiers of Optometry: First International Congress* 1984. London: British College of Ophthalmic Opticians (Optometrists). Vol. 2, pp. 26–34

CAMPBELL, F.W. and ROBSON, J.G. (1959) High-speed infrared optometer. *J. Opt. Soc. Am.*, **49**, 268–272

CHARMAN, W.N. (1976) A pioneering instrument. The Collins electronic refractionometer. *Ophthal. Optn*, **16**, 345–348, 484

CHARMAN, W.N. (1980) Reflection of plane-polarized light by the retina. *Br. J. Physiol. Optics*, **34**, 34–39

CHARMAN, N. and HERON, G. (1975) A simple infra-red optometer for accommodation studies. *Br. J. Physiol. Optics*, **30**, 1–12

CHARMAN, W.N. and JENNINGS, J.A.M. (1976) Objective measurement of the longitudinal chromatic aberration of the human eye. *Vision Res.*, **16**, 999–1005

COLLINS, G. (1937) The electronic refractionometer. *Br. J. Physiol. Optics*, **11**, 30–42

CORNSWEET, T.N. and CRANE, H.D. (1970) Servo-controlled infrared optometer. *J. Opt. Soc. Am.*, **60**, 548–554

CREWTHER, D.P., MCCARTHY, A., ROPER, J. and COSTELLO, K. (1987) An analysis of eccentric photorefraction. *Clin. Exp. Optom.*, **70**, 2–7

DAVIS, B., COLLINS, M. and ATCHISON, D. (1993) Calibration of the Canon Autoref R-1 for continuous measurement of accommodation. *Ophthal. Physiol. Opt.*, **13**, 191–198

EHRLICH, D.L., ANKER, S. and BRADDICK, O.J. (1994) On- and off-axis refraction of infants. *Invest. Ophthalmol. Vis. Sci.*, **35** (suppl, abs 2571),1806

EHRLICH, D. (1996) MDA reports on autorefractors. *Optom. Today*, **36**(16), 38

EHRLICH, D.L., ANKER, S., ATKINSON, J., BRADDICK, O.J., WEEKS, F. and WADE, J. (1995) Infant photorefraction and cycloplegic retinoscopy of 'poor accommodators'. Poster at *The British College of Optometrists Centenary Conference*, Cambridge, UK.

FITZKE, F.W., HOLDEN, A.L. and SHEEN, F.H. (1985) A Maxwellian-view optometer suitable for electrophysiological and psychophysical research. *Vision Res.*, **25**, 871–874

FLETCHER, R.J. (1954) Near vision astigmatism. *Optician*, **127**, 341–345, 350

FRENCH, C. and WOOD, I.C.J. (1982) The Dioptron II's validity and reliability as a function of its three accuracy indices. *Ophthal. Physiol. Opt.*, **2**, 57–74

FRY, G.A. (1937) An experimental analysis of the accommodation–convergence relation. *Am. J. Optom.*, **14**, 402–414

GHOSE, S., NAYAK, B.K. and SINGH, J.P. (1986) Critical evaluation of the NR-1000F Auto Refractometer. *Br. J. Ophthal.*, **70**, 221–226

GRIFFITHS, G. (1988) Autorefractors – their use and usefulness. *Optician*, **196**(5178), 22–29

HENSON, D.B. (1996) *Optometric Instrumentation*, 2nd edn. Oxford: Butterworth-Heinemann

HODI, S. (1994) Screening of infants for significant refractive error using videorefraction. *Ophthal. Physiol. Opt.*, **14**, 310–313

HODI, S. and WOOD, I.C.J. (1994) Comparison of the techniques of videorefraction and static retinoscopy in the measurement of refractive error in infants. *Ophthal. Physiol. Opt.*, **14**, 20–24

HOWLAND, H.C. (1980) The optics of photographic skiascopy. *Acta Ophthal.*, **58**, 221–227

HOWLAND, H.C. (1985) Optics of photoretinoscopy: results from ray tracing. *Am. J. Optom.*, **62**, 621–625

HOWLAND, H.C., ATKINSON, J. and BRADDICK, O. (1979) A new method of photographic refraction of the eye. *J. Opt. Soc. Am.*, **69**, 1486

HOWLAND, H.C., BRADDICK, O., ATKINSON, J. and HOWLAND, B. (1983) Optics of photorefraction: orthogonal and isotropic methods. *J. Opt. Soc. Am.*, **73**, 1701–1708

HOWLAND, H.C. and HOWLAND, B. (1974) Photorefraction: a technique for the study of refractive state at a distance. *J. Opt. Soc. Am.*, **64**, 240–249

JASCHINSKI-KRUZA, W. (1988) Technical note: a hand optometer for measuring dark focus. *Vision Res.*, **28**, 1271–1275

KAAKINEN, K. (1979) A simple method for screening of children with strabismus, anisometropia or ametropia by simultaneous photography of the corneal and the fundus reflexes. *Acta Ophthal.*, **57**, 161–171

KNOLL, H.A. and MOHRMAN, R. (1972) The Ophthalmetron, principles and operation. *Am. J. Optom.*, **49**, 122–128

KNOLL, H.A., MOHRMAN, R. and MAIER, W.L. (1970) Automatic objective refraction in an office practice. *Am. J. Optom.*, **47**, 644–649

KRUGER, P.B. (1979) Infrared recording retinoscope for monitoring accommodation. *Am. J. Optom.*, **56**, 116–123

LONG, W.F. (1974) A mathematical analysis of multi-meridional refractometry. *Am. J. Optom.*, **51**, 260–263

LONG, W.F. (1981) The accuracy of multimeridional refraction. *Am. J. Optom.*, **58**, 1161–1173

LOVASIK, J.V. (1983) A simple continuously recording infrared optometer. *Am. J. Optom.*, **60**, 80–87

McBRIEN, N.A. and MILLODOT, M. (1985) Clinical evaluation of the Canon Autoref R-1. *Am. J. Optom.*, **62**, 786–792

McCAGHREY, G.E. and MATTHEWS, F.E. (1993) Clinical evaluation of a range of autorefractors. *Opthal. Physiol. Opt.*, **13**, 129–137

McDEVITT, H.I. JR. (1977) Automatic retinoscopy: the 6600 Auto-Refractor. *Optician*, **173**(4485), 33, 37, 40, 42

MOSES, R.A. (1971) Vernier optometer. *J. Opt. Soc. Am.*, **61**, 1539

MUNNERLYN, C.R. (1978) An optical system for an automatic eye refractor. *Opt. Eng.*, **17**, 627–630

NAYAK, B.K., GHOSE, S. and SINGH, J.P. (1987) A comparison of cycloplegic and manifest refraction on the NR-1000F (an objective Auto Refractometer). *Br. J. Ophthal.*, **71**, 73–75

POLSE, K.A. and KERR, K.E. (1975) An automatic objective optometer. *Archs. Ophthal., N.Y.*, **93**, 225–231

PUGH, J.R. and WINN, B. (1988) Modification of the Canon AutoRef R-1 for use as a continuously recording infra-red optometer. *Ophthal. Physiol. Opt.*, **8**, 460–465

ROTH, N. (1962) Recording infrared coincidence optometer. *Am. J. Optom.*, **39**, 356–361

SAFIR, A., KOLL, H. and MOHRMAN, R. (1970) Automatic objective refraction: report of a clinical trial. *Trans. Am. Acad. Ophthal. Oto-lar.*, **74**, 1266–1275

SCHAEFFEL, F., FARKAS, L. and HOWLAND, H.C. (1987) Infrared photoretinoscope. *Appl. Opt.*, **26**, 1505–1509

SCHAEFFEL, F., HOWLAND, H., WEISS, S. and ZRENNER, E. (1993) Measurement of the dynamics of accommodation by automated real time photorefraction. *Invest. Ophthalmol. Vis. Sci.*, **34**(2968), 1306

SEARLE, C.M., MILLER, R.C., BOURNE, K.M. and CRAMPTON, A.M. (1990) Evaluation report – the Cambridge Video Refractor. *Aust. Orthopt. J.*, **26**, 13–18

SLOAN, P.G. and POLSE, K.A. (1974) Preliminary clinical evaluation of the Dioptron. *Am. J. Optom.*, **51**, 189–197

STRANG, N.C., GRAY, L.S., WINN, B. and PUGH, J.R. (1997) An evaluation of automated infra-red optometers. *Optom. Today*, **37**(1), 41–44

WETZEL, P.A., GERI, G.A. and PIERCE, B.J. (1996) An integrated system for measuring static and dynamic accommodation with a Canon Autoref R-1 refractometer. *Ophthal. Physiol. Opt.*, **16**, 520–527

WOOD, I. (1982) A comparative study of autorefractors. *Ophthal. Optn*, **22**, 221–225

WOOD, I. (1988) Computerized refractive examination. In *Optometry* (Edwards, K. and Llewellyn, R., eds), pp. 92–110. London: Butterworths

WOOD, I.C.J. and FRENCH, C.N. (1981) The Dioptron II – in theory. *Optician*, **181**(4702), 7–11

WOOD, I.C.J., PAPAS, E., BURGHARDT, D. and HARDWICK, G. (1984) A clinical evaluation of the Nidek autorefractor. *Ophthal. Physiol. Opt.*, **4**, 169–178

19

Vision screening, new subjective refractors and techniques

Vision screening

There are many occasions when it is desirable to check the visual ability of large numbers of people. For example, the presence of significant refractive errors or anomalies of binocular vision will handicap the visual and mental performance of young children; visual comfort and efficiency at work may be poorer than normal; routine checks on the vision of employees, new applicants for jobs, recruits to the Armed Forces and drivers are all sensible if not compulsory.

There are not enough suitably qualified practitioners to give a full eye examination to all those requiring such a check. Moreover, the large proportion of normal people renders such a procedure both expensive and time-wasting. Hence, some type of vision screening is required to identify those people who should be referred for a full eye examination and/or be rejected for certain occupations.

Visual screening may be classified under various headings of complexity:

(1) simple vision tests,
(2) mechanical vision screeners,
(3) simplified or partial routine examination.

In general, such screening is for visual requirements, and no check is made on the ocular health.

Simple vision tests

Screening is often undertaken by means of visual acuity tests alone, often with a conventional Snellen chart. The appropriate type of chart should be used for young children, for example Stycar or Ffooks. Virtually all myopes and people with medium or high astigmatism and amblyopia will be detected. Unfortunately, some with significant astigmatism may be missed because the unaided vision for the clear well-spaced lettering of the Snellen chart may be quite reasonable. Absolute hypermetropia will also be detected, but the young person with significant hypermetropia may well be able to read the 6/6 (20/20) line or better with ease since the duration of the test is so short. Visual comfort for prolonged viewing, especially in near vision, will nevertheless be

poor. A supplementary check for hypermetropia with a lens of appropriate plus power to verify that vision blurs is to be strongly recommended. Suggested strengths are +2.00 DS for ages up to 20, +1.50 DS for 20–35 years and +1.00 DS for higher ages up to 50. Similarly, the near vision, with spectacles if possessed, should be measured for people over 40 years of age.

Binocular vision problems such as pronounced heterophoria and poor convergence will be missed unless the appropriate extra tests are added.

Mechanical vision screeners

These are stereoscope-type instruments presenting a sequence of tests and are designed for operation by nonprofessional staff. The stereoscope design allows the separate measurement of both binocular and monocular functions. Binocular visual acuity (or vision) is tested by presenting identical slides to each eye. Words of decreasing size, illiterate Es and checkerboard patterns are used in different manufacturers' instruments. Monocular vision may be checked by presenting the acuity test to each eye in turn. In some instruments, these vision tests are mounted on a background giving stereoscopic relief, in which case the vision test will be superimposed on the respective side only. If checkerboard patterns are used, the eye not being tested will be shown uniformly grey or finely stippled diamonds. These two types of background give a binocular lock, stabilizing convergence and hence accommodation.

Heterophoria may be checked by showing a line to one eye and a tangent scale to the other, separate tests being needed for horizontal and vertical phorias. A simpler screening test is to present a dot to one eye and a rectangle to the other eye. The subject passes if the heterophoria is within normal limits but fails if the dot appears to lie outside the rectangle, which demonstrates the presence of, say, more than 1Δ of vertical phoria, 3Δ of esophoria or 6Δ of exophoria.

Tests may also be provided for colour vision, stereopsis and suppression. The presence of low amounts of hypermetropia can be tested on some instruments which automatically insert weak plus spherical lenses or position the slide farther from the collimating lenses. If the test detail can still be seen, hypermetropia exists.

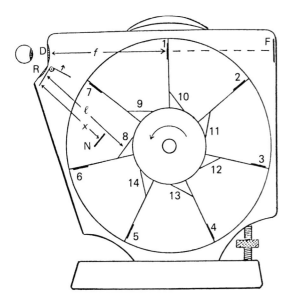

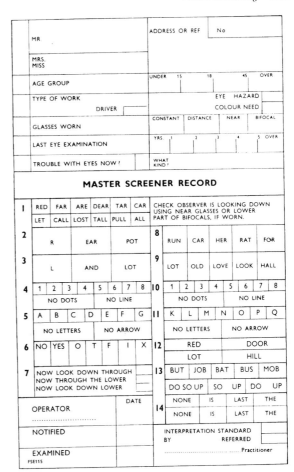

Figure 19.1. The Master Vision Screener (Mavis): 1–7 distance targets; 8–14 near vision targets; D the distance collimating lens and *f* its focal length; F fogging charts, viewed through aperture in l; R near vision lens with object distance *ℓ* for targets to be imaged at 330 mm and *x* for target N to be imaged at 200 mm. Note shutter for lenses D and R. (Reproduced by kind permission of Professor R.J. Fletcher, from *Ophthalmics in Industry*, 1961.)

Figure 19.2. The Mavis record card. (Reproduced by kind permission of British American Optical Co. Ltd.)

Some of the tests may be repeated in near vision (with different slides to avoid memorizing), either by positioning the test nearer or by viewing through weaker stereoscope lenses. In some instruments these are positioned to allow comfortable viewing through the near portion of bifocals (*Figure 19.1*).

The results are recorded on a special card, for example that shown in *Figure 19.2*, by ticking the relevant boxes. These cards are then passed to professional staff, who can interpret the standard of vision in relation to the requirements for the particular occupation or medical check. Anyone not meeting the standard is then referred for a full eye examination. An alternative procedure is for the professional adviser to draw up lists of standards for particular tasks. These requirements can be marked on a transparent plastic sheet to form a template which can be laid on top of the individual's record, thus allowing non-professional staff to decide whether or not to refer.

Note should be taken of the proximal or instrument accommodation (Chapter 7) induced in young patients, particularly children under 10 years. It may lead to false referrals from mechanized screening because emmetropes and low hypermetropes could apparently show reduced vision through pseudo-myopia.

Patients with strabismus may well need to have their better eye occluded before their strabismic eye's vision can be measured.

The test plates in some instruments are not enclosed in an instrument case and so are illuminated by the general room lighting. This means that the visual acuity results especially could vary from one testing location to another. Other instruments have totally enclosed test panels and rely on internal illumination. The operator should ensure that the illuminance is both uniform and compatible with the ambient lighting in the workplace. A very high test-chart illuminance may not identify those people whose vision will be inadequate if the work illuminance is poor. Conversely, a low test-panel illuminance may result in failure for a subject whose vision out of doors in daylight is (legally) adequate for driving. Rossi (1992) gives a recent review of vision screeners.

Automated vision screeners

The French firm Essilor have introduced automation into screening by incorporating a voice synthesizer to give instructions to the subject, together with computerized recording. Their simpler model named Optivision measures the right and left monocular acuities, and includes a fogging test to detect hypermetropia over 1 D and a bichromatic test to identify lower degrees. A fan chart to detect astigmatism, a heterophoria screening test and a test for binocular visual acuity are also incorporated.

In addition to the above automatic tests, the Ergovision model has many extra features for testing occupational vision, the appropriate functions being used as indicated. To reproduce the lighting conditions at work, the tests can be undertaken with a surround luminance of 15, 150 and 300 cd/m^2, while vision under mesopic conditions can be assessed with an acuity chart at 4 cd/m^2. Night vision can be further assessed by measuring the recovery time from glare, and driving vision checked by tests of kinetic visual acuity and the field of vision. Provision is also made for estimating binocular visual acuity at intermediate distances and also with a low-contrast chart in distance vision. Ishihara colour vision plates, a more accurate heterophoria test and tests for stereoscopic vision and fixation disparity have also been added.

The Canon Auto Acuitometer also uses a voice synthesizer and computer recording to allow the subject to test his own acuity automatically. Landolt ring charts are provided for this purpose.

The autorefractors in general, but particularly those incorporating test charts, could also be used as vision screeners for refractive errors. They are not able to examine other functions such as binocular co-ordination, for which they were not intended.

Computerized screening for DSE users

In Europe, workers who spend a significant amount of time viewing display screen equipment (DSE – visual display units/terminals) are entitled to regular eye examinations, partly to ensure their comfort and performance while working. For employers with large numbers of such employees, it is economically beneficial to screen to identify those who would benefit from a full eye examination, those whose discomfort may be equipment or environmentally related and those who are both symptom-free and visually normal.

While optical screening instruments of the types described above may be employed, they do not necessarily provide a suitable combination of tests for DSE users. Programs for use at the worker's display unit have the advantage of testing at the actual viewing distance and angle habitually used. They can include questions on screen size and viewing distance (for calibration for acuity and oculo-motor balance), on problems such as lighting levels, reflections off the screen and the ergonomic comfort of the layout, as well as an appropriate selection of vision screening tasks.

Two such programs available in the UK are the City University Vision Screener for VDU Users* (Thomson, 1994) and the Keeler Vutest† (Scheinman, 1993).

Like the optical screeners, these include visual acuity, oculo-motor balance and fixation disparity tests. The City University test also includes a subjective comfort rating for the legibility of print, search tasks to check whether ocular performance drops with a longer duration task, and a simple central visual field check. The Vutest uses a combination search and visual field test and an Amsler chart (*see* page 252) to investigate the central fields. Both will print out a report of the visual screening, while the City University program will also offer advice on any workstation problems elicited by the questions. Advice on both the DSE regulations and layout is given in *Display screen equipment work – guidance on regulations* (1992), published by the UK Health and Safety Executive.

For conventional optometric examination, the UK Association of Optometrists recommends the following standards for comfortable DSE work, which are reproduced here with their kind permission:

(1) The ability to read N6 throughout the range 70–33 cm with adequate visual acuity for any task undertaken at a greater distance, if this is an integral part of the work.
(2) Well-established monocular vision or good binocular vision. Phorias at working distances should be corrected unless well compensated or deep suppression is present.
(3) No central (20°) field defects in the dominant eye.
(4) Near point of convergence normal.
(5) Clear ocular media checked by ophthalmoscopy.

They point out that these criteria are intended to increase the level of operator comfort and efficiency, but are not inflexible and should *not* be used to exclude persons from working with DSE.

Simplified examination routines

In view of the disadvantages of both lay-person and mechanical-instrument screening, a much reduced version of a normal eye examination by professional staff has much to recommend it. A suggested scheme for older school children and adults would cover:

(1) Distance vision, with spectacles if possessed, monocularly and possibly binocularly.
(2) Cover test in distance vision.
(3) Near vision, with the patient's own spectacles, again monocularly and binocularly, at the required working distance.
(4) Near cover test and near point of convergence.
(5) Retinoscopy sufficient to identify the presence of significant uncorrected hypermetropia, astigmatism or anisometropia. Myopia will show both here and by reduced distance vision.
(6) Ophthalmoscopy.
(7) Colour-vision testing, where appropriate. In primary schools where colour coding is used in teaching arithmetic, colour-deficient children need to be identified, despite the greater difficulty of assessment at that age. For older children, when careers advice is given.
(8) Stereopsis – for some industrial tasks. It can also be used as a test for the quality of binocular vision.

Screening of young children

The purpose of screening very young children, about 1 year old, is to try to identify those at risk of developing strabismus and/or amblyopia. About 3.7% of the infants of this age reported upon in a study by Ingram *et al.* (1986b) showed a significant refractive error. Ingram (1977) had earlier found that while over 50% of chil-

---

* Available from City Visual Systems Ltd, Citybridge House, 235–245 Goswell Road, London, EC1V 7JD.
† Available from Keeler Ltd, Clewer Hill Road, Windsor, Berks SL4 4AA.

dren presenting either of these conditions had a family history of strabismus or amblyopia, over 70% had an abnormal refraction defined as an error exceeding 2.00 D in the least hypermetropic meridian of either eye or 1.00 D or more of spherical or cylindrical anisometropia. Although Atkinson *et al.* (1987) concluded that refractive correction at this age had a beneficial effect in reducing the incidence of strabismus and amblyopia, Ingram *et al.* (1985) found no evidence that spectacles significantly altered the child's prospect of avoiding either of these conditions. Ingram *et al.* (1986a) further suggested that screening at age $3\frac{1}{2}$ is too late to be effective in combating amblyopia. While this may well be true for deep amblyopia, optometric opinion would certainly not agree with this view when initial acuities of 6/24 or better are obtained.

For large-scale refractive screening of infants, the computerized isotropic photorefractor has undoubted possibilities, as shown, for example, by Atkinson *et al.* (1987). Should acuities be required, forced-choice preferential looking or some other objective technique will be needed (*see* pages 38–39).

With slightly older children the appropriate acuity tests should be used. Dynamic retinoscopy with a small picture or miniature toy animal or car as fixation object may give more reliable results, at least for astigmatism and anisometropia, than static retinoscopy, though this should be attempted to verify the absence of marked hypermetropia. The child's mother may need to flash a pen torch on and off in order to obtain a reasonable distance fixation. Mohindra near retinoscopy is another possible option.

The presence of fusion may be confirmed by observing compensatory eye movements when a prism of 20Δ base out is held before one eye. With the prism held in turn before both eyes, adduction of the eye behind the prism with no movement of the other eye should occur. The presence of suppression – and hence, probably, of strabismus – is demonstrated by no movement of either eye when the prism is held before the weak eye, and binocular version movements when the prism is placed before the dominant eye. No response from either eye could indicate lack of attention or possibly too strong a prism. Only 15Δ base out should be used with a child under 18 months and 10Δ base out with a child under 1 year down to 3 months old (Bishop, A., pers. comm., 1983).

The presence or absence of stereopsis (*see* Chapter 11) may also be used for evaluating the quality of binocular vision. The present author feels that, while a positive response to a stereopsis test is an indicator of binocular vision, a negative response may merely be a lack of interest or understanding by a young child. Thus Broadbent and Westall (1990) found that 50% of their sample of 6–12-month-old infants responded to the Lang test (e.g. by patting or pointing to one of the hidden objects), rising to 75% of the children aged over 1 year, while the 3 or 6 mm plates of the Frisby test were identified by about 20% of the 6–12-month group, rising to 85% by the age of 24 months. The TNO test, needing the child to wear red–green goggles, was unsuccessful until about 2 years of age.

While Ingram *et al.* (1986a) suggested refraction and possibly the cover test for screening at age $3\frac{1}{2}$, Dholakia (1987) proposed that lay staff could use the 20Δ prism test, 7-letter Stycar chart (*see* page 33) and near point of convergence for 3 year olds, leaving out the last for 4 and 5 year olds. To increase sensitivity to possible defects, the high acuity standard of 6/6 was chosen as a criterion. This might be thought a very high level of acuity for the younger age groups.

A simplified routine such as the above is of great value, both in organized screening sessions and also as an occasional procedure for young children when the practitioner is examining parents or older siblings.

Imaged refraction systems

Introduction

Both the trial frame and refractor head (phoropter) require the correcting lenses to be placed in front of the patient's eye, hindering the refractionist's view of the face. The trial frame system is relatively heavy but does allow the patient to move his head. The refractor head is supported mechanically, but the patient must keep his head pressed firmly against it to maintain the correct vertex distance. A better view for the practitioner and possibly a greater sense of freedom for the patient would be achieved if the lenses were moved away from the eyes.

As demonstrated in a paper by Reiner (1966), it is possible to reproduce the refractive effect of a contact lens on the eye by removing the real lens to some convenient distance and forming an optical image of it on the cornea itself. The optical system used for this purpose consists of two lenses of equal positive power, separated by twice their focal length to form an inverting afocal system of unit magnification ($m = -1$). In this arrangement, an object (the contact lens) placed in the anterior focal plane of the first lens is imaged in the posterior focal plane of the second lens, positioned to coincide with the observer's eye.

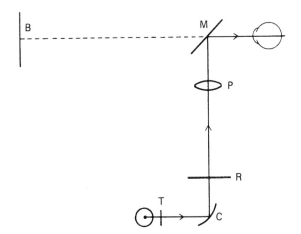

Figure 19.3. A Reiner imaged refraction system. B black screen against which test images are viewed, C collimating mirror, presumably toroidal to counteract oblique astigmatism; M glass plate mirror; P projection lens; R refractor head; T test slide.

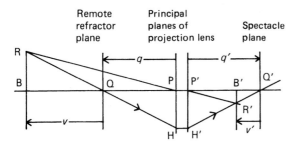

Figure 19.4. Optical principle of remote refraction: the remote refractor plane is made conjugate with the spectacle plane.

Figure 19.3 shows another imaged (or remote) refraction system subsequently designed by Reiner. The patient has a wide view of the room through a plate glass beam splitter, while the test charts seen through the refraction system appear superimposed on the black screen. The optical principles can be derived from *Figure 19.4* which shows a projection lens of power F_p forming an image Q' of an object Q with a magnification m_q equal to q'/q. The test slide is at RB.

From the two pairs of similar triangles QBR, QPH and $Q'B'R'$, $Q'P'H'$, an expression identical to equation (12.7) can be derived. Using the symbols appropriate to the present system it becomes

$$m_q V' = V/m_q + F_p \qquad (19.1)$$

For the special case in which $m_q = -1$, this expression reduces to

$$V = V' + F_p \qquad (19.2)$$

If Q' is regarded as being in the spectacle plane and Q in the remote plane in which the refractor head lenses are placed, V is the lens power needed in this plane to give a vergence V' or F_{sp} in the spectacle plane. Thus, with $m_q = -1$ and $F_p = +10$ D, a lens of power $(+10 + F_{sp})$ would be needed in the refractor head to 'correct' an ametrope.

Guyton *et al.* (1987) suggests various optometric uses for imaged refraction systems, while Freeman (1992) described the use of a pair of nominally identical camera lenses, mounted front elements towards each other, to provide a simulation system providing excellent visual performance over a 6 mm diameter pupil and a visual field of ±8°.

The Humphrey Vision Analyser

The first commercially available system using remote refraction was the Humphrey Vision Analyser, introduced in the mid-1970s. Though it is no longer in production, it introduced so many new concepts that it is still described here. The positive powered imaging system is a concave mirror of 30 cm diameter, placed at about 2.5 m from the patient, in which he sees the test object by reflection (*Figure 19.5*). The mirror's centre of curvature C is in a mid-way position, approximately in the patient's spectacle plane and in the effective plane of the correction lens unit L. The image W'X' formed by the

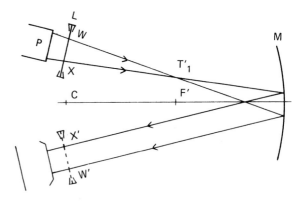

Figure 19.5. The remote-refraction system of the Humphrey Vision Analyser: C and F' centre of curvature and principal focus of mirror M; L effective position of trial correction (aperture WX) images at W'X' in the spectacle plane. The ray path shown is for emmetropia (trial lens power zero). In myopia, the minus trial correction moves image T'_1 further from the projector.

mirror of the correction lens aperture WX is therefore of the same size as WX and situated in the patient's spectacle plane.

For an emmetrope, the image of T'_1 of the test object T must be projected by the system P into the mirror's focal plane through F' so as to give rise to parallel pencils after reflection. The image T'_2 is then formed at infinity. In order to compensate for image aberrations caused by the slightly oblique incidence, the surface of the mirror is made fractionally toroidal.

If a low-powered negative lens is introduced at L, the test object will be imaged nearer the mirror, resulting in a divergent beam reaching the eye. A negative lens of slightly higher power will put the aerial image on to the mirror, so that the vergence at the eye is $-1/2.5$ or -0.40 D. A steady increase in negative power will push the aerial image towards the eye, providing an effective test object for any degree of myopia.

Any positive correcting lens at L will cause the first aerial image T'_1 to lie between the projector and the mirror's principal focus, so that the second image T'_2 by reflection is formed behind the patient's head. This is illustrated in *Figure 19.6*, in which the dotted lines show the ray paths when the system is at zero for an emmetrope. The unbroken lines are the ray paths from W and X through T'_1. After reflection, they necessarily

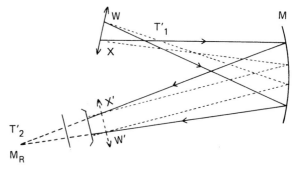

Figure 19.6. Humphrey Vision Analyser: ray path with positive trial-lens power in operation for correction of hypermetropia.

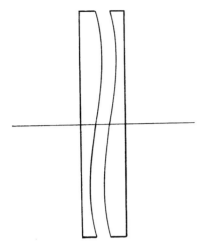

Figure 19.7. Central cross-section of the Alvarez two-element variable-power lens.

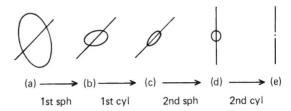

Figure 19.8. Refraction steps with the Humphrey Vision Analyser: patient's astigmatic meridians at 70° and 160°. (a) Initial blur ellipse, (b) blur ellipse with best sphere, (c) blur ellipse aligned with test line object by first cylindrical adjustment, (d) blur circle with second spherical adjustment, (e) point focus with second cylindrical adjustment.

pass through W′ and X′ to form the image T′₂ behind the patient's eye, thus simulating the effect of a plus correcting lens placed in the spectacle plane.

A second breakthrough of the Humphrey Vision Analyser was to replace conventional trial lenses with continuously variable optical systems. Spherical power is provided by a two-element Alvarez lens formed by two identical components in reverse orientation (*Figure 19.7*). Placed in contact in the zero setting, they would form a flat parallel plate without focal power. If the left-hand component in the diagram were moved upwards and its fellow downwards, the result would be to generate minus power – surprisingly uniform over the whole area of overlap. The magnitude of the power is directly proportional to the travel of the components. Relative movement in the opposite direction would produce plus power. The complex geometry of the refracting surfaces is lucidly explained in the patent specification (Alvarez, 1967) and by Charman (1994). The astigmatic components are provided by systems invented by Humphrey (1973). In effect, they are cylinders of variable power by sliding adjustment, not by rotation as in the optically equivalent Stokes lens. The mean spherical power remains at zero, so that adjustment does not alter the position of the circle of least confusion relative to the retina.

A third innovation was a new technique for measuring astigmatism, called 'astigmatic decomposition' – a concept originated by Humphrey from the theory of obliquely crossed cylinders as described in Chapter 5. It is based on the fact that a plano-cylinder of any given power and orientation can be replaced by two plano-cylindrical components in contact, with their respective axes in *any* specified meridians. Both plus and minus cylinder components are needed to cover all possibilities. The equivalent combination does, however, generate a spherical component in accordance with equation (5.10). A general demonstration of the basic theorem with numerical examples has been given by Bennett (1977).

In a similar way, a cross cylinder (as used in refraction) of given power and orientation is replaceable by a combination of two such lenses with their respective axes at any specified orientation. In this case, however, no added spherical power is generated by the combination because the mean spherical power of any cross cylinder is zero.

Although in the Humphrey Vision Analyser a combination of variable power cross cylinders is used at fixed orientations 0°/90° and 45°/135°, the theory of the method is explained most simply by reducing them to simple cylinders, plus or minus as required, at axes 0° and 45° respectively. In effect, the correcting cylinder is replaced by a combination of these two components, adjusted in turn to the appropriate power.

The patient initially looks at a line in the 135° meridian of about 1 minute of arc subtense in width and adjusts the variable spherical lens system to give the best view obtainable of the line. If astigmatism is present, the line can be seen quite clearly only if the axis of the correcting cylinder is at 45°. By adjusting the power of the axis horizontal cylinder component, the ocular astigmatism is then modified so that it becomes correctable by a cylinder at axis 45°. Only then can the line at 135° be seen in its sharpest focus. The patient accordingly adjusts the power of the 90°/180° cross cylinder until this result is achieved.[*]

This process is shown diagrammatically in *Figure 19.8* which represents the *patient's* view of the test lines with the projected retinal blur ellipses (due to a point object) superimposed on them. In *Figure 19.8(a)*, the test line is at 135° and the major axis of the blur ellipse is at 70°, corresponding to one of the astigmatic meridians of the eye under test. The sharpest focus of this line is obtained by spherical adjustment to place the most favourable cross-section of the astigmatic pencil on the retina. This occurs when the retinal blur presents the least width perpendicular to this line, as in *Figure 19.8(b)*. The major axis of the ellipse is now at 160°, at right-angles to its original orientation. Adjustment of the axis horizontal cross cylinder is then made so as to align the major axis of the resultant blur ellipse with the 135° line, as shown in *Figure 19.8(c)*.

The oblique line test object is now replaced by a verti-

---

[*] Accuracy is enhanced by showing a fan of three lines. The middle one should appear sharpest with the two outer ones equally blurred, somewhat similar to the Maddox v test.

cal line, and the spherical power system readjusted to provide the best view obtainable Since the resulting astigmatic error at this stage is at axis $45°$, the clearest view of the vertical line occurs when the circle of least confusion is on the retina (*Figure 19.8d*). Adjustment of the $45°/135°$ cross cylinder should then bring it into sharp focus, as indicated in *Figure 19.8(e)*.

A built-in computer calculates and displays in spherocylindrical form the result of the spherical and two cross-cylinder components. A print-out can also be obtained.

A notable feature of this system is that it obviates the prior need to locate the astigmatic axis of the subject's eye. Thus, instructions to the patient and the decisions required are simplified. Moreover, there are no confusing side-effects sometimes attendant on other routines. It is immaterial in which order the line test objects are presented, provided that the correct cross-cylinder system is adjusted on both occasions.

To enable binocular examination to be made, two projection and correcting lens systems are provided side by side. Crossline targets are projected on to the patient's face to allow accurate horizontal centration for each eye by means of a sliding-mirror assembly. Vertical adjustment is by the height of the patient's chair. The vertex distance is set by a supplementary projector from the side. It can be adjusted to zero to obviate the need for effectivity allowances when contact-lens patients are being refracted. Over-refraction through the patient's own spectacles, a useful expedient when they are of high power, presents no difficulties.

As with a refractor head or phoropter, the patient must keep his head still and firmly pressed up against the rest. Especially in cases of anisometropia, lateral or vertical head movements will generate relative prism, while a head tilt may also cause axis errors significant in high astigmatism. In this sense, the trial frame retains its superiority, but the clear view of the patient's face with the remote refraction of the Humphrey Vision Analyser means that head movement can easily be seen.

Monocular refraction may be performed either by switching off one of the projector bulbs, or, more usually, by introducing excess positive spherical power to fog the eye. Conventional bichromatic and Snellen charts may be presented. Prismatic elements can be introduced to correct fixation disparity revealed by the special slides. Since separate channels are used for each eye, no analysing visor is necessary.

The eyes' performance in near vision can be examined by lowering a mounted periscope, thus permitting depressed gaze as well as convergence.

Since the test slides are viewed by reflection in a mirror instead of by projection on to a metallized screen as with conventional test chart projectors, only low-powered bulbs need to be used. High contrast is obtained in full room illumination.

With both the Reiner and the Humphrey systems, the patient can change fixation and view the room surroundings unaided. While this does not stimulate accommodation in a myope, there is a possibility that the hypermetrope could then accommodate and not relax sufficiently on returning his attention to the chart.

Other methods of measuring astigmatism

Axis determination

The Crisp–Stine test

This test is essentially the same as the conventional cross-cylinder method of axis determination, except that a cross is used, rotated to be at $45°/135°$ to the trial cylinder axis. If the trial cylinder is at the correct axis, the two limbs of the cross will be equally clear. Introduction of a cross cylinder with its axes parallel to the cross will cause equal blurring of the two arms in both positions. If the trial cylinder is at an incorrect axis, then, as shown in *Table 6.3* on page 103, there is a resultant error of refraction at an axis outside the angle enclosed between the trial cylinder and true axis. One limb of the cross will thus appear clearer than the other. Introduction of the cross cylinder will either aggravate or reduce the difference in clarity of the limbs. The trial cylinder and cross are then rotated towards the negative (or positive) cylinder axis of the cross cylinder in its preferred position, depending on whether negative (or positive) trial cylinders are used.

To the present writers, the technique seems to make the subjective examination even more complicated for the patient than the standard cross-cylinder technique. He is required to assess which of two positions shows less difference between two unclear limbs.

The Raubitschek arrow or paraboline chart

The writer's modification of the Maddox V and blocks used with the standard fan chart was described on page 104. The new V is a simplification of the Raubitschek arrow introduced by him in 1929 and later described in 1952. The arms of the arrow are curved, being almost parallel near the apex and curving away from each other as the base is approached (*Figure 19.9*). This parabolic form explains the alternative name of paraboline chart.

When the Raubitschek arrow is well off-axis, a length of one of the curves will appear sharp. As the arrow is turned away from the clearer limb, the sharp portion will pass up towards the apex of the arrow. The axis setting is correct when an equal portion of each limb appears clear.

Power determination

In the version of the Raubitschek arrow or paraboline chart produced by the American Optical Corporation, a dashed cross is superimposed to enable the power of the cylindrical lens to be determined, in a manner similar to (but less decisive than) the conventional blocks.

An alternative technique in which the Raubitschek arrow is used was described by Dunscombe (1933) and

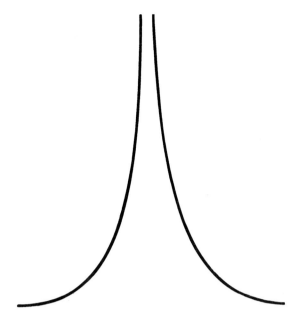

Figure 19.9. The Raubitschek arrow or paraboline chart.

O'Leary (1988). It relies on the fact that the axis of the resultant of two obliquely crossed cylinders of equal power and like sign lies mid-way between their axes. Thus, if the indicated minus cylinder axis were 20°, a trial cylinder would be placed at, say, axis 40°. The true cylinder correction at axis 20° may be regarded as correcting an ocular plus cylinder at axis 20°, which is astigmatically the same as a minus cylinder at axis 110°. Since the resultant axis of equally powered cylinders at axes 110° and 40° is 75°, the arrow tip should be pointed at 75°. Trial cylinders are then added at axis 40° until the two limbs of the Raubitschek arrow are equal. The cylinder is then turned back to 20°, and the usual fogging lens removed.

Laser-speckle refraction

When a broad divergent beam of coherent light from a laser falls on a roughly diffusing surface, an irregular speckled pattern will be seen. On moving the head, the speckle will appear to move 'with' or 'against' the head movement, depending upon the state of refraction of the observer's eye. This may be explained with the aid of *Figure 19.10*.

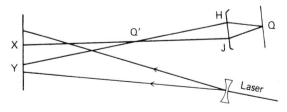

Figure 19.10. Laser-speckle refraction: relevant fringe formation is in the plane through Q′ conjugate with the retina.

---

* The diameter XY will depend both upon the pupillary aperture and the position of Q′.

A retinal element Q of the observer's eye having its image Q′ in the plane conjugate with the retina will receive light reflected from a large number of points in the area of the surface bounded by XY.* The individual wavefronts from each of these reflecting points retain constant-phase relationships with each other and are therefore capable of constructive or destructive interference. The fringe spacing due to any two points will depend upon their individual separation, but the eye sees the summation of countless fringe patterns giving the appearance of an irregular speckle in the retinal conjugate plane through Q′.

Consequently, for the myopic eye illustrated in *Figure 19.10*, a head movement will result in an against movement of the speckle pattern. To a hypermetropic observer, the fringe pattern becomes a virtual object apparently moving with the head movement. When the retina is conjugate with the surface, the speckle appears stationary.

Instead of moving the head, it is simpler to move the surface by using a drum rotating slowly at between 1 and 10 revolutions per hour. In this case, the plane of 'stationarity' (zero movement) is not the surface of the drum but lies between the surface and the axis of rotation. Its distance x_s from the latter is given by Charman and Chapman (1980) as

$$x_s = \frac{r \cos \phi \, (p + r \cos \phi)}{p \, (1 + \cos \phi) + r \cos^2 \phi} \tag{19.3}$$

where r is the radius of curvature of the drum (regarded as positive), p the radius of curvature of the incident wavefront (regarded as positive) and ϕ, the angle of incidence of the wavefront relative to the direction of observation.

For a plane incident wavefront, equation (19.3) reduces to

$$x_s = \frac{r \cos \phi}{1 + \cos \phi} \tag{19.4}$$

For a patient who is hypermetropic with respect to the plane of zero movement, the speckle moves 'against' the direction of the drum movement, while for a myopic patient the speckle moves 'with'.

Expressed in terms of the observer's viewpoint, the speckle moves with an apparent angular velocity Ω given by Charman and Chapman (1980) as

$$\Omega = \frac{-\omega r (K - V)}{V (r - x_s)} \tag{19.5}$$

where ω is the angular velocity of drum and V is the dioptric distance of the plane of zero movement from the plane of the observer.

The speckle velocity is thus proportional to the ametropia relative to the plane of zero movement.

The negative sign was prefixed to Charman and Chapman's expression to maintain the sign convention for angles. If the drum rotates anticlockwise, a with movement of the speckle results in a clockwise movement relative to the observer's position.

For conventional refraction purposes, the drum could be mounted at 6 m and the speckle movement eliminated (or reduced to random motion) by placing trial lenses before the eye. The rotation of the drum allows only the meridian perpendicular to its axis to be investigated at any one time. In the presence of an astigmatic error whose principal meridians are oblique to the drum, the perceived speckle motion will not be parallel to the motion of the drum surface but oblique. There is no simple way, however, of using the laser and drum to determine the axis of the astigmatic error. If this is first determined by conventional subjective techniques, the laser speckle can be used to measure the two meridional corrections, the drum being placed consecutively in these two positions. When the first meridian has been corrected, the speckle may appear to move along the drum axis.

Alternatively, multi-meridional refraction can be used. The apparent ametropia is measured in three or more regularly spaced meridians and an average sphero-cylindrical ametropia calculated to fit the results, a process similar to that used in some of the automatic objective optometers.

It was established experimentally by Haine *et al.* (1976) that meridional refraction by laser speckle measured the quantity $(S + C \sin^2 \theta)$ in the given meridian (*see* page 352). The six-meridian method was found to yield an accuracy comparable with that of subjective refraction. A similar conclusion was reached by Phillips *et al.* (1976).

Whitefoot and Charman (1980) compared the results of conventional subjective and laser-speckle refraction using both the multi-meridional method in six orientations and a twin-drum arrangement set parallel and perpendicular to the subjective astigmatic axis. The latter technique allowed the subject to observe both meridians almost simultaneously because sphero-cylindrical corrections were used. A detailed analysis of the experimental results from the two speckle refraction methods showed very little difference between them and close agreement with the conventional refraction.

Morrell *et al.* (1991) point out that the term plane of stationarity may be a misnomer when laser speckle is generated by a rotating drum if viewed from a close distance or in a Badal optometer system. If a large area of the drum is exposed, then the 'plane' of stationarity is probably curved so that the observation distance will depend upon which part of the area is viewed.

A disadvantage of the laser system is that a small proportion of patients are unable to perceive the speckle, possibly because their media are too irregular to allow the constructive/destructive interference to take place in their eyes. Another is that the light is necessarily monochromatic, requiring an allowance to be made for the longitudinal chromatic aberration of the eye[*] (Gilmartin and Hogan, 1985). The luminance of the speckle may also be much lower than that recommended for a conventional chart.

From a research standpoint, speckle refraction has several advantages over other subjective optometer systems for monitoring the accommodative state of the eye. For example, unlike Scheiner disc systems, it allows the whole pupil area to be utilized and gets around the difficulty of deciding upon the position of sharpest focus. Aberrations may, however, affect the laser refraction, since the central zones of the pupil could be giving an against movement and relatively more myopic peripheral zones a with motion; this could explain the random speckle motion seen at reversal.

It was frequently suggested that as the laser-speckle pattern did not act as a stimulus to accommodation, the duration of any exposure in monitoring accommodation response was of little importance. Hogan and Gilmartin (1984) showed, however, that an exposure shorter than the accommodative reaction time was needed to ensure consistent results. They recommended a duration of 300 ms.

Possible research uses include the investigation of instrument or proximal myopia, inadequate stimulus myopias and the accuracy of the accommodative response. References to some of these researches are made in Chapter 7 and in Charman and Chapman (1980).

Instruments based on laser speckle have been marketed to allow prospective patients to screen themselves on the need for (new) spectacles or a correction for night myopia when driving. Rubinstein (1987) found that laser-speckle refraction was not a reliable screening test for ametropia in children. It has been generally reported that patients with media opacities find the speckle difficult to perceive.

Some practical aspects of this test are brought out in Exercise 19.4.

Modifying Palmer's (1976) suggestion of using a finely ground glass screen, Bahuguna *et al.* (1984) have put forward an alternative system for speckle refraction. A slowly rotating drum carrying a series of torch bulbs illuminates a reflecting screen through an aperture which allows only one bulb at any instant to shine on to the screen. This is made from aluminium foil that has been pressed on to emery cloth, thus forming a rough reflector. Unlike the laser-speckle instrument, the pattern that is seen is not formed by interference fringes but by the distorted wavefronts from the individual reflection points.

Exercises

19.1 In laser-speckle refraction, a plane wavefront is incident, along the subject's visual axis, on a drum of radius *r*. What is the position of the plane of stationarity?

19.2 In laser-speckle refraction, the drum rotates at 0.01 revolutions per minute. If *r* is 100 mm, x_5 50 mm, the uncorrected refractive error −3.00 DS and the working distance −4 m, what is the apparent angular speed of movement of the speckle pattern? What does this speed become if a −2.00 DS trial lens is held before the eye?

19.3 A remote refractor system incorporates a projector lens of power +10 D effectively situated 300 mm in front of the patient's spectacle plane. From the simple paraxial relationship, calculate the power of the lens needed in the remote refractor plane to correct: (a) an emmetropic eye, (b) an eye −5.00 D

---

[*] Miller (1987) drew attention to the uncertainties about the eye's longitudinal chromatic aberration and the wavelength for which the eye was assumed to be in focus when viewing objects in white light. He concluded that research reports should provide basic technical information but leave it to individual readers to make whatever adjustment they deem appropriate. A useful list of references is given.

myopic, (c) an eye +5.00 D hypermetropic. Assume the test object to be at infinity. Verify your answers using equation (19.1).

19.4 A laser-speckle device is observed by a presbyope from a distance of 2 m while wearing his distance correction. Comment on (a) whether the speckle would appear to be stationary and (b) whether the 3-metre observation distance recommended is feasible for a device placed in a practice window.

References

ALVAREZ, L.W. (1967) Two-element variable-power spherical lens. US Pat. 3,305,294

ATKINSON, J., BRADDICK, O.J., DURDEN, K., WATSON, P.G. and ATKINSON, S. (1987) Screening for refractive errors in 6–9 month old infants by photorefraction. *Br. J. Ophthal.*, **68**, 105–112

BAHUGUNA, R.D., HALACARA, D. and SINGH, K. (1984) White-light speckle optometer. *J. Opt. Soc. Am. A*, **1**, 132–134

BENNETT, A.G. (1977) Some novel optical features of the Humphrey Vision Analyser. *Optician*, **173**(4481), 8–16

BROADBENT, H. and WESTALL, C. (1990) An evaluation of techniques for measuring stereopsis in infants and young children. *Ophthal. Physiol. Opt.*, **10**, 3–7

CHARMAN, W.N. (1995) Shearing systems with variable power. *Optician*, **209**(5490), 38–40

CHARMAN, W.N. and CHAPMAN, D. (1980) Laser refraction and speckle movement. *Ophthal. Optn*, **20**, 41–51

DHOLAKIA, S. (1987) The application of a comprehensive visual screening programme to children aged 3–5 years. Can a modified procedure be devised for visual screening for ancillary staff? *Ophthal. Physiol. Opt.*, **7**, 469–476

DUNSCOMBE, K.O. (1933) A new and remarkably sensitive test for astigmatism. *Br. J. Physiol. Optics*, **7**, 112–128

FLETCHER, R.J. (1961) *Ophthalmics in Industry*. London: Hatton Press

FREEMAN, M.H. (1992) A binocular simulator for visual experiments. *Ophthal. Physiol. Opt.*, **12**, 86

GILMARTIN, B. and HOGAN, R.E. (1985) The magnitude of longitudinal chromatic aberration of the human eye between 458 and 633 nm. *Vision Res.*, **25**, 1747–1753

GUYTON, D.L., ALLEN, J., SIMONS, K. and SCATTERGOOD, K.D. (1987) Remote optical systems for ophthalmic examination and vision research. *Appl. Opt.*, **26**, 1517–1526

HAINE, C., LONG, W. and READING, R. (1976) Laser meridional refractometry. *Am. J. Optom.*, **53**, 194–204

HOGAN, R.E. and GILMARTIN, B. (1984) The choice of laser speckle exposure duration in the measurement of tonic accommodation. *Ophthal. Physiol. Opt.*, **4**, 365–368

HUMPHREY, W.E. (1973) Variable astigmatic lens and method for constructing lens. US Pat. 3,751,138

INGRAM, R.M. (1977) Refraction as a basis for screening children for squint and amblyopia. *Br. J. Ophthal.*, **61**, 8–15

INGRAM, R.M., HOLLAND, W.W., WALKER, C., WILSON, J.M., ARNOLD, P.E. and DALLY, S. (1986a) Screening for visual defects in preschool children. *Br. J. Ophthal.*, **70**, 16–21

INGRAM, R.M., WALKER, C., WILSON, J.M., ARNOLD, P.E. and DALLY, S. (1986b) Prediction of amblyopia and squint by means of refraction at age 1 year. *Br. J. Ophthal.*, **70**, 12–15

INGRAM, R.M., WALKER, C., WILSON, J.M., ARNOLD, P.E., LUCAS, J. and DALLY, S. (1985) A first attempt to prevent amblyopia and squint by spectacle correction of abnormal refractions from age 1 year. *Br. J. Ophthal.*, **69**, 851–853

MILLER, R.J. (1987) The chromatic aberration adjustment in laser optometry. *Ophthal. Physiol. Opt.*, **7**, 491–494

MORRELL, A., WHITEFOOT, H.D. and CHARMAN, W.N. (1991) Ocular chromatic aberration and age. *Ophthal. Physiol. Opt.*, **11**, 385–390

O'LEARY, D. (1988) Subjective refraction. In *Optometry* (Edwards, K. and Llewellyn, R., eds), pp. 111–139. London: Butterworths

PALMER, D.A. (1976) Speckle patterns in incoherent light and ocular refraction. *Vision Res.*, **16**, 436

PHILLIPS, D.E., McCARTER, G.S. and DWYER, W.O. (1976) Validity of the laser refraction technique for meridional measurement. *Am. J. Optom.*, **53**, 447–450

RAUBITSCHEK, E. (1952) The Raubitschek arrow test for astigmatism. *Am. J. Ophthal.*, **35**, 1334–1339

REINER, J. (1966) Prüfung der Mehrstärken-Kontaktlinsen. *Klin. Mbl. Angenheilk*, **149**, 556–559

ROSSI, A. (1992) A review of vision screeners. *Optician*, **25** Sept., 14–18

RUBINSTEIN, M. (1987) Laser optometry. *Optometry Today*, **27**, 94–96

SHEINMAN, J. (1993) Screening made simple. *Optician*, **206**(5422), 22–28

THOMSON, D. (1994) A new approach to screening VDU users. *Optician*, **207**(5438), 23–28

WHITEFOOT, H.D. and CHARMAN, W.N. (1980) A comparison between laser and conventional subjective refraction. *Ophthal. Optn*, **20**, 169–173

WOO, G.C. and WOODRUFF, M.E. (1978) The AO SR III subjective refraction system: comparison with phoropter measures. *Am. J. Optom.*, **55**, 591–596

20

Measurement of ocular dimensions

Principal methods of measurement

General considerations

The ocular dimensions considered in this chapter are those affecting the eye's optical system. Various techniques of measurement have been applied to them. Although research is one motive, there are also clinical reasons for making certain measurements. For example, the change in corneal thickness may need to be monitored in contact lens practice. The depth of the anterior chamber is significant in potential closed-angle glaucoma and the axial length of the eye is an invaluable guide in the fitting of intra-ocular lenses. Certain simplifications may need to be made, as in the construction of schematic eyes. Most dimensions can nevertheless be determined to a satisfactory standard of accuracy.

Optical methods

Optical methods utilize the image-forming properties of the eye and its Purkinje images. One complication arises from the fact that a direct view of the eye's internal refracting surfaces cannot be obtained. What is seen or photographed is the image of the particular feature formed by all the eye's refracting surfaces lying in front of it. An error in the determination of one dimension, especially of the anterior corneal radius of curvature, may thus have repercussions when this quantity is used in the calculation of other dimensions. For simplicity, the eye is generally treated as a chosen three-surface schematic eye, such as the Bennett–Rabbetts model.

X-ray methods

X-ray methods are now in disfavour for safety reasons. Before this hazard was realized, they were successfully used in a number of investigations. They depend on the fact that X-rays can penetrate the eye and surrounding structures without being deflected and can stimulate the retina in its dark-adapted state. In 1938, Rushton described an apparatus he had devised for measuring the axial length of the eye. A narrow X-ray beam, in a plane perpendicular to the optical axis, is passed through the eye from the temporal side, a short distance in front of its posterior pole. Its intersection with the retina gives rise to the sensation of a luminous ring. As the beam is moved closer to the posterior pole, the diameter of the ring decreases. When it finally disappears, or only a very small disc is seen, the distance of the beam from the plane of the corneal vertex gives the eye's axial length.

An ingenious use of X-ray methods to determine the equivalent power of the eye was later devised by Goldmann and Hagen (1942). It is particularly simple when applied to emmetropic eyes. Two very narrow X-ray beams separated by 5.2 mm were directed into the eye from below at an angle of about 15° from the horizontal. To the subject they gave the impression of two luminous vertical lines which could be brought into apparent coincidence with two movable line markers when projected on to a screen or wall at a known distance. The separation between the markers was then measured. In emmetropia, the distance from the second nodal point to the retina (the reciprocal of the eye's equivalent power) could then be determined without significant error from the known dimensions. Goldmann and Hagen extended the same technique to ametropic eyes, the subject wearing a spectacle correction. It was then necessary to determine the axial length of the eye, for which purpose Rushton's method was used. From the data then available it was possible to calculate not only the equivalent power of the eye but also that of the crystalline lens.

Ultrasonography

Ultrasonography is a technique of spatial location or probing, particularly suited to the determination of axial dimensions of the eye. It is based on measuring the 'elapsed' or total time taken by an ultrasonic wave reflected from a boundary surface or obstruction to return to its point of origin. In ophthalmic applications, the wave frequencies commonly used are 10–20 MHz, well above the range of human audibility.

The choice of frequency is governed by conflicting considerations. A higher frequency has better resolution and will reveal thinner tissues than a lower one. For example, 20 MHz detects the posterior surface of the cornea, which 10 MHz fails to do. On the other hand, lower frequencies have more penetration and depict the vitreous/retina boundary more strongly.

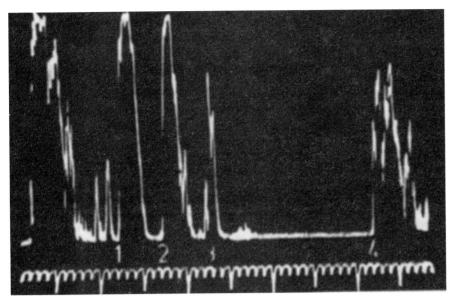

Figure 20.1.   An ultrasonic A-scan of an eye with advanced cataract. The transducer was dipped into a saline column held above the eye with a contact lens. Echoes beyond those of the transducer (far left) and bubbles in the saline are: 1 cornea, 2 anterior lens, 3 posterior lens and 4 retina. Some extra echoes caused by the cataract are seen between the principal lens echoes 2 and 3. (Reproduced by kind permission of the late Dr J.K. Storey, 1981.)

The ultrasonic waves are generated by a small transducer, which is activated by voltage pulses. The reflected waves are then amplified and rectified, the negative phases of the waveform being either suppressed or integrated with the positive by reversing their polarity. The resulting signal drives an oscilloscope display.

Ultrasonography can be performed in various ways. In the A-mode (time-amplitude), the direction of the ultrasonic beam is fixed. For measuring axial distances it would be aligned with the subject's visual axis. The oscilloscope display (with a 10 MHz frequency) then takes the form shown in the photograph in *Figure 20.1*. It is virtually a graph in which the amplitude of the reflected wave is plotted against elapsed time. The graduated scale shows time intervals in microseconds (μs). From left to right, the four numbered wave disturbances indicate the anterior cornea, the outer surfaces of the crystalline lens and the retina. Measurement should be taken from the beginning of each wave-form. In the photograph, the time interval between the cornea and anterior lens surface is approximately 5.0 μs, but this has to be divided by 2 because elapsed time includes the outward as well as the return travel. To convert time differences into distances requires a knowledge of the velocity of the ultrasonic waves in the medium in which they are travelling. These velocities are sensitive to temperature changes. The following values at 37°C are accepted generally:

Medium	Velocity (m/s)
Cornea	1550
Humours	1532
Crystalline lens	1641

Thus, from the photograph, the depth of the anterior chamber is approximately

$$(5.0/2) \times 10^{-6} \times 1532 \times 10^3 = 3.8 \text{ mm}$$

Accuracy in determining time intervals can be improved in various ways described in the literature. The most satisfactory is probably the use of an electronic interval counter.

Comparison of optical and ultrasonography measurements of the thickness of the crystalline lens led Koretz *et al.* (1989a,b) to suggest that the velocity of ultrasound in the lens was approximately linearly dependent on age and was given by the expression:

velocity (m/s) = $1733 - 2.830 \times$ age (years)

Current clinical instruments are stated to be accurate within ±0.1 mm to ±0.2 mm in the measurement of axial length, leading to possible errors up to 0.25 D and 0.50 D respectively in the calculation of refractive errors.

If the transducer is placed close to the eye, various disturbing effects are produced. They can largely be obviated if the beam is first made to traverse a column or tube of water held in contact with the cornea. Originally, this meant that the patient had to be supine, which is undesirable because the crystalline lens may then be axially displaced by gravity. A number of different 'stand-off' devices have since been designed. They not only allow the patient to be seated but also incorporate a means of controlling the fixation so that the beam can be accurately aligned.

The B-mode (intensity modulation) of ultrasonography is extensively used in the wide field of medicine for diagnostic and other purposes. It is capable of making a two-dimensional survey of soft tissue by scanning. The echo signals are processed in the same way as for the A-mode but the regulation of the oscilloscope display is different. In each direction of scan, any echo modulates the oscilloscope's electron beam so as to produce a spot proportional in intensity to the amplitude of the echo. If

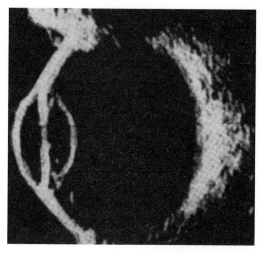

Figure 20.2. An ultrasonic B-scan of an eye. (Reproduced from part of a photograph by Dr G. Baum, 1965.)

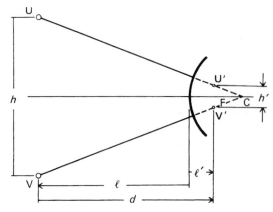

Figure 20.3. The principle of keratometry: formation by the cornea of a virtual image U′V′ at a predetermined distance d from the object UV.

no echo is received, the electron beam is suppressed. In effect, the display shown in *Figure 20.1* would be reduced to four spots, on a dark ground, denoting the positions of the corneal vertex, the poles of the crystalline lens and the retina.

As the direction of scan is varied by moving or rotating the transducer, the new intersections of the ultrasonic beam with the boundary surfaces are similarly plotted, rather as in a radar display. A complete cross-sectional view of the eye in the meridian scanned is thus built up (*Figure 20.2*). It bears a striking resemblance to the familiar diagram of the schematic eye. Unfortunately, it cannot be taken in its entirety as a true geometrical plan; in any direction of scan, the separation between surfaces represents time intervals, not distances. Because of the higher velocity of ultrasonic waves in the crystalline lens, the origins of echo waves passing through it are displaced forwards from their true positions.

There is now an extensive literature on ocular ultrasonography and its biometric applications. For further information, reference should be made to one of the specialized texts, such as the work by Coleman *et al.* (1977).

Corneal radii and power

Basic principle of the keratometer

Instruments designed to measure corneal radii or curvature are becoming generally known as keratometers.[*] An older term, 'ophthalmometer', is less suitable because it has a wider connotation, though it has been adopted in the International Standard, ISO 10343.

The keratometer was first used, in the 1840s, as a laboratory instrument for acquiring data on corneal curvature. Suitably adapted, it was then extensively used in the late nineteenth and early twentieth century as

an aid to refraction, especially of the astigmatic eye. For this purpose, an additional calibration in terms of corneal power was of greater utility. The instrument's main use now is in contact lens practice.

Keratometers utilize the reflected image (Purkinje I) formed by the anterior corneal surface.[†] As long ago as 1619, Scheiner had suggested a method of estimating the corneal radius from a set of glass spheres of known size. The examiner merely found which of them gave a reflected image of the same size as Purkinje I when held beside the subject's eye. A facing window was the test object. Whether Scheiner, a notable experimenter, himself used this technique is not stated. Subsequent progress, briefly reviewed by Stone (1975), has substituted accurate measurement for visual comparison.

In *Figure 20.3*, U and V represent the ends of an extended object, of height h, whose images U′ and V′ lie just short of the focus for reflection F of the cornea. In the standard paraxial expression for refraction,

$$\frac{n'}{\ell'} = \frac{n}{\ell} - \frac{n'-n}{r} \tag{2.1}$$

n' may be replaced by $-n$ to obtain the following expression for reflection:

$$\frac{1}{\ell'} + \frac{1}{\ell} = \frac{2}{r} \tag{20.1}$$

The magnification m for reflection is given by

$$m = h'/h = -\ell'/\ell \tag{20.2}$$

On multiplying equation (20.1) throughout by ℓ and using equation (20.2), we get

$$\ell = (m-1)r/2m$$

Similarly, on multiplying equation (20.1) throughout by ℓ', we get

$$\ell' = (1-m)r/2 = (m-m^2)r/2m$$

The positive distance d from object to image is therefore

$$d = -\ell + \ell' = (1-m^2)r/2m$$

---

[*] This name has also been given to a much simpler device (the Wessely keratometer), designed mainly for measuring vertex distances and visible iris diameters.

[†] Strictly, the pre-corneal tears film, assumed to be of negligible thickness.

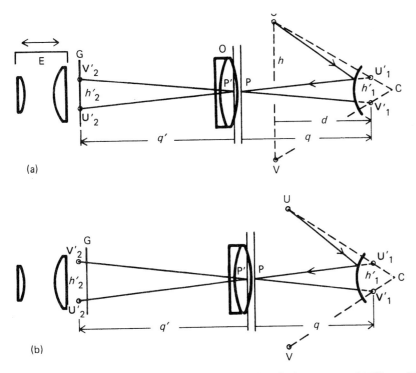

(a)

(b)

Figure 20.4. (a) Formation of the aerial image within the keratometer. (b) Effects of focusing error.

which gives

$$r = \frac{2dm}{1 - m^2} \qquad (20.3)$$

$$\approx 2dm \approx 2dh'/h \qquad (20.3a)$$

since m is small (0.03 to 0.04) and m^2 very small.

The position of the image $U'V'$ within the cornea prevents its direct measurement by superimposing a scale. Consequently, the keratometer incorporates a long-focus microscope (or short-focus telescope) whose objective O forms a second image in a plane accessible for measurement. The principle of the arrangement is illustrated in *Figure 20.4(a)*. To ensure that the magnification q'/q of the objective remains constant, a fixed graticule (reticle) G is placed in the predetermined image plane at a distance q' from the second principal point P'. The conjugate object distance q from the first principal point P is thereby also fixed. In use, the keratometer is moved bodily along the subject's visual axis until the second image $U'_2V'_2$ is seen in sharp focus on the graticule. Since the test object UV is fixed to the instrument and moves with it, the distance d attains its predetermined value simultaneously with q and q'. To bring the graticule crossline or other markings into sharp focus for the observer, the eyepiece E (of high power and small depth of field) can be adjusted independently. This adjustment must always be checked *before* the instrument is used.

The radii of curvature of an astigmatic cornea should be recorded as in the example

7.80 along 15/7.65 along 105

or

7.80 mer (or m) 15/7.65 mer (or m) 105

To prevent misunderstanding, the meridian along which the radius is measured should not be recorded as an 'axis', since the axis of an astigmatic lens is at right-angles to the meridian.

The same notation should also be used to record corneal powers. For example, assuming the calibration index to be 1.332, the above would become (after rounding off)

+42.50 along 15/+43.37 along 105

The corneal power could thus be considered to incorporate a +0.87 D cylinder at axis 15, but in terms of the correction needed the corneal astigmatism is −0.87 DC axis 15.

The effect of a focusing error is shown in *Figure 20.4(b)*. The eyepiece has not been adjusted and is in focus (for the user) for a plane behind the graticule. To see the mire images clearly, the user is obliged to move the instrument closer to the patient's eye. This has two consequences. First, the mires (a special pattern representing the test object) subtend a larger angle at C, the corneal centre of curvature, so that the image height h'_1 is increased. Secondly, the magnification by the objective is increased because the object distance q is shorter and the image distance q' longer. Thus, both errors increase the image height h'_2 and the radius of curvature recorded is too large.

A somewhat similar expedient may rarely be employed to extend the range of an instrument. If a lens of about +1.25 D is placed in front of the objective, then the instrument will have to be brought closer to the cornea, thus enlarging the image, and hence extending the range to smaller radii. Conversely, a negative powered lens will extend the range towards flatter radii.

Calibration graphs would need to be drawn from measurements of test spheres with the lens in place.

The doubling principle

Because of the patient's involuntary eye movements, the image height cannot be read off against a scale on the eyepiece graticule. Instead, the image size is measured by the lateral displacement of a doubled image. The principle of doubling and one practical method of producing it are both illustrated in *Figure 20.5*. A plano prism placed over one half of the objective can be moved along the optical axis. Rays passing through the prism are deviated by an amount proportional to the distance of the prism from the image. For simplicity, the diagrams show only the pencil initially directed towards the extremity V'_2 of the image. The deviated portion of it forms the doubled image point. In *Figure 20.5(a)* the image displacement δ of that part of the pencil intercepted by the prism is greater than the image size. There is hence a separation between the doubled images. In *Figure 20.5(c)*, the prism is much closer to the image. The displacement is smaller than the image size and so the doubled images overlap. At a certain intermediate position shown in *Figure 20.5(b)*, the displacement is exactly equal to the image size, so that the doubled images are just in contact. In various forms, this is the criterion used in keratometry for determining image size. It is not affected by eye movements because both images move together.

Mandell (1960) brought to light the fact that Jesse Ramsden, the English optician and instrument maker, constructed the first keratometer with a doubling device. It was described in 1796.

Keratometry of the astigmatic cornea not only requires measurement of the differing radii of curvature in its two principal meridians, but also a prior means of locating them. The instrument must therefore be rotatable about its optical axis. To locate the eye's astigmatic meridians, advantage is taken of the 'scissors' distortion arising on reflection from an astigmatic surface as well as on refraction by it. This has already been discussed on pages 234–236.

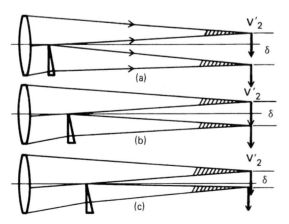

Figure 20.5. The doubling principle using a prism travelling along the axis. V'_2 is the upper extremity of the image $V'_2U'_2$ in *Figure 20.4*. Note: in this and subsequent figures up to 20.11 the ray path through the instrument is from left to right.

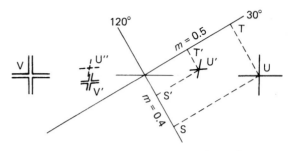

Figure 20.6. The position of the images U′ and V′ when the mires U and V are reflected by an astigmatic cornea. U″ is the doubled image formed by the keratometer.

The extended test object is often represented only by its extremities U and V in the form of special patterns called 'mires' (from the French, in which *mire* denotes a sighting mark). In one design, U is a fine cross and V a hollow cross into which the fine cross would be seen to fit symmetrically when the instrument was correctly adjusted. The doubling is effected in a direction parallel to the meridians containing U and V. For brevity, this meridian will be referred to as the measuring line.

Figure 20.6 shows the relative positions of U and V and of their reflected images U′ and V′ when the measuring line is horizontal but the cornea is astigmatic with its principal meridians at 30° and 120°. For the purpose of this scale drawing, the magnifications of the cornea for reflection were taken as 0.5 along 30° and 0.4 along 120°, both values considerably larger and with a greater proportional difference than in reality. Referred to the astigmatic axes, the co-ordinates of the centre of the single cross are SU and TU, while those of its image are S′U′ and T′U′ such that

$$S'U' = 0.5\, SU \text{ and } T'U' = 0.4\, TU$$

The position of U′ is thereby determined, and the same process was used to locate the extremities of the cross-line image. The image of the hollow cross is formed in the symmetrically equivalent position as shown.

Two points of note arise. First, the images U′ and V′ are on opposite sides of the measuring line. Consequently, the doubled image of U′ will appear in the position indicated by the dashed cross U″, out of register with the image of the hollow cross. Secondly, both images exhibit some degree of scissors distortion. The first effect is the more marked of the two and immediately indicates that the astigmatic meridians of the eye are oblique to the measuring line. The latter is then rotated, in this example to the 30° meridian. Both mire images then fall on the measuring line and are also free from scissors distortion. Adjustment of the doubling will bring them into correct register.

In some instruments, the mire consists of a complete circle surrounding the telescope housing, with external coincidence marks in the form of plus and minus signs as shown later in *Figure 20.11*. With an astigmatic cornea, the circle is imaged as an ellipse with its major axis parallel to the principal corneal meridian of longer radius. This is not always readily detectable, but the scissors distortion and displacement of the plus signs in off-axis settings operate essentially as shown in *Figure 20.6*.

Table 20.1 Classification of typical keratometers

Characteristics	Variable mire separation	Fixed mire separation			
Doubling	Fixed	Variable			
Position	Two	Two			One
Objective aperture	Full	Full	Divided		Divided
Typical instrument	Javal–Schiötz	Zeiss Ophthalmometer	Rodenstock	Zeiss CL 110	Bausch & Lomb
		G, H Gambs	Zeiss keratometer		
Doubling arrangement	Wollaston prism (bi-prism)	beam splitter and transversely moving lenses	Helmholtz inclined plates	Risley prism?	Axially travelling prisms

The height h'_2 of the image formed on the eyepiece graticule is that of the Purkinje image h'_1 multiplied by the fixed magnification q'/q of the objective (*Figure 20.4*). Doubling systems can be divided into two main types: fixed and variable. In the fixed type, the height h of the test object or the distance between the mires is adjusted to make h'_2 equal to the fixed amount of doubling. In variable doubling systems, h is fixed and the corresponding image height h'_2 is determined by the amount of doubling required.

It is possible to produce systems in which variable doubling can be effected simultaneously in two mutually perpendicular meridians. When these have been rotated into coincidence with the eye's astigmatic meridians, measurement of the two radii can be made in this one setting. Instruments using such systems are known as 'one-position' keratometers. The first (*see* Emsley, 1946) was designed by J.H. Sutcliffe, a former Secretary of the British Optical Association. Instruments with dou-

bling in one meridian only, requiring two separate settings for astigmatic eyes, are known as 'two-position' keratometers.

Some doubling systems require the telescope objective to be divided into separate areas, each transmitting only a portion of the incident reflected beam. In others, the doubling is effected with the aid of a full-aperture beam-splitting device. *Table 20.1* classifies many of the current makes of keratometers according to the characteristics of the doubling system used. We shall now look at six representative models in the following sections.

Some representative models

The Javal–Schiötz keratometer

This instrument (*Figure 20.7*) has changed little in essentials since its introduction in 1880 and the design is still popular. The doubling is fixed and the separation of

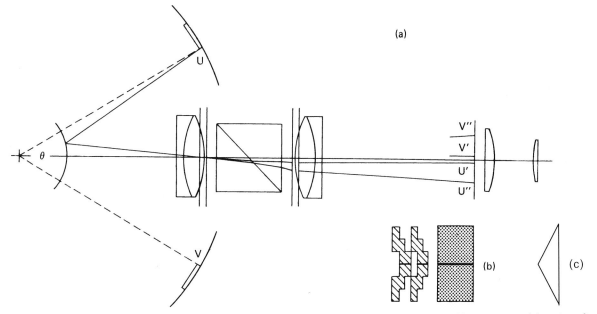

Figure 20.7. (a) Optical system of the Javal–Schiötz keratometer with fixed doubling. The variable separation of the mires alters their angular subtense θ at the corneal centre of curvature. (b) Pattern of the traditional mires, usually one green, one red. (c) The simpler bi-prism doubling system.

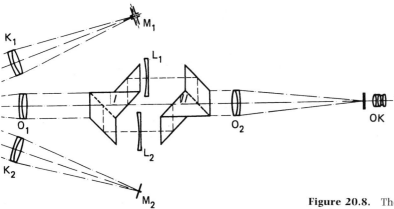

Figure 20.8.   The Zeiss (Oberkochen) Ophthalmometer
(Models G and H). (Illustration kindly supplied by Zeiss Ltd.)

the mires is varied by moving them symmetrically round a circular path approximately concentric with the cornea under test. A single control effects this movement. The fixed doubling is provided by a Wollaston double-image prism.* It is mounted between the two achromatic doublets comprising the telescope objective, so that the light passing through it is collimated. If a parallel pencil of rays is incident on such a prism, it emerges as two separated parallel pencils at a small fixed angle to each other.

The diagram shows the path of the chief ray of the pencil from the inner side U of one mire. After refraction by the second doublet of the objective, the two pencils emerging from the prism are focused on the eyepiece graticule to form the doubled images U′ and U″. Similarly, the inner extremity V of the other mire gives rise to the images V′ and V″. The separation of the mires has to be adjusted so as to make U′ and V′ coincide. As shown in the diagram, it is too great.

The traditional pattern of the mires is shown in *Figure 20.7(b)*. One is usually red and the other green, any overlap producing yellow. The steps on one of the mires give an approximate indication of corneal astigmatism. If the mires are set in apposition for the flatter meridian, an overlap of each step when the instrument has been rotated to measure the steeper meridian corresponds to 1 dioptre of astigmatism.

When the measuring line is in an off-axis position with respect to the cornea, the black central line of one mire image becomes out of alignment with its fellow on the other mire. Scissors distortion of the mires may also be apparent.

Cheaper copies of this instrument utilize a bi-prism instead of the Wollaston prism. As shown in *Figure 20.7(c)*, this would have its dividing line positioned on the optical axis, orientated perpendicular to the plane of the diagram. As this divides the objective aperture into two, errors caused by poor focusing are liable to be worse with this design than the original.

---

* A detailed description of this device, which depends on the bi-refringence of quartz, can be found in most textbooks on optics.

The Zeiss (Oberkochen) ophthalmometers G and H

These instruments (*Figure 20.8*), like the similarly designed Gambs instrument, are no longer in production. Their sophisticated optical design is free from the focusing errors discussed on page 381, and so is worth describing. The mires, which are of the pattern shown in *Figure 20.6*, are separately imaged at infinity by collimating lenses mounted with a fixed angle between their optical axes. By this means the size and separation of the Purkinje images are unaffected by errors in the intended working distance.

The objective of the observation system comprises two achromatic lenses O_1 and O_2. The first, acting as a collimating lens, is followed by a full-aperture beam-splitting prism which produces parallel intermediate optical axes. A weak lens of minus power (L_1, L_2) is placed on each of these axes in the plane containing the posterior principal focus of the lens O_1 after passage of the light through the prism. Variable doubling is produced by a lateral displacement of both lenses, in opposite directions, from the zero position in which their optical centres lie on the intermediate optical axes. The prismatic effects thereby created give rise to a variable angle between the two emergent beams. These are then recombined by another beam-splitting prism so as to pass through the second component O_2 of the objective to the fixed eyepiece OK.

The magnification of the objective system is constant by virtue of the fact that its two components O_1 and O_2 are separated by the sum of their focal lengths. It thus forms an afocal system. In all such systems, a parallel incident pencil emerges as a parallel pencil. The transverse magnification h'/h for an object at any finite distance is hence unchanged. Moreover, the afocal property of the objective system is unaffected by the doubling lenses L_1 and L_2 because they are situated at the common focal plane of O_1 and O_2.

Thanks to these main features of the design, the keratometer can be used both by emmetropes and ametropes without eyepiece adjustment. If the instrument itself is not correctly focused, some blurring may result but the readings will not be affected.

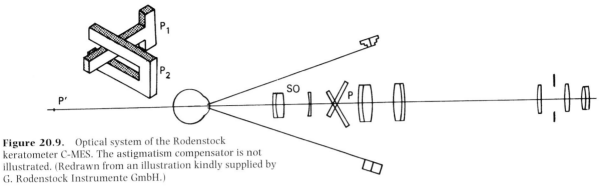

Figure 20.9. Optical system of the Rodenstock keratometer C-MES. The astigmatism compensator is not illustrated. (Redrawn from an illustration kindly supplied by G. Rodenstock Instrumente GmbH.)

The Rodenstock keratometers CES and C-MES

These are two-position variable-doubling instruments (*Figure 20.9*) in which the doubling is effected by tilted plates, a method first used by Helmholtz in 1854. They operate in a similar manner to those in the pachometer (*see* pages 309–310), the image displacement being dependent on their obliquity. The central plate P_1 tilts in one direction and the outer one P_2 in the opposite direction. Unless it is in accurate focus, the image formed by rays passing through the top and bottom sections of this plate will be doubled because the twin apertures act like a Scheiner disc. This out-of-focus doubling must not be confused with the measuring doubling.

In the current C-MES instrument, focusing errors are eliminated by a secondary objective system SO mounted in front of the Helmholtz plates to form a real image P', behind the patient's head, of the telescope entrance pupil P. If the instrument is moved too close to the eye under test, the mires subtend too large an angle. This is compensated by the greater distance of the Purkinje image from the effective entrance pupil P'. Because the Helmholtz plates effect a lateral and not an angular displacement, the doubling produced is not affected by changes in the object distance. An astigmatism compensator, adjusted to the corneal radius, neutralizes the astigmatism generated by the oblique path of the diverging beams through the plates.

The Zeiss keratometer attachment

This instrument (*Figure 20.10*) was designed as an attachment for certain of the same firm's slit lamps, but is no longer in production. It replaced the first or collimating objective of the microscope (*see Figure 16.4*). Collimated mires are used, as in the Zeiss ophthalmometer already described, but the doubling is effected by Helmholtz tilting plates. The combination eliminates focusing errors from this instrument also, since the tilting plates give the same sideways displacement irrespective of small changes in object distance. The images are viewed by the left eye, and the scale (not shown) by the right eye, the remaining part of the microscope system being used for this purpose.

The Zeiss CL110 ophthalmometer

This currently available instrument (*Figure 20.11*), like the Zeiss ophthalmometer already described, uses collimated mires to help avoid errors caused by poor focusing. The doubling system is placed in the second focal plane of the first objective, O_1, and hence is imaged at infinity behind the patient's eye, also contributing to the error-free design. The doubling is probably produced by Risley prisms D (see *Figure 11.20* and *Figure 20.11b*), with an outer annulus providing prismatic effect in one direction, and the central zone in the opposite direction. Filters R provide a red beam, possibly to reduce chromatic aberration from the prisms. The iris diaphragm A can be used to occlude the outer annulus, thus giving a single image for use with an accessory for measuring contact lens diameters. By employing the ends instead of the centre of the specially designed mires, measurement of soft lenses in a saline bath may be made without needing to convert the scale readings. Because the surface reflectance is low, this measurement requires a lot of light. The lamps of the mire system are therefore focused by condenser lenses C and projector lenses P on to the cornea. The instrument can measure over the radius range from 4.0 to 13.0 mm.

The Bausch and Lomb keratometer

The Bausch and Lomb keratometer, introduced in 1932, is the typical one-position instrument in current use (*Figure 20.12a*). It has been extensively copied in recent years.

A lamp bulb illuminates the circular mire M by means of the concave reflector A, inclined mirror BB and annular condenser C. This latter does not impinge on the reflected beam used for observation. A mask S behind the objective system O reduces it into four separated circular areas as shown in *Figure 20.12(b)*. Behind apertures 1 and 2 respectively are a horizontal and a vertical achromatic prism, producing independent variable doubling by movement parallel to the optical axis as in *Figure 20.5*. To equalize the optical path lengths, parallel plates of glass are mounted immediately behind apertures 3 and 4, which are used to form an undeviated image. Three images of the mire are thus seen in the eyepiece, a central one and two others doubled in mutually perpendicular directions, as shown in *Figure 20.12(c)*. Unless in correct focus, the central image will itself appear slightly doubled because of the Scheiner disc effect of apertures 3 and 4, which should not be confused with measuring doubling.

The plus and minus signs forming part of the mire pattern are used as fiducial marks. In any off-axis setting

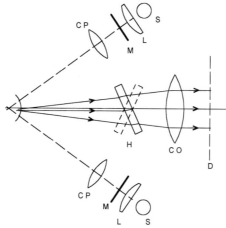

Figure 20.10. The Zeiss keratometer attachment. S lamp, L condenser lens, M mire, CP collimating projector lens, H Helmholtz tilting plate, CO collimating objective, D dividing line between the keratometer attachment and the Gallilean turret and remainder of the slit lamp microscope. (Redrawn from an illustration kindly supplied by Zeiss Ltd.)

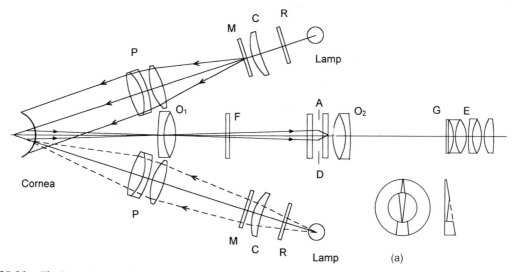

Figure 20.11. The Zeiss CL110 ophthalmometer. Key: mire projection system: R red filter, C condenser, M mire, P projection lens. Observation system: O_1, O_2 objective, F fixation stimulus, D doubling device, A aperture stop, G graticule for centration, E eyepiece. Inset (a) plan view and vertical cross-section of one element of the assumed variable prism doubling device. (Redrawn from an illustration kindly supplied by Zeiss Ltd.)

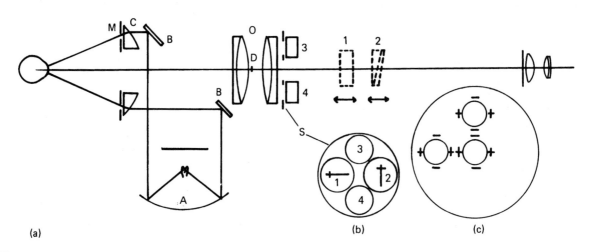

Figure 20.12. (a) The Bausch and Lomb keratometer. The dotted rectangle and prism in the main figure are the doubling prisms, positioned in front of and behind the plane of the diagram. The plane parallel compensating plates behind apertures 3 and 4 are shown behind plate S. (b) Subdivided areas of the objective. (c) Appearance in the eyepiece when correctly focused, but with too much doubling in both meridians.

of the measuring directions relative to the astigmatic meridians of the cornea, the radial limbs of the two adjacent plus signs will be out of register for the reason illustrated in *Figure 20.6*. When correct meridional alignment has been established, the two radius settings can be made in sequence by adjusting the doubling so as to bring adjacent plus and minus signs into exact coincidence.

A small mirror D mounted centrally between the objective lenses provides a fixation point for the patient, who sees a reflection of his own eye. Though theoretically superior to a fixation light since it ensures that the patient's eye is positioned on or very close to the instrument axis, this system is unsatisfactory if the patient has more than a small refractive error.

A ring-type mire as in the Amoils Astigmometer may also be used during cataract surgery to minimize induced corneal astigmatism.

A Drysdale-type keratometer

An accurate method of measuring short radii of curvature of optical surfaces is known after its originator as Drysdale's principle. It is used in the radiuscope or optical microspherometer, an instrument described in many textbooks on contact lenses. In brief, light from an illuminated object is reflected by a semi-silvered mirror behind the objective of a microscope to form an aerial image at the focus of the objective. When the focus is placed at the centre of curvature of the surface, the rays forming the image are normal to the surface and will thus be reflected back along their own paths. If the microscope is then moved away from the surface (assuming it to be convex), the convergent beam as a whole will be reflected back along its path when the focus is positioned at the surface with normal incidence. The object's reflection will therefore be seen in sharp focus through the microscope in these two settings, the distance travelled between them being the radius of curvature.

Applied to a keratometer, this arrangement would have the disadvantage that the subject's head could move between settings. It has been overcome in a keratometer designed by Douthwaite (1987). Simultaneous observation of both settings is achieved by placing a cylindrical lens, or a Stokes lens, behind the microscope objective which converges the incident beam. Two separated astigmatic line images are thus created. When the instrument has been moved so as to place the more remote image at the centre of curvature of the cornea, the other is then placed at the surface by axially moving the cylindrical lens or adjusting the Stokes lens. Experimental trials have given promising results.

Since only a small circular area of the cornea is covered in any one measurement, this instrument could readily be adapted for use in topographical keratometry.

Calibration of keratometers

In the keratometer, the image-forming rays are reflected from the cornea at a height of at least 1 mm from its vertex. Since the catoptric focal length of the typical cornea is approximately 4 mm, an effective aperture of 2 mm is large enough for spherical aberration to become significant. As a result, equation (20.3) derived from paraxial relationships cannot be used. In the design stage, calibration is presumably by exact ray tracing, subsequently checked with precision steel or glass balls. Instruments in clinical use should periodically be checked with a precision spherical surface, both for accuracy of radius and absence of skew or astigmatic misalignment.

Corneal power calibration

If the refractive index of the cornea is taken as 1.376, division of the anterior radius of curvature into 376 will give the dioptric power of its front surface. To find the equivalent power of the cornea as a whole would require a knowledge of its posterior radius of curvature and axial thickness.

Many keratometers, however, have a useful second calibration giving an approximate value of the corneal power. In Gullstrand's No.1 schematic eye, the equivalent power is +43.05 D and the anterior radius of curvature 7.7 mm. A single-surface cornea of this radius would have an equivalent power of +43.05 D if the refractive index of the aqueous humour were 1.3315. Moreover, the same figure would be obtained for other corneal dimensions, provided that the anterior and posterior radii were in the same proportion as in the Gullstrand eye, namely 7.7–6.8. The rear surface would then neutralize the same proportion of front-surface power in each case. This is the basis on which Olsen (1987) advocated 1.3315 as the notional index for power calibration. There is, however, a scarcity of data on posterior corneal radii which leaves the question in some uncertainty.

The calibration index adopted by current manufacturers varies from 1.332 (Zeiss) to 1.3375 (Haag–Streit and many others). This latter value, first chosen by Javal and Schiötz, was probably influenced by the fact that 7.5 mm corresponds exactly to 45 D. Interestingly, this same index is also obtained if the back vertex power of the Gullstrand cornea *in situ* is to be given by a surface of radius 7.7 mm. Intermediate values for the calibration index include 1.336 (American Optical). The writers consider this to be the best choice because it is the accepted value for the refractive index of the aqueous humour, and of tears, thus simplifying many contact lens calculations.

For average radii and small amounts of astigmatism, a useful rule of thumb is that a radius difference of 0.2 mm indicates approximately 1 D of corneal astigmatism. This rule may also be used to estimate the power of the tear lens trapped between a rigid contact lens and the cornea, and for the power change required on such a lens if the Back Optic Zone Radius (base curve) is altered.

The approximate calibration formula

$$r = 2\,dh'/h$$

suggests that for a variable doubling instrument, where h is fixed and h' measured, the radius scale is linear. In fact, although precise calibration results in a different relationship, it is still a linear one (Bennett, 1966). Conversely, in an instrument with fixed doubling and *h* variable, the power scale is uniform because curvature $R(1/r)$ is proportional to *h*.

Separation of measurement areas

In *Figure 20.4*, the chief ray leaving the upper mire U is shown being reflected off the cornea at a height slightly smaller than the height of the image U′. The approximate calibration formula shows that the image height *h*′ is proportional to the corneal radius. For variable doubling instruments, the two small zones utilized for measurement are therefore separated by a variable distance, approximately proportional to the radius. For a typical instrument, these areas may be separated by about 2.4 mm for a radius of 6.0 mm, increasing to 2.9 mm at 7.5 mm and 3.4 mm at 9.0 mm. Some instruments, however, measure across a smaller chord, for example the Gambs instrument utilizes around 2.2 mm at 7.5 mm, while the Bausch and Lomb keratometer spans almost 3.2 mm (Lehmann, 1967; Stone, 1994). Thus, apart from calibration errors, use of different instruments may result in slightly different readings for an aspheric surface. It must be emphasized that the keratometer does not measure the very centre of the cornea, but samples from zones just peripheral to the apex.

For a fixed doubling system, the mire separation *h* is adjusted to give a constant image height. There is thus only a very small variation in the separation of the reflection areas for the Haag–Streit instrument with increasing radius. Lehmann found a separation of around 3.5 mm at 7.0 mm, decreasing to 3.3 mm at 9.0 mm.

Measurement of contact lens radii

The keratometer can be used to measure the radii of curvature of contact lens surfaces. Normally, it is only the concave surface which requires to be checked because it affects the fit and also the power of the liquid lens formed between the contact lens and the eye. To dull the unwanted reflection from the convex surface, the lens is placed on a drop of water, with the light from the mires reflected downwards by a front-surface silvered or similar mirror. The lens mount and mirror are attached to the instrument's headrest.

To measure a soft lens, one method is to place it concave-side down in a cell filled with a saline solution and mounted on top of a 45° prism which reflects the light upwards. Because of the small difference in refractive index between the lens material and the solution, little light is reflected from the lens surfaces, so that a keratometer with a bright source is needed. Moreover, since light is reflected from both surfaces of the lens, relatively fine mires are necessary to allow the two sets of reflections to be distinguished. On a minus lens, the back surface is the steeper one and will produce the smaller image. The indicated radius of curvature has to be multiplied by the refractive index *n* of the saline, which reduces the true radius *r* to its 'equivalent mirror' value *r/n* (*see* Exercise 20.12).

If the mires are collimated, the keratometer readings

given for convex surfaces apply equally to concave surfaces. In other designs, an adjustment has to be made. Tables published for the Bausch and Lomb keratometer show that the radius recorded for a concave surface has to be increased by an allowance ranging from 0.02 mm on the shortest radii to 0.05 mm on the longest. For other instruments, a calibration graph could be plotted by measuring a number of contact lenses whose radii have previously been determined with a radiuscope. Quesnel and Simonet (1994) similarly recommend that for soft lens verification a calibration graph be drawn from PMMA lenses measured in saline. This overcomes the re-calibration for both the index of the saline and the measurement of the concave surface. The Zeiss CL110 ophthalmometer incorporates special mires enabling the normal scale reading to be employed for soft lens verification.

As pointed out by Stone (1962), the practice of specifying contact lens radii in terms of surface power based on a notional keratometer index is inadvisable because it wrongly assumes all keratometers to be calibrated for the same refractive index. For example, a +42 D power corresponds to a radius of 7.90 mm if the index used is 1.332, but 8.04 if the index is 1.3375.

Errors in keratometry

The accuracy of keratometry depends largely on the care with which the instrument to cornea distance is adjusted. This, in turn, requires accurate focusing of the eyepiece upon its graticule. To provide a diffusely illuminated background for this operation, the patient could be asked to close his eyes. The eyepiece is then screwed outwards to its most hypermetropic setting and then moved slowly inwards until the graticule markings just become clear. When the patient opens his eyes, the mire images should be brought into the centre of the field of view and the whole instrument moved back and forth to obtain the best focus.

Despite the provision of external sights to align the instrument with the patient's eye, this is not always easy because of the small field of view. Stone (1975) suggested shining a torch down the instrument from behind the eyepiece, so that a patch of light falls on the patient's face. The instrument is then moved to bring the light patch on to the eye.

While it is often stated that the conventional keratometer measures the central corneal radius, the instrument utilizes pencils reflected from small areas each situated not less than 1 mm and up to about 1.7 mm from the centre. Because of the peripheral flattening it is probable that the keratometer readings are slightly longer than the vertex radius. It is difficult to generalize, but the error would probably not exceed 0.05 mm on a normal eye.

Those instruments with doubling systems based on isolated areas of the objective aperture have an exit pupil of corresponding formation of possibly 3 mm overall diameter. Marked spherical aberration or irregular refraction of the examiner's eye will upset the apparent instrument focus, especially if the head is moved. In one-position instruments, uncorrected astigmatism of the observer's eye may similarly affect the focus.

While a local distortion of the cornea in the region of the reflection area or areas will cause a corresponding distortion of the mire, it can also render uncertain the focusing of those instruments with Scheiner disc doubling. The mire can then appear clear but double, or single but blurred: or, if of circular form, part may be single and part doubled. Since the keratometry image is formed by reflection from the tear layer, variations in this may affect both the quality of the image and its size. Relative movement between the two mire images immediately after a blink is a frequent occurrence while the tear layer stabilizes. If the patient is requested to blink, then to stare and refrain from blinking, the duration after the blink until the mire image distorts is an indicator of tear quality – one of several techniques to evaluate the non-invasive tear break-up time (NIBUT). Cronje-Dunn and Harris (1996) found that artificial tears on a plastics artificial cornea increased the variance of keratometry readings considerably. Being viscous, they are, however, unlikely to wet the plastic corneas as uniformly as natural tears do the real eye.

Charman (1972) investigated the limits set by diffraction on the precision of radiuscopes and keratometers, other sources of error being excluded. He found that for typical keratometers the limit on reproducibility could not be lower than about 0.2 D, corresponding to a spread of about +0.04 mm on average radii, though scale graduations finer than this are frequently provided.

From a review of experimental findings, Clark (1973a) suggested an average figure of 0.015 mm for the standard deviation of a series of radius readings. Since 95% of a normal distribution probably lies within two standard deviations from the mean value, Clark's estimate is in reasonable agreement with Charman's findings.

The Humphrey Auto-keratometer

This is an automated instrument of an entirely new and sophisticated design, providing information beyond the scope of the conventional keratometer. It measures corneal curvature by projecting three beams of near infrared light on to the cornea in a triangular pattern within an area about 3 mm in diameter. After reflection, they are received by directional photo-sensors which effectively isolate rays making a predetermined angle with the instrument's optical axis. In principle, although the ray paths are reversed, this recalls a variable doubling keratometer in which the mires subtend a constant angle at the cornea.

Figure 20.13 shows a simplified scheme of ray paths in one of the three beams. The source S is a light-emitting diode (LED) focused by condenser L to form an image S′ on the instrument's axis. This image, in turn, acts as an object for projector lens P which forms a second image S″ behind the patient's eye. One ray RH of the reflected beam – not necessarily the central one through L – passes into the detector D at the predetermined angle.

The precise location of the reflection point R on the cornea is determined by the position of the rotating chopper C which sweeps across all three beams and is imaged in the plane of the cornea by projector lens P. Since the image S″ lies on the axis at a known position, the angle at which the incident ray GR meets the cornea can also be determined. From the information provided by all three beams, the principal radii and meridians of the cornea on the visual axis can then be calculated by the internal computer.

At the start, the patient fixates a central red LED while the instrument is aligned approximately by the operator and accurately by its own monitoring and servo-systems. The two beams in the same horizontal plane are then positioned on each side of the visual axis, with the third beam below it. In general, skew reflections occur unless the corneal astigmatic meridians are exactly horizontal and vertical.

Peripheral readings are then taken with the subject's fixation directed in turn at 13.5° to either side of the central fixation mark. Their purpose is to provide the additional data needed to determine the quasi-ellipsoidal surface giving the best fit to the cornea. The parameter e^2 defining the 'shape' of this hypothetical surface in its horizontal meridian is included in the print-out, together with the estimated position of its apex relative to the visual axis. The calculated principal radii and meridians at the apex of this surface are also recorded in addition to those measured on the visual axis of the true cornea.

A more detailed account of this instrument is given by Rabbetts (1985).

The Canon and Topcon Auto-keratometers

Canon produce both a separate auto-keratometer, the K-l, and another, the RK-l which is combined with an auto-refractor. Descriptions have been given by Port (1985) and Stockwell (1986). An annular lens projects collimated light from a ring mire on to the cornea. The eye is viewed by means of an internal television system which enables the reflected mire image to be focused and centred within a ring displayed on the TV monitor. The operator then triggers an electronic flash positioned behind the ring mire. Another image of the mire reflection is projected on to a photo-detector system consisting of five 72° sectors. From the light distribution on each of these sectors the computer is able to calculate the corneal radii. A central fixation light is normally used, but for peripheral keratometry further lights are provided to enable fixation to be displaced by 10° in any of the four cardinal directions. The diameter of the

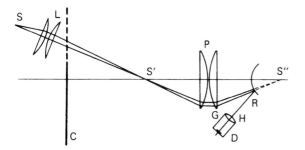

Figure 20.13. Principle of the Humphrey Auto-keratometer. (Drawn from information kindly supplied by Humphrey Instruments Inc.)

measuring zone was shown by Ehrlich and Tromans (1988) to be slightly larger than that of the Bausch and Lomb (manual) instrument. Other auto-keratometers are manufactured by Nidek and Topcon. The Topcon instrument employs an optical system similar to that introduced by Mandell and St. Helen (1971). In this, the observation system is telecentric, a pinhole aperture in the posterior focal plane of the objective restricting the rays reflected from the cornea to paths parallel to the instrument's axis.

Multi-meridional keratometry

If the misalignment of the mire images in the direction perpendicular to the doubling system is ignored, keratometry readings may be taken in meridians positioned between the principal astigmatic ones. If these readings are plotted against keratometer orientation, they will lie on or very close to a $\sin^2 \theta$ curve, where θ is the angle between the keratometer orientation and the steeper principal meridian. Conversely, measurements in three or more meridians enables the corneal curvature to be calculated without initially determining the orientation of the principal meridians. This is similar to the determination of ocular refractive error from an analysis of the refractive error measured in three oblique meridians – *see* pages 352–353. Royston *et al.* (1989b) and Rosenfield and Portillo (1996) have suggested this technique of keratometry may provide acceptable results. It is possible that some of the automated keratometers employ this principle.

The keratometer and ocular astigmatism

Keratometer readings of power and astigmatism assume the anterior and posterior corneal radii to be in a fixed ratio. If astigmatism is present, the principal meridians of the two surfaces are assumed to be in alignment, with the fixed ratio in operation in both of them. With effectivity taken into account, the back surface will then neutralize just over one-ninth of the front-surface astigmatism. Should these assumptions not hold good for any given eye, the keratometer reading of astigmatism will become inaccurate as a measure of the total corneal astigmatism. Such errors are seldom likely to be significant.

Non-corneal factors contributing to ocular astigmatism are the two surfaces of the crystalline lens and astigmatism due to oblique incidence. This may be caused by a tilt of the crystalline lens or of the cornea, so that its apex is decentred with respect to the visual axis. Nevertheless, since the cornea is the dominant element of the eye's refracting system, a highly astigmatic cornea is likely to result in a similarly astigmatic ocular refraction.

Javal's rule

During the period when the keratometer was used as an aid to refraction, Javal (1890) formulated a tentative statistical relationship between corneal and ocular astigmatism. If the latter is represented by the power C of the correcting cylinder in the spectacle plane, and the corneal astigmatism A by the keratometer reading, Javal's rule (with all quantities in dioptres) can be expressed as

$$C = 1.25A - 0.50 \tag{20.4}$$

The corneal astigmatism A is regarded as positive when with the rule and negative when against. Expressions similar to Javal's were arrived at by other researchers. Javal emphasized that the coefficients in his expression were approximations and that further terms may need to be added in the light of advancing knowledge and improved methods of refraction, among which he included retinoscopy. Though no longer of clinical use, Javal's rule throws an interesting light on the sources of ocular astigmatism.

Cylinder effectivity

Javal's rule raises the question of effectivity, the change in vergence from the spectacle plane to the cornea or vice versa. Unless the mean spectacle refraction M (sphere + half-cylinder) and the cylinder power C are both quite small, vergence changes become significantly different in the two principal meridians. This is best demonstrated by a numerical example. Suppose the spectacle correction is

$$+5.00/-2.00 \times 90$$

at a vertex distance of 14 mm. The ocular refraction K in the two principal meridians can be found as follows:

Vertical meridian

	D			mm
F_{sp}	+5.00	$\rightarrow$	f'_v	+200
			$-d$	−14
K	+5.38	$\leftarrow$		+186

Horizontal meridian

	D			mm
F_{sp}	+3.00	$\rightarrow$	f'_v	+333.33
			$-d$	−14
K	+3.13	$\leftarrow$		+319.33

Ocular refraction: $+5.38/-2.25 \times 90$

In this example, M is $+4.00$ D. For all positive values of M, the spectacle cylinder is smaller than the ocular astigmatism. The reverse applies when M has a negative value.

If the vertex distance is denoted by d and the ocular astigmatism by Ast, use of equation (2.12) leads quickly to the close approximation

$$C \approx (1 - 2dM)\text{Ast} \tag{20.5}$$

Crystalline lens

Javal's rule implies that the eye's total astigmatism includes a contribution of 0.50 D against the rule, unaccounted for by the keratometer reading. It *could* arise from a tilt of the crystalline lens about a vertical axis, but *Figure 12.3* shows that the tilt would need to be about 14°, twice the amount of actual tilt regarded as normal (*see* page 209).

From a limited number of measurements made by Tscherning (1924), showing the posterior corneal radius in the vertical meridian to be disproportionately short, he tentatively suggested that this might be a contributory element to the 0.5 D of astigmatism against the rule in Javal's expression.

It is possible that marked corneal astigmatism is accompanied by astigmatism of the same type, though smaller in degree, of one or both surfaces of the crystalline lens. This was Javal's own explanation of the coefficient 1.25 in his rule.

Javal intended his expression to apply only when the eye's principal meridians are approximately horizontal and vertical. If the corneal and lenticular components are at different axes, the resultant ocular astigmatism will have its axis in yet another direction in accordance with the theory of obliquely crossed cylinders. Extensive tables and graphs by Neumueller (1953) give the summation effects of corneal and non-corneal astigmatism at differing axes.

Decentration of corneal apex

As shown in *Figure 20.14* (and explained more fully on page 208), if the cornea resembles a conicoid with its apex at A, the surface becomes astigmatic at all other points. Suppose the visual axis passes through P, a point in the vertical meridian above A. At this point, the (tangential) radius of curvature PC_T in the vertical meridian is longer than the (sagittal) horizontal radius PC_S. A keratometer reading from this area would therefore show against the rule astigmatism. On the other hand, unless the angle of incidence were quite small, a pencil of parallel rays *refracted* at this point would become *more* convergent in the tangential than in the sagittal meridian, producing an element of with the rule astigmatism. A similar but opposite reversal would result from a horizontal displacement of the corneal apex.

An excess of tangential over sagittal power for oblique pencils is a common feature of converging surfaces and lenses. As shown by *Figure 15.10*, it is exhibited by the eye as a whole, making the final tangential image shell more steeply curved than the sagittal.

It is now recognized that decentration of the corneal apex is common. In an early study of eight subjects, Mandell and St. Helen (1969) found a mean difference

of the order of 0.35 D between readings taken along the visual axis and at the corneal apex. No directional pattern of displacement emerged. On this evidence, apical decentration can be regarded as contributing a random element to the total ocular astigmatism. Mandell *et al.* (1995) examined 20 eyes with videokeratography (*see* page 394), to find that the corneal apex fell below the visual axis in 18 eyes, with slightly more lying nasally than temporally, with a mean displacement of 0.82 mm and a mean difference in radius of 0.06 mm.

Rigid contact lenses with spherical surfaces substantially neutralize the corneal astigmatism as indicated by the keratometer reading. Hence, any residual astigmatism with the contact lens in use should be predictable by comparing the keratometer reading with the spectacle correction found by refraction, after allowing for effectivity. Decentration of the corneal apex may account for those cases in which the residual astigmatism is found to differ significantly from the amount predicted.

Corneal topography

Introduction

The study of corneal topography presents many complications, not only experimental. To simplify it at the outset while providing a basis for elaboration, it is convenient to assume the corneal profile in any meridian to be a conic section. The curvature would thus vary continuously from the centre outwards. Except near the limbus, this must be so because any discontinuity, even if physically smooth, would seriously affect the cornea's optical imagery. For this reason, the notion of a 'corneal cap', a central area of some 4 mm diameter having uniform spherical or toroidal curvature, can be misleading. It would be more correct to say that within such an area the effects of curvature variation are too small to be detected with certainty by the conventional keratometer.

The revolution of a conic about an axis of symmetry generates a conicoid. In *Figure 20.14*, the conic is an ellipse with its apex or vertex at A and its axis of symmetry AA'. The point C_0 is the centre of curvature of the surface at A, the distance AC_0 being the vertex radius r_0. For practical purposes, the apex can be defined as the point of maximum curvature or shortest radius. The curved line C_0E is one branch of the evolute of the conic, formed by the intersection of neighbouring normals to the surface from points on the opposite side of the axis. Every normal meets the evolute tangentially.

At any point $P(x, y)$ other than the vertex, the surface is astigmatic, having two principal radii of curvature in mutually perpendicular meridians. In the tangential meridian, coinciding with the plane of the diagram, the centre of curvature is at C_T where the normal touches the evolute. In the sagittal section, perpendicular to the tangential and containing the normal, the centre of cur-

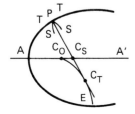

Figure 20.14. (a) Observer's view of an astigmatic cornea. (b) Principal radii of curvature at a peripheral point P on a conicoid: centres of curvature C_S (sagittal) and C_T (tangential). Arcs SS and TT are in the mutually perpendicular sagittal and tangential sections.

---

* For a fuller treatment of the mathematics of conic sections in relation to the cornea and contact lenses, the reader is referred to the papers by Burek (1987) and Bennett (1988a).

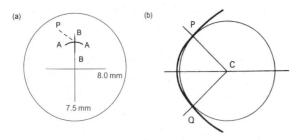

Figure 20.15. (a) Observer's view of a toric cornea showing with the rule astigmatism; central radii 8.00 along 180° by 7.50 along 90°. Radii along AA 8.04 mm, along BB 7.64 mm. (b) Cross-section through a spherical and an ellipsoidal surface having common normals at P and Q and hence giving the same keratometer readings. The radius of curvature of the spherical surface is the sagittal radius of the ellipsoid at P and Q.

vature is at C_S where the normal intersects the axis. As stated on page 208, the equation to a conic[*] can be put in the form

$$y^2 = 2r_0 x - px^2 \qquad (12.1)$$

Instead of the parameter p, some writers use Q for $(p - 1)$, some the 'eccentricity' e for $(1 - p)^{1/2}$, and others the confusingly named shape factor for $e^2 = (1 - p)$.

The sagittal radius of curvature r_S (PC$_S$) is given by

$$r_S = \{r_0^2 + (1 - p)y^2\}^{1/2} \qquad (20.6)$$

and the tangential radius r_T (PC$_T$) by

$$r_T = r_S^3 / r^2 \qquad (20.7)$$

For example, taking a typical value of 0.7 for p and $y = 1.5$ mm, equations (20.6) and (20.7) give $r_S = 8.04$ and $r_T = 8.13$ mm when $r_0 = 8$ mm and $r_S = 7.54$ and $r_T = 7.64$ mm for $r_0 = 7.5$ mm. As shown by Bennett and Rabbetts (1991), and confirmed experimentally by Douthwaite and Burek (1995), the dimension measured by the conventional keratometer is effectively the sagittal radius of curvature at the reflection point (*Figure 20.15*). Even though it is the tangential image that is aligned by the doubling system, the tangential radius cannot be measured because its centre of curvature does not lie on the axis of observation (*Figure 20.14*).

For similar curves of a higher order, *Figure 20.14* applies in principle but the values of r_S and r_T need to be determined by the methods of differential calculus. For a cornea that is not a surface of revolution, the terms sagittal and tangential are perhaps ill chosen, and the terms axial (denoting the distance along the normal to the axis) and instantaneous are preferable. *Figure 20.15(a)* shows the observer's view of an astigmatic cornea with apical radii of 8.0 along the horizontal meridian and 7.5 mm along the vertical. At a peripheral point P, the radius of arc BB will be the instantaneous (tangential) radius, say 7.64 mm, as in *Figure 20.14*. Along AA, however, the radius will be the axial (sagittal) radius appropriate to the horizontal meridian, i.e. 8.04 mm. When the keratometer is aligned to measure the vertical meridian, the radius determined is that of the circle centred at C, radius 7.54 mm, as shown in *Figure 20.15(b)*.

The aim of corneal topography is to obtain a close approximation to the corneal surface in a mathematical formulation. This may be an equation to the surface or of its profile in different meridians. Another approach is to define the surface in terms of its departure from a reference sphere in contact with its apex. For example, one method would be to specify the difference Δz in the sags of the two surfaces at a given distance y from the axis. This is a quantity of great interest in contact-lens fitting. Alternatively, the distance between the two surfaces could be measured along a normal to the corneal surface making a specified angle with the axis. This was the method used by Bonnet (1964) in his work on corneal topography. In a critical review of these various systems, Clark (1973b) advocated a modification of Bonnet's. In his view, the distance between the corneal surface and a touching reference sphere, not necessarily of radius r_0, is more conveniently measured along the normal to the reference sphere, not to the corneal surface.

Topographical keratometry

An instrument designed for peripheral as well as central keratometry was described in 1964 by its inventor, R. Bonnet. It was manufactured by Guilbert–Routit & Co. of Paris but is now out of production. An essential feature was that only one of the two small mires was used for peripheral measurements, so as to restrict the reflection area to a minimum. A different doubling system was then operated to make one end of the single mire image coincide with the opposite end of its duplicated image.

Following the work of Mandell (1962) a number of conventional keratometers can now be supplied or fitted with attachments for topographic use. Some provide a range of fixation points to control ocular rotation, while others allow central fixation by means of supplementary mires subtending a larger angle at the cornea. The reflection points are thus at a greater distance from the visual axis.

The results need to be processed to obtain the most useful information. Wilms and Rabbetts (1977) have detailed two different systems of measurement and calculation. One, which is of general application, enables the p (or e) parameter of the matching conic to be determined for each of the two principal meridians of an astigmatic cornea. Thus, by providing a fixation point 30° below the instrument's axis, the radius along an arc such as AA in *Figure 20.15(a)* may be determined. Correcting this value by the difference in the central astigmatic corneal radii gives an approximate value for the sagittal radius for the vertical meridian, and hence the p-value. The other system is for specific use with the Rodenstock keratometer and its topographical accessories.

A radically different approach was made by Douthwaite and Sheridan (1989). The idea was to measure the corneal radius at two known different apertures, without eccentric fixation. From the results it is possible to calculate the corneal asphericity in terms of the parameter p in equation (12.1). For this purpose, a Bausch and Lomb keratometer was modified by increasing the distance between the minus signs on the mire (*see Figure 20.12c*) and maintaining correct calibration by altering the power of the travelling prism for that meridian. By this means the diameter of the zone measured was increased to about 6 mm, approximately double the normal value. In use, the corneal curvature is first measured conventionally in the meridian using the plus signs on the mire. The instrument is then rotated through 90° and the same meridian measured with the larger mire. The results[*] were found to be in good agreement with those given by the Guilbert–Routit topographical keratometer and the PEK (described in the section immediately following).

General reviews of the subject have been given by Mandell (1981), Sheridan (1971, 1989) and Stone (1994).

Keratoscopy and photokeratoscopy

Introduction

The keratoscope is a device for studying the corneal contour over a relatively large area, whether for clinical purposes or for investigating corneal topography. Its origins and evolution have been researched by Levene (1965). Its simplest practical form is the hand-held Placido disc introduced in 1880. This consists of a flat disc with a series of concentric black and white rings. It is illuminated by a light placed above or beside the patient's head, the corneal reflections of the bright rings being examined through a central aperture furnished with a magnifying lens. Since the outer ring subtends a larger angle at the patient's eye than the mires of a keratometer, visual inspection can be made of a central corneal area 4–6 mm in diameter. The Klein keratoscope is a similar device but is internally illuminated.

Marked astigmatism causes the reflected rings to appear elliptical, while surface irregularities due to scars or keratoconus produce distorted or asymmetrical reflections, as in *Figure 20.16*. Controlled displacement of the patient's fixation allows the regularity of peripheral areas to be assessed, or, in keratoconus, the approximate position of the corneal apex, at which point the reflected rings show the least asymmetry. As Levene (1962) has pointed out, a keratoscope must be held normal to the line of sight, otherwise a false impression of corneal toricity is given.

The keratoscope may be converted into a quantitative instrument by attaching a camera to photograph the images. It is then called a photokeratoscope. The earlier models had a flat ring surface like the Placido disc, but

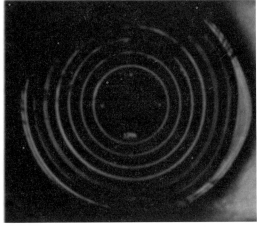

(a)

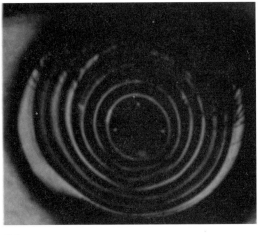

(b)

Figure 20.16. Photographs produced with the Photo-electronic Keratoscope: (a) a normal cornea, (b) a cornea with keratoconus. (Reproduced by kind permission of Mr A.G. Sabell, 1983, and the British Contact Lens Association.)

this design has two disadvantages: it restricts the corneal area that can be examined and gives a curved image surface, making it impossible to obtain a photograph with all the rings in sharp focus. A hemispherical object surface concentric with the cornea provides much larger coverage and was found to give a flatter image. A further step forward was the demonstration by Ludlam and Wittenberg (1966) that the system giving the flattest images was a series of rings arranged to lie on an ellipsoidal surface. For certain applications, there are also advantages in the use of Polaroid 'instant' photography.

The data provided by the measured dimensions of the ring images needs to be processed to yield the information desired. One requirement is to determine, for a given point on any ring image, the location of the associated reflection point on the cornea, which is related to the sagittal radius of curvature at that point. This may be seen from *Figure 20.15*, in which the normals to an ellipsoidal surface from the opposite points P and Q are the same as those for the inscribed sphere with its centre at C and of radius PC, which is also the sagittal radius of curvature of the ellipsoid at the point P (com-

---

[*] Although their calculations were based on the assumption that the keratometer measured the tangential radius of curvature, Douthwaite and Burek's (1995) data shows that there is very little difference in the apical radius derived from this or from the basis of sagittal measurement. There is a marked difference, however, in the p-values depending on the basis of calculation. Lam and Douthwaite (1994) present a computer program to solve for r_0 and p, given the normal and widely separated mire K-readings and the ray incidence heights on the cornea.

pare with *Figure 20.14*). The same principle applies to keratometry with central fixation.

Calibration with a set of steel balls, though useful as a check, is inadequate if the asphericity of the cornea is to be deduced. For this purpose, a number of different mathematical procedures have been evolved by various researchers including Wittenberg and Ludlam (1966), Townsley (1967), and El Hage (1971). These and others are appraised in a review by Clark (1973c) which evoked a rejoinder (Townsley and Clark, 1974). A review of more recent techniques is given by Fowler and Dave (1994).

An instrument designed specifically for contact-lens practice was the Wesley-Jessen Photoelectronic Keratoscope (PEK) described by Bibby (1976). It had seven rings on an ellipsoidal surface, the smallest reflected from a corneal zone approximately 3 mm in diameter and the largest from a 9 mm diameter zone. From an enlargement of the original Polaroid transparency, the relevant dimensions of the reflected rings were determined by photoelectronic scanning. The results obtained were then computer processed to locate the two principal meridians and a series of points on the profile of each of them. The position of the corneal apex relative to the visual axis was also determined, together with the vertex radius and 'shape factor' e^2 (or $[1 - p]$), defining the conic with the best matching profile for each of the two principal meridians.

An auto-collimating photokeratoscope, claimed to give greater accuracy than then obtainable by other means, was designed and described by Clark (1972). The mathematical theory and operational procedure were also explained in detail.

Much light on corneal topography has been thrown by some extensive studies carried out with these instruments.[*] Using the Wesley-Jessen PEK, Townsley (1970) examined the eyes of 350 contact lens patients. The conic sections giving the best corneal fit in the horizontal and vertical meridians were then determined. For normal eyes, the curve was found to be elliptical with *p*-values ranging from 0.84 to 0.19, the mean being 0.70.

Over the entire sample, the range of *p*-values was from 1.49 to −0.96, the mean being 0.80 in the horizontal and 0.84 in the vertical meridian. Values of *p* less than 0.2, including negative values (which denote hyperbolas) generally indicated keratoconus. A small number of eyes were found to have *p*-values in excess of unity, denoting a prolate ellipsoid (formed by revolution about the minor axis) with peripherally *steepening* curvature.

Using Clark's auto-collimating instrument, Kiely *et al.* (1982) examined 176 healthy eyes of 49 male and 39 female subjects aged 16–80. For the best-fitting conic they found a range of *p*-values from 1.47 to 0.24. The highest value is nearly the same as Townsley's, while the absence of values below 0.24 is explained by the fact that no cases of keratoconus were included in the sample. The mean *p*-value was 0.70, very close to Town-

sley's. Further topics investigated by this team were the variation in asphericity in different meridians of the same eye and the effect of peripheral flattening on the eye's spherical aberration.

More recently, Guillon *et al.* (1986) examined 200 healthy eyes of 65 females and 45 males covering a wide range of ages and refractive errors. The instrument used was the PEK keratoscope. As in previous studies, a large spread of *p*-values was found. In the flattest corneal meridian, 30.9% of the total fell within the range 0.7–0.8 and 30.5% within the range 0.8–0.9. In the steepest corneal meridian, the corresponding percentages were 21.4% and 33.6%. Chinese eyes have been studied by Lam and Loran (1991) and Lam and Douthwaite (1996). Both sets of workers found the mean keratometry readings to be similar to those of Caucasians, but with higher *p*-values, 0.82 in the horizontal, 0.86 in the vertical meridian, indicating less peripheral flattening.

Some other methods of investigating corneal topography are described by Kawara (1979) who used moiré fringe techniques and de Cunha and Woodward (1993) who illuminated the cornea obliquely from the nasal and temporal sides with vertical planes of light. Fluorescein dye in the tear film enabled the intersection of the planes with the cornea to be photographed electronically, and the resulting data processed by computer. This technique is claimed to be superior to other methods for investigating irregular corneas. A somewhat similar technique is provided in a commercially available instrument, the PAR corneal topography system: in this, a grid of light is projected on to the cornea from one side, and the resulting intersection pattern photographed obliquely from the side. Two of the advantages listed by Belin *et al.* (1995) are that the instrument does not have to be positioned along the visual axis, and can provide results even if the corneal surface is non-reflective.

Computerized videokeratography

The development of relatively inexpensive personal computers has enabled the introduction of many instruments in which the image of the keratoscope rings are recorded electronically, and fed directly to the computer for measurement and subsequent processing – a technique called videokeratography. These videokeratoscopes, or videokeratometers, enable the corneal shape to be analysed very quickly and to be presented graphically upon the computer screen. They usually have more rings situated closer together than the Wesley-Jessen PEK and therefore should give better detail.

The mathematical treatment presented here mostly follows that of Doss *et al.* (1981) and Klyce (1984). To simplify the discussion, the rings of the keratoscope faceplate are assumed to lie in a flat plane perpendicular to the instrument's axis – the actual position of the rings in the typical curved array can be allowed for by merely changing the co-ordinates in some of the equations, while Fowler and Dave (1994) assume a hemispherical faceplate whose centre of curvature is coincident with the centre of curvature of the cornea.

The first step in the analysis is to find the centre of the

---

[*] Results were given in different parameters, but to facilitate comparison have been converted into *p*-values as used in equation (12.1) and illustrated in *Figure 12.1*.

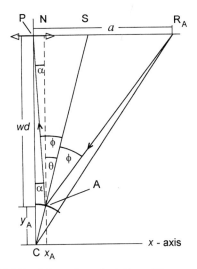

Figure 20.17. Scheme for calculation of the co-ordinates of the point A where the chief ray from ring R_A is reflected into the photographic system at P.

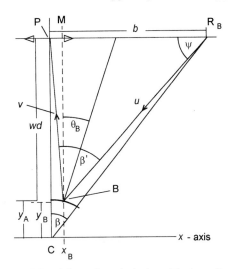

Figure 20.18. Scheme for calculation of the co-ordinates of the point B where the chief ray from the next ring R_B is reflected into the photographic system at P.

image of the smallest ring, since this gives the origin from which all image measurements are made. The radius of this image is initially used to calculate the central corneal radius. In *Figure 20.17*, the origin of the x and y co-ordinates is taken to be the centre of curvature C of the central cornea in the meridian investigated. The first principal point P of the objective is assumed to lie in the same plane as the faceplate, with the first ring R_A of radius a lying a working distance wd from the cornea. Unlike keratometry where the mire's image height is investigated, we are now interested in the position of the point A on the cornea where the ray from the mire R_A is reflected to enter the objective at P. If the co-ordinates of this point are x_A and y_A, then the distance CP is given by:

$$CP = y_A + wd$$

if the tiny difference between y_A and the corneal radius for this ring is ignored. The radius of the first ring image, divided by the instrument's magnification, gives the x_A co-ordinate of the reflection point.

If the reflected ray entering the objective subtends the angle α at P, then:

$$\tan \alpha = x_A/wd$$

while the angle $R_A\hat{A}N$ equalling $(2\phi - \alpha)$ is given by:

$$\tan (2\phi - \alpha) = (a - x_A)/wd$$

If CAS is the normal to the cornea at the reflection point, angle $S\hat{A}N$ is given by:

$$\phi = \theta + \alpha$$

which can be rearranged to give

$$\theta = \tfrac{1}{2}(2\phi - \alpha - \alpha)$$

From the small triangle at the origin,

$$x_A = y_A \tan \theta$$

whence

$$y_A = x_A/\tan \tfrac{1}{2}\{\arctan [(a - x_A)/wd] - \arctan (x_A/wd)\}$$

and the central radius can be calculated from

$$r_A = x_A/\sin \theta$$

The next step is to obtain an estimated value for the y-ordinate for the reflection point B of the next ring R_B, situated at radius b from P. In *Figure 20.18*, the distance b subtends an angle β at the centre of curvature of the cornea. The angles of incidence and reflection will be approximately $\beta/2$, and as an initial trial, this value is also taken for the angle θ_B. *Figure 20.19* shows the small section of the cornea in the zone AB. The point D has co-ordinates x_A, y_B so the distance DB or Δx equals $(x_B - x_A)$, while distance DA equals $-\Delta y$ or $-(y_B - y_A)$. If tangents are drawn to the cornea at A and B, they will make the same angles θ_A and θ_B with the x-axis as the normals to the cornea do with the y- or instrument axis.

A geometrical construction enables the value for Δy to be predicted from the difference Δx. A line is drawn through B parallel to the tangent at A, and then perpendiculars to it are dropped from A and D to meet it at E and G respectively, with DG continuing to intersect the tangent through A at H.

Then, from triangle DBG,

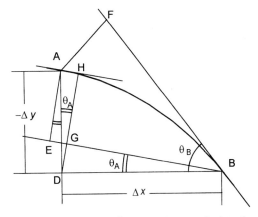

Figure 20.19. Geometrical construction to calculate the difference Δy in the y-ordinate from Δx, the change in the x-co-ordinate of the reflection point from one ring to the next.

$$GB = \Delta x \cos \theta_A$$

and, from triangle ADH,

$$AH = -\Delta y \sin \theta_A$$

and as AE and HGD are parallel,

$$AH = EG$$

so

$$EB = \Delta x \cos \theta_A - \Delta y \sin \theta_A$$

By drawing a tangent to the corneal profile at B and dropping the perpendicular to it from A to meet it at F, it may similarly be shown that

$$FB = \Delta x \cos \theta_B - \Delta y \sin \theta_B$$

For the small length of arc AB, the lengths EB and FB are similar. Thus equating the two equations and solving:

$$y_B = y_A - \frac{(x_A - x_B)(\cos \theta_A - \cos \theta_B)}{\sin \theta_A - \sin \theta_B} \qquad (20.8)$$

Returning to *Figure 20.18*, this initial value for y_B may now be substituted to determine a more accurate value for the angles β' and θ_B. Thus if

$$d_A = wd + y_A$$

and if u and v are the lengths of the raypaths R_BB and BP,

$$u^2 = (b - x_B)^2 + (d_A - y_B)^2$$

$$v^2 = (d_A - y_B)^2 + x_B^2$$

and by the cosine rule from the triangle R_BBP

$$\beta' = \arccos \left[(b^2 - u^2 - v^2)/(-2uv) \right]$$

From triangle R_BBM, where M is the normal to the faceplate from B,

$$180° = \pi \text{ radians} = \pi/2 + \beta'/2 + \theta_B + \psi$$

and

$$\psi = \arctan \left[(d_A - y_B)/(b - x_B) \right]$$

so that

$$\theta_B = \pi/2 - \beta'/2 - \arctan \left[(d_A - y_B)/(b - x_B) \right]$$

By substituting this value for θ_B into equation (20.8), a refined value for y_B can be obtained. This iteration is continued until a negligible change in y_B occurs.

The whole process is then repeated for each ring in turn to the edge of the keratoscope image. Since the peripheral radii are calculated as a function of the central radius, any errors in this will result in errors of scale for the periphery.

The corneal radius at B may be calculated in at least three ways. First, it may be regarded as that of the inscribed circle tangential to the cornea at B – see *Figure 20.15* – giving the axial radius (*see page 392*) as

$$r_B = x_B/\sin \theta_B$$

Secondly, *Figure 20.20* assumes a small section of the cornea to have the same radius r_i at three neighbouring reflection points, E, F and G. The co-ordinates (h, k) of the instantaneous centre of curvature C_i can be calculated from the equations given in Klyce (1984) and the

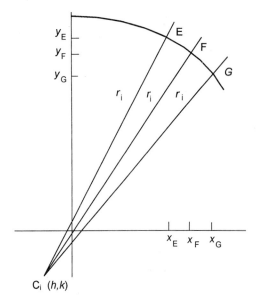

Figure 20.20. One method for calculating an approximate value for the instantaneous radius of curvature r_i of the cornea at reflection point F.

radius for the central point F from

$$r_i = \sqrt{(x_F - h)^2 + (y_F - k)^2}$$

Because both these methods give a discontinuous profile to the cornea with an abrupt change corresponding to each ring, Klein (1992) developed equations and a simple computer program generating a smooth curve. The instantaneous radius can also be obtained by fitting a curve to the x- and y-co-ordinates of the cornea, and then differentiating this twice. Chan *et al.* (1995) found that the elliptical model chosen for the normal corneal curve was unable to provide accurate values for the instantaneous radius for keratoconic eyes.

By repeating the whole process for meridians at 1–2° intervals, these instruments can determine the corneal toricity, and display central 'keratometry readings' generated by the mean radii along the principal meridians over the central 3 mm diameter reflection zone, and the orientation of the principal meridians in peripheral zones of the cornea. The equations derived above require that the incident and reflected rays both lie in the same plane as each other and with the instrument's axis, an impossibility for all except the principal meridians of an astigmatic cornea. Halstead *et al.* (1995) approached the problem from the opposite direction. Rather than trying to calculate the corneal shape from the image dimensions, they used trial and error in the form of computer iteration to model the corneal shape that gave the image. Skew refraction could then be incorporated.

These computerized videokeratoscopes also display the corneal profile in terms of power maps. In general, they are often programmed to convert radius to power by the simple paraxial equation $F = 337.5/r$. This assumes that the ray bundle is incident normally on the corneal surface, something definitely untrue for the peripheral cornea where oblique incidence will give rise to spherical aberration. To some extent, spherical aberration can be incorporated by calculating the point of intersection with the instrument axis of a ray incident initially parallel with the axis. This, however, ignores the effects of aberrations from the crystalline lens, and can hardly be reconciled with a conversion for the instantaneous radius. This use of power rather than radius may result from the preference in the USA to give keratometry readings in terms of corneal power rather than radius. Thus Salmon and Horner (1995) recommend that these power maps should be interpreted as dioptric curvature maps, while Applegate *et al.* (1995), like Bonnet and Clark (*see* page 392), recommend that the elevation of the cornea relative to a spherical surface may be the best method for portraying corneal shape.

Typical plots and the use of the instrument in contact lens practice are given by, for example, Burnett Hodd and Ruston (1993) and Stevenson (1992, 1995). The interested reader is referred to the November 1995 and 1997 issues of *Optom. Vis. Sci.*, **72** and **74**, which are devoted to computer-assisted corneal topography.

Angle alpha

The angle alpha between the optical and visual axes is conveniently measured with apparatus similar to Tscherning's ophthalmophakometer. This consisted of a graduated circular arc, supported on a stand, with an observing telescope T mounted in a central aperture of the arc (*Figure 20.21*). For various purposes, lamps and fixation objects could be attached to the arc and moved along it, the subject's eye being placed at its centre of curvature.

To measure the angle alpha, two lamps are placed one above and one below the telescope, so as to give rise to separated pairs of Purkinje images I, III and IV. With the subject initially fixating the telescope, the effect of angle alpha is to displace the images horizontally by various amounts so that they appear out of alignment to the observer. A small fixation object F is then moved along the arc until the six Purkinje images are brought into the best vertical alignment obtainable. The axis of the telescope is now assumed to coincide with the eye's optical axis, so that the angular scale reading at F gives the angle alpha. If the whole apparatus is rotated through 90°, the vertical component of angle alpha can be determined by the same procedure.

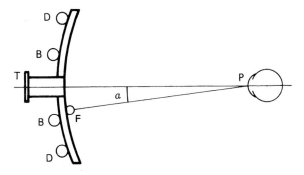

Figure 20.20. Basic features of Tscherning's ophthalmophakometer and its use in measuring angle alpha.

Tscherning (1924) found it to be generally of the order of 2–3°, with the visual axis in object space upwards from the optical axis. Like Tscherning, Dunne *et al.* (1993) found the visual axis to lie 5° temporal to the optical axis, intersecting the nasal retina. They also measured the objective refraction for the nasal and temporal retina. The plot of astigmatism, surprisingly, fell to a minimum around 9° nasal to the fovea. They concluded that this difference was produced by asymmetries in the ocular refracting surfaces.

As indicated by its name, the ophthalmophakometer can also be used, as described by Tscherning, to measure the radii of curvature of the crystalline lens surfaces, the thickness of the lens and the depth of the anterior chamber.

Corneal thickness

A comprehensive review of methods of measuring corneal thickness has been given by Ehrlers and Hansen (1971). Some in which the slit lamp is used were described on pages 309–310. Ehrlers and Hansen considered the Jaeger pachometer method to be not only simple but also the most accurate. All optical methods require the anterior corneal radius r_1 to be determined and a value for the corneal refractive index n to be assumed. From a mathematical analysis of the possible errors arising from an error in measuring r_1 and a variation in the value of n, Patel (1981) considered the Jaeger method with illumination normal and viewing oblique to be marginally superior to the others. The relative error of each method was expressed as the ratio $\delta t/t$. When the value of 40° is assigned to the obliquity of observation θ in Jaeger's method, Patel's expression reduces to

$$\delta t/t = 4.8\,\delta a + (3.6 \times 10^{-3})\,\delta r_1 + 0.87\,\delta n \qquad (20.9)$$

where a is the oblique width of the slit lamp section as in *Figure 16.11*.

Depth of the anterior chamber

Slit-lamp methods were described on pages 309–310. The pachometer has the merit of convenience, though ultrasonography will simultaneously provide other axial separations that might be needed. An ingenious method devised by Lindstedt was improved by Stenström (1953). A well-corrected objective is masked by a plate with four radial slits, one in each half of the 45° and 135° meridians. Rays from a small light source pass through the 135° slits to form one image of the source. Rays passing through the 45° slits are first intercepted by a narrow minus lens of low power, thus forming a second image at a greater distance from the objective than the first. Measurement of the apparent depth of the anterior chamber is obtained by adjusting the apparatus and the axial position of the auxiliary minus lens so that the two images fall simultaneously on the poles of the cornea and anterior lens surface respectively.

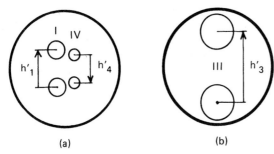

Figure 20.22.   Purkinje images of a double light source: (a) shows the first and fourth images, (b) the third image.

Phakometry

Radii of curvature

The theory of equivalent mirrors applied to a three-surface schematic eye provides the simplest basis for the calculations involved in phakometry (*see* pages 217–220). In the three-surface eye, it is the second surface which gives rise to Purkinje III and the third surface to Purkinje IV. These images are used to determine the radii of curvature of the relevant equivalent mirrors. There are two different techniques for measuring their relative sizes.

Comparison phakometry

Two circular sources in the same vertical plane are arranged so as to give rise to twin Purkinje images I and IV as shown in *Figure 20.22(a)*. The distances between their centres, h'_1 and h'_4, can each be regarded as the height of a single Purkinje image of the same extended object of height h. Applied to the three-surface schematic eye, equation (12.21) gives

$$r'_3 = r_1(h'_4/h'_1) \tag{20.10}$$

in which r'_3 is the radius of the equivalent mirror corresponding to the posterior lens surface.[*]

The ratio (h'_4/h'_1) is determined by photographing the images, which are almost in the same plane. Since r_1 is known from keratometry, the value of r'_3 can be found from equation (20.10).

Similarly, the radius r'_2 of the equivalent mirror corresponding to the anterior lens surface is given by

$$r'_2 = r_1(h'_3/h'_1) \tag{20.11}$$

Because the Purkinje III image is about 7 mm behind the plane of I and IV, a second photograph is taken with Purkinje III brought into sharp focus to measure h'_3 (*Figure 20.22b*). The value of h'_1 is taken from the first photograph.

---

[*] Smith and Garner (1996) point out that equations (20.9) and (20.10) assume a distant test object. It may be more convenient to have the light sources closer to the eye, either at a fixed distance from the eye or attached to the camera. Corrected equations are given for these conditions, while Garner (1997) gives an iterative computer scheme.

Tscherning's method

Tscherning's method, suited to his ophthalmophakometer, is the inverse of the comparison method. Two bright lamps BB (*Figure 20.21*) are fixed in position so that their Purkinje images III are visible to the observer. The positions of two dimmer lamps DD are then adjusted so that their twin Purkinje I images have the same separation between centres as the Purkinje III pair. To give images h'_1 and h'_3 of the same size, the conjugate object sizes h_1 and h_3 must be inversely proportional to the equivalent mirror radii r_1 and r'_2. Accordingly,

$$r'_2 = r_1(h_1/h_3) \tag{20.12}$$

Applied to Purkinje image IV, the same method gives

$$r'_3 = r_1(h_1/h_4) \tag{20.13}$$

Experimental difficulties in phakometry with particular reference to Purkinje III images have been discussed in detail by Fletcher (1951).

Determination of actual radii

To determine the actual radius r_2 corresponding to the equivalent mirror radius r'_2 it is necessary to know the apparent depth d'_1 of the anterior chamber in addition to its real depth d_1 as given by the pachometer reading or otherwise. The apparent depth can be found from the conjugate foci relationship, which gives

$$d'_1 = \frac{d_1}{n_2 - d_1 F_1} \tag{20.14}$$

where d_1 is the true depth of the anterior chamber, n_2 is the refractive index of the aqueous humour and F_1 the power of the single-surface cornea.

In *Figure 20.23*, A'_2 is the vertex of the equivalent mirror, C'_2 its centre of curvature, and r'_2 its radius of curvature $A'_2C'_2$. From the diagram,

$$A_1C_2 = d_1 + r_2$$

and

$$A_1C'_2 = d'_1 + r'_2$$

Since C_2 and C'_2 are conjugate by refraction at the

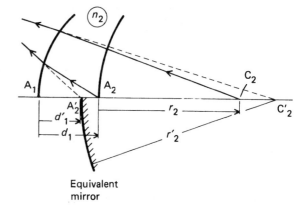

Figure 20.23.   True and apparent depths of the anterior chamber, and the equivalent mirror corresponding to the front surface of the lens.

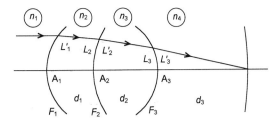

Figure 20.24. Step-along method for calculation of crystalline lens surface powers.

cornea,

$$\frac{n_2}{d_1 + r_2} - \frac{1}{d'_1 + r'_2} = F_1 \qquad (20.15)$$

From which r_2, the only unknown, can be determined.

The more complicated operation of determining the posterior radius r_3 from the equivalent mirror radius r'_3 has been detailed by Bennett (1961). It is, however, unnecessary even to measure r'_3 if the ocular refraction K is known and the eye's axial dimensions have been found from ultrasonography. In this event, phakometry can be confined to the anterior surface, thus arriving at its surface power F_2. To find the power F_3 of the posterior surface, an axial pencil from the eye's far point is traced through the eye by the step-along method (*Figure 20.24*). The vergence L_3 at the posterior lens surface is thereby determined, while the value of L'_3 required to focus the pencil on the retina can be found from

$$L'_3 = n_4/d_3$$

where n_4 is the refractive index of the vitreous and d_3 the distance from the posterior pole of the lens to the retina. Finally,

$$F_3 = L'_3 - L_3 \qquad (20.16)$$

Dunne's method, avoiding measuring Purkinje III

An alternative scheme for calculating the optical components of the eye was suggested by Dunne (1992) to avoid using Purkinje III. This was for three reasons: Purkinje III is poor since it is formed by reflection at the shagreen-like anterior lens surface; a separate photograph is required since the image lies deeper in the eye than the others, and Dunne was interested in recording Purkinje II, and equipment for generating the two corneal images is inappropriate for forming an image from the anterior lens surface.

If the posterior corneal radius is ignored, then keratometry, ultrasonography and photography of Purkinje I and IV are needed. A hypothetical trial value for the anterior lens power F_2 is initially assumed. As shown in *Figure 20.24*, a ray trace through the eye enables the vergence of light L_3 incident on the back surface of the lens to be calculated, while the vitreous depth gives the image vergence L'_3, and hence an initial trial value for the posterior lens back surface power. By calculating the image positions of the posterior pole A_3 and centre of curvature C_3 formed by the anterior lens and cornea,

the equivalent mirror radius r'_3 is found, and hence the ratio r'_3/r_1. If this ratio does not agree within a stipulated tolerance with the figure determined experimentally from the photograph of Purkinje IV and I, a new trial value for F_2 is needed. Computer iteration or a graphical solution can be used to find an optimum value for F_2, which then gives the correct value for F_3. For the Bennett–Rabbetts schematic eye, the ratio r'_3/r_1 is -0.789.

Equivalent power of the crystalline lens

When its radii of curvature and axial thickness are known, the surface powers of the crystalline lens and its equivalent power F_L can be calculated from the expressions given on page 211.

If neither radius is known, a close approximation to the equivalent powers of the lens and also of the eye itself can be calculated from a method devised by Bennett (1988b). This is based on the assumption that the shape of the crystalline lens of the relaxed schematic eye is a reasonable approximation to that of the subject's own lens, and hence that the principal points of the real crystalline may be located to a sufficient accuracy by those of a schematic lens of the same thickness. The data required are the spectacle refraction (F_{sp}) at a specified vertex distance (v), the corneal power (F_1) obtained from keratometry, and the axial separations of the refracting surfaces and retina, found from ultrasonography.

The thickness of the crystalline lens is known. If the positions of its principal points P_2 and P'_2 can reliably be conjectured, the two separate surfaces can then be ignored and the lens replaced by its theoretical Gaussian equivalent of power F_L (*Figure 20.25*).

Let us assume that values have been allotted to e_2 and e'_2. Since the eye's far point M_R is conjugate with the retina, a paraxial pencil from M_R must, after emerging from the lens, be focused at the axial point M'. All the required axial distances are known, and so the vergences L_2 and L'_2 can be calculated by the normal procedure. The rest then follows.

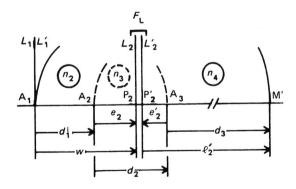

Figure 20.25. The crystalline lens of the schematic eye replaced by its Gaussian equivalent of power F_L, the positions of the principal points P_2 and P'_2 having been conjectured. The value of F_L is given by the vergences L_2 and L'_2, found from the axial ray trace as explained in the text.

The required values of e_2 and e'_2 can be determined as follows. From the equations given on page 254 we can write

$$e_2 = A \cdot d_2$$

where

$$A = (n_2/n_3)(F_3/F_L) \qquad (20.17)$$

and

$$e'_2 = -B \cdot d_2$$

where

$$B = (n_4/n_3)(F_2/F_L) \qquad (20.18)$$

If the lens of the schematic Bennett–Rabbetts eye is taken as the norm, the numerical values will become

$$e_2 = 0.599\, d_2$$

and

$$e'_2 = -0.353\, d_2$$

It will be seen from the above equations that the ratio B/A is equal to F_2/F_3, which means that the positions of the principal points vary with the form or profile of the lens. This can also be expressed as the quantity Q defined by

$$Q = F_2/F_L$$

indicating the proportion of the total lens power contributed by its front surface. For the Bennett–Rabbetts eye, $Q = 0.375$.

If the actual but unknown Q-value of a real eye is not 0.375, the values of A and B produced by the computing scheme will be incorrect for that eye. The resulting errors in the calculated values of F_L and F_e are directly proportional to the difference between the real and assumed Q-values and will be quite small in most cases. At both ends of the range of actual Q-values from 0.28 to 0.48, which is thought to cover all but exceptional lens configurations, the error in F_L would not exceed ± 1.0 D, and the consequential error in the value of F_e would not exceed ± 0.5 D. From this point of view, the new method compares favourably with phakometry. This was confirmed by Royston *et al.* (1989a), but may no longer be true with more precise techniques of ophthalmophakometry (Mutti *et al.*, 1992). Their use of video-recording meant that several photographs of the image could easily be taken and averaged. They also used collimated mires and a narrower angle between these and the camera to improve accuracy.

A possible computing scheme is set out below.

1. $L_1 = F_{sp}/[1 - vF_{sp}]$
2. $L'_1 = L_1 + F_1$
3. $e_2 = 0.596\, d_2$
4. $e'_2 = -0.358\, d_2$
5. $w = d_1 + e_2$
6. $L_2 = L'_1/[1 - (w/n_2)L'_1]$
7. $\ell'_2 = -e'_2 + d_3$
8. $L'_2 = n_4/\ell'_2$
9. $F_L = L'_2 - L_2$
10. $F_e = F_1 + F_L - (w/n_2)F_1F_L$

Thus, if an eye has the following measurements:

$$F_{sp} = +6.00 \text{ DS}$$

at a vertex distance of 16 mm

$$F_1 = +41.75 \text{ D}$$

(keratometry reading of 8.05 mm and assuming an index of 1.336)

Anterior chamber depth,	$d_1 = 3.4$ mm
Lens thickness,	$d_2 = 4.0$ mm
Vitreous depth,	$d_3 = 14.9$ mm

the power of the eye is calculated as follows.

The ocular refraction is given by:

$$K = L_1 = +6.00/(1 - 0.016 \times 6.00) = +6.637 \text{ D}$$

Therefore the vergence L'_1 leaving the cornea is:

$$L'_1 = +6.637 + 41.75 = +48.387 \text{ D}$$

$$e_2 = 0.599 \times 4.0 = 2.396 \text{ mm}$$

and

$$e'_2 = -0.353 \times 4.0 = -1.412 \text{ mm}$$

and the distance w to the first principal point of the lens is given by:

$$w = 3.4 + 2.396 = 5.796 \text{ mm}$$

Hence

$$\ell'_1 = 1336/ + 48.387$$
$$= +27.611 \text{ mm}$$
$$-w = -5.796 \text{ mm}$$
$$\ell_2 = +21.815 \text{ mm}$$

giving

$$L_2 = +61.242 \text{ D}$$

The final image distance is given by

$$\ell'_2 = -e'_2 + d_3 = 1.412 + 14.9 = 16.312 \text{ mm}$$

so

$$L'_2 = 1336/16.312 = +81.903 \text{ D}$$

Therefore, the equivalent power of the crystalline lens, F_L, is given by

$$F_L = L'_2 - L_2 = +20.66 \text{ D}$$

while the equivalent power of the eye, F_e is given by

$$F_e = +41.75 + 20.66 - (5.796/1.336) \times 41.75 \times 20.66$$
$$= +58.67 \text{ D}$$

The posterior corneal radius

Phakometry can also be employed to measure the radius of curvature of the posterior corneal surface. The thinness and similarity in curvature of the two surfaces means that Purkinje I and II are very similar in size. Small, widely separated sources of light enable the two images to be resolved. Royston *et al.*'s (1990) mean findings (for the vertical meridian) were 7.77 mm for the anterior radius, 6.40 mm for the posterior. The latter is significantly steeper than the figure of 6.8 mm adopted in the Gullstrand schematic eye.

Slit-lamp determination of radii and thickness

The photographic slit lamp can be employed to measure the corneal thickness and radius of curvature of its surfaces. Thus, much as in *Figure 16.11(a)*, the slit lamp can record the apparent cross-section of the cornea. If a scale, held in focus and perpendicular to the camera, is subsequently photographed, then the magnification of the system, including any subsequent enlarging, can be determined. From these scaled measurements, equations (16.3) and (16.1) allow the true thickness to be calculated, though more accurate results should be given by the equations in the appendix of Brennan *et al.* (1989). The radius of curvature of the anterior surface may be found in one of three ways. First, for a given chord, the apparent sag can be measured. This is then corrected for the obliquity of view, also by equation (16.3), and hence the radius of curvature found from the sag formula:

$$r = \frac{y^2 + s^2}{2s}$$

where y is half the length of the chord and s is the sag, assuming a circular profile.

Alternatively, curves of known radii can be photographed obliquely, and templates drawn from the resultant negatives used to match to corneal photographs, while Brown (1972b) cites a method of Fisher's for directly determining the apparent radius from the photographs.

A similar process was also used by Royston *et al.* (1990) to measure the posterior radius, obtaining results agreeing with their phakometric measurements.

Scheimpflug photography

The normal photoslit lamp cannot be used to measure the crystalline lens because its thickness is too great to have both the anterior and posterior surfaces in focus, let alone the cornea. Brown (1969, 1972a,b) adopted the principle of Scheimpflug photography. In one version of this method (*Figure 20.26*) the subject, with pupils widely dilated, fixates the slit beam which is directed through the centre of the pupil while the eye is photographed from 45° to the side. The cornea is closer to the camera than the posterior lens, and is therefore imaged much closer to the camera lens. The film plane is therefore tilted approximately 60° towards the slit lamp. Because of the varying conjugates across the field of view, the magnification on the negative is not linear. The intersection of the slit beam with the anterior surface of the lens is therefore always positioned in the centre of the field, and measurements taken in relation to calibration photographs. For more details, the reader is referred to the original articles, and to the more recent papers by Koretz *et al.* (1987, 1989a,b) and Cook and Koretz (1991). If the pupils do not dilate suffi-

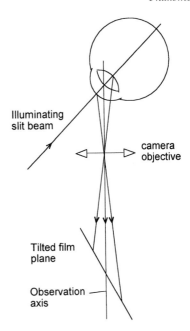

Figure 20.26. The tilted image plane technique of Scheimpflug photography.

ciently to allow the whole of the cornea and lens to be photographed, the slit lamp may be displaced sideways in the direction away from the camera. Sparrow *et al.* (1993) have published equations to correct for the resulting change in apparent lens thickness.

A similar photographic system has been used to monitor the lens changes in cataract – *see*, for example, Sparrow *et al.* (1990) and Magno *et al.* (1994).

The astigmatic eye

The foregoing discussion has tacitly assumed the various refracting surfaces to be spherical. In large-scale surveys, such as those by Sorsby *et al.* (1961), phakometry is usually carried out either in the vertical or the horizontal meridian, and the ocular dioptrics are then determined as though for a section of a spherical eye in the chosen meridian. If the ocular refraction has a cylindrical component, the 'notional' cylinder power in the selected meridian is calculated from the expression

$$C_\theta = C \sin^2 \theta \qquad (20.19)$$

where θ is the angle between the cylinder axis and the selected meridian. The same procedure is applied to corneal astigmatism at an oblique axis. Thus, a corneal power equivalent to

$$+42.00 \, DS / -3.00 \, DC \text{ axis } 60$$

would be considered to have a notional power of $(+42 - 0.75)$ or $+41.25 \, D$ in the vertical meridian (*see* pages 352–353).

Axial length and equivalent power of the eye

At present, direct measurement of the eye's axial length is possible only by X-ray methods or by ultrasonography. If the three surface powers, depth of anterior chamber d_1, axial thickness of lens d_2 and ocular refraction are all known, a ray trace from the eye's far point will determine the vergence L_3' at which the pencil emerges from the lens. The corresponding value of ℓ_3' is the axial distance d_3 needed to determine the eye's overall length $(d_1 + d_2 + d_3)$.

The simplest method of calculating the eye's equivalent power from its known dimensions is given on page 211.

Pupillometry

A difficulty inherent in pupillometry is to prevent pupillary reaction caused by or occurring during the process of measurement. A change in luminance, involuntary accommodation and pupillary reaction by the fellow eye could all affect the result. Since the pupil can be viewed or scanned only through the cornea, any measurement by such means refers to the eye's entrance pupil, not to the natural pupil.

Simple methods

For most clinical purposes only a modest standard of accuracy is required, attainable by various simple methods. Direct comparison with a graduated series of circles or circular apertures is one such method. A scale with a lens and telecentric stop, such as the Wessely keratometer, is possibly more accurate. A very old method, reintroduced from time to time in various embodiments, is based on the Scheiner (twin pinhole) disc. If held close to the eye, two entoptic images of the pupillary aperture will be seen. They may be separated or partially overlapping but will just touch if the pupil diameter is equal to the distance between the pinhole centres. Small amounts of ametropia have only a negligible effect but the pupil may dilate with the occlusion. A simple device which obviates this drawback consists of a thin transparent plate on which two strips of coloured transparent material are mounted. Their inner edges touch at the top and are separated by 8–10 mm at the bottom. Looking between the two coloured strips near their junction, the subject views a distant spotlight while fogged by about $+3.00\,\mathrm{DC}$ axis vertical. The lateral edges of the blurred image of the pinhole initially appear coloured. The plate is then slowly raised until these coloured borders just disappear. The distance between the strips at this level gives the pupil diameter.

Experimental methods

By way of contrast, an extremely high standard of accuracy is demanded of pupillometers used in visual and psychological researches. The requirements may include a continuous recording of pupillary size at time intervals of the order of 0.01 second. Motion-picture photography with infra-red radiation was originally the only basis for pupillometry of this kind and was considered by Taylor (1977) in his review of techniques to be the only one applicable to normal viewing situations.

In the mid-1950s, electronic scanning of the pupil in conjunction with closed-circuit television was pioneered by Lowenstein and Loewenfeld (1958). Various improvements and refinements have since been introduced. Both analogue and digital display systems have been used, and the pupillary area may also be recorded instead of or in addition to its diameter. Developments in this field are briefly reviewed in the papers by Saladin (1978) and Watanabe and Oono (1982) in which their own designs are described.

A pupillograph using infra-red radiation to examine both eyes simultaneously was constructed by Clarke *et al.* (1966).

Doubling methods

The recent use of doubling devices to measure pupillary diameter to a higher standard of accuracy (about 0.1 mm) than the simpler methods already noted has been reviewed by Charman (1980). A much earlier and simpler doubling method devised by Landolt was described by Sous (1881) as the most accurate of existing pupillometers. A bi-prism producing equal horizontal deviations in opposite directions is movable along a graduated bar having a viewing aperture for the examiner at one end and an adjustable support to rest on the subject's cheek at the other. The examiner slides the bi-prism along the bar until the doubled images of the pupil are just in contact. The pupil diameter is a simple function of the power of the bi-prism and its distance from the eye under test.

Exercises

20.1 When a tower at a distance of 500 m is viewed through a bi-prism with its line of junction horizontal, the two images of the tower just appear to touch end to end. The power of each prism is 4 Δ. Find the height of the tower and draw a diagram showing the path of the rays by which the two images are seen.

20.2 In a certain keratometer, the test object consists essentially of a circle and its diameter, the latter coinciding with the direction of doubling. Show, by means of a diagram drawn to scale, the appearance seen by an examiner when using the instrument on an astigmatic cornea, the principal radii of which are 7.50 mm along 150° and 8.25 mm along 60°, the direction of doubling being (a) horizontal, (b) along 60°, (c) along 150°. What would be the astigmatism recorded by the instrument if the index of calibration were 1.3375?

20.3 The arc of a certain Javal–Schiötz type keratometer has a radius of curvature of 480 mm. A point Q on one of the mires is 200 mm from the vertex of the arc, measured along it. Find: (a) the height from the axis at which a ray from Q would be incident on the cornea and, after reflection, pass through the vertex of the arc; (b) the angle which this reflected ray would make with the axis. Assume that the arc containing the mires is concentric with the cornea, the latter having a radius of 8 mm.

20.4 A certain astigmatic cornea has its principal meridians horizontal and vertical. In the horizontal, the radius of curvature of the front surface is 7.50 mm and that of the back surface 6.50 mm, the radii in the vertical meridian each being 10% longer than the corresponding horizontal radius. Assuming refractive indices of 1.376 and 1.336 for the corneal substance and aqueous humour respectively, find: (a) the total corneal astigmatism, (b) the astigmatism that should be recorded by a keratometer calibrated for a refractive index of 1.3375.

20.5 (a) The astigmatism of a certain eye as recorded by a keratometer is −4.00 DC axis 30°. Estimate the distance correction, given that the 'best sphere' placed 15 mm from the cornea is: (a) −10.00 D, (ii) +10.00 D. State clearly any assumptions made. (b) In general, if S is the power of the best sphere at a distance d from the cornea and if A is the astigmatism recorded by the keratometer, find an approximate expression for C, the power of the correcting cylinder needed at the same distance d.

20.6 An aphakic eye has a spectacle refraction of +10.00 D in the horizontal meridian at a vertex distance of 12 mm. What is the spectacle refraction in the other meridian if the keratometry readings are 7.60 along 180° by 8.10 along 90°? Assume a refractive index for calibration of 1.3375.

20.7 Assuming a keratometer calibration index of 1.3375, what is the power difference corresponding to the following radii differences:

7.0–7.2; 7.5–7.7; 8.0–8.2; 8.5–8.7?

(Note: it is interesting to draw a Heine double scale – two columns to scale – in which the left is the radius in 0.05 mm steps, the right power in dioptres. Most keratometers have this on the dual-radius power calibration.)

20.8 A patient's spectacle prescription is

$-5.00/-5.50 \times 170$ at 15 mm

and the keratometer reading 7.50 m 170 by 6.95 m 80. Compare the ocular with the corneal astigmatism, assuming the keratometer to be calibrated for index 1.3375. What residual astigmatic error would you expect to find when a rigid contact lens with spherical surfaces is placed on the eye?

20.9 A contact lens surface of radius 7.8 mm is ordered on the assumption of a keratometry index of 1.3375. If the lens is erroneously produced on the basis of a notional index of: (a) 1.336, (b) 1.332, what radius would the manufacturer use?

20.10 A model keratometer has an objective of power +20.00 D and a single eyepiece lens of conventional magnification 16×. The objective magnification when the instrument is correctly positioned is −1.0×. If the mires are in the plane of the objective, what percentage error in radius is made if the eyepiece is positioned 1 mm behind its correct plane, and to what dioptric error does the eyepiece maladjustment correspond?

20.11 A keratometer based on the Zeiss ophthalmometers G and H has objectives of focal length f'_1 and f'_2 separated by the distance $f'_1 + f'_2$. Using Newton's relation for paraxial imagery, show that the linear magnification of the aerial image formed by this system is $-f'_2/f'_1$ and is independent of object distance x_1. Show also that if a prismatic deviation Δ is introduced in the coincident focal plane of the objectives, the image displacement is $f'_2\Delta$ and is also independent of object distance x_1.

20.12 (a) Show that for a contact lens in saline, the apparent radius is r/n where r is the true radius of curvature and n the refractive index of the saline. Assuming n to be 4/3, for what range of corneal radii should the keratometer be calibrated to measure surfaces of true radii from 7.5 to 9.5 mm? (b) What is the reflection factor for perpendicularly incident light on: (i) tears of refractive index 1.333; (ii) PMMA of index 1.490 and (iii) the surface of a soft lens in saline, refractive indices 1.43 and 1.333 respectively? The reflection factor is $(n'-n)^2/(n'+n)^2$.

20.13 An ellipsoidal cornea of vertex radius 7.8 mm has a parameter p of 0.7. Tabulate the sagittal and tangential radii at distances y from the axis of 1.0, 1.5, 2.0 and 2.5 mm. Which radius, r_s or r_t, does the keratometer measure?

20.14 (a) In his *Physiologic Optics*, Tscherning gives the following corneal radii in mm for three patients:

Radius	A		B		C	
	Hor	Vert	Hor	Vert	Hor	Vert
Anterior	7.98	7.60	7.78	7.90	8.29	8.33
Posterior	6.22	5.55	5.66	5.11	6.17	5.87

For each meridian, calculate the ratio of the anterior to the posterior radius. (Compare these results with the ratio of 1.283

given in Tscherning's schematic eye.) (b) Calculate the equivalent power of each cornea in both meridians, assuming a thickness of 0.5 mm and a refractive index of 1.376, the aqueous index being 1.333. Compare the resulting astigmatism with that given by a keratometer calibrated for an index of 1.336.

20.15 A Javal–Schiötz keratometer has its mires mounted on a circular arc assumed to be concentric with the corneal centre of curvature. The included angle θ subtended at this point by the mires is adjusted so that the image height is equal to the fixed amount of doubling. (a) Show that this angle is approximately proportional to the power of the cornea. (b) Calculate the amount of doubling required such that θ in degrees corresponds to half the corneal power. (c) Which of the scales, power or radius, is approximately uniform?

20.16 In the presence of oedema, the refractive index of the cornea probably decreases. Assuming a new value of 1.371, calculate the equivalent power of the cornea with: (a) radii of curvature and thickness of the Gullstrand No. 1 schematic eye (+7.7, +6.8 and 0.5 mm), (b) radii +7.5, +6.7, thickness 0.55 mm. Compare these with the equivalent power of the Gullstrand cornea of normal index (1.376), taking the aqueous index as 1.3333 in all cases.

20.17 Adopting the axial dimensions of the Bennett–Rabbetts schematic eye but modified to include a cornea of thickness of 0.5 mm, calculate the time intervals in ultrasonography between the echoes from the cornea and (a) anterior lens, (b) posterior lens, (c) retina. Assume the velocities given in the text. (d) Also calculate the extra time taken if the axial length were 1 mm greater.

20.18 Light from one mire of a keratometer is reflected from a point on the cornea 1.5 mm from the optical axis, the angle of incidence i being 10°. The vertex radius of the cornea is 7.8 mm and its form is assumed to be (a) spherical, (b) paraboloidal. Find the sagittal and tangential image distances (s' and t') from the standard expressions

$$1/s' = (2\cos i)/r - 1/s$$

$$1/t' = 2/(r\cos i) - 1/t$$

in which s and t are the sagittal and tangential object distances (measured along the incident ray path), in this case both equal to −80 mm.

20.19 Using Dunne's method (*see* page 399) for the determination of crystalline lens dimensions, calculate the ratio r_1/r'_3 for an eye with the anterior lens surface power of +8.25 D, assuming all axial dimensions and the corneal curvature to be the same as in the Bennett–Rabbetts schematic eye. Assuming a linear relation between this ratio and the anterior lens surface power, estimate the anterior surface power of an eye showing a ratio of −0.80.

20.20 A myopic eye with ocular refraction −6.00 DS has a corneal radius of 7.9 mm, anterior chamber depth of 3.8 mm, lens thickness of 3.9 mm and axial length of 26.0 mm. Using Bennett's scheme (page 400), calculate the eye's equivalent power.

References

APPLEGATE, R.A., NUÑEZ, R., BUETTNER, J. and HOWLAND, H.C. (1995) How accurately can videokeratographic systems measure surface elevation? *Optom. Vis. Sci.*, **72**, 785–792

BAUM, G. (1965) A synopsis of ophthalmic ultrasonography. *Wissenschaftliche Zeitschrift der Humboldt-Universitaet zu Berlin: Mathematisch-Naturwissenschaftliche Reihe*, **14**(1), 51–62

BELIN, M.W., CAMBIER, J.L., NABORS, J.R. and RATLIFF, C.D. (1995) PAR corneal topography system (PAR CTS): the clinical application of close-range photogrammetry. *Optom. Vis. Sci.*, **72**, 828–837

BENNETT, A.G. (1961) Appendix D. The computation of optical dimensions. In *Sorsby et al.* (1961), pp. 55–64 (*see* separate reference)

BENNETT, A.G. (1966) The calibration of keratometers. *Optician*, **151**, 317–322

BENNETT, A.G. (1988a) Aspherical and continuous curve contact lenses. *Optometry Today*, **28**, 11–14, 140–142, 238–242, 433–444, 630–632

BENNETT, A.G. (1988b) A method of determining the equivalent powers of the eye and its crystalline lens without recourse to phakometry. *Ophthal. Physiol. Opt.*, **8**, 53–59

BENNETT, A.G. and RABBETTS, R.B. (1991) What radius does the conventional keratometer measure? *Ophthal. Physiol. Opt.*, **11**, 239–247

BIBBY, M.M. (1976) Computer-assisted photokeratoscopy and contact lens design. *Optician*, **171**(4423), 37–43; (4424), 11–17; (4425), 22–23; (4426), 15–17

BONNET, R. (1964) *La topographie Cornéenne*. Paris: Desroches

BRENNAN, N.A., SMITH, G., MACDONALD, J.A. and BRUCE, A.S. (1989) Theoretical principles of optical pachometry. *Ophthal. Physiol. Opt.*, **9**, 247–254

BROWN, N. (1969) Slit-image photography. *Trans. Ophthalmol. Soc. UK*, **89**, 397–408

BROWN, N. (1972a) An advanced slit-image camera. *Br. J. Ophthalmol.*, **56**, 624–631

BROWN, N. (1972b) Quantitative slit-image photography of the lens. *Trans. Ophthalmol. Soc. UK*, **92**, 303–317

BUREK, H. (1987) Conics, corneae and keratometry. *Optician*, **194**(5122), 18, 21, 23, 24, 26, 29, 33

BURNETT HODD, N.F. and RUSTON, D.M. (1993) The Eyesys Corneal Analysis System. *Optom. Today*, **33**(17), 12–22

CHAN, J.S., MANDELL, R.B., BURGER, D.S. and FUSARO, R.E. (1995) Accuracy of videokeratography for instantaneous radius in keratoconus. *Optom. Vis. Sci.*, **72**, 793–799

CHARMAN, W.N. (1972) Diffraction and the precision of measurement of corneal and other small radii. *Am. J. Optom.*, **49**, 672–679

CHARMAN, W.N. (1980) Measurement of pupil diameter by image-doubling. *Optician*, **179**(22), 24–28

CLARK, B.A.J. (1972) Autocollimating photokeratoscope. *J. Opt. Soc. Am.*, **62**, 169–176

CLARK, B.A.J. (1973a) Keratometry: a review. *Aust. J. Optom.*, **56**, 94–100

CLARK, B.A.J. (1973b) Systems for describing corneal topography. *Aust. J. Optom.*, **56**, 48–56

CLARK, B.A.J. (1973c) Conventional keratoscopy – a critical review. *Aust. J. Optom.*, **56**, 140–153

CLARKE, W.B., KNOLL, H.A. and NELSON, C. (1966) A binocular infrared pupillograph. *Archs Ophthal. N.Y.*, **76**, 355–358

COLEMAN, D.J., LIZZI, F.L. and JACK, R.L. (1977) *Ultrasonography of the Eye and Orbit*. Philadelphia: Lea & Febiger

COOK, C.A. and KORETZ, J.F. (1991) Acquisition of the curves of the human crystalline lens from slit lamp images: an application of the Hough transform. *Appl. Optics*, **30**, 2088–2099

CRONJE-DUNN, S. and HARRIS, W.F. (1996) Keratometric variation: the influence of a fluid layer. *Ophthal. Physiol. Opt.*, **16**, 234–236

DE CUNHA, D.A. and WOODWARD, E.G.(1993) Measurement of corneal topography in keratoconus. *Ophthal. Physiol. Opt.*, **13**, 377–382

DOSS, J.D., HUTSON, R.L., ROWSEY, J.J. and BROWN, D.R. (1981) Method for calculation of corneal profile and power distribution. *Arch. Ophthalmol.*, **99**, 1261–1265

DOUTHWAITE, W.A. (1987) A new keratometer. *Am. J. Optom.*, **64**, 711–715

DOUTHWAITE, W.A. and BUREK, H. (1995) The Bausch and Lomb keratometer does not measure the tangential radius of curvature. *Ophthal. Physiol. Opt.*, **15**, 187–193

DOUTHWAITE, W.A. and SHERIDAN, M. (1989) The measurement of the corneal ellipse for the contact lens practitioner. *Ophthal. Physiol. Opt.*, **9**, 239–242

DUNNE, M.C.M. (1992) Scheme for the calculation of ocular components in a four-surfaced eye without need for measurement of the anterior crystalline lens surface Purkinje images. *Ophthal. Physiol. Opt.*, **12**, 370–375

DUNNE, M.C.M., MISSON, G.P., WHITE, E.K. and BARNES, D.A. (1993) Peripheral astigmatic asymmetry and angle alpha. *Ophthal. Physiol. Opt.*, **13**, 303–305

EHRLERS, R. and HANSEN, F.K. (1971) On the optical measurement of corneal thickness. *Acta Ophthal.*, **49**, 65–81

EHRLICH, D.L. and TROMANS, C. (1988) The Canon RK-1. Poster session, British Contact Lens Association International Contact Lens Centenary Congress, London

EL HAGE, S.G. (1971) Suggested new methods for photokeratoscopy. A comparison of their validities. Part I. *Am. J. Optom.*, **48**, 897–912

EMSLEY, H.H. (1946) *Visual Optics*, 4th edn, pp. 309–310 (not in subsequent editions). London: Hatton Press

FLETCHER, R.J. (1951) The utility of the third Purkinje image for studies of change of accommodation of the human eye. In *Int. Opt. Congr. 1951*, pp. 121–136. London: British Optical Association

FOWLER, C.W. and DAVE, T.N. (1994) Review of past and present techniques of measuring corneal topography. *Ophthal. Physiol. Opt.*, **14**, 49–58

GOLDMANN, H. and HAGEN, R. (1942) Zur direkten Messung der Totalbrechkraft des lebenden menschlichen Auges. *Ophthalmologica, Basel*, **104**, 15–22

GUILLON, M., LYDON, D.P.M. and WILSON, C. (1986) Corneal topography: a clinical model. *Ophthal. Physiol. Opt.*, **6**, 47–56

HALSTEAD, M.A., BARSKY, B.A., KLEIN, S.A. and MANDELL, R.B. (1995) A spline surface algorithm for reconstruction of corneal topography from a videokeratographic reflection pattern. *Optom. Vis. Sci.*, **72**, 821–827

JAVAL, E. (1890) *Mémoires d'Ophtalmométrie*, p. 131. Paris: Masson

KAWARA, T. (1979) Corneal topography using moiré contour fringes. *Appl. Optics*, **18**, 3675–3678

KIELY, P.M., SMITH, G. and CARNEY, L.G. (1982) The mean shape of the human cornea. *Optica Acta*, **29**, 1027–1040

KLEIN, S.A. (1992) A corneal topography algorithm that produces continuous curvature. *Optom. Vis. Sci.*, **69**, 829–834

KLYCE, S.D. (1984) Computer-assisted corneal topography. High-resolution graphic presentation and analysis of keratoscopy. *Invest. Ophthalmol. Vis. Sci.*, **25**, 1426–1435

KORETZ, J.F., KAUFMAN, P.L., NEIDER, M.W. and GOECKNER, P.A. (1989a) Accommodation and presbyopia in the human eye – aging of the anterior segment. *Vision Res.*, **29**, 1685–1692

KORETZ, J.F., KAUFMAN, P.L., NEIDER, M.W. and GOECKNER, P.A. (1989b) Accommodation and presbyopia in the human eye. 1: Evaluation of *in vivo* measurement techniques. *Appl. Optics*, **28**, 1097–1102

KORETZ, J.F., NIEDER, M.W., KAUFMAN, P.L., BERTASSA, A.M., DEROUSSEAU, C.J. and BITO, L.Z. (1987) Slit-lamp studies of the Rhesus monkey eye. I. Survey of the anterior segment. *Exp. Eye Res.*, **44**, 307–318

LAM, A.K.C. and DOUTHWAITE, W.A. (1996) Derivation of corneal flattening factor, *p*-value. *Ophthal. Physiol. Opt.*, **14**, 423–427

LAM, A.K.C. and DOUTHWAITE, W.A. (1994) Application of a modified keratometer in the study of corneal topography on Chinese subjects. *Ophthal. Physiol. Opt.*, **16**, 130–134

LAM, C.S.Y. and LORAN, D.F.C. (1991) Designing contact lenses for Oriental eyes. *J. Br. Contact Lens Assoc.*, **14**, 109–114

LEHMANN, S.P. (1967) Corneal areas used in keratometry. *Optician*, **154**, 261–264

LEVENE, J.R. (1962) An evaluation of the hand keratoscope as a diagnostic instrument for corneal astigmatism. *Br. J. Physiol. Optics*, **19**, 123–138, 237–251

LEVENE, J.R. (1965) The true inventors of the keratoscope and photo-keratoscope. *Br. J. Hist. Sci.*, **2**, 324–342

LOWENSTEIN, O. and LOEWENFELD, I.E. (1958) Electronic pupillography: a new instrument and some clinical applications. *A.M.A. Archs Ophthal.*, **59**, 352–363

LUDLAM, W.M. and WITTENBERG, S. (1966) Measurements of the ocular dioptric elements using photographic methods. Part II: Cornea – theoretical considerations. *Am. J. Optom.*, **43**, 249–267

MAGNO, B.V., FREIDLIN, V. and DATILES, M.B. III (1994) Reproducibility of the NEI Scheimpflug cataract imaging system. *Invest. Ophthalmol. Vis. Sci.*, **35**, 3078–3084

MANDELL, R.B. (1960) Jesse Ramsden: inventor of the ophthalmometer. *Am. J. Optom.*, **12**, 633–638

MANDELL, R.B. (1962) Reflection point ophthalmometry. A method to measure corneal curvature. *Am. J. Optom.*, **39**, 513–537

MANDELL, R.B. (1981) *Contact Lens Practice*, 3rd edn, pp. 62–87. Springfield, Ill.: Thomas

MANDELL, R.B., CHIANG, C.S. and KLEIN, S.A. (1995) Location of the major reference points. *Optom. Vis. Sci.*, **72**, 776–784

MANDELL, R.B. and ST. HELEN, R. (1969) Position and curvature of the corneal apex. *Am. J. Optom.*, **46**, 25–29

MANDELL, R.B. and ST. HELEN, R. (1971) Mathematical model of the corneal contour. *Br. J. Physiol. Opt.*, **26**, 183–197

MUTTI, D.O., ZADNIK, K. and ADAMS, A.J. (1992) A video technique for phakometry of the human crystalline lens. *Invest. Ophthalmol. Vis. Sci.*, **33**, 1771–1782

NEUMUELLER, J. (1953) Optical, physiological and perceptual factors influencing the ophthalmometric findings. *Am. J. Optom.*, **30**, 281–291

OLSEN, T. (1987) On the calculation of power from curvature of the cornea. *Br. J. Ophthal.*, **70**, 152–154

PATEL, S. (1981) Some theoretical factors governing the accuracy of corneal thickness measurement. *Ophthal. Physiol. Opt.*, **2**, 193–203

PORT, M. (1985) New instrumentation and techniques. The Canon Auto-Keratometer K-1. *J. Br. Contact Lens Assoc.*, **8**, 79–85

QUESNEL, N.-M. and SIMONET, P. (1994) Precision and reliability study of a modified keratometric technique for measuring the radius of curvature of soft contact lenses. *Ophthal. Physiol. Opt.*, **14**, 320–325

RABBETTS, R.B. (1985) The Humphrey Auto-keratometer. *Ophthal. Physiol. Opt.*, **5**, 451–458

ROSENFIELD, M. and PORTILLO, J.K. (1996) Multi-meridional keratometry. *Ophthal. Physiol. Opt.*, **16**, 83–85

ROYSTON, J.M., DUNNE, M.C.M. and BARNES, D.A. (1989a) Calculation of crystalline lens radii without resort to phakometry. *Ophthal. Physiol. Opt.*, **9**, 412–414

ROYSTON, J.M., DUNNE, M.C.M. and BARNES, D.A. (1989b) An analysis of three meridional keratometric measurement of the anterior corneal surface. *Ophthal. Physiol. Opt.*, **9**, 322–323

ROYSTON, J.M., DUNNE, M.C.M. and BARNES, D.A. (1990b) Measurement of the posterior corneal radius using slit lamp and Purkinje image techniques. *Ophthal. Physiol. Opt.*, **10**, 385–388

RUSHTON, R.H. (1938) The clinical measurement of the axial length of the living eye. *Trans. Ophthal. Soc. UK*, **58**, 136–142

SABELL, A.G. (1983) Keratoconus in the contact lens wearer – some clinical observations. *J. Br. Contact Lens Assoc.*, **6**, 104–109

SALADIN, J.J. (1978) Television pupillometry via digital time processing. *Invest. Ophthal. Visual Sci.*, **17**, 702–705

SALMON, T.O. and HORNER, D.G. (1995) Comparison of elevation, curvature, and power descriptors for corneal topographic mapping. *Optom. Vis. Sci.*, **72**, 800–808

SCHEINER, C. (1619) *Oculus sive fundamentum opticum.* Oenoponti (Innsbruck): Daniel Agricola

SHERIDAN, M. (1971) Corneal contour and refractive error of the human eye. *Master's thesis*, University of Bradford

SHERIDAN, M. (1989) Keratometry and slit lamp biomicroscopy. In *Contact Lenses*, 3rd edn (Philips, A.J. and Stone, J., eds), pp. 243–259. London: Butterworths

SMITH, G. and GARNER, L. (1996) Determination of the radius of curvature of the anterior lens surface from the Purkinje images. *Ophthal. Physiol. Opt.*, **16**, 135–143

SORSBY, A., BENJAMIN, B. and SHERIDAN, M. (1961) Refraction and its components during the growth of the eye from the age of three. *Spec. Rep. Ser. Med. Res. Coun.*, No. 301. London: HMSO

SOUS, G. (1881) *Traité d'Optique*, 2nd edn, pp. 452–454. Paris: Octave Doin

SPARROW, J.M., BROWN, N.A.P., SHUN-SHIN, G.A. and BRON, A.J. (1990) The Oxford modular cataract image analysis system. *Eye*, **4**, 638–648

SPARROW, J.M., PHELPS BROWN, N.A. and BRON, A.J. (1993) Estimation of the thickness of the crystalline lens from on-axis and off-axis Scheimpflug photographs. *Ophthal. Physiol. Opt.*, **13**, 291–294

STENSTRÖM, S. (1953) An apparatus for the measurement of the depth of the anterior chamber, based on the principle of Linstedt. *Acta Ophthal.*, **31**, 265–270

STEVENSON, R. (1992) Corneal topographic modelling systems. *Optician*, **204**(5376), 16–22

STEVENSON, R. (1995) New developments in corneal topographic analysis. *Optician*, **210**(5520), 20–28

STOCKWELL, H.J. (1986) From old ophthalmometers to new keratometers. *Optician*, **191**(5041), 18–24

STONE, J. (1962) The validity of some existing methods of measuring corneal contour compared with suggested new methods. *Br. J. Physiol. Optics*, **19**, 205–230

STONE, J. (1975) Keratometry. In *Contact Lens Practice* (Ruben, M., ed.). London: Baillière Tindall

STONE, J. (1994) Keratometry and specialist optical instrumentation (revised by R. Rabbetts). In *Contact Lens Practice*, 2nd edn (Ruben, M. and Guillon, M., eds), pp. 277–306. London: Chapman and Hall

STOREY, J.K. (1981) The Marton Lecture: ultrasound in ophthalmic optics. *Ophthal. Physiol. Opt.*, **1**, 133–157

TAYLOR, S. (1977) Techniques for measuring pupil size. *Optician*, **174**(4510), 19–20, 29

TOWNSLEY, M.G. (1967) New equipment and method for determining the contour of the human cornea. *Contacto*, **11**(4), 72–81

TOWNSLEY, M.G. (1970) New knowledge of the corneal contour. *Contacto*, **14**(3), 38–43

TOWNSLEY, M.G. and CLARK, B.A.J. (1974) Conventional keratoscopy – a critical review. Comment. *Aust. J. Optom.*, **57**, 118–126

TSCHERNING, M. (1924) *Physiologic Optics*, 4th edn, pp. 150–154 (trans. C. Weiland). Philadelphia: Keystone Publishing Co.

WATANABE, T. and OONO, S. (1982) A solid-state television pupillometer. *Vision Res.*, **22**, 499–505

WILMS, K.H. and RABBETTS, R.B. (1977) Practical concepts of corneal topography. *Optician*, **174**(4502), 7–13

WITTENBERG, S. and LUDLAM, W.M. (1966) Derivation of a system for analyzing the corneal surface from photokeratoscopic data. *J. Opt. Soc. Am.*, **56**, 1612–1615

21

Distribution and ocular dioptrics of ametropia

Distribution of ametropia

Three large-scale surveys

Practice and hospital records provide useful information about the demand for ophthalmic services but throw less light on the incidence of ametropia in the general population. For this purpose, unselected samples are required. 'Captive' samples, such as Army recruits and school children, are the most amenable to large-scale surveys.

In classifying ametropia into spherical power groups, astigmatism presents a difficulty. Different investigators have adopted various means of dealing with it, which slightly affects comparison of their results. Though it does not affect low-power groupings, another point of difference is whether the results are recorded in terms of spectacle or ocular refraction.

Table 21.1 summarizes the distribution of ametropia (in terms of spherical power) found in three notable studies by Strömberg (1936), Stenström (1946) and Sorsby *et al.* (1960). Strömberg's subjects were 2616 Swedish Army conscripts (20-year-old males). Both eyes were refracted, giving a total of 5121 after 111 eyes had been excluded. The figures in the table refer to the results as amended by Stenström to convert them into ocular refraction.

In Stenström's own study, the sample consisted of patients of the Eye Clinic of the University of Uppsala (Sweden), colleagues and nurses and cadet officers of the army and air force. The first and third of these groups were considered to form a balance, having, respectively, a larger and smaller proportion of appreciable refractive errors than the general population. Potential subjects with astigmatism at axes more than 30° from the horizontal or vertical were excluded. All the subjects were aged 20–35 years. The right eye only was examined, giving a total sample of 1000 eyes. Ametropia was recorded in terms of the ocular refraction in the principal meridian nearer to the horizontal.

In the study by Sorsby and colleagues, the subjects were 1017 young men in the United Kingdom called up for National Service in an army unit accepting refractive errors from +8 D to −6 D. In addition, the survey

Table 21.1 Distribution of ametropia: summary of three studies (the figures denote percentages of the total sample)

Ocular refraction (D)	Strömberg males (5121 eyes)	Stenström		Sorsby et al. males (2066 eyes)
		Males (685 eyes)	Females (315 eyes)	
over −8	0.1	0.7	1.6	0.4
−8 to −7	0.2	0.3	1.0	0.2
−7 to −6	0.2	0	1.6	0.4
−6 to −5	0.3	0.3	2.5	0.4
−5 to −4	0.3	1.6	2.9	0.4
−4 to −3	0.7	2.2	3.2	0.9
−3 to −2	1.1	2.7	5.1	1.5
−2 to −1	1.9	5.3	4.8	2.4
−1 to 0	4.1	11.5	11.4	5.1
0 to +1	64.9	56.9	46.3	40.0
+1 to +2	23.8	12.6	14.6	33.4
+2 to +3	1.6	2.0	1.3	6.4
+3 to +4	0.3	1.0	0.3	4.0
+4 to +5	0.2	0.6	1.3	1.7
+5 to +6	0.2	0.7	0.9	1.2
+6 to +7	0.1	0.7	0	0.9
over +7	0.1	0.9	1.3	0.7

included 16 case records selected at random from men who had been rejected because of refractive errors, 13 of them myopes and the remainder hypermetropes. All the subjects were aged 20–27 years and 91% of them were under 23. Subjective refraction following retinoscopy was performed under mild cycloplegia. The vertex distance was measured so that the results could be expressed in terms of ocular refraction.

If the astigmatism did not exceed 0.50 D, the ametropia was taken to be the mean refractive error, equal to the sphere plus half the cylinder. In higher degrees of astigmatism, the figure tabulated was the refractive error in the less ametropic principal meridian. Results were presented both for the total sample of 2066 eyes and also for the 1033 subjects as persons on the basis of the better eye. Very little difference was shown between the two sets of tabulations.

Despite differences, the three studies considered agree in showing that hypermetropia is much more common than myopia. For the male samples, 70% or more of all eyes fall into the range of hypermetropia up to +2.00 D, while the most common refractive state for both sexes is hypermetropia less than +1.00 D. The distribution of myopia is also skewed because it extends to far higher degrees of error than hypermetropia.

Table 21.1 is restricted to young adults. Changes in ametropia with age are considered on pages 411–417.

Unaided and corrected vision

Before the outbreak of war in 1939, some 90 000 young men between the ages of 20 and 21 had been medically examined under the Military Training Act of that year. The medical records, which included the unaided vision, were later analysed by the Statistical Research Unit of the Medical Research Council and a report was prepared by Martin (1949). The sample, though not strictly random, was considered to be representative of the young men throughout the UK.

The results showed that 65.9% of the total sample obtained unaided vision of 6/6 or better in both eyes, while a further 13.3% achieved this standard in their better eye. About 80% could thus be considered to possess high-grade vision. Only 9.4% fell below the standard of 6/12 in at least one eye.

A regional analysis confirmed the popular view that countrymen enjoy better vision than city dwellers. Some 73% of the subjects from rural areas achieved 6/6 or better in both eyes as against 65% from elsewhere. In this analysis the London area was excluded because of its complex character. A separate tabulation of the overall figures for England, Scotland and Wales showed only trifling differences in the percentages reaching the highest category.

In the 1960 study by Sorsby and colleagues referred to previously, the unaided and corrected visual acuities were also recorded. In general, the results for the unaided vision were very similar to those found in 1939. Of the 1033 subjects, 67.7% reached 6/6 or better in at least one eye and a further 12.9% reached 6/7.5 (20/25). Those falling below 6/12 in at least one eye totalled only 10.0%.

Figures for the corrected visual acuity in at least one eye gave 88.9% with 6/6 or better and a further 8.1% with 6/7.5 or better – a total of 97%. Only 0.4% remained worse than 6/12 and no one below 6/24.

Data on ophthalmic prescribing

The most comprehensive survey of ophthalmic prescribing on record is undoubtedly that undertaken by the Ministry of Health (now the Department of Health and Social Security) in 1962.[*] A random sample of prescriptions totalling about 0.25% of the annual local demand was taken from every administrative area of England and Wales. About one-sixth of the prescriptions

---

[*] In the UK, all but an insignificant fraction of ophthalmic dispensing in 1962 was carried out under the National Health Service.

Table 21.2 Distribution of ametropia (analysis of 9163 distance prescriptions from a Ministry of Health survey in 1962)

Mean refractive error (D)	Percentage of total		
	R eye	L eye	Overall
over −6.00	2.65	2.54	2.6
−3.12 to −6.00	5.36	5.39	5.4
−1.12 to −3.00	8.43	8.37	8.4
−0.62 to −1.00	4.04	3.94	4.0
−0.37 to −0.50	2.52	2.80	2.7
−0.12 to −0.25	2.76	3.08	2.9
0 to +0.25	8.43	8.73	8.6
+0.37 to +0.50	7.03	6.98	7.0
+0.62 to +1.00	15.01	14.30	14.6
+1.12 to +2.00	20.10	19.74	19.9
+2.12 to +4.00	17.40	17.65	17.5
+4.12 to +8.00	5.90	6.08	6.0
over +8.00	0.38	0.39	0.4

had been issued by ophthalmic medical practitioners, the remainder by ophthalmic opticians (optometrists). By permission of the Ministry of Health, an analysis of the technical data was published by Bennett (1965). It included a tabulation of the 21 042 single-vision lenses in the sample. Up to 6.00 DS and 4.00 D every lens power was shown separately, all the astigmatic prescriptions having been recorded in the plus cylinder transposition. This information provided an accurate indication of the relative demand at that time for different single-vision lens powers.

Table 21.2 shows the distribution of ametropia, in terms of mean refractive error, according to the 9163 distance prescriptions in the same Ministry of Health survey. The separate tabulations for right and left eyes confirm the well-known tendency for fellow eyes to have similar refractions. Near vision prescriptions were omitted from this analysis to avoid introducing a plus bias in the spherical element.

Because many young hypermetropes do not wear a correction until the approach of presbyopia, data obtained from records of prescribing will tend to show a larger proportion of myopes than is found in the general population. For example, *Table 21.2* indicates a total of 26%. This is over twice the proportion revealed by the study of Sorsby *et al.* (1960).

In *Table 21.3*, the sample of distance prescriptions analysed in *Table 21.2* has been classified into arbitrary ametropic groups in which the two eyes of each pair have been taken into account.

Sex differences in ametropia

In 1950, a comprehensive survey of visual defects was made by Giles, who summarized the data then available from American and British sources. General agreement was found that women tend to be somewhat more prone to myopia than men, from childhood onwards. A corresponding difference was found in various studies of unaided vision.

The same sex difference is revealed in Stenström's findings (*Table 21.1*) which show myopia among 24.6% of the 685 men in the sample and 34.1% of the 315

Table 21.3 Classification of ametropia into arbitrary groups (same sample as *Table 21.2*)

Ametropic group*	Percentage of total sample
High myopia: over −6.00 D in worse eye	3.2
Moderate myopia: −0.62 D to −6.00 D in worse eye	17.3
Near emmetropia: −0.50 D to +1.00 D in both eyes	28.7
Hypermetropia: over +1.00 D to +8.00 D in worse eye	47.4
Marked hypermetropia or aphakia: over +8.00 D in worse eye	0.5
Antimetropia (other than in near emmetropia)	2.9

* Determined by the mean refractive error.

Table 21.4 Incidence of astigmatism (analysis of 12 916 prescriptions for distance or for near vision only from a Ministry of Health survey in 1962)

Power of correcting cylinder (D)	Percentage of total sample	Percentage of astigmatic lenses
0	32.0	
0.25–0.50	34.6	50.9
0.75–1.00	17.7	26.0
1.25–2.00	9.8	14.4
2.25–3.00	3.8	5.6
3.25–4.00	1.5	2.2
over 4.00	0.6	0.9

women. Both these figures are substantially higher than those in the other two studies summarized. This may be due, in part, to the nature of the sample. A noteworthy feature of Stenström's results is that the preponderance of female myopes in his sample occurs only in errors exceeding −2.00 D, for which the percentages are 7.8 for men and 17.9 for women.

From various studies cited by Giles it emerged that women made, in general, a greater demand than men for ophthalmic services. This is certainly true in the UK, as shown by official statistics analysing the 'sight tests' (i.e. eye examinations) carried out under the National Health Service in 1959. In proportion to their relative numbers, the demand by women exceeded the men's at all ages. Except in the age group 0–14 years, the difference was never less than 25 per thousand and usually over 30 per thousand of the relevant population. The greatest difference occurred in the age group 15–19, in which over 140 per thousand women but less than 80 per thousand men sought an eye examination (Bennett, 1973).

From his own practice records, Slataper (1950) found that during the 5-year period from age 45–50, the decline in the amplitude of accommodation was about 0.6 D greater for women than for men. He attributed it to menopausal effects.

Ethnic differences in ametropia

From the inadequate data available it would appear that the distribution of ametropia in different ethnic populations conforms to a broadly similar pattern. Differences are mainly in the incidence of myopia. The conclusion that it is slightly more common among Jewish people is well founded, but there is a dearth of information about adult populations in China and Japan. The few available studies do suggest, however, that the incidence of myopia in these countries, especially China, is appreciably though not dramatically greater than in the Western world.

The literature on this general topic, including many studies on small or isolated ethnic groups, has been ably summarized in a dissertation by Eisenstadt (1983).

Incidence of astigmatism

General pattern of distribution

Analysis of the data obtained by the Ministry of Health survey in 1962 gives an accurate idea of the incidence of astigmatism in the spectacle-wearing population of England and Wales. *Table 21.4* shows the picture given by 12 916 prescriptions for distance vision or for near vision only.

Nearly one-third of all the individual lenses were spherical. Of the astigmatic lenses, about one-half had cylinder powers of either 0.25 or 0.50 D, while a further quarter had cylinder powers of 0.75 or 1.00 D. Less than 1% had cylinders over 4.00 D.

A more detailed analysis of the raw data again confirms a general similarity between the two eyes of a pair. Over 22% of all the prescriptions in this sample were for spherical lenses in both eyes, while another 22% were for sphero-cylinders with cylinders up to 0.50 D in both eyes.

In the 1960 study by Sorsby and colleagues, the refraction of the 1033 subjects is classified to show the incidence of astigmatism. A total of 38.6% were found to have astigmatism less than 0.2 D, while as many as 90.2% had astigmatism, if any, not exceeding 1.00 D. No support was found for the suggestion that high degrees of astigmatism tend to be associated with high spherical components.

In his analysis of the Ministry of Health sample, Bennett (1965) also found astigmatism of all degrees to be fairly evenly distributed over the range of spherical powers up to plus and minus 8.00 D. Beyond these limits, which substantially define the boundaries of the study by Sorsby and co-workers, a marked association of high astigmatism with high spherical errors was found.

Variations in astigmatism with age are discussed on pages 412 and 415.

Table 21.5 Distribution of cylinder axis orientations (analysis of 7594 astigmatic single-vision distance lenses from a Ministry of Health survey in 1962)

Cylinder power (D)	Percentage distribution of axis orientation in each cylinder power		
	With the rule	Against the rule	Axis oblique
0.50	36	34	30
1.00	34	34	32
1.50	35	31	34
2.00	38	24	38
2.50	50	18	32
3.00	54	17	29
3.50	49	17	34
4.00	50	15	35
over 4.00	58	13	29

Table 21.6 Worked example of the use of Humphrey notation to determine the mean of three astigmatic corrections

Sphero-cylinder notation			Humphrey notation		
S sphere	C cylinder	$\theta°$ axis	MRE	C_o	C_{45}
+2.00	−3.00	60	+0.50	+1.50	−2.60
−1.00	+5.00	70	+1.50	−3.83	+3.21
+3.00	−2.00	140	+2.00	−0.35	+1.97
Sum			+4.00	−2.68	+2.58
Mean			+1.33	−0.89	+0.86

Sphero-cylinder equivalent +1.95 DS/−1.24 DC axis 158°

Axis direction

The Ministry of Health survey provided interesting data on the distribution of cylinder axis directions. In his 1965 analysis of this material, Bennett regarded any axis within 15° of the horizontal or vertical as with or against the rule (as appropriate) and all others as oblique. On this basis, only 38% of the astigmatic single-vision distance lenses in the sample indicated with the rule astigmatism. The remainder was made up of 30% against the rule and 32% oblique. In *Table 21.5*, abridged from Table 7 in Bennett's analysis, the division into the three categories of axis direction is shown as percentages of the total within each separate cylinder power listed. Although the percentage of oblique directions remains fairly constant, there is a marked increase of with the rule in cylinder powers over 2.00 D.

Method of analysis

As explained in Chapter 5, the principle of 'astigmatic decomposition' can usefully be applied to the statistical analysis of any number of ophthalmic prescriptions. Those with an astigmatic component would first be transposed into what might be termed Humphrey notation, in which the three elements C_o, C_{45} and M are defined by equations (5.13), (5.14) and (5.16) respectively. In the present context, the mean power M is renamed the mean refractive error (MRE). Purely spherical prescriptions would also be entered under this heading.

When tabulated in this notation, all cylinders are put on a common basis in which a component either with or against the rule is combined with an oblique component, plus or minus, at the neutral oblique axis 45°. A numerical example is set out in *Table 21.6* which is modelled on *Table 5.1* On dividing the sum of the three components by the number of prescriptions, the mean of the entire sample is obtained in Humphrey notation. Re-conversion into its orthodox equivalent then requires the three steps defined by equations (5.17), (5.18a) and (5.19).

Corneal astigmatism could also be analysed by this new method. For this purpose it would be necessary to transpose the keratometer power readings into a sphero-cylindrical form. A more detailed treatment of this subject has been given by Bennett (1984).

Methods similar to those of Harris cited in Chapter 5 were employed by McKendrick and Brennan (1996) to find the mean astigmatic error of 198 young adult patients' eyes to be Right −0.17 DC × 14 and Left −0.24 DC × 180. Because astigmatic errors against the rule tend to cancel out those that are with the rule, a value for the mean error determined this way does not imply that the mean cylindrical power is only around 0.25 DC when the axes are ignored.

Components of refraction

The four main variables which collectively determine the refractive state of an eye are the corneal power, the depth of the anterior chamber, the equivalent power of the crystalline lens and the eye's axial length. Subject to a proviso concerning the axial length, the spread of all four dimensions follows a normal distribution curve. They will now be considered in turn.

Cornea

For statistical purposes the corneal radii and power are taken as the keratometer readings, generally in a specified meridian. Different instruments may use slightly different notional refractive indices for converting anterior corneal radii of curvature into powers (*see* page 387).

In his 1946 study, Stenström found the range to be from 7.0 to 8.65 mm, with a mean for all subjects of 7.86 mm (7.90 mm for males and 7.77 for females). In about 84% of all eyes, the radius was between 7.5 and 8.2 mm. The upper age limit of the subjects in this sample was 35 years. Significant changes in corneal curvature which begin to occur at about this age are discussed on pages 415–416.

In considering Stenström's results it should be borne in mind that they refer to readings in the principal meridian nearer to the horizontal. With the rule corneal astigmatism would result in somewhat shorter radii of curvature in the meridian nearer the vertical. Converted into corneal powers, Stenström's findings show a spread from about +39 to +48 D, with an overall mean

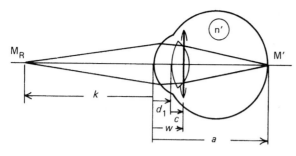

Figure 21.1. Replacement of the crystalline lens by a hypothetical thin lens of the same equivalent power, placed near the principal points of the original schematic lens. A simplified relationship between ametropia and the individual components of refraction can then be deduced from the ray path illustrated.

of +42.75 D (+42.50 D for males and +43.25 for females). Some 85% of all eyes fell within the range +41 to +45 D.

The ocular refraction K is the reciprocal of the distance k to the eye's far point M_R which is conjugate with the retina (*Figure 21.1*). Since the cornea is the last refracting element traversed by a pencil of rays diverging from the retina, it follows that a change ΔF_1 in the corneal power would result in an equal but opposite change ΔK in the ocular refraction. Expressed mathematically,

$$\Delta K = -\Delta F_1 \tag{21.1}$$

Thus, an increase of 1 dioptre in the corneal power would alter the ocular refraction by 1 dioptre in the direction of myopia. Strictly, the distance k should be measured from the first principal point of the eye, about 1.5 mm behind the corneal vertex.

Depth of anterior chamber

In this context, the depth of the anterior chamber is taken to include the corneal thickness. Stenström found a range from 2.8 to 4.6 mm, with an overall mean value of 3.68 mm (3.70 mm for males and 3.61 for females). About 84% of all eyes fell within the range 3.2–4.0 mm.

From a study of 144 subjects whose ages were fairly evenly spread over 4–70 years, except two aged 75 and 85, Calmettes *et al.* (1958) found the anterior chamber depth to increase slightly from age 4, reaching a maximum at about age 20. The peak values averaged 3.80 mm for men and 3.73 mm for women. Because of the subsequent gradual decrease in this dimension, to be discussed on page 415, the mean figure for the entire sample fell to 3.58 mm.

In the emmetropic Bennett–Rabbetts schematic eye, a reduction of 1 mm in the anterior chamber depth would result in myopia of −1.32 D if the axial length remained constant. An increase of 1 mm would produce hypermetropia of +1.29 D. For smaller displacements the resulting ametropia would be pro rata. Accordingly, if the variation in depth is denoted by Δd_1 (in mm),

$$\Delta K \approx 1.4 \Delta d_1 \tag{21.2}$$

Thus, the smaller depth in the average female eye, all

other dimensions remaining unchanged, would result in myopia of somewhat less than −0.12 D.

Among other aspects investigated by Calmettes and colleagues was the relationship between anterior chamber depth and ametropia. A scattergram of their results showed that whereas the values were evenly spread about a mean figure in all degrees of myopia, there was a progressive reduction in depth with increasing hypermetropia, averaging roughly 0.17 mm per dioptre. A similar trend is discernible in Table A1 of the report by Sorsby *et al.* (1957).

Crystalline lens

In Stenström's procedure the equivalent power F_L of the crystalline lens (and also of the eye) was calculated from the experimental data on the assumption that the lens was of zero thickness and situated at the front vertex of the true lens. To compensate for the errors thereby introduced, an addition of +3.00 D to all the calculated values of F_L was suggested. Though the amended values can be regarded only as approximate, a reliable picture of the spread of values is obtained.

With the +3.00 D added, the range was found to be from about +15.5 to +25 D, with a mean value of +20.35 D (+20.25 D for males and +20.56 for females). Some 91% of the total fell within the range +18 to +23 D. It is noteworthy that the total spread of powers, about 9.5 D, is slightly greater than that of the cornea.

If the equivalent power of the crystalline lens is varied by ΔF_L, its centre thickness and all other ocular dimensions being unchanged, the approximate effect on the eye's refractive state can be found from the expression

$$\Delta K \approx -0.65 \Delta F_L \tag{21.3}$$

This was derived from the Bennett–Rabbetts emmetropic schematic eye.

Axial length of the eye

Stenström determined the axial length by the X-ray method of Rushton. He found a range from 20 to 29.5 mm, with a mean value of 24.00 mm (24.04 mm for males and 23.89 for females). Although no extreme myopes were included in the sample, the distribution of axial lengths is clearly not symmetrical but shows a pronounced 'tail' on the long side. In fact, axial lengths over 40 mm have been reported. Nevertheless, Stenström found that if eyes showing the conus or myopic crescent usually associated with pathological myopia were excluded from his sample, the remaining results did conform to a normal distribution.

For the Bennett–Rabbetts emmetropic schematic eye, calculation shows that the approximate effect ΔK of a variation Δa (in mm) in the axial length is expressed by

$$\Delta K \approx -2.7 \Delta a \tag{21.4}$$

for values of Δa up to about ±1 mm. For $\Delta a = +3$ mm, the coefficient in equation (21.4) would become −2.4, while for $\Delta a = -3$ mm it would be −3.1.

Equivalent power of the eye

For the reason already mentioned, Stenström suggested an addition of $+1.50$ D to his calculated values for the equivalent power of the eye. When thus amended, the values he found ranged from $+54$ to $+65$ D, with a mean of $+59.63$ D ($+59.32$ D for males and $+60.23$ D for females). Just over 90% of all the eyes fell within the range $+57$ to $+63$ D. Once again, a normal distribution pattern is revealed.

A very similar sex difference was found in the study by Sorsby *et al.* (1961) of 628 boys and 717 girls aged from 4 to 14 years (girls to 15 years). In most of the yearly age groups the difference fell between 1.0 and 1.4 D, the mean for the whole sample being about 1.2 D. In the 14-year-old age group, the difference was 1.0 D. The mean equivalent powers for this group, $+59.1$ D for the boys and $+60.1$ D for the girls, are about 0.50 D higher than Stenström's amended figures for his adult sample. They refer, however, to the vertical meridian, whereas Stenström's refer to the horizontal.

Ocular refraction

For an accurate determination of a given eye's refractive state or ametropia, the surface powers and axial thickness of the crystalline lens are needed in addition to the four main components of refraction. For purposes of statistical analysis, however, a simplified scheme can be adopted without introducing serious errors. It requires the equivalent power of the crystalline lens to have been determined accurately. A hypothetical 'thin' lens of this power is then considered to be situated at a distance c from the anterior pole of the true lens (*Figure 21.1*), such that it lies at or near the mean position of the principal points of the true lens. For the Bennett–Rabbetts schematic eye the appropriate value of c is 2.3 mm.

Let F_1 denote the corneal power, d_1 the depth of the anterior chamber, $w = (d_1 + c)$, F_L the equivalent power of the true crystalline lens, a the overall axial length of the eye and n' the refractive index of humours. Then an axial pencil of rays diverging from the fovea can be traced through the eye by the step-along method. After refraction by the cornea, this pencil must converge to (or apparently diverge from) the eye's far point. Its vergence L_2' is therefore equal to $-K$, where K now denotes the ametropia measured at the corneal vertex. This approach leads almost directly to the approximation

$$K = \frac{n' - (a - w)F_L}{a - (w/n')(a - w)F_L} - F_1 \qquad (21.5)$$

where the linear dimensions are all in metres.

If the value assigned to a is varied or in error by ±0.1 mm, the resulting change in the value of K is approximately ±0.12 D.

Co-ordination of components

Since all the components of refraction (subject to the reservation about axial length) are normally distributed,

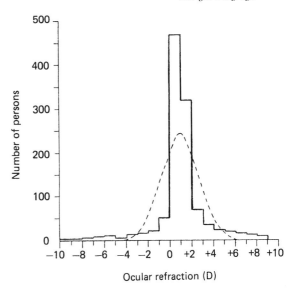

Figure 21.2. Histogram showing the distribution of ametropia in 2066 young adult males. A normal distribution curve (dashed line) is superimposed. (Redrawn from Sorsby *et al.*, 1960.)

a large sample of eyes in which each component is selected at random from the available range could also be expected to show a normal distribution of refractive errors. A conclusive statistical exercise on these lines was carried out by Sorsby *et al.* (1981). The fact that the actual distribution of ametropia takes a very different pattern is shown by *Figure 21.2*. The histogram depicts the findings of Sorsby *et al.* (1960) summarized in *Table 21.1*, while the dashed line is the normal distribution curve. (Because of the nature of the sample, the histogram does not show the myopic tail found in the general population.)

The concentration of refractions in the neighbourhood of emmetropia proves the typical eye to have a co-ordinated optical system. Moreover, since the axial length of the full-term neonate eye is approximately 18 mm, the equivalent power must be of the order of $+75$ D. There is thus considerable scope for large refractive errors to occur during the period of growth. A study of this process discloses the optical adjustments by which the necessary co-ordination is effected.

The growing eye

The infantile phase

In their study of 1000 neonate eyes refracted under atropine, Cook and Glasscock (1951) found about 57% to be hypermetropic up to $+4$ D, with a further 18% hypermetropic beyond this degree up to $+12$ D. The remaining 25% were myopic, the limiting value being -12 D. The mean for the entire sample was hypermetropia of about $+1.50$ D. These findings are not far removed from a normal distribution with slight skewness.

Changes in refraction during the first 3 years are largely uncharted. Gwiazda *et al.* (1993) measured the refraction in a longitudinal study in a sample of 72 children, perhaps biased as over 60% of the parents were

Table 21.7   Changes in ocular refraction and its components between the ages of 3 and 14 (or 15) (data from Sorsby *et al.*, 1961)

Dimension	Boys		Girls		
	53 *aged 3*	40 *aged 14*	36 *aged 3*	75 *aged 14*	34 *aged 15*
Corneal power (D)	+42.6	+42.9	+43.8	+43.8	+43.5
Anterior chamber (mm)	3.4	3.5	3.3	3.5	3.5
Power of lens (D)	+21.8	+19.9	+21.4	+20.7	+20.5
Axial length (mm)	23.2	24.0	22.5	22.5	23.7
Power of eye (D)	+60.4	+59.1	+62.0	+60.6	+60.1
Ocular refraction (D)	+ 2.2	+1.0	+2.7	+ 0.8	+ 0.7

myopic. In infancy, their results showed a similar distribution to, but were more negative than, those of Cook and Glasscock, probably because Mohindra near retinoscopy without cycloplegia was used. The mean spherical equivalent error was slightly negative at 3 months, rising to about +0.50 D at age 1 year, which was maintained till age 8 when it moved towards myopia again. Plotting the results separately for the initially myopic eyes and for those with ≥ +0.50 D, the graphs converge by the age of 1 year, demonstrating the emmetropization process; while the initially hypermetropic group remained hypermetropic, the myopic group's mean returned to myopia at the age of 8. The emmetropization process is also shown by the spread of refractions: if the standard deviation is taken as the indicator, it fell from ±2.0 D in infancy to around ±1.0 D at 1 year and to a minimum of about 0.75 D at age 6 years.

New methods have enabled astigmatism to be measured in the very young. For example, Mohindra *et al.* (1978) made a study of 276 full-term infants aged from birth up to 50 weeks. Astigmatism over 1 D was found in 45% of the infants, including 12% with 3 D or more. A follow-up study was made of 28 of the infants who had shown over 2 D of astigmatism when 3–6 months old. Re-examined when 50 weeks old, 14 had lost their astigmatism and 7 showed a reduction of 1–2 D. The remaining 7 showed no change. Further reductions continued in the second year, and astigmatism once lost was not found to return. No sign of meridional amblyopia (*see* page 42) was detected before the end of the third year.

Similar findings of high astigmatism were reported in a study by Howland *et al.* (1978) of 93 children aged from 1 day to 12 months, using the technique of photorefraction. No fewer than 60% were found to have astigmatism over 1.00 D, including 23% with over 2.00 D. The work by Gwiazda and colleagues also showed a similar reduction with age. Thirty-five percent of their infants had 2 D or more of astigmatism, 15% at 1 year and none at age 4; the proportion showing errors up to 2 DC remained at about 30% until 30 months, then falling to less than 10% by the age of 5 onwards.

The juvenile phase

Considerable light on the growing eye and the ocular dioptrics of ametropia has been thrown by the researches of the late Arnold Sorsby and his associates

(Sorsby *et al.*, 1957, 1961, 1970). Because their experimental procedure included phakometry, they were able to determine the axial length of the eye as accurately by calculation as by the radiological method. A full account of the apparatus and methods of calculation used is given in their 1961 report.

The following summary of these investigations is limited to the main findings and conclusions. In the first of the studies, the sample population comprised 341 adults aged 20–60 years, with mainly spherical ocular refractions ranging from −21 to +12 D. The 90 subjects with ametropia not greater than ±0.50 D were regarded as emmetropes. This group was found to have a wide range of optical dimensions: corneal powers from +38 to +48 D, lens powers from +17 to +26 D, and axial lengths from 21 to 26 mm, mainly 22–26 mm. From these results it was concluded that co-ordination, not conformity, is the essential feature of emmetropia.

With few exceptions, the same ranges of component values were also found in ametropia up to ±4.00 D. Within these limits, the myopes tended to have longer axial lengths and higher corneal powers than the emmetropes, while the opposite was shown by hypermetropes. Nevertheless, ametropia of both kinds up to 4.00 D should be regarded as resulting from an imperfect co-ordination of a normal spread of component values. A study of correlations revealed that while corneal and lens powers were both well correlated with axial length, the correlation of corneal power was particularly high among the emmetropes. The cornea thus appeared to play a greater role than the lens in co-ordinating the eye's optical system. In ametropia greater than ±4.00 D, the factor of axial length was undoubtedly the major determinant. For example, no myopic eye in this range had an axial length less than 25 mm, and no hypermetropic eye a length greater than 22 mm.

Growth of the eye is most rapid during the first 3 years, at the end of which the adult size has almost been reached. Unfortunately, examination during this period presents such difficulties that little information on the components of refraction is available. The second major undertaking by Sorsby and his team was a cross-sectional study of children aged 3 years and upwards, mainly drawn from day nurseries and London schools. Approximately equal numbers, usually from 50 to 60 of each sex, were examined in every yearly age group up to 14 years for boys and 15 years for girls. The total sample comprised 671 boys and 761 girls.

In the published report, the mean dimensions given for each age group were determined after exclusion of 43 boys and 44 girls whose ocular refractions differed by more than two standard deviations from the mean of their own age group. *Table 21.7* gives the figures for the first and final age group. The report also gives the mean values of ocular refraction (only) when the entire sample is taken into consideration. For boys, the mean refraction change over the whole period was from +2.33 to +0.93 D, and for girls from +2.96 to +0.64 D. The average change is thus in the direction of myopia, amounting to about 1.4 D for boys and 2.3 D for girls.

To supplement the cross-sectional study, a limited follow-up was made on 440 of the children to assess rates of change in the variable quantities. The interval between the two examinations was from 2 to 6 years. Because of inconsistencies in the findings, the number of results analysed was reduced to 386. In brief, it was found that the rate of growth gradually decreases with age and that development is usually complete by the age of 14. No evidence for a spurt of growth at puberty was found. The crucial factor determining the refractive state is the extent to which power changes, particularly of the crystalline lens, compensate for increases in the axial length. Annual rates of increase varied from less than 0.1 to over 0.5 mm, with an average of about 0.2 mm per annum.

Because of inadequate compensation, some 13% (17 boys and 33 girls) of the total sample became myopic or showed an increase in myopia during the 2–6-year period between examinations. Nevertheless, even among those children whose axial length increased at double the average rate, power-change compensations still played an important role. Of a group of 21 children whose ametropia changed by over 2.00 D between examinations, invariably in the direction of myopia, the average amount of compensation was approximately 1.4 D. Without this, the ametropia would have changed on average by 3.9 instead of by 2.5 D. Two of these children were already myopic, and 11 became myopic, but the remaining 8 had their hypermetropia reduced. A more detailed study of this group reveals that the amount of compensation, though inadequate in some cases, was generally proportionate to the full amount needed. For example, the girl whose axial length increased the most (by 2.1 mm) had the corresponding myopic change decreased by as much as 3.3 D.

Further observations were subsequently made on 129 of the children in the follow-up study and on 12 others first seen at the age of 14–16 years. These investigations formed the basis of the 1970 report by Sorsby and Leary. Though adding much detail to the picture, they did not change its general outlines.

A longitudinal study of school children in California revealed changes in refraction similar in pattern to those found by the Sorsby team. From comparison of refractions at the age of 5 or 6 and at 13 or 14, Hirsch (1964) concluded that the following generalized predictions would be warranted:

Ametropia at age 5 or 6	Predicted ametropia at 13 or 14
Myopia of any degree	Increased myopia
0 to +0.50 D	Probably myopia
+0.50 to +1.50 D	Best chance of emmetropia
Over +1.50 D	Little change in
(especially over +2.00)	hypermetropia

A separate report (Hirsch, 1963) had shown that astigmatism over 0.12 D was found in 55% of the children at the initial examination but in 66% at the final examination. The percentage having astigmatism with the rule remained at a little under 40%, while against the rule increased from 17 to 27%. This variety occurred most frequently among myopes. Citing Gullstrand in support, Hirsch expressed the view that against the rule astigmatism in the young is more likely to result in symptoms than the more common form.

Exhaustive studies have been made on myopia in the hope that it might be prevented, cured or moderated. These researches, which are beyond the scope of the present work, are summarized in the text by Borish (1970).

The adult and ageing eye

Age norms of refraction

From cross-sectional analyses of large numbers of case records in a single practice, it is possible to construct a picture of what Slataper (1950) termed 'age norms of refraction'. The upper curve in *Figure 21.3*, in which mean refractive error is plotted against age, is a smoothed version of the graph in his well-known study.

The relationship between cross-sectional studies of refraction and studies based on longitudinal case histories was analysed by Saunders (1986a). He concluded that large-scale studies of both types should lead to statistically identical conclusions, and that a large-scale cross-section study is preferable to a small-scale longitudinal one.

Age-norm graphs do not purport to represent the general population but only those members of it who seek optical assistance in the given locality, a distinction which almost disappears in the presbyopic age groups.

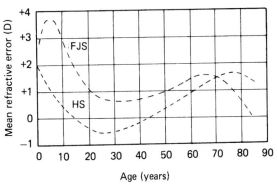

Figure 21.3. Age norms for refraction. (Curve FJS from the data of Slataper, 1950. Curve HS reproduced by kind permission of Mr H. Saunders, 1981.)

There are, of course, many individual exceptions to the broad pattern of ametropic change presented.

Whereas Sorsby and his colleagues found that hypermetropia was already declining by the age of 3, when the mean values were $+2.33$ D for boys and $+2.96$ D for girls, Slataper's graph shows it to increase to a peak value of about $+4$ D at the age of 6. It could be that many of his very young patients had been brought to him because they were showing a tendency to esotropia as a result of excessive hypermetropia.

A more recent study by Saunders (1981)[*] of his own case records led him to the conclusion that the graphs of his findings for all patients could be fitted very closely by the cubic equation

$$MRE = 2.036 - 0.227x + 5.847(10^{-3})x^2$$
$$- 3.871(10^{-5})x^3 \qquad (21.6)$$

in which MRE is the mean refractive error (or 'equivalent sphere') and x the age in years.

For the separate sexes the following equations were also given:

Females

$$MRE = 2.205 - 0.238x + 6.053(10^{-3})x^2$$
$$- 3.963(10^{-5})x^3 \qquad (21.7)$$

Males

$$MRE = 1.831 - 0.214x + 5.666(10^{-3})x^2$$
$$- 3.838(10^{-5})x^3 \qquad (21.8)$$

From the above analysis the following equation was later derived (Saunders, 1984b) to give the predicted MRE (S_x) at age x, knowing the MRE (S_a) at age a:

$$S_x = S_a - 0.227(x - a) + 5.847(10^{-3})(x^2 - a^2)$$
$$- 3.871(10^{-5})(x^3 - a^3) \qquad (21.9)$$

For the separate sexes, the coefficients in this expression should be replaced by those in equations (21.7) or (21.8), whichever applies.

A series of age-norm graphs had previously been published by Gasson (1932). Separate graphs were given for hypermetropes and myopes as well as for the entire sample of 3436 patients. This latter graph, plotted in terms of the mean refractive error, is similar in outline to Slataper's and Saunders' in *Figure 21.3* and would occupy an intermediate position between them. The same applies to the graph constructed by Freeman (1956) from his own practice records. In a later paper (1935), Gasson analysed the relative demand for eye examination in different age groups and also published age norm graphs for males and females separately. All these investigations agree in showing a steady drift towards hypermetropia from about age 25 or 30, reaching a peak between 65 and 75 years. There is then a reversal which often takes the form of a fairly steep descent towards myopia. A reason for this overall pattern of

change must first be sought in the effects of ageing on the components of refraction.

Individual variations from the typical course of development are revealed in longitudinal studies, such as those by Freeman (1956) and Elliott (1971). Elliott plotted annual rates of change in the mean refractive error. Separate graphs showed these rates for 260 right eyes and 257 fellow left eyes, each subdivided into those initially myopic, emmetropic and hypermetropic. Little difference was found between the last two groups. In the myopic group, however, the swing towards hypermetropia after the age of about 30 appeared to be less marked and to reach its peak several years earlier than the average. It was also found, particularly in the hypermetropic group, that rates of change for the left eye of a pair were significantly smaller than for the right eye and that the peak of the hypermetropic drift was reached 10 or more years later.

Prognosis of future refraction

The separate forms of equation (21.9) were later tested by Saunders (1985) against 47 case histories from another practitioner. Over a short interval the error in prediction did not exceed 0.25 D in nearly 60% of the cases and 0.50 D in 92% of them. These margins of error were approximately doubled in long-term predictions. The greatest uncertainty was in cases of medium and high myopia.

Freeman (1956) found that moderate myopia tends to stabilize at about the age of 20, when it rarely exceeds -6 D. Higher degrees of myopia, fortunately rare, are the result of abnormal lengthening of the globe. Such cases become noticeable at a very early age and progress rapidly through school life and beyond.

Discussing this question, Goss (1987) divided childhood and young adult myopia into three categories. In the first, adult stabilization, the myopia tends to settle at about -6 D by the age of 15 or so, though it may continue at a very slow rate of progress until the middle twenties. About 68% of males and 87% of females in the sample examined were in this category. In the adult continuation category, which included 25% of the males and 13% of the females, the progress of myopia slows down appreciably by the age of about 18 and then continues at a slower rate. In adult acceleration, which applied to 6% of the males and none of the females, myopia progresses at a faster rate after adolescence. Various factors having a possible bearing on the different rates at which myopia progresses in childhood and young adulthood were identified.

Practitioners are frequently asked by parents of very young myopes to give a long-term prognosis. Caution is advised by both Goss (1987) and Saunders (1986b, 1986c, 1987b), who recommended that it should not be attempted without knowing at least two refractive findings over a period of several years.

Recent work on myopia

Recent investigations have used keratometry and ultrasonography to measure the components of refraction of

---

[*] Table 7 in this paper was later corrected (Saunders, 1984a).

groups of emmetropes and myopes. Typical findings are those of Bullimore *et al.* (1992) who found the vitreous depths in groups of late-onset (after the age of 15) and early-onset myopes were both longer than in emmetropes. In general, findings show that early-onset myopes have longer axial lengths than late-onset myopes, but Grosvenor and Scott (1991) pointed out that the early-onset group usually are more myopic than the late-onset group. Choosing sets matched for equal refractive error, no significant differences in the components of refraction were found. Of the original 79 subjects, 53 were re-measured 3 years later (Grosvenor and Scott, 1993). Statistically significant slight increases in vitreous depths and axial lengths were found in the myopic groups, while the emmetropes' lenses became slightly thicker. There was no change in the mean corneal power for any of the groups who were in their early twenties, while the mean equivalent spherical power became mildly more myopic (by ≤ 0.25 D, though with a larger scatter towards both hypermetropia and myopia for the initially emmetropic group).

A group of 87 children of mean age 11 years was followed by Goss and Jackson (1995), who compared the mean spherical refractive error and ocular dimensions of those who remained emmetropic (defined as plano to $+0.25$ DS) with those who became myopic. They found three suggestive pointers to identify those who were to become myopic, the simplest being a refractive error of less than $+0.25$ D. Secondly, 87% of the boys who became myopic showed keratometry readings in the nearer horizontal meridian of 7.85 mm or less, 64% of the girls 7.60 mm or less. Thirdly, the ratio of axial length measured with ultrasonography under cycloplegia to horizontal corneal radius of greater than 3.00.

Gwiazda *et al.* (1993) found that children who were myopic in the first few months of life, as demonstrated by Mohindra near retinoscopy, were most likely to become myopic later, especially if initially showing against the rule astigmatism. Those who had no astigmatism in infancy tended, as a group, to become myopic later, at around age 11, while the with the rule group remained emmetropic. There was an increased risk of myopia in children with two, compared with none or one, myopic parents.

Crystalline lens changes

One reason for the hypermetropic drift shown by age-norm graphs is the continued growth of the crystalline lens throughout life. Between the ages of 20 and 65 the axial thickness of the crystalline lens increases by about 1 mm, and it may be assumed for calculation that both its radii of curvature are lengthened by 0.5 mm. During the same period the lens moves forward into the anterior chamber, reducing its depth by about 0.6 mm. If the Bennett–Rabbetts emmetropic schematic eye is modified accordingly, a reverse axial ray trace from the retina shows it to have become hypermetropic by just under $+1.00$ D. An increase in lens thickness of 1.2 mm with corresponding radius changes and the same forward displacement of 0.6 mm would produce hypermetropia just over $+1.25$ D.

This has been the accepted view for many years. Recently, however, evidence has been put forward by Brown (1987) to suggest that the radii of the external lens surfaces become shorter with age, not longer. If so, the effect would be to make the eye relatively more myopic. This would deprive the hypermetropic drift of the only explanation based on changes observed hitherto. The only plausible explanation would be that the myopia induced by the suggested shortening of the lens radii is more than neutralized by refractive index changes within the lens (*see* page 416).

The transmittance of the crystalline lens decreases with age but not uniformly over the visible spectrum (Said and Weale, 1959). Their graphs show, for example, that for blue light the transmittance is approximately 70% at age 21 but only 40% at age 63. For yellow light the figures are about 80% and 60%, which incidentally explains the yellowish tinge of the ageing lens. Over the same period of time there is also a marked reduction in pupil diameter (*see* page 26). Both changes demonstrate the importance of good illumination to the elderly patient.

Changes in corneal curvature

Although the corneal radius changes very little after the age of 3 years until much later in life, it appears to increase slowly to a peak value in the second or third decade. There is then a decrease which begins to flatten out after the age of 70. The dashed line M in *Figure 21.4(a)* plots the probable variation with age of the typical mean corneal radius. It was constructed as a composite of the experimental findings of Heim (1941) and Saunders (1982), together with unpublished keratometric records provided by Rabbetts. Data from this latter source were also used to construct the dashed

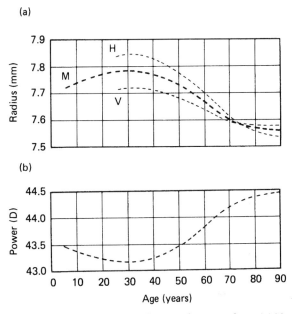

Figure 21.4. The corneal radius as a function of age. (a) M denotes the mean radius compiled from the data of Heim (1941), Saunders (1982) and Rabbetts. H and V denote the substantially horizontal and vertical radii of Rabbetts' sample. (b) Corneal power corresponding to the mean radius M.

lines H and V in *Figure 21.4(a)*, representing mean horizontal and vertical radii. They were based on an analysis of 383 eyes whose meridians of corneal astigmatism were within 20° of the horizontal and vertical.

Figure 21.4(a) clearly shows the well-known trend away from astigmatism with the rule from early years onwards. Several researchers have shown that whereas over 90% of astigmatic corneae are with the rule in infancy, the percentage falls to below 80 by the age of 50 and declines rapidly after 60. It is also apparent from the graph that although the vertical radius decreases from its peak value in the young adult, the horizontal radius decreases at a faster rate. This fact may throw some light on the cause of differential curvature changes. Keratometry on Hong Kong Chinese by Goh and Lam (1994) and Lam *et al.* (1994) similarly showed the preponderance of with the rule astigmatism in the young (over 85% of under 40-year olds) declining to almost equal proportions of with, against and oblique at age 47 to less than 15% with and more than 55% against at ages over 60.

Little detail is known about the variation with age of the intra-ocular element of total ocular astigmatism. In a study reported in 1954, Tait compared the corneal and ocular astigmatism of 1600 eyes, making the appropriate allowance for effectivity. The difference between them was taken to be the intra-ocular astigmatism. His total sample was equally divided among four age groups, the oldest of which was 50–65 years. In each group, the majority of eyes showed 0.50 or 0.75 D of intra-ocular astigmatism against the rule, the mode in all four being 0.50 D. Nevertheless, the older age groups showed a wider spread of values, with more eyes having 1.00 or 1.25 D. With the rule intra-ocular astigmatism, mainly of 0.25 D, was found in only a few eyes.

Because of the intra-ocular component, the overall percentage of prescriptions for against the rule astigmatism is not much lower than for with the rule. There is, however, a considerable variation with age, reflecting the change in corneal astigmatism. This is shown by *Figure 21.5*, reproduced from the study by Saunders (1981). In this analysis of 1817 prescriptions for the right eye, astigmatism was regarded as with or against the rule if the minus cylinder axis was not more than 22.5° from the horizontal or vertical as appropriate. Astigmatism at oblique axes was subdivided into with the rule (minus axis at $22\frac{1}{2}$ to 45° or 135 to $157\frac{1}{2}°$) and against the rule (minus axis at 45 to $67\frac{1}{2}°$ or $112\frac{1}{2}$ to 135°). Except in the first two decades, the total percentage of oblique axes remained in the vicinity of 20–25%. It will be noted that the two main varieties become equal at about age 45. Apart from a somewhat higher percentage of oblique axes, a very similar pattern of distribution was found by Jackson in 1933. A wide-ranging investigation into the manner in which the cylinder axis changes from a with the rule into an against the rule orientation was made in further studies by Saunders (1986d, 1987a, 1988).

Refractive-index changes

Despite the lack of hard evidence, it is tempting to invoke refractive-index changes to explain a puzzling feature of the age-norm graph. *Figure 21.4(b)* shows the corneal power corresponding to the mean radius in the upper part. It increases by about +0.75 D between the ages of 30 and 65, during which the growth of the lens possibly produces a change towards hypermetropia of the order of +1.00 D. The net result would be a change of only +0.25 D in the direction of hypermetropia. On the other hand, Slataper's graph shows a change of about +1.00 D. The balance of +0.75 D remains to be explained.

An increase in the refractive index of the vitreous humour would produce relative hypermetropia for two reasons: it would not only shorten the 'reduced' distance of the retina from the back surface of the lens but also reduce the power of that surface. Calculation shows that an increase of 0.006 in the vitreous index would make the Bennett–Rabbetts schematic eye hypermetropic by the amount required. An increase of 0.006 is not inconceivable. The swing towards myopia after the age of 65 or so, sometimes referred to as senile myopia, can be accounted for by the increase in corneal power. Another factor is probably a slight increase in the refractive index of the lens nucleus. As pointed out by Weale (1982), this quantity shows a considerable increase with age in the bovine eye, though only a slight upward tendency in the human eye during adult life. More determinations after the age of 60 would be enlightening. On the basis of Gullstrand's No. 1 schematic eye, an index change in the lens nucleus of only +0.005 need be postulated to account for a myopic change of −1.00 D. This suggests that only a small change in the complex refractive index structure of the real lens would be needed to produce a similar result. The rapid and considerable myopic changes shown by some elderly patients are undoubtedly the result of index changes caused by nuclear sclerosis of the lens.

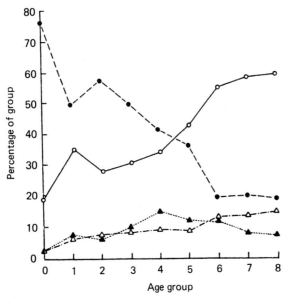

Figure 21.5. Type of astigmatism as a percentage of the total in each age group: ● with the rule, ○ against the rule, ▲ oblique (with the rule), △ oblique (against the rule). (Reproduced by kind permission of Mr H. Saunders, 1981. Copyright © Pergamon Press.)

The normal growth of the lens with age, particularly if the surfaces steepen, would suggest that its power would increase even in the absence of nuclear sclerosis. Although further work needs to be done to establish agreement on the precise mechanism, Pierscionek (1990), Smith *et al.* (1992) and Hemenger *et al.* (1995) postulate a change in the gradient of the refractive index within the lens rather than a change in the index itself as the stabilising factor (*see also* page 213).

Another subject for investigation is the extent, if any, to which the eye's axial length diminishes in the elderly. The advent of ultrasonography opens up wide possibilities for research of this kind. Thus Lam *et al.* (1994), among others, has shown an apparent shortening of axial length with age, their regression line suggesting by 0.02 mm per year. Grosvenor (1991) cites personal communications from Borish and Hofstetter as pointing out that cross-sectional studies may be misleading: younger people tend to have greater stature than their elders, so their eyes may also be longer in proportion, hence erroneously suggesting shrinkage with age. An increase in the velocity of ultrasound in the hardening elderly lens may also suggest a decrease in axial length.

Changes in visual acuity and functions

Slataper's age norms of corrected visual acuity included in his 1950 paper provide a basis for the following generalizations. Visual acuity begins to decline after the age of 50, at first very slowly. It does not fall below 20/20 until about 65. After this age the decline is more rapid: 20/25 (6/7.5) at 70 and 20/40 (6/12) at 80. These norms do not apply to patients with incipient cataract or other pathology. With the same exclusions, about 50% of those aged 70 and 15% of those aged 80 can expect to retain the 20/20 standard of acuity.

A survey by Elliott (1971) of 2000 case records has shown that there is a wide spread of corrected as well as uncorrected acuities at all age levels. In general, her figures are consistent with Slataper's data, as were those of Taylor's (1990) sample of 950 patients.

A 2-year study of the unaided vision and visual acuity of the elderly in a small market town was made by Lavery *et al.* (1988). Controlled tests were made on over 500 subjects, a representative sample of the population over the age of 75.

In respect of unaided vision, the males were more fortunate than the females, only 0.9% of whom had 6/6, as against 2.4% of the males. Those with 6/12 or better were 25.8% of the males and 17.3% of the females. Nevertheless, the mode for each sex was 6/36 (M 26.5%, F 28.5%). Vision poorer than 6/60 was shown by 13.9% of the males and 19.9% of the females.

The corrected acuity was ascertained for 156 of the males and 318 of the female subjects. In the age groups 76–79, 80–84, and 85+, the percentage of males attaining 6/12 or better in the better eye was 86.8, 78.8 and 77.3 respectively; for the females it was 81.8, 69.9 and 53.9 respectively. For all age groups combined, only 2.6% of the males and 4.4% of the females had acuities lower than 6/36. An overall total of 73.8% of the subjects attained a binocular acuity of 6/12 or better.

Examination of near visual acuity in test conditions showed that 88% of the subjects could read N8 or better. Many of them would not have reached this standard at home because of inadequate lighting. Much of the other information given should be of value to those concerned with social welfare in other localities.

Stokes (1991), in a sample of 400 patients requiring domiciliary visits of whom over 40% had cataract or macular degeneration, found 81% could manage 4/12 and N8 or better, though the percentage fell to 78% for the 80 and over age group and to 57% for the over 90s.

While data including patients with identifiable ageing changes is a valid indication of the capabilities of patients seeking optometric advice, better VAs occur if all such patients are excluded. Thus Elliott *et al.* (1995), using logMAR charts illuminated to $160\,\mathrm{cd/m^2}$, showed their scatter plots could be fitted by the regression line:

$$\mathrm{logMAR} = +0.0021 \times \mathrm{age} - 0.20$$

with an acuity of -0.10 or better (6/4.8) up to the 55–59 age group, deteriorating to -0.02 (6/6+) at age 75 or more. Further analysis showed that although their data could, like Slataper's, also be fitted with two lines, suggesting a constant acuity up to age 50 followed by a decline, a better fit was obtained by two lines intersecting at age 29. That for ages up to 29 shows a small improvement in acuity with age:

$$\mathrm{logMAR} = -0.049 \times \mathrm{age} - 0.025$$

followed by a slow decline:

$$\mathrm{logMAR} = +0.0029 \times \mathrm{age} - 0.250$$

They concluded that the concept that the average, optimally corrected visual acuity is 6/6 was incorrect. Causes of such a measurement may be poor luminance and contrast, especially if projector charts are employed, and for mean data, charts terminating at the 6/6 or 6/5 line, a point also made by Lovie-Kitchen (1988).

Other visual functions also deteriorate with age. Detailed treatments are given in specialized texts by Hirsch and Wick (1960), Weale (1982) and Rosenbloom and Morgan (1986).

Surgery for refractive error

Of the four variables governing an eye's refractive error, neither the depth of the anterior chamber nor the axial length of the eye can be altered surgically. In order, however, to prevent further lengthening of the globe in progressive myopia, reinforcement of the posterior sclera with tissue from other parts of the body has been proposed (Nesterov and Libenson, 1970).

The crystalline lens can be removed, but as it provides about one-third of the total refractive power of the eye, the patient would need to be about $-16\,\mathrm{D}$ myopic to benefit (*see* Figure 12.17). This operation was proposed by Fukala but is no longer advocated because both myopia and aphakia increase the probability of retinal detachment. Should cataract extraction become necessary in a highly myopic eye, an intra-ocular implant might be inserted, even of very low power, because this lessens the subsequent risk of a retinal detachment. It is possible, however, to insert a negatively powered anterior chamber implant, similar in construction to those used in pseudo-phakia, into the phakic myopic eye.

The cornea is the most accessible part of the eye for surgery, and as equation (21.7) shows, a change in corneal power has an equal and opposite effect on the refractive error. There are various possible techniques for the surgical modification of corneal curvature (or refractive keratoplasty):

(1) keratomileusis   (5) radial keratotomy
(2) epikeratophakia   (6) laser keratoplasty
(3) keratophakia   (7) intra-stromal ring
(4) corneal grafting

Keratomileusis

This method, described by Barraquer (1964), was originally proposed by him in 1949. A circular trephine is used to cut part of the way through the central cornea. A disc of anterior stroma together with its epithelium is then removed, frozen, and the rear surface turned on a lathe. To correct myopia, the surface is steepened so that when the disc is thawed and sutured back on the eye, a shallower front surface results. The disc is about 7 mm in diameter and initially about $\frac{1}{3}$ mm thick. As Bowman's layer is undisturbed, the corneal epithelium should recover quickly.

Epikeratophakia

In this operation, the central corneal epithelium is removed, and a shallow annular groove made in the cornea. A pre-shaped graft from a donor cornea is then placed on the cornea and sutured into the groove. It is not possible to make either small or precise changes to the corneal power, so that a minimum change of about 8 D is indicated. The technique is useful where contact lenses are rejected both in keratoconus and by aphakics who have not or cannot be given an implant. Myopes may also benefit. A review is given by Halliday (1988).

Keratophakia

As in keratomileusis, a lamella of anterior stroma is removed. A thinner lenticule of positive meniscus form, pre-shaped from a donor cornea, is then inserted to become embedded within the stroma when the original lamella is sutured back in place. It may become possible to use an oxygen-permeable synthetic plastics material for the lenticule. A solution to the complicated optics involved in this technique has been provided by Churms (1979).

Corneal grafting

While epikeratophakia is a form of corneal grafting, a whole-thickness or penetrating graft may be needed when the patient is suffering from severe keratoconus, or the cornea has been damaged by trauma or disease.

Radial keratotomy

In this technique, a series of radial incisions are made in the peripheral cornea. This then bulges forward slightly, while the central cornea flattens. This operation is therefore suitable only for myopes, though it has also been claimed to be applicable to astigmatism. Steele (1988) points out that the principles were discussed by Lans as long ago as 1898. Before the importance of damage to the corneal endothelium was realized, both anterior and posterior corneal incisions were used by Sato in Japan in the 1950s. The person most credited with promoting the technique is Fyodorov in the USSR.

The correction obtained depends on the number of incisions and the area of the central cornea left undisturbed. Steel considers the diameter of this area to be between 2.5 and 5 mm, the incisions not quite reaching the limbus. It appears possible to treat an initial error of up to about −6 D. Even after healing, flare from light scattered by the incisions can be disturbing at night, while any residual refractive error can fluctuate during the day for about 6 months after the operation. Because of the unusual corneal profile – flat centrally with steepening periphery – subsequent fitting of contact lenses to correct any residual error is difficult.

The interested reader is referred to the many papers published in the USA on the Study on the Prospective Evaluation of Radial Keratotomy (PERK), for example in *Archives of Ophthalmology*, **105**(1), 1987.

Laser keratoplasty (keratotomy, keratectomy)

At the time of writing, this technique is gradually becoming accepted, but is still under development. An excimer laser, mentioned on page 312, ablates (removes) a uniform layer of the anterior corneal surface with each flash. By progressively reducing the circular area ablated, more tissue can be removed centrally than peripherally in order to flatten the corneal curve. Marshall (1988) suggests that the maximum depth of stroma that can be removed without causing subsequent corneal haze is 50 μm (0.05 mm).

The degree of myopia that can be corrected is found as follows. If the maximum area to be treated is 5 mm in diameter and the initial corneal radius is 7.8 mm, the sag over this chord is given by

$$\text{sag} = r - \sqrt{r^2 - y^2}$$
$$= 0.411 \text{ mm}$$

The minimum sag after ablation of 0.050 mm will therefore be 0.361 mm, which, over the 5 mm chord, corresponds to a new radius of 8.83 mm. Taking the value of 1.376 for the refractive index of the cornea, the change in power is from 48.21 to 42.58 D or 5.63 D. A similar calculation would be appropriate for keratomileusis and epikeratophakia. Although chord diameters of up to 7 mm are now treated, a non-uniform power change is made in the peripheral zones to taper the newly flattened central zone into the untreated periphery.

Astigmatic corneas may be treated by preferential ablation. Surprisingly at first sight, a larger chord has to be ablated in the flat meridian than the steeper. Thus, if a patient has a refractive error of −2.00/−3.00 × 180 and a cornea of radii 7.8 mm along 180° by 7.3 mm along 90°, the new corneal radius for emmetropia is approximately 8.18 mm. If a zone of 5 mm were ablated in the horizontal meridian, a depth of 0.019 mm would be removed, resulting in a zone only 3.2 mm diameter in the vertical.

This can be achieved by projecting the laser beam on to the cornea through a simultaneous combination of decreasing sized rectangular and circular apertures, by placing a thin astigmatic mask in the system which has to be eroded before the beam strikes the cornea, or by using a scanning beam rotating in a spiral with a controlled variable intensity.

Although Bowman's membrane is lost, the stromal surface that is left by the laser is so smooth that the epithelium regenerates very uniformly. For this reason, the instrument shows promise for treating the irregular surfaces of scarred corneae.

LASIK

For larger refractive errors, laser ablation tends to leave a mildly scarred, hazy cornea. The modified technique of Laser Assisted Stromal Interstitial Keratectomy leaves the anterior cornea and Bowman's membrane intact. A central zone of the cornea is partially excised and hinged up to allow the laser to treat the base stroma; the anterior layers are then hinged back into place.

Laser thermokeratoplasty

Hypermetropia appears less amenable to treatment than myopia, the cornea tending to regress to its original shape. In this experimental technique, a holmium YAG laser is used to create a ring of laser burns within the peripheral corneal stroma, causing peripheral shrinkage and a steepened central cornea.

The intra-stromal ring

In this experimental method, two semi-circular springs of PMMA are inserted by rotation into the peripheral cornea concentric with the pupil. Low degrees of myopia may be treated, while, theoretically, the procedure is reversible since the arcs can be removed.

Exercises

21.1 In Stenström's simplification of the eye, the crystalline lens was replaced by a thin lens placed at the anterior pole of the real lens. If the Bennett–Rabbetts schematic eye were thus modified: (a) what thin lens power would be required to produce emmetropia, (b) what would be the equivalent power of the eye? By what amounts do these results differ from the corresponding values in the Bennett–Rabbetts schematic eye?

21.2 Repeat the calculations in Exercise 21.1, but with the hypothetical thin lens now placed near the mean position of the principal points of the schematic lens, i.e. 2.3 mm behind its anterior pole.

References

BARRAQUER, J.I. (1964) Queratomileusis para la correcion de la miopia. *Archivos de la Sociedad Americana de Oftalmologia y Optometria*, **5**(1–2), 27–48

BENNETT, A.G. (1965) Lens usage in the Supplementary Ophthalmic Service. *Optician*, **149**, 131–137

BENNETT, A.G. (1973) Some vital ophthalmic statistics. *Ophthal. Optn.*, **13**, 62–64, 69–70

BENNETT, A.G. (1984) A new approach to the statistical analysis of ocular astigmatism and astigmatic prescriptions. In *The Frontiers of Optometry: First International Congress 1984*, Vol. 2, pp. 35–42. London: British College of Ophthalmic Opticians

BORISH, I.M. (1970) *Clinical Refraction*, 3rd edn, Vol. 1, pp. 83–114. Chicago: Professional Press

BROWN, N.P. (1987) How can the eye remain emmetropic with age? *Optician*, **193**(5089), 35–37

BULLIMORE, M.A., GILMARTIN, B. and ROYSTON, J.M. (1992) Steady-state accommodation and ocular biometry in late-onset myopia. *Doc. Ophthalmologica*, **80**, 143–155

CALMETTES, DEODATI, HURON and BÉCHAC (1958) Etude de la profondeur de la chambre antérieure. *Archs Ophthal. Rev. gén. Ophthal.*, **18**, 513–542. (English translation by Pitts, D. A. and Millodot, M. (1966). *Am. J. Optom.*, **43**, 765–794

CHURMS, P.W. (1979) The theory and computation of optical modifications to the cornea in refractive keratoplasty. *Am. J. Optom.*, **56**, 67–74

COOK, R.C. and GLASSCOCK, R.E. (1951) Refractive and ocular findings in the newborn. *Am. J. Ophthal.*, **34**, 1407–1413

EISENSTADT, M.D. (1983) Racial differences in refractive conditions. *Student dissertation*. London: The City University

ELLIOTT, D.B., YANG, K.C.H. and WHITAKER, D. (1995) Visual acuity changes throughout adulthood in normal, healthy eyes: seeing beyond 6/6. *Optom. Vis. Sci.*, **72**, 186–191

ELLIOTT, P.E. (1971) Changes in refraction and vision with age. *Master's thesis*. London: City University

FREEMAN, P. (1956) An investigation into ametropia. *Optician*, **132**, 289–292, 341–346, 393–395

GASSON, W. (1932) A survey of refractive errors. *Optician*, **83**, 37–41, 57–59, 75–76

GASSON, W. (1935) The nature of ametropic errors in the general community. *Br. J. Physiol. Optics*, **7**, 85–103

GILES, G.H. (1950) The distribution of visual defects. *Br. J. Physiol. Optics*, **7**, 179–208, 216

GOH, W.S.H. and LAM, C.S.Y. (1994) Changes in refractive trends and optical components of Hong Kong Chinese aged 19–39 years. *Ophthal. Physiol. Opt.*, **14**, 378–382

GOSS, D.A. (1987) Matters arising. Cessation age of childhood myopia progression. *Ophthal. Physiol. Opt.*, **7**, 195–196

GOSS, D.A. and JACKSON, T.W. (1995) Clinical findings before the onset of myopia in youth. 1. Ocular optical components. *Optom. Vis. Sci.*, **72**, 870–878

GROSVENOR, T. (1991) Changes in spherical refraction during the adult years. In *Refractive Anomalies, Research and Clinical Applications* (Grosvenor, T. and Flom, M.C., eds), pp. 131–145. Boston: Butterworth-Heinemann

GROSVENOR, T. and SCOTT, R. (1991) Comparison of refractive components in youth-onset and early adult-onset myopia. *Optom. Vis. Sci.*, **68**, 204–209

GROSVENOR, T. and SCOTT, R. (1993) Three-year changes in refraction and its components in youth-onset and early adult-onset myopia. *Optom. Vis. Sci.*, **70**, 677–683

GWIAZDA, J., THORN, F., BAUER, J. and HELD, R. (1993) Emmetropization and the progression of manifest refraction in children followed from infancy to puberty. *Clin. Vis. Sci.*, **8**, 337–344

HALLIDAY, B.L. (1988) Alternatives to contact lens wear: epikeratophakia. *Trans. Br. Contact Lens Ass. Int. Contact Lens Centenary Congr.*, 43–46

HEIM, M. (1941) Photographische Bestimmung der Tiefe und des Volumens der menschlichen Vorderkammer. *Ophthalmologica, Basel*, **102**, 193–220

HEMENGER, R.P. GARNER, L.F. and OOI, C.S. (1995) Change with age of the refractive index gradient of the human ocular lens. *Invest. Ophthal. Vis. Sci.* **36**, 703–707

HIRSCH, M.J. (1963) Changes in astigmatism during the first eight years of school – an interim report from the Ojai longitudinal study. *Am. J. Optom.*, **40**, 127–132

HIRSCH, M.J. (1964) Predictability of refraction at age 14 on the basis of testing at age 6 – interim report from the Ojai longitudinal study of refraction. *Am. J. Optom.*, **41**, 567–573

HIRSCH, M.J. and WICK, R.E. (eds) (1960) *Vision of the Ageing Patient*. An optometric symposium. Philadelphia: Chilton

HOWLAND, H.C., ATKINSON, J., BRADDICK, O. and FRENCH, J. (1978) Astigmatism measured by photorefraction. *Science*, **202**, 331–333

JACKSON, E. (1933) Changes in astigmatism. *Am. J. Ophthal.* **16**, 967–974

LAM, C.S.Y., GOH, W.S.H., TANG, Y.K., TSUI, K.K., WONG, W.C. and MAN, T.C. (1994) Changes in refractive trends and optical components of Hong Kong Chinese aged over 40 years. *Ophthal. Physiol. Opt.*, **14**, 383–388

LAVERY, J.R., GIBSON, J.M., SHAW, D.E. and ROSENTHAL, A.R. (1988) Vision and visual acuity in an elderly population. *Ophthal. Physiol. Opt.*, **8**, 390–393

LOVIE-KITCHEN, J.E. (1988) Validity and reliability of visual acuity measurements. *Ophthal. Physiol. Opt.*, **8**, 363–370

MCKENDRICK, A.M. and BRENNAN, N.A. (1996) Distribution of astigmatism in the adult population. *J. Opt. Soc. Am. A*, **13**, 206–214

MARSHALL, J. (1988) Potential of lasers in refractive surgery. *Trans. Br. Contact Lens Ass. Int. Contact Lens Centenary Congr.*, 43–46

MARTIN, W.J. (1949) The physique of young adult males. *Medical Research Council Memorandum No 20*. London: HMSO

MOHINDRA, I., HELD, R., GWIAZDA, J. and BRILL, S. (1978) Astigmatism in infants. *Science*, **202**, 329–331

NESTEROV, A.P. and LIBENSON, N.B. (1970) Strengthening the sclera with a strip of fascia lata in progressive myopia. *Br. J. Ophthal.*, **54**, 46–50

PIERSCIONEK, B.K. (1990) Presbyopia – effect of refractive index. *Clin. Exp. Optom.*, **73**, 23–30

ROSENBLOOM, A.A. and MORGAN, M.W. (1986) *Vision and Aging: General and Clinical Perspectives*. New York: Professional Press

SAID, F.S. and WEALE, R.A. (1959) The variation with age of the spectral transmissivity of the living human crystalline lens. *Gerontologia*, **3**, 213–231

SAUNDERS, H. (1981) Age-dependence of human refractive errors. *Ophthal. Physiol. Opt.*, **1**, 159–174

SAUNDERS, H. (1982) Corneal power and visual error. *Ophthal. Physiol. Opt.*, **2**, 37–45

SAUNDERS, H. (1984a) Matters arising. Age-dependence of human refractive errors. *Ophthal. Physiol. Opt.*, **4**, 107

SAUNDERS, H. (1984b) Age-dependence of human refractive errors. *Ophthal Physiol. Opt.*, **4**, 281

SAUNDERS, H. (1985) Prognosis of refractive corrections. *Ophthal. Physiol. Opt.*, **5**, 391–395

SAUNDERS, H. (1986a) A longitudinal study of the age dependence of human ocular refraction – I. Age-dependent changes in the equivalent sphere. *Ophthal. Physiol. Opt.*, **6**, 39–46

SAUNDERS, H. (1986b) A longitudinal study of the age dependence of human ocular refraction – II. Prediction of future trends in medium and high myopia by means of cluster analysis. *Ophthal. Physiol. Opt.*, **6**, 177–186

SAUNDERS, H. (1986c) Correspondence. Age of cessation of the progression of myopia. *Ophthal. Physiol. Opt.*, **6**, 243–244

SAUNDERS, H. (1986d) Correspondence. Changes in the orientation of the axis of astigmatism associated with age. *Ophthal. Physiol. Opt.*, **6**, 343–344

SAUNDERS, H. (1987a) A longitudinal study of the age dependence of human ocular refraction – III. The mediation of changes from direct to inverse astigmatism examined by means of matrices of transition probabilities. *Ophthal. Physiol. Opt.*, **7**, 175–186

SAUNDERS, H. (1987b) Author's reply. Cessation age of childhood myopia progression. *Ophthal. Physiol. Opt.*, **7**, 195–197

SAUNDERS, H. (1988) Changes in the axis of astigmatism: a longitudinal study. *Ophthal. Physiol. Opt.*, **8**, 37–42

SLATAPER, F.J. (1950) Age norms of refraction and vision. *Archs Ophthal., N.Y.*, **43**, 468–481

SMITH, G., ATCHISON, D.A. and PIERSCIONEK, B.K. (1992) Modeling the power of the aging human eye. *J. Opt. Soc. Am. A*, **9**, 2111–2117

SORSBY, A. and LEARY, G.A. (1970) A longitudinal study of refraction and its components during growth. *Spec. Rep. Ser. med. Res. Coun.*, No. 309. London: HMSO

SORSBY, A., BENJAMIN, B. and BENNETT, A.G. (1981) Steiger on refraction: a reappraisal. *Br. J. Ophthal.*, **65**, 805–811

SORSBY, A., BENJAMIN, B., DAVEY, J.B., SHERIDAN, M. and TANNER, J.M. (1957) Emmetropia and its aberrations. *Spec. Rep. Ser. med. Res. Coun.*, No. 293. London: HMSO

SORSBY, A., BENJAMIN, B. and SHERIDAN, M. (1961) Refraction and its components during the growth of the eye from the age of three. *Spec. Rep. Ser. med. Res. Coun.*, No. 301. London: HMSO

SORSBY, A., SHERIDAN, M. and LEARY, G.A. (1960) Vision, visual acuity, and ocular refraction of young men. *Br. Med. J.*, **1**, 1394–1398

STEELE, A.D. MCG. (1988) Radial keratotomy today. *Trans. Br. Contact Lens. Ass. Int. Contact Lens Centenary Congr.*, 79–82

STENSTRÖM, S. (1946) Untersuchungen über die Variation und Kovariation der optischen Elemente des menschlichen Auges. *Acta Ophthal.*, suppl. 26. (Also English translation by Woolf, D., *Am. J. Optom.*, **25**, 218–232, 1948)

STOKES, T.J. (1991) How good is vision in old age? *Optician*, **201**(5297), 46

STRÖMBERG, E. (1936) Ueber Refraktion und Achsenlänge des menschlichen Auges. *Acta Ophthal.*, **14**, 281–293

TAIT, E.F. (1954) Relationship between corneal and total astigmatism. *A.M.A. Archs Ophthal.*, **52**, 167–169

TAYLOR, S. (1990) An analysis of vision and VA in patients attending for eye examination. *Optician*, **199**(5256), 15–17

WEALE, R.A. (1982) *A Biography of the Eye*. London: H. K. Lewis

Further reading

CURTIN, B.J. (1985) *The Myopias*. Philadelphia: Harper & Row

Entoptic phenomena

Introduction

The eye's function is to form an inverted image of the external scene and to convert this to a pattern of neural signals for the brain to interpret. Visual sensations can also arise from shadows of opacities within the eye, mechanical pressure on the globe and a variety of other causes. These sensations not directly due to the formation of an optical image by the refracting system of the eye are called entoptic phenomena (from the Greek, meaning things perceived within vision).

These phenomena may be subdivided as follows:

Optical
(1) (a) shadows due to objects or opacities in the media,
    (b) the blood vessel silhouette,
(2) haloes and diffraction patterns,
(3) Haidinger's brushes,
(4) Maxwell's spot.

Physiological, in the restricted sense of non-optical stimulation of the retina:
(5) phosphenes,
(6) blue arcs,
(7) after-images,
(8) Troxler effect.

Sensations or perceptions arising in the visual cortex, for example the scintillations or fortification spectra seen in migraine, or complete scenes as in dreaming, are excluded.

Entoptic phenomena are occasionally used to verify the macula function in patients with cataract before operation. The shadows of the retinal vessels or circulation of white blood corpuscles within the smaller capillaries are mentioned by Hurst *et al.* (1993).

Entoptic phenomena due to opacities or objects in the media

Basic principles

Unless an opacity is either nearly the same size as the pupil or close to the retina, it will not cause a noticeable shadow. This is analogous with the shadow of objects in a room lit by a single window. In order to make a shadow both denser and more sharply defined, a small

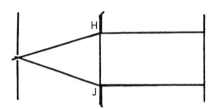

Figure 22.1. An illuminated pinhole disc placed in the anterior focal plane of the eye. The cylindrical column of light reaching the retina is ideal for demonstrating opacities.

source of light is required. In ophthalmic work, a pinhole disc is the simplest means of producing well-defined shadows of opacities or refractive irregularities in the media.

If the strongly illuminated pinhole is placed in the anterior focal plane of the eye, the parallel beam of light within the vitreous will have the same cross-sectional shape and size as the exit pupil (*Figure 22.1*). Crenellations due to irregularities in the pupil margin, and fluctuations in size with alterations of pupil diameter will be readily visible. The consensual pupil reaction due to changes in the illumination of the fellow eye will also be evident. Entoptic appearances (if any) will be seen within the illuminated fundus patch. A small pinhole (0.25 mm or less) gives well-defined retinal shadows.

If the ocular media were perfectly clear and the surfaces without blemish, the patch of light on the retina would be featureless. Any defect affecting the uniform transmission of light will, however, cast a shadow on the retina, giving rise to an entoptic phenomenon. The obstruction need not necessarily be opaque, but could be translucent or merely a clear but refractive disturbance, for example, a tear globule on the front surface of the cornea or a vacuole in the crystalline lens.

Using a slit lamp at maximum brightness positioned at 45–50° from the fixation axis, Johnson *et al.* (1987) took photographs of corneal striae following soft contact lens wear. They proved to be very similar to the entoptic view as drawn by the subjects. Light scattered in the normal cornea appears as a uniform white haze.

Orientation and location of obstruction

If a pinhead is placed between the pinhole and the eye, as in *Figure 22.2*, the shadow cast on the retina will be

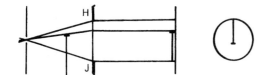

Figure 22.2.   The erect retinal shadow of a pin, placed between the pinhole and the eye, appears inverted.

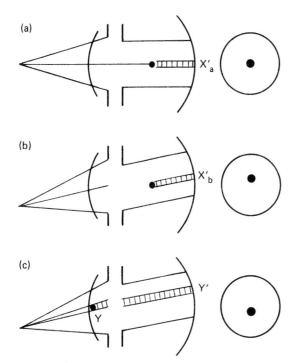

Figure 22.3.   The use of parallax to locate the site of an opacity. The circles on the right represent the entoptic field and the apparent relative position of a central opacity as seen by the subject. (a) Opacity behind pupil, pinhole central. (b) Effect on (a) of downward movement of pinhole. (c) Opposite effect of pinhole shift when opacity is in front of pupil.

erect and an apparently inverted pin will thus be seen. If the pinhead is placed on the opposite side of the pinhole from the eye, it will appear the correct way up because the usual imagery then applies.

The position of the obstruction relative to the pupil may be indicated by parallax. Thus, *Figure 22.3(a)* shows an axial opacity behind the exit pupil casting a shadow X'_a on the retina in the centre of the illuminated retinal area.

In *Figure 22.3(b)*, the pinhole source S is lowered and the shadow X'_b moves downwards relative to the patch of light on the retina. The shadow therefore appears to move upwards within the entoptic field, showing an against movement relative to that of the source.

In *Figure 22.3(c)*, an axial opacity Y lies in front of the entrance pupil. When the pinhole is again displaced downwards, the shadow Y' now appears to move downwards in the entoptic field, thus showing a with movement.

This may easily be confirmed by experiment. The entoptic view of eyelashes shows a with movement, but most other entoptic features, for example lenticular or

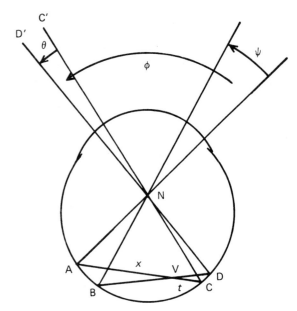

Figure 22.4.   Use of the entoptic shadow of a retinal blood vessel V to determine its distance t from the percipient layer (not to scale). The retinal elements A and B illuminated from the right cast shadows of the vessel at C and D, seen entoptically by projection in the directions C' and D'.

vitreous opacities, show an against movement because they lie behind the exit pupil.

As the obstruction approaches the retina, or approaches the source if in front of the entrance pupil, the amount of parallactic movement increases. Listing (cited by Helmholtz, 1924, Vol. I) showed in 1845 that it was therefore possible to estimate the approximate position of an obstruction.

This technique may be used to measure the position of the blood vessels in the eye relative to the retinal receptors. The shadows of the retinal vessels are often seen by the patient when ophthalmoscopy[*] or slit-lamp examination is performed in a dark room. Because the appearance is similar to the twigs and branches of a tree silhouetted against the sky, the phenomenon is often termed the 'retinal tree'. It was first described by Purkinje in 1819 (cited by Helmholtz, 1924, Vol. I). In normal conditions, light passes through the patient's pupil to form a shadow of the blood vessels on the retinal receptors immediately behind them. These receptors and related neural cells adapt to the lower illumination, so that the external scene is perceived without vascular shadows. The ophthalmoscope beam, however, strikes one region A of the retina (*Figure 22.4*). This illuminated area acts as a fresh source of light, causing a shadow of vessel V to fall on retinal receptors C. Since this is not the normal position for the vascular shadow, it may be perceived (in the direction CC'), although the receptors soon adapt to the reduced stimulus, so causing the perception to fade. If the ophthalmoscope beam is now moved to illuminate region B, the vessel shadow will now fall on yet another group of retinal receptors D.

---

[*] Before commencing ophthalmoscopy at a patient's first examination, it is worth mentioning that any such pattern, if seen, is normal.

From a knowledge of the geometry of the eye, it is possible to estimate the distance of the blood vessels from the percipient layer of the retina. For this purpose, transillumination of the anterior sclera will allow direct measurement of the distance AB. The projected angular separation ϕ between source and vessel shadow, and the angular displacement θ from C$'$ to D$'$ will need to be measured (Muller, 1849, cited by Helmholtz, 1924, Vol. I).

Thus, in *Figure 22.4* in which $t =$VC and $x =$ AV,

$$t/\mathrm{CD} \approx x/\mathrm{AB}$$

Assuming that the radius of curvature ρ of the posterior part of the globe equals the distance between the nodal point and the retina,

$$x \approx 2\rho \sin(\phi/2)$$

where ϕ is the projected angular separation between the source of light and vascular shadow. Also

$$\mathrm{CD} = 2\rho \sin(\theta/2)$$

Hence, the distance t between the vessel and the percipient layer is

$$t \approx \frac{4\rho^2 \sin(\phi/2)\sin(\theta/2)}{\mathrm{AB}} \tag{22.1}$$

If the source of light does not transilluminate the sclera but is imaged through the eye's optical system, then AB in equation (22.1) can be replaced by

$$2\rho \sin(\psi/2)$$

leading to

$$t \approx \frac{2\rho \sin(\phi/2)\sin(\theta/2)}{\sin(\psi/2)} \tag{22.2}$$

In a more precise form derived by Jago (1864), the source of light was considered to alternate symmetrically from one side of the optical axis to the other through an angle ψ while the vessel's shadow jumped through an angle θ, giving the expression

$$t = \rho\left\{1 - \frac{\cos\frac{1}{4}(\psi+\theta)}{\cos\frac{1}{4}(\psi-\theta)}\right\} \tag{22.3}$$

Zeffren *et al.* (1990) and Bradley *et al.* (1992) describe a technique for visualizing the retinal vessels near the fovea.

The Brewster–Donders method for the depth of opacity

Although Listing's method using the movement of the light source will demonstrate the relative depth of an opacity within the eye, a more exact method is due to Brewster (1843) in the form modified by Donders (1847), both cited by Helmholtz (1924) Vol. I. A Scheiner disc SD with two small pinholes about 2 mm apart is held as near as possible to the anterior focal plane of the eye (*Figure 22.5*). The field of view is then bounded by two overlapping circles H$'_1$J$'_1$ and H$'_2$J$'_2$, the points H and J being the borders of the eye's exit pupil Ex.

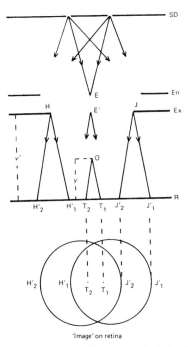

Figure 22.5. The Brewster–Donders method of determining the depth of an ocular opacity.

Because of the two sources, an opacity O at a distance y from the retina R casts two shadows T$_1$ and T$_2$. By similar triangles,

$$y/v' = \mathrm{T_2T_1}/\mathrm{J'_2J'_1} \tag{22.4}$$

The points T$_2$, T$_1$, J$'_2$ and J$'_1$ as projected can be marked on the screen S and the ratio y/v' found from equation (22.4). An estimated value must be given to the distance v' from the exit pupil to the retina, about 20.3 mm in the standard emmetropic eye. It is essential that fixation does not move, otherwise the projected images will also move.

Causes of entoptic shadows

These shadow entoptic phenomena may be caused by opacities or refractive irregularities anywhere in the media. Commonly observed effects are due to:

(1) Lashes, lid margins, and their associated tears prisms.
(2) Mucous or oil globules, etc., in the tears layer. These appear as spots of light generally appearing to move downwards (in reality, upwards). The globules are pushed down on blinking but return slowly upwards during the interval between blinks.
(3) Rubbing or pressing on the eye, which disturbs the corneal integrity and causes an entoptic effect of mottling.
(4) Lens sutures.
(5) Lens opacities. Tscherning (1924) suggests that 'an intelligent patient can thus follow step by step the

development of his cataract', perhaps questionable advice to give to many patients.

(6) Vitreous floaters, as distinct from
(7) Muscae volitantes. These are delicate, somewhat lacy or chain-like shadows which can often be seen without the aid of a pinhole because they are due to fine opacities positioned close to the retina. They move with the gaze, but tend to overshoot and come back when ocular movement stops, as though tethered to the retina. It is the jelly-like nature of the vitreous, however, which limits the motion of the floaters. The Latin name given to these shadows means flying gnats, which aptly described their flitting nature.

Muscae volitantes were often assumed to be shadows of strings of red blood corpuscles. White and Levatin (1962) measured the apparent size of 'corpuscular' floaters and found it to be about 25–40 µm, much larger than the 8.5 µm diameter of a blood corpuscle. Analysis suggested that the 'shadows' were actually diffraction patterns formed by blood corpuscles suspended about 250–350 µm (microns) in front of the foveal cones. Their apparent tendency to drop when the eye is stationary means that the corpuscles are in fact rising. White and Levatin suggest that as the main body of the vitreous descends, the more fluid vitreous close to the retina consequently rises.

It must be pointed out that the blurred image of a small source of light viewed by an uncorrected ametrope or artificially defocused emmetrope also allows many of these irregularities in the media to be perceived.

An artificial obstruction in the form of a wire across the pupil may be used as a subjective test. Velonoskiascopy, as this technique is called, was introduced by Holth in 1904 and further developed by Trantas (1921) and Lindner (1926). If the wire is mounted across a trial frame, the head can be rocked to traverse the wire across the pupil. As noted on pages 73–74, the direction of movement of the entoptic shadow across the retinal blur may be used to distinguish between hypermetropia and myopia. To correct the eye, lenses are added until the shadow disappears. The recommended object is a white line, orientated parallel to the wire and subtending about 3 minutes of arc, mounted on a red ground. Although methods for examination of astigmatism were introduced, the present writers have been unable to confirm their efficacy.

Entoptic phenomena and cataract

Entoptic phenomena generated in the retina could, in theory, be used to verify reginal integrity behind a cataract. First, as already mentioned, shadows of the retinal vessels may be seen if an intense light transilluminates the sclera. In another suggested technique, the retina is strongly illuminated with blue light. The slit lamp can be used as the light source, aimed directly at the pupil. To provide a larger field of illumination, a ground-glass diffuser held immediately in front of the eye may be needed. The patient should be able to see moving bright spots which are thought to be white blood cells in the retinal vessels, the red corpuscles absorbing the light. The same effect can be observed while reclining and looking upwards into a cloudless bright blue sky. There is no doubt that the methods of verifying retinal integrity described on pages 44–45 are far superior.

Haloes and coronas

The cornea and crystalline lens are not homogeneous but fibrous, as may be seen in life with the slit-lamp microscope. As a result, a small portion of the light passing through the eye is scattered. It may be scattered irregularly or form a pattern on the retina, in which case it could be perceived as an entoptic phenomenon, given suitable observation conditions. The usual effect of all such stray light is to reduce the contrast of the retinal image (*see* pages 295–298).

The corneal corona

The cornea is composed of layers of very fine collagen fibrils between 19 and 34 nm in thickness, laid down in lamellae which are 1.5–2.5 µm thick and 90–260 µm wide. It is possibly the boundaries of these lamellae that are visible in the slit-lamp beam, although Maurice (1962) postulated that some of the light was scattered by the nuclei of the stromal cells.

The healthy cornea scatters about 10% of the incident light. Maurice compared the fibrils of each corneal lamellae with a three-dimensional diffraction grating.* Because the inter-fibril separation is much less than the wavelength of light, light scattered by one fibril cannot interfere constructively with light scattered by the neighbouring fibril, so that no diffraction spectra can be formed. Moreover, any scattered light will interfere destructively with non-scattered light owing to the phase change on reflection. As a result, the incident beam must pass unattenuated through each lamella.

If the corneal stroma becomes oedematous, through contact-lens wear or raised intra-ocular pressure, for example, the regularity of the stromal fibrils becomes disturbed and the normal destructive interference of scattered light no longer takes place. Similarly, if the epithelium becomes oedematous, the intra-cellular spacing may increase to more than 0.5 µm with globules (mostly of water) also giving rise to scattering of light.

Any particular globule in the cornea will scatter light in all directions. Destructive interference, however, will occur if the path difference from opposite sides of the globule is an odd number of half wavelengths (*Figure 22.6*). In monochromatic light, the appearance will be that of an Airy disc and ring. In white light, the first minimum will occur at an increasing angle from the centre as wavelength increases. The white centre will then be surrounded by a subtraction spectrum, with the first minimum for blue giving a reddish-yellow ring,

---

* A diffraction grating is any two- or three-dimensional array of lines or dots showing periodic variations of either transparency or of refractive index. Physics textbooks often illustrate clear and occluded transmission gratings (such as Foucault gratings), but many natural structures are phase gratings.

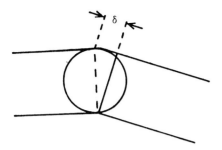

Figure 22.6. Diffraction by a globule: the relative path difference is δ.

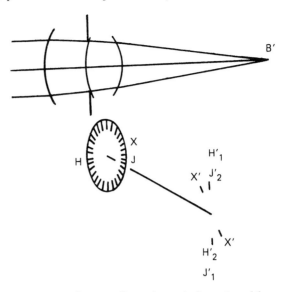

Figure 22.7. The upper figure shows the formation of the normal or zero-order diffraction image, while the lower figure in isometric form shows the positions of the first-order diffraction images arising from the fibres at H, J and X.

then the green minimum giving purple, and so on. Irregular shaping of a particular globule will cause an irregular halo, but summation over the whole pupillary area generates a symmetrical (but perhaps less well-defined) corona around a light. Similar coronas will be seen if a light is viewed through spectacle lenses or a window steamed up with fine condensation, through a blood smear on a slide or lycopodium powder.

The corneal corona was first observed by Descartes in 1637 (cited by Simpson, 1953).

A similar halo is seen by the very occasional patient with a nuclear sclerosis type of cataract, light being scattered by the brown discoloured lens nucleus (Elliot, 1921). The authors have met very few such patients.

The lenticular halo

The crystalline lens gives a somewhat similar halo, but the origin is quite different. With the exception of the zonule and anterior cellular layer, the lens is composed of fibres which pass in an approximately radial manner from the anterior to the posterior sutures. These fibres are about 8–12 μm wide by 2 μm thick in the outer layers of the lens.

The axial part of the crystalline lens appears to be relatively uniform, no lens halo being observed with a pupil less than about 3 mm in diameter. When the pupil is dilated, however, either under conditions of low illumination or especially with a mydriatic, the effects of the peripheral zones become very marked. The lens may be regarded as a strong positive lens on whose periphery is superimposed a radial diffraction grating. In *Figure 22.7*, an element H of the radial grating will form the zero order image B' at the primary focus of the lens (ignoring aberrations) while first-order diffraction images will form above and below the focus at H'_1, H'_2. Similarly, the diametrically opposite element J will form images J'_1 and J'_2 in the same place as H'_1 and H'_2. Various other zones of the lens will form diffraction images on the radius perpendicular to the zone orientation (such as X) so that the complete effect is one of a circular corona.

The diameter or spacing of the lens fibres is not completely uniform so that the resultant halo is not absolutely circular but somewhat erratic. Thinner fibres in a particular direction produce longer spectra than thicker fibres elsewhere.

Although the lens fibres may not be truly radial since they are directed at the lens sutures rather than the axis, any tilt in the orientation of the fibres – at H, say, of *Figure 22.7* – will rotate the first-order spectra H'_1 and H'_2 around the principal image, but at the same distance from it. Thus the approximate circularity of the corona remains undisturbed, although variations in intensity are generated.

The lens halo and the corona arising from corneal oedema have the similar appearance of circular rings, although the order of colours is different. Since corneal oedema can arise from pathological causes such as an increase in intra-ocular tension in angle-closure glaucoma, whereas the lens halo is a physiological effect, it is important to be able to differentiate between the two sites of origin.

Corneal oedema causes small-body diffraction, each element scattering light equally in all meridians. If a stenopaeic slit is held before the eye to restrict the light entering to a small zone of the entrance pupil, the corneal halo is merely dimmed. Passage of light through a particular strip of the crystalline lens generates a specific double section of the lenticular halo. Moving a vertical stenopaeic slit across the pupil therefore gives moving sectors of light, as indicated in *Figure 22.8*. This is the Emsley–Fincham test (1922) for differentiating corneal from lenticular haloes, a development of Druault's test of 1899 which used the edge of an occluder.

If glaucoma is suspected as the cause of a halo, then the intra-ocular tension can be measured with a tonometer. The pressure at the time of measurement might be normal, in which case the patient could perform the Fincham test if the halo should ever reappear. A fuller ocular investigation initially would be advisable. Mueller's (Sattler's or Fick's) veil occurring in contact-lens wear may need to be distinguished from the crystalline lens halo or to flare from contact-lens edges or transitions.

(a)

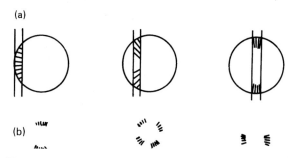

(b)

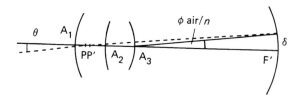

Figure 22.9. Derivation of the Druault coefficient for light scattered near the posterior pole A_3 of the crystalline lens.

Figure 22.8. (a) The Emsley–Fincham test for distinguishing a lenticular halo. The stenopaeic slit is passed across the pupil, isolating differently orientated groups of lens fibres responsible for the sections of the halo shown in (b).

Table 22.1 Conversion factors giving the true angle of diffraction ϕ_{air} corresponding to the subjective angular subtense θ

Source	Conversion factor	
	Accurate	Approximate
Cornea	0.909	0.925
Anterior lens surface	1.092	1.087
Centre of lens	1.200	1.195
Posterior lens surface	1.326	1.326

The ciliary corona

Most people observe the ciliary corona, a spread of light around an isolated bright source such as a street lamp. This is due to diffraction by particles within the eye, the angle of scatter being lower than that for the first Airy minimum so that only the central disc or aureole is perceived. Thus, no coloured fringes are seen, the scattered light remaining white for a white source. The intensity of the central aureole falls as the angle of scatter increases (*see Figure 3.4*). If the source luminance is increased, the intensity at some particular angle from the image will also increase, possibly from below to above threshold. The diameter of the aureole thus depends upon the source brightness (and background darkness). If the light is bright enough, the corona fills the lenticular halo, the radius of which subtends about 3–$4°$.

Simpson (1953) showed that the diameter of the diffracting particles must be less than $10\ \mu m$. This follows from the Airy disc equation (3.2) when the value of θ exceeds $4°$.

Unlike the corneal corona caused by oedema, the ciliary corona is a normal phenomenon. It may appear to be composed of fine moving dots and lines. This form in which it is perceived may arise from the processing of the neural signal by elements higher in the visual system.

Theoretical analysis

For a grating-like source of diffraction such as the crystalline lens, the angle of diffraction in air, ϕ_{air}, to the first maximum is

$$\phi_{air} = \lambda/d \qquad (22.5)$$

where d is the grating element.

For diffraction by approximately spherical bodies, such as the glaucomatous halo, the first maximum outside the central disc occurs for

$$\phi_{air} = 1.638\lambda/d \qquad (22.6)$$

where d is now the body diameter.

For the second maximum,

$$\phi_{air} = 2.666\lambda/d \qquad (22.7)$$

In a medium of refractive index n, the angle of diffraction becomes ϕ_{air}/n.

Druault (1899) introduced the principle of position coefficients relating the apparent diameter of the entoptic haloes to the position of their source within the eye. For example, consider light scattered at the posterior lens surface. In *Figure 22.9*, the deviation δ at the retina is given by

$$\delta = A_3F'(\phi_{air})/n \qquad (22.8)$$

Projected into object space through the principal points, the apparent angular subtense of the halo is given by

$$\theta = (n/P'F')\{A_3F'(\phi_{air})/n\}$$
$$= A_3F'(\phi_{air})/P'F'$$

which gives

$$\phi_{air} = P'F'(\theta/A_3F') \qquad (22.9)$$

If refraction by the crystalline lens is ignored, a similar equation can be derived for light scattered in the cornea:

$$\phi_{air} = P'F'(\theta/A_1F') \qquad (22.10)$$

A more accurate result can be derived by finding the position of the virtual image A_1' of the corneal vertex A_1 formed by the crystalline lens, giving

$$\phi_{air} = P'F'(\theta/A_1'F') \qquad (22.11)$$

Table 22.1 gives these conversion factors, both approximate and accurate, based on the Bennet–Rabbetts schematic eye.

Haidinger's brushes

Haidinger's brushes, first described in 1844, is the name given to an hour-glass or propeller-like figure seen in polarized light near the fixation point. In white light, both blue and yellow brushes are seen, at right angles to each other. The blue brushes lie in the plane of vibration* of the polarized light. They are best seen, however, when a uniformly illuminated white screen is viewed through a rotating polarizer and blue filter (an

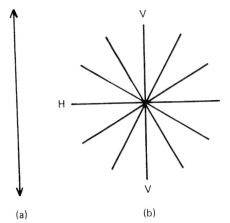

Figure 22.10. A radial analyser's selective absorption of plane polarized light: (a) plane of vibration of incident light, (b) radial analyser.

instrument known as a Cüpper's co-ordinator), when the yellow brushes appear as dark shadows. In the purple light transmitted by a cobalt blue filter, the phenomenon appears as dark shadows and light reddish-orange brushes.

There are many theories as to the cause of the brushes. One possibility is that some structure of the eye acts as a radial analyser for blue light. *Figure 22.10* shows incident light with vertical vibrations falling on a radial analyser. The horizontal section along HH has its plane of transmission at right-angles, or 'crossed' with respect to the incident light so that blue light is absorbed. In white light a yellow brush would then be seen in this direction by colour subtraction. Conversely, the vertical elements VV will transmit more blue light than average for the macular area so that a blue brush would be seen. As the plane of polarization of light reaching the eye is rotated, the 'bright' brushes would successively fall in different planes to give the subjective appearance of rotation. This effect of absorption of light polarized in one direction and transmission in the plane at right-angles, as in Polaroid sheet, is known as dichroism.

Many suggestions have been made as to the position of the analysing structure in the eye. Since aphakics can see the brushes, the crystalline lens is not the site. Stanworth and Naylor (1950a,b) have shown that although the cornea is birefringent,[†] which slightly alters the quality of polarization of transmitted light, it is not responsible for the brushes. Helmholtz (1924, Vol. II) postulated that the cause lay in the radial structure of the supporting neuroglial fibres of Müller, while another possibility is the neural outer plexiform layer

(Henle's fibres). There is no evidence, however, that either of these fibres is dichroic. Because of its absorption of blue light and the similar location and subtense of Haidinger's brushes and Maxwell's spot (see below), a more probable explanation is the yellow macular pigment. Naylor and Stanworth (1954) and Stanworth and Naylor (1955) found excellent agreement in a comparison of the visibility of Haidinger's brushes in light of various wavelengths and the spectral absorption of xanthophyll, a yellow carotenoid pigment which is similar to, if not identical with, the macular pigment. They confirmed previous findings that Haidinger's brushes were not visible in light of wavelength longer than about 560 nm. They suggested therefore that a proportion of the yellow macular pigment was orientated along the supportive tissues to act as a radial analyser. If the pigment was dichroic, then Haidinger's brushes would be explained. Their data conflicted with the suggestion that the blue receptors had a selective response depending upon the plane of polarization of the incident light.

Although the macula pigment theory appears the most probable, Hallden (1957) postulated that the brushes were caused by an interference effect. If the retina contained a layer of birefringent substance arranged with its optic axis at a constant angle to the radially analysing receptors, then coloured brushes rotating with the plane of vibration of the incident light would be seen. He suggested that the birefringent Henle's fibres might constitute the retarding plate, while the analysing structure was not necessarily the blue receptors.

If a viewing screen is observed through a rotating polarizer, and a half-wave plate (e.g. Cellophane about 40 μm thick or polyethylene sheet) placed between the polarizer and the eye, the direction of rotation of the Haidinger's brushes is reversed. If the polarizer is kept still and the half-wave plate rotated, the brushes appear to rotate in the same direction as the half-wave plate but at twice the angular speed. Both these effects can be explained in terms of alterations in the plane of vibration of the light external to the eye.

Haidinger's brushes are of clinical importance since they are formed only at the fovea. If a patient with normal fixation looks through a Cüpper's co-ordinator and fixates a mark on the viewing screen, Haidinger's brushes will be seen to rotate around the fixation point. If the patient's eye normally fixates with an eccentric part of the retina, the brushes appear to rotate about a point displaced from fixation. This readily measurable discrepancy is the angle of eccentricity. Stanworth and Naylor (1955) suggested that the visibility of Haidinger's brushes was useful in assessing retinal function in patients with macular changes such as degeneration or oedema.

Maxwell's spot

The yellow pigment of the macula lutea has already been mentioned in relation to Haidinger's brushes. This yellow pigment may also be seen entoptically as Maxwell's spot (1856) but not under normal conditions.

---

[*] Helmholtz stated that the yellow brush was in the plane of polarization, but the convention for the plane of 'polarization' was subsequently changed to that of the electrical vibration direction of the electromagnetic radiation. This is at right-angles to the original notation.

[†] Birefringent: a simplified explanation is that refraction of light inside the substance will produce an ordinary and an extraordinary ray with vibration planes at right-angles, the two rays having different velocities (cf. the Wallaston prism in the Javal–Schiötz keratometer on page 383).

The absorption of blue light by the pigment would be expected to cause a slight blue shadow around the fixation point, but the blue receptors in the macula adapt by increasing their sensitivity. As a result, Maxwell's spot is not normally noticeable, exactly like the Purkinje retinal tree.

Maxwell's spot may be seen by viewing a brightly illuminated white surface or the blue sky alternately through a purple (e.g. cobalt blue) and grey filter. An irregularly shaped dark-red spot will be seen through the purple filter subtending about 6Δ.

The yellow macular pigment cannot be seen with the normal ophthalmoscope. It can, however, be seen in the red-free light of mercury illumination with the indirect ophthalmoscope (Ballantyne and Michaelson, 1965) or by photography with a blue filter.

Physiological entoptic phenomena

The physiological entoptic phenomena will be discussed only briefly since they are not of optical origin.

Phosphenes

Phosphenes are vague visual sensations arising when the retina is stimulated by energy other than light. Since the optic nerves and pathways end in the occipital cortex, any response by the retina will give the specific sensation of vision. The retina is very sensitive to luminous energy but much larger amounts of non-luminous energy are required for stimulation to occur. Hence, the eye must usually be dark adapted to see phosphenes. The somewhat inappropriate term 'inadequate stimulus' is often used to describe non-luminous stimulation.

X-rays can stimulate the retina and have been used in measurements of the axial lengths and focal power of the eye (*see* page 378), but their excessive use can cause serious side-effects. Their wavelength, 100 nm to 0.01 nm, is very much shorter than the wavelength of light. Medical X-rays are nearer the short end of the range.

Mechanically induced phosphenes may be of internal or external origin. The separating or 'detaching' retina is a cause with serious consequences that must immediately be investigated should a patient complain of flashing lights. Similar phosphenes may occur with a fluid vitreous and with some other pathological states of retina and choroid. Direct pressure on the globe with a finger will stimulate the underlying receptors, giving a projected phosphene on the opposite side to the finger. Version movements of the eyes from side to side may well give dull phosphenes due to the traction of the lateral and medial rectus muscles on the globe. A ring phosphene has been reported on accommodating (Czermak, cited by Tscherning, 1924).

The blood circulation may also give rise to phosphenes.* These are perhaps more optical than physiological since they are best seen against a blue sky and appear as tiny bright specks in the field of view moving along a short path and then disappearing. Barrett (1906) suggested that these were due to white blood corpuscles moving along the retinal capillaries.

Some other phosphenes have recently been described by Tyler (1978).

The blue-arcs phenomenon

If a moderately dark-adapted eye views a small source of red light positioned one or two degrees from the fixation point, a dim bluish arc may be seen extending from the coloured source. These arcs, which follow the route of the post-ganglionic nerve fibres towards the optic disc, were noted by Purkinje.

For an account of recent work on this phenomenon, *see* Moreland (1968, 1969).

After-images

A comprehensive discussion of the physiology of after-images is given by Lott Brown (1965) in the work by Graham and in other texts on physiology.

Because the after-image is fixed in relation to the retina, and will therefore be projected in a fixed position with respect to the eye, after-images may be used in orthoptics to verify binocular retinal correspondence and in the treatment of amblyopia (Caloroso, 1972; Mallett, 1975).

The Troxler effect

Even when a specific object is steadily fixated, the eye is constantly moving slightly. There is a high-frequency tremor of up to 1 minute of arc superimposed on larger drifting and saccadic movements. The image is therefore moving constantly over the retina so that the stimulation of the receptors is also varying. Thus on–off effects occur in the neural pathways and retinal adaptation is reduced.

If fixation is maintained as steadily as possible for 30 s or more, objects in the periphery of the field of vision appear to dim, a phenomenon noted by Troxler. Because the size of the integrated receptor fields increases from the central retina outwards, small eye movements produce less fluctuation in illumination and retinal stimulation in peripheral areas. Hence, adaptation occurs first in the periphery and results in the dimming of perception. The shadow of the retinal vascular system is nullified by sensory adaptation in an even more striking manner.

Much quicker fading of the visual field can be produced if the image is stabilized on the retina. One method uses a rigid contact lens fitting tightly on the sclera. It can carry either a test object and collimating lens or a 45° mirror and telescope assembly of angular magnification 0.5. Alternatively, electronic systems can be used to monitor the eye movements and hence adjust the object position on a video display. Techniques using after-images have also been devised.

---

* This phenomenon, like many others, was first noted by Purkinje in the 1820s. Some recent American authors, such as Priestley and Foree (1955), have named it after Scheerer who investigated it in 1924.

Exercises

22.1 Show that if a pinhole is held at the anterior focal plane of the eye, the projected shadow of a vitreous opacity is magnified by d/f_e, where f_e is the anterior focal length of the eye and d the distance at which the projected shadow is measured.

22.2 In Helmholtz's technique of velonoskiascopy, an occluder is passed downwards across the pupil. In uncorrected hypermetropia, does the perceived blur appear to shrink from bottom or top?

22.3 In Lindner's technique with a white line on a red ground, why does the shadow of the wire appear red?

22.4 In Lindner's technique, a myope observes an upright line with a vertical occluding wire mounted in the trial frame. (a) Does the shadow appear to move with or against when the head (together with the trial frame) is turned to the right? (b) What is the horizontal retinal blur width, given an eye of dioptric length +60 D with a residual refractive error of 0.50 D? Assume the diameters of wire and pupil to be 1 and 4 mm respectively. (c) Compare this with the basic image width of a test line object subtending 0.1Δ.

22.5 (a) Calculate the Druault coefficient for diffraction in the plane of the geometrical centre of the crystalline lens. (Hint: determine the position of the image of this point formed by the posterior lens surface, assuming the constants of the Gullstrand–Emsley eye.) (See Appendix B.) (b) Given that the diameter of the lens halo is $6°$ in sodium light ($\lambda = 589$ nm) and assuming grating-type diffraction, calculate the grating element (fibre size).

References

BALLANTYNE, A.J. and MICHAELSON, I.C. (1965) *Textbook of the Fundus of the Eye*, pp. 1–30. Edinburgh: E. & S. Livingstone

BARRETT, W.F. (1906) On entoptic vision, or the self-examination of objects within the eye. *Scient. Proc. R. Dubl. Soc.*, **11**, 43–88, 111–136 + plates III–VIII, 1905–1908

BRADLEY, A., APPLEGATE, R.A., ZEFFREN, B.S. and VAN HEUVEN, W.A.J. (1992) Psychophysical measurement of the size and shape of the human foveal avascular zone. *Ophthal. Physiol. Opt.*, **12**, 18–23

BROWN, J.L. (1965) Afterimages. In *Vision and Visual Perception* (Graham, C.H., ed.), pp. 479–503. New York: Wiley

CALOROSO, E. (1972) After-image transfer: a therapeutic procedure for amblyopia. *Am. J. Optom.*, **49**, 65–69

DRUAULT, A. (1899) Sur les anneaux colorés que l'on peut voir autour des flammes à l'état normal ou pathologique. *IX Int. Ophthal. Gngr. (Utrecht)*, pp. 196–219

ELLIOT, R.H. (1921) The haloes of glaucoma. *Br. J. Ophthal.*, **5**, 500–502

EMSLEY, H.H. and FINCHAM, E.F. (1922) Diffraction haloes in normal and glaucomatous eyes. *Trans. Opt. Soc. Lond.*, **23**, 225–240

HALLDEN, U. (1957) An explanation of Haidinger's brushes. *A.M.A. Archs Ophthal.*, **57**, 393–399

HELMHOLTZ, H. VON (1924) Physiological Optics, Vol. I, pp. 204–225 (optically based phenomena); Vol. II, pp. 301–311 (other phenomena). English translation ed. Southall, J.P.C. New York: Optical Society of America. (Reprinted 1962 by Dover Publications, New York.)

HOLTH, M.S. (1904) Nouveau procédé pour déterminer la réfraction. *Ann. Oculist.*, **131**, 418–438

HURST, M.A., DOUTHWAITE, W.A. and ELLIOTT, D.B. (1993) Assessment of retinal and neural function behind a cataract. In *Cataract, Detection, Measurement and Management in Optometric Practice* (Douthwaite, W.A. and Hurst, M.A., eds), pp. 49–51. Oxford: Butterworth-Heinemann

JAGO, J. (1864) *Entoptics, With Its Uses in Physiology and Medicine*, pp. 135–137. London: Churchill

JOHNSON, M.H., RUBEN, C.M. and PERRIGEN, D.M. (1987) Entoptic phenomena and reproducibility of corneal striae following contact lens wear. *Br.J. Ophthal.*, **71**, 737–741

LINDNER, K. (1926) Beiträge zur subjektiven Bestimmung des Astigmatismus. *Z. Augenheilk.*, **60**, 346–360

MALLETT, R.F.J. (1975) Using after-images in the investigation and treatment of strabismus. *Ophthal. Optn.*, **15**, 727–729

MAURICE, D.M. (1962) The cornea and sclera. In *The Eye*, Vol. 1 (Davson, H., ed.), pp. 312–322. New York and London: Academic Press

MORELAND, J.D. (1968) On demonstrating the blue arc phenomenon. *Vision Res.*, **8**, 99–107

MORELAND, J.D. (1969) Retinal topography and the blue arcs phenomenon. *Vision Res.*, **9**, 965–976

NAYLOR, E.J. and STANWORTH, A. (1954) Retinal pigment and the Haidinger effect. *J. Physiol.*, **124**, 543–552

PRIESTLEY, B.S. and FOREE, K. (1955) Clinical significance of some entoptic phenomena. *A.M.A. Archs Ophthal.*, **53**, 390–397

SIMPSON, G.C. (1953) Ocular haloes and coronas. *Br. J. Ophthal.*, **37**, 449–486

STANWORTH, A. and NAYLOR, E.J. (1950a) The polarization optics of the isolated cornea. *Br. J. Ophthal.*, **34**, 201–211

STANWORTH, A. and NAYLOR, E.J. (1950b) Haidinger's brushes and the retinal receptors. *Br. J. Ophthal.*, **34**, 282–291

STANWORTH, A. and NAYLOR, E.J. (1955) The measurement and clinical significance of the Haidinger effect. *Trans. Ophthal. Soc. UK*, **76**, 67–79

TRANTAS, M. (1921) La velonoskiascopie et son utilité surtout pour la détermination des principaux méridiens de l'astigmie. *Bull. Mém. Soc. Fr. Ophthal.*, **34**, 273–293

TSCHERNING, M. (1924) *Physiologic Optics*, 4th edn, pp. 178–179. (trans. Weiland, C.). Philadelphia: Keystone Publishing Co.

TYLER, C.W. (1978) Some new entoptic phenomena. *Vision Res.*, **18**, 1633–1639

WHITE, H.E. and LEVATIN, P. (1962) Floaters in the eye. *Scientific American*, **206**(6), 119–123, 125, 127

ZEFFREN, B.S., APPLEGATE, R.A., BRADLEY, A. and VAN HEUVEN, W.A.J. (1990) Retinal fixation point location in the foveal avascular zone. *Invest. Ophthalmol. Vis. Sci.*, **31**, 2099–2105

Appendix A: a suggested routine examination procedure

(1) *Symptoms and history* (including health and medication)

(2) *Distance vision*

If the patient is an habitual spectacle wearer, measure the vision of R and L eyes through spectacles and possibly the unaided vision. If not an habitual wearer, measure the R and L vision and also the binocular vision as this may be significantly better.

(3) *Near vision*

With test types.

(4) *Cover test*

In distance vision, with spectacles if habitually worn. Also in near vision, but perhaps omit if patient would need to don reading spectacles.

(5) *Near point of convergence*

(6) *Motility test*

(7) *Refraction*

(a) *Distance procedures*

Objective.

Subjective, including binocular refraction or balancing when appropriate.

Distance visual acuity.

Distance oculo-motor balance, for example, cover test (and/or Maddox rod) and fixation disparity.

*Suppression tests.

(b) *Near procedures*

Amplitude of accommodation or reading addition.

Accommodative lag: near bichromatic test or dynamic retinoscopy.

Oculo-motor balance, for example, cover test and fixation disparity.

*Suppression tests.

*Stereopsis.

(c) *Supplementary procedures*

*Cycloplegic refraction.

*Orthoptic investigation.

(8) *Colour vision*

On first examination or if an acquired defect suspected.

(9) *Ocular health*

(a) *Basic procedures* (These may conveniently be performed here, or before the refraction, according to the practitioner's preference.)

Pupil reactions: direct, consensual and near.

†Hand slit-lamp examination.

Ophthalmoscopy.

†Confrontation test.

(b) *Further procedures*

Tonometry on patients over 40 years, or younger where indicated.

Major slit-lamp (biomicroscope) examination.

Visual-fields examination.

Amsler chart investigation.

Mydriasis, possibly with indirect ophthalmoscopy (head mounted or with slit-lamp).

---

* Tests undertaken only when indicated or advisable.
† The procedures in section 9b are preferable.

Appendix B: the Bennett–Rabbetts schematic eye, relaxed and accommodated 10 D and, for historical reference, the Gullstrand–Emsley relaxed schematic eye (in italics)

Quantity		Gullstrand–Emsley	Relaxed	Accommodated (10.0 D)
Radii of curvature				
cornea	r_1	+7.80	+7.30	+7.80
crystalline: first surface	r_2	+10.00	+11.00	+5.20
crystalline: second surface*	r_3	−6.00	−6.47515	−4.750
Axial separations				
depth of anterior chamber	d_1	3.6	3.60	3.21
thickness of crystalline	d_2	3.6	3.70	4.09
depth of vitreous body	d_3	16.69	16.79	16.79
Overall axial length†		23.89	24.09	24.09
Mean refractive indices				
air	n_1	1	1	1
aqueous humour	n_2	1.3333	1.336	1.336
crystalline	n_3	1.4160	1.422	1.422
vitreous humour	n_4	1.3333	1.336	1.336
Surface powers				
cornea	F_1	+42.73	+43.08	+43.08
crystalline: first surface	F_2	+8.27	+7.82	+16.54
crystalline: second surface	F_3	+13.78	+13.28	+18.10
Equivalent powers				
crystalline	F_L	+21.76	+20.83	+33.78
eye	F_o	+60.49	+60.00	+71.12
Equivalent focal lengths of eye				
first (PF)	f_o	−16.53	−16.67	−14.06
second (P′F′)	f'_o	+22.04	+22.27	+18.79
Distances from corneal vertex				
first principal point	A_1P	+1.55	+1.51	+1.87
second principal point	A_1P'	+1.85	+1.82	+2.23
first nodal point	A_1N	+7.06	+7.11	+6.60
second nodal point‡	A_1N'	+7.36	+7.42	+6.95
entrance pupil	A_1E	+3.05	+3.05	+2.68
exit pupil	A_1E'	+3.69	+3.70	+3.25
first principal focus	A_1F	−14.98	−15.16	−12.19
second principal focus	A_1F'	+23.89	+24.09	+21.01
Refractive state (principal point)	K	0	0	−10.00
Distance of near point from corneal vertex				−98.1

All linear dimensions are in millimetres and powers in dioptres. See *Table 12.1* for intermediate values of accommodation – values for accommodated eyes should be regarded as provisional until further data become available.

* This radius is specified to three or more places of decimals solely to 'fine-tune' the resulting refractive state, and does not imply that an eye has to be constructed to this degree of precision.

† The accurate value of 24.0859 was used in the reversed ray traces for the accommodating and elderly Bennett–Rabbetts eyes.

‡ Rounding errors explain the apparent differences between PP′ and NN′ for the various eyes.

General bibliography

This bibliography is divided by subject matter into five sections. Except for a number of classic and older texts, all the works listed are in print at the time of writing. In each section the works are given in alphabetical order of author's or editor's name.

Classic texts and general works

CRONLY-DILLON, J. (ed.) (1991) *Vision and Visual Dysfunction* (17 vols). Basingstoke: Macmillan. The following volumes are particularly relevant: 1: *Visual Optics and Instrumentation* (Charman, W.N., ed.); 9: *Binocular Vision* (Regan, D., ed.)

DONDERS, F.C. (1864) *Anomalies of Refraction and Accommodation of the Eye*. London: New Sydenham Society. Reprinted in facsimile: London: Hatton Press, 1952

DUKE-ELDER, W.D. (ed.) (1958 onwards) *System of Ophthalmology* (15 vols). Edinburgh: Churchill Livingstone. The following volumes are particularly relevant: IV: *The Physiology of the Eye and Vision*; V: *Ophthalmic Optics and Refraction*; VI: *Ocular Motility and Strabismus*; VII: *The Foundations of Ophthalmology*

HELMHOLTZ, H. VON (1856–66) *Physiological Optics*. English translation: J.P.C. Southall. New York: Optical Society of America, 1924. Reprinted: New York: Dover Publications, 1962

MILLODOT, M. (1997) *Dictionary of Optometry*, 4th edn. Oxford: Butterworth-Heinemann

TSCHERNING, M. (1898) *Physiologic Optics*. English translation: C. Weiland, 4th edn, 1924. Philadelphia: Keystone Publishing Co.

Ophthalmic practice and instrumentation

BALL, G.V. (1982) *Symptoms in Eye Examination*. London: Butterworths

BORISH, I.M. (1970) *Clinical Refraction*, 3rd edn (2 vols). Chicago: Professional Press

CURTIN, B.J. (1985) *The Myopias*. Philadelphia: Harper and Row

EDWARDS, K.H. and LLEWELLYN, R.D. (1989) *Optometry*. London: Butterworths

GROSVENOR, T. and FLOM, M.C. (1991) *Refractive Anomalies. Research and Clinical Applications*. Boston: Butterworth-Heinemann

HENSON, D.B. (1996) *Optometric Instrumentation*, 2nd edn. Oxford: Butterworth-Heinemann

MICHAELS, D.D. (1985) *Visual Optics and Refraction*, 3rd edn. St Louis: C.V. Mosby Co.

PHILLIPS, A.J. and SPEEDWELL, L. (eds) (1997) *Contact Lenses*, 4th edn. Oxford: Butterworth-Heinemann

PITTS, D.G. and KLEINSTEIN, R.N. (1993) *Environmental Vision. Interactions of the Eye, Vision, and the Environment*. Boston: Butterworth-Heinemann

TUNNACLIFFE, A.H. (1997) *Introduction to Visual Optics*, 4th edn. London: Association of British Dispensing Opticians

Geometrical and physical optics

BENNETT, A.G. (1985) *Optics of Contact Lenses*, 5th edn. London: Association of Dispensing Opticians

DOUTHWAITE, W.A. (1995) *Contact Lens Optics and Design*, 2nd edn. Oxford: Butterworth-Heinemann

FREEMAN, M.H. (1995) *Optics*, 10th edn. Oxford: Butterworth-Heinemann

FRY, G.A. (1969) *Ophthalmic Optics*. Philadelphia: Chilton

SOUTHALL, J.P.C. (1933) *Mirrors, Prisms and Lenses*, 3rd edn. New York: Macmillan. Reprinted 1964: New York: Dover Publications

TUNNACLIFFE, A.H. and HIRST, J.G. (1996) *Optics*, 2nd edn. London: Association of British Dispensing Opticians

Physiological optics and visual perception

COREN, S. and GIRGUS, J.S. (1978) *Seeing is Deceiving: The Psychology of Visual Illusions*. Hillsdale, N.J.: Lawrence Erlbaum Associates

DAVSON, H. (1990) *Physiology of the Eye*, 5th edn. London: Macmillan

GREGORY, R.L. (1974) *Eye and Brain*, 3rd edn. London: Weidenfeld

HART, JR, W.M. (1992) *Alder's Physiology of the Eye*, 9th edn. St Louis: Mosby Year Book

Binocular vision and orthoptics

EVANS, B.J.W. (1997) *Pickwell's Binocular Vision Anomalies*, 3rd edn. Oxford: Butterworth-Heinemann

OGLE, K.N. (1950) *Resources in Binocular Vision*. Philadelphia: W.B. Saunders Co. Reprinted: New York: Hafner, 1964

OGLE, K.N., MARTENS, T.G. and DYER, J.A. (1968) *Oculomotor Imbalance in Binocular Vision and Fixation Disparity*. Philadelphia: Lea and Febiger

VON NOORDEN, G.K. (1995) *Binocular Vision and Ocular Motility*, 5th edn. St Louis: C.V. Mosby Co.

WALSH, F.B. and HOYT, W.F. (1982) *Clinical Neuro-Ophthalmology*, Vol. 1, 4th edn. Baltimore: Williams and Wilkins

Answers

Chapter 2

2.1 (a) $+6.38\,D$ (b) $-7.14\,D$
2.2 $5.16°$; $0.9\,m$
2.3 Entrance pupil 2.49 mm behind cornea, $m = +1.11$
Exit pupil 3.07 mm behind cornea, $m = +1.03$
2.4 $A_1P = -37.5$, $A_2F' = +50$, $PP' = +22.5$, $F'B' = +31.25$, $PB = -625$ (all in mm)
2.5 $P'A_1 = -e' - t$, $A_2B' = -e' + \ell$, $PP' = -e + t + e'$, $B'P = -\ell' - e' - t + e$, $BB' = -\ell - e + t + e' + \ell'$
2.6 $n = 1.440$, $r = 7.3333$

Chapter 3

3.1 6/14 (20/47), 6/7 (20/23), 6/4.7 (20/16)
3.2 (a) 6/16
3.3

	6-metre letter	4-metre letter
(a)	8.48 and 8.98 mm	5.57 and 6.07 mm
(b)	6.73 and 7.23 mm	4.42 and 4.88 mm
(c)	1.66 and 1.84 mm	1.04 and 1.28 mm

3.4 15.0 mm, 1.07
3.5 Yes
3.6 68.75 m
3.7 7, 24
3.8 $N5 \approx 6/9$ (20/30), $N48 \approx 6/84$ (20/280)
3.9 1.51 M
3.10 83.6%
3.11 (a) 0.012 mm (b) 0.019 mm (c) 0.048 mm
3.12 0.67, 1.33, 0.17
3.13 6/12 (20/40), 6/24 (20/80), 6/18 (20/60), 6/30 (20/90)

Chapter 4

4.1 (a) $\pm 400\,mm$ (b) $\pm 200\,mm$ (c) $\pm 133\frac{1}{3}\,mm$ (d) $\pm 100\,mm$
4.2 (a) $+2.16\,D$ (b) emmetropia (c) $-10.39\,D$ (d) 2.79 D
4.3 One dioptre corresponds to $\approx -3/8$ mm variation in axial length
4.4 $K = -8.94\,D$
4.5 Ocular refraction ranges from $-15.63\,D$ to $+18.98\,D$
4.6 $+3.25\,D$
4.7 (a) (i) $-11.72\,D$ (ii) $-12.30\,D$
(b) (i) $+15.46\,D$ (ii) $+14.56\,D$
4.8 (a) $+55.44\,D$ (b) -0.075 mm
4.9 Object is virtual, 200 mm *behind* principal point and 1.3 mm high
4.10 -0.242 mm in the given eye, -0.237 in the emmetropic eye, ratio (relative spectacle magnification) 1.021
4.11 $h'_2 = \dfrac{-w}{F_{sp} + F_e - dF_{sp}F_e}$
4.12 (a) $4\frac{1}{6}$ mm (b) 4.5 mm
4.13 Blur circle diameter 0.172 mm, basic heights -0.025 and -0.251 mm
4.14 Projected circular blur patches are each of 60 mm diameter, their centres separated by 180 mm. The upper patch appears red
4.16 (a) -0.0993 mm (b) -0.437 mm
4.17 (a) 15.625 mm per dioptre
(b) (i) -0.246 mm (ii) -0.291 mm
4.19 Hypermetrope: blur ratio -4, myope: blur ratio $+8$
4.20 Blur ratio decreases for all except low myopes
4.21 3.91 mm per dioptre
4.22 $-5.00\,D$
4.23 (a) 3.29 (b) 8.06 D

Chapter 5

5.1 Horizontal focal line: 20.87 mm from P and 0.1875 mm long
Vertical focal line: 21.55 mm from P and 0.1935 mm long
Circle of least confusion: 21.21 mm from P and 0.0952 mm diameter
Blur ellipse: 0.2 mm horiz. and 0.4 mm vert.
5.2 Blur ellipse on retina: 0.5 mm horiz. and 0.1 mm vert. Projected size of blur: 180 mm horiz. and 36 mm vert.
5.3 Basic height of retinal image: $-1\frac{2}{3}$ mm
Size of blur ellipse: 0.2 mm along $45°$ and 0.5 mm along $135°$
5.4 Since the circle of least confusion lies on the retina, the Scheiner disc will give rise to two circular patches on the retina. Also, since the rays cross over vertically but not horizontally, the alignment of them is: (a) horizontal, A lying outwards (b) vertical, A lying below (c) along $135°$, A lying below
5.5 Rays in a vertical plane reach the pinhole parallel but rays in a horizontal plane are converged towards the pinhole. The retinal image of every point is therefore a long horizontal focal line, which when projected extends across the lens (Maxwellian view)
5.6 Spectacle refraction: $-1.20\,DS/-2.70\,DC$ axis 180
Ocular refraction: $-1.18\,DS/-2.52\,DC$ axis 180
5.7 $-9.07\,DS/-3.24\,DC$ axis 120
5.8 (a) $+11.76/-5.17 \times 90$ (b) $+10.25/-4.25 \times 90$
5.9 (a) $-5.50/-3.19 \times 180$ (b) $-6.00/-3.75 \times 180$
5.12 $+0.50/+2.00 \times 40$

Chapter 6

6.1 Axis shift varies from $28°$ for trial cylinder power 0.50 D to $3.5°$ for cylinder power 6.00 D
6.2 $+11.76\,D$, $+13.17\,D$, $+26.57\,D$, $+28.57\,D$; $+1.41\,D$ and $+2.00\,D$
$-8.70\,D$, $-9.44\,D$, $-14.79\,D$, $-15.38\,D$; $-0.74\,D$ and $-0.59\,D$
6.4 (a) $-1.25\,DS$ (b) $+0.75\,DC \times 180$ (c) $-0.75/-0.50 \times 80$ (d) $+1.25/-1.00 \times 95$
6.5 (a) (i) 0.0625 mm (ii) 0.0833 mm (iii) 0.0417 mm
6.6 $+1.07/-1.15 \times 162\frac{1}{2}$

Chapter 7

7.1 (a) Infinity to $-133\frac{1}{3}$ mm (b) Real part: infinity to -500 mm; virtual: $+364$ mm to infinity (c) $+308$ mm to $+1000$ mm (virtual) (d) $-83\frac{1}{3}$ to -62.5 mm
7.2 (a) Spectacle accommodation 3.00 D; ocular accommodation 2.40 D (b) 3.00 D and 3.52 D respectively
7.3 (i) 2.75 D (ii) 2.77 D
7.4 (a) 14.19 D (b) 11.44 D (c) 12.10 D
7.5 (a) 667 down to 250 mm (b) 1000 down to 222 mm
7.6

	Additions			
	+2.00	+2.25	+2.50	+2.75
(a)	422 mm	382 mm	348 mm	321 mm
(b)	500	444	400	364
(c)	617	535	472	422

(d) 195 mm, 124 mm (e) 29 mm more on the distal side
7.7 44 mm
7.8 R $-2.53\,D$, L $-2.86\,D$
7.9 0.33 D
7.10 $+6.05\,D$
7.11 9.3 and 39 minutes of arc, 3.99 mm (between N18 and N24)
7.12 For 56 mm PD: 2.7, 2.3, 2.0, 1.8 and 1.6 mm

Chapter 9

9.1   6.8 ΔD
9.2   (a) -1.50 D   (b) yes, if accommodation sufficient
9.3   (a) $+1.00$ D   (b) only if under-corrected hypermetrope
9.4   slight over-convergence (esophoria)

Chapter 10

10.1   Distance 9 Δ esophoria, near 16.5 Δ esophoria
10.2   (a) Optical centre distance may be up to 15 mm wider than PD but image defects may then be apparent, (b) optical centre distance should not exceed PD but may be somewhat smaller
10.3   (a) R 1 mm up, L 1 mm down   (b) R 2.5 mm down, L 2.5 mm up
10.4   Distance 2.4 Δ base out, near 5.4 Δ base out
10.5   0.96 Δ R hyperphoria
10.6   1/3 Δ, 0.056 mm
10.8   (a) 64 mm, 1.2 Δ base out
    (b) 63 mm, 0.9 Δ base out
10.9   63.2 mm, 2.4 Δ base out

Chapter 11

11.1 ±0.03, 0.19, 0.75, 18.7, 74.7, 298.7, 672.1, 1867 and 7468 mm
11.2   (a) 6.2 seconds of arc   (b) 7.2 seconds of arc
11.3   At $10\times$, 2.9 μm; at $20\times$, 1.5 μm
11.4   The collimating objective may be under-powered for blue in relation to yellow – typical of the secondary spectrum of an achromatic doublet
11.5   (a) 1.3 Δ (b) 16 Δ
11.6   (a) 71.4 mm   (b) 48.2 mm
11.7   (a) 16.8   (b) 3.8
11.8   (a) (i) 21.74 Δ, (ii) 10.39 Δ (b) (i) 7.24, (ii) 3.46
11.10   (a) $\eta/4$ (b) $\eta/2$
11.11   (a) 10 Δ each eye   (b) 260 mm
11.12   Crossed, C 284.4 mm, D 277.4 mm; uncrossed, C 455.0 mm, D 474.0 mm

Chapter 12

12.1   (a) $+59.97$ D. (b) First principal point P $+1.37$ mm from first lens; second principal point P$'$ $+1.13$ mm from first lens (note that principal planes are crossed). (c) 17.81 mm
12.2   (a) Near point 286.5 mm in front of corneal vertex, (b) equivalent power increased by $+4.14$ D
12.3 $K = -4.75$ D, $K' = +55.25$ D, -209.12 mm from corneal vertex
12.4   25.05 mm
12.5 -1.34 D, denoting 1.34 D of accommodation
12.6   Principal values $F_o = +60.23$ D, $F_L = +21.55$ D, axial length $+24.01$ mm
12.7 -5.04 D
12.8   3.23 mm behind corneal vertex, 5.13 mm diameter
12.9 -17.63 D
12.10   Moved forward 30.56 (or 209.44) mm
12.11   First principal point (P) -3.74 mm from cornea; second principal point (P$'$) -5.14 mm from cornea (note that principal planes are crossed)
12.12   1.31 m
12.13 $K = +22.59$ D, $+31.0$ D
12.14   (a) $+9.10$ D, (b) 24.8% increase

Chapter 13

13.1   (a) 1.068   (b) 1.097
13.2   (b) 0.940   (c) (i) 0.986, (ii) 1.083, (iii) 1.024
13.3   0.992 along 150° and 0.944 along 60°
13.4   Spectacle refraction -6.00 D, ocular refraction -5.45 D
13.5   0.342 mm along 45° by 0.326 mm along 135°
13.7   Spectacle lens 10.58 mm^2, contact lens 12.23 mm^2
13.8   Areas ratio of pre-aphakic to corrected aphakic 0.60. Illumination ratio 1.08

13.9   (a) (i) 1.51° anticlockwise, (ii) 1.51° clockwise   (b) (i) 0.26° clockwise, (ii) 0.26° anticlockwise
13.10 -500 mm
13.11   Continuous rotation with scissors movement
13.12   9.14 Δ downwards
13.13   Total convergence 15.04 Δ (R 6.82 Δ, L 8.22 Δ)
13.14   R 37.9 Δ downwards, L 42.4 Δ downwards
13.15   1.23, 1.07, 1.00, 0.94, 0.89, 0.84 and 0.76 Δ
13.19   e.g. $d = 0$, $A = 4$ D, $M = 3.0$
    $d = 10$ cm, $A = 2$ D, $M = 2.1$
    $d = 20$ cm, $A = 0$ D, $M = 2.0$
13.20   (a) 1.054   (b) 0.75   (c) (i) 1.75, (ii) 1.45
13.21 $+5.00$ D
13.22 -4.25 DS
13.23   (a) $+2.00$ D, (b) $+4.00$ D
13.24   (a) Range -58.82 to -66.67 or 7.85 mm. (b) Range -162.83 to -170.64 or 7.81 mm
13.25   Spectacle telescope 31.3°, contact-lens telescope 51.7°
13.26   (a) $4.37\times$, (b) (i) $2.08\times$, (ii) $2.45\times$, (iii) $2.65\times$
13.27   Without
13.29   (a) $\pm0.6\%$, $\pm1.5\%$ (b) $\pm1.3\%$, $\pm3.1\%$

Chapter 14

14.3   R 1.5 Δ base down
14.4   (a) Decentre both lenses 3 or 4 mm upwards from horizontal centre line. (b) Work optical centres 1 mm above segment tops to divide vertical prismatic imbalance equally between distance and near visual points
14.5   1.33° excyclophoria
14.6   R 3.1% × 82, L 2.1% × 172
14.7   (a) Ratio 1/1.111
14.8   (a) 5.78   (b) 4.67

Chapter 15

15.1   (a) 0.015 mm   (b) -294 to -625 mm
15.2   (a) ±4.44 D   (b) -67 mm

Chapter 16

16.1   6.7 μm, $7\times$
16.2 ±0.2 mm, ±0.5 mm
16.3   1.25 mm
16.4   2.15 mm
16.5   (a) $+8.33$ D   (b) -12.50 D
16.6   2.91 D
16.7   (a) $+15.56\times$, 2.57 mm   (b) $+16.67\times$, 2.40 mm
16.8   With: 1.85 mm, $13.33\times$, without: 1.45 mm, $18.65\times$
16.9   Horizontal: $13.36\times$, vertical: $16.85\times$
16.10   0.37%
16.11   (a) $+3.64$ mm from cornea, height 0.182 mm
    (b) $+3.45$ mm from cornea, height 0.276 mm
16.12   (a) 375 mm behind condenser   (b) 77.4 mm from condenser, -5.72 mm   (c) $-3.20\times$
16.13   71.4 mm, 8.4 mm
16.14   (a) $1\frac{1}{3}$ mm   (b) (i) $-5\times$, (ii) $-4.58\times$
16.15   7.33 mm
16.17   (a) (i) $-3.84\times$, (ii) 32.3°
    (b) (i) $-3\times$, (ii) 43.6°
    (c) (i) $-2.14\times$, (ii) 51.1°

Chapter 17

17.1   (a) 0.51 mm   (b) 0.35 mm   (c) 0.37 mm
17.2   (a) 42.4 mm   (b) 7.36 mm   (c) 27.2 mm
17.4   (a) Instantaneous disappearance, (b) against movement, (c) against movement in an apparently vertical direction
17.5   (a) 3.0, 2.0, 6.0 and 5.0 mm   (b) 5.5, 7.0, 11.0 and 7.5 mm   (c) 8.0, 12.0, 4.0 and 0 mm
17.6   (a) -0.36 rad (against)   (b) $+0.138$ rad (with)
17.7 $+4\times$ (with), $+2\times$ (with), $-4\times$ (against)
17.8   (a) Speed increased by 57.0 times   (b) by 8.07 times
17.9   (a) (i) 2.14 mm, 0.00369 sr; (ii) 1.15 mm, 0.00107 sr;
    (b) (i) 2.14 mm, 0.000052 sr; (ii) 1.15 mm, 0.000015 sr
17.10   R 2.15°, L 7.97°

17.11 17.9°
17.12 (a) $K = 2W(a/g)$

g (mm)	$a = 1$ mm	$a = 2$ mm	$a = 3$ mm
2	-1.50 D	-3.00 D	-4.50 D
4	-0.75	-1.50	-2.25
6	-0.50	-1.00	-1.50

17.13 (a) 0.53 D, 0.97° (b) 0.64 D, 1.13° (c) 0.73 D, 1.33°
17.15 e.g. (i): (a) $+5.45$ D, (f) $+0.21$ D; (ii): (a) $+9.14$ D, (f) $+0.24$ D

Chapter 18

18.2 (a) 36 mm (b) 7.58 mm

Chapter 19

19.1 $x_s = r/2$
19.2 $-79.2°$ per minute, $-21.6°$ per minute
19.3 (a) $+20.00$ D (b) 0 (c) $+40.00$ D

Chapter 20

20.1 40 m
20.2 -4.10 DC axis 60
20.3 (a) 1.654 mm (b) 0.20°
20.4 -4.02 DC axis 90 (b) -4.09 DC axis 90
20.5 (a) (i) $-7.45/-5.30 \times 30$, (ii) $+11.41/-2.90 \times 30$
20.6 $+12.06$ DS
20.7 1.34, 1.17, 1.03 and 0.91 D
20.8 Ocular ast -4.42 DC axis 170; corneal ast -3.56 DC axis 170; residual ast -0.86 DC axis 170
20.9 (a) 7.765 mm (b) 7.673 mm

20.10 Image 3% too large, interpreted as radius 3% too small; $+3.85$ D
20.12 (a) From 5.625 to 7.125 mm (b) (i) 2.0%, (ii) 3.8%, (iii) 0.12%
20.13

$y = 1$ mm	$y = 1.5$ mm	$y = 2$ mm	$y = 2.5$ mm
$r_s = 7.82$ mm	7.84 mm	7.88 mm	7.92 mm
$r_t = 7.86$	7.93	8.03	8.16

20.14 (a) Ratios in order: 1.283, 1.369, 1.375, 1.546, 1.344, 1.419
(b) Calculated ast: (A) -1.54×180 (B) -1.54×90 (C) -0.57×90
(c) Keratometry: (A) -2.10×180 (B) -0.66×90 (C) -0.19×90
20.15 2.94 mm
20.16 (a) $+42.735$ D (increase of $+0.072$ D)
(b) $+43.951$ D (increase of $+1.288$ D)
20.17 (a) 4.69 μs (b) 9.08 μs (c) 30.87 μs (d) 1.31 μs
20.18 (a) $s' = 3.773$; $t' = 3.665$ (b) $s' = +3.839$; $t' = +3.860$

Chapter 21

21.1 (a) $+16.47$ D (b) $+57.63$ D (c) respectively 4.36 D and 2.37 D weaker than in the Bennett–Rabbetts eye
21.2 (a) $+20.25$ D (b) $+59.47$ D (c) respectively 0.58 D and 0.53 D weaker than in the Bennett–Rabbetts eye

Chapter 22

22.2 From bottom
22.4 (a) With (b) 1/120 mm (c) 1/60 mm
22.5 (a) 1.197 (b) 9.4 μm

Index

Richard Sellers

Richard Sellers